Acute Care Physical Therapy

A CLINICIAN'S GUIDE

SECOND EDITION

Acute Care Physical Therapy

A CLINICIAN'S GUIDE

SECOND EDITION

Daniel J. Malone, PT, PhD, CCS

Associate Professor
Physical Therapy Program
Department of Physical Medicine and Rehabilitation
University of Colorado School of Medicine
Aurora, Colorado

Kathy Lee Bishop, PT, DPT, CCS

Cardiovascular and Pulmonary Clinical Specialist
Program Manager
Emory St. Joseph's Cardiac Rehabilitation Program
Program Director
Emory University Acute Care Residency Program
Assistant Professor
Interim Assistant Director of Clinical Education
Doctor of Physical Therapy Program
Emory University School of Medicine
Atlanta, Georgia

Routledge
Taylor & Francis Group
NEW YORK AND LONDON

Acute Care Physical Therapy: A Clinician's Guide, Second Edition includes ancillary materials specifically available for faculty use. Included are PowerPoint Slides. Please visit www.routledge.com/9781032956961 to obtain access.

First published in hardback 2024

First published 2020 by SLACK Incorporated

Published 2024 by Routledge
605 Third Avenue, New York, NY 10158

and by Routledge
4 Park Square, Milton Park, Abingdon, Oxon OX14 4RN

Routledge is an imprint of the Taylor & Francis Group, an informa business

Publisher's Note
The publisher has gone to great lengths to ensure the quality of this reprint but points out that some imperfections in the original copies may be apparent.

Cover Artist: Christine Seabo

Library of Congress Cataloging-in-Publication Data

Names: Malone, Daniel Joseph, editor. | Bishop, Kathy Lee, editor.
Title: Acute care physical therapy : a clinician's guide / [edited by] Daniel J. Malone, Kathy Lee Bishop.
Description: Second edition. | Thorofare, NJ : SLACK Incorporated, [2020] | Includes bibliographical references and index.
Identifiers: LCCN 2019022882 (print) | ISBN 9781617119866 (paperback)
Subjects: MESH: Physical Therapy Modalities | Acute Disease--therapy
Classification: LCC RM700 (print) |NLM WB 460 | DDC 615.8/2--dc23

LC record available at https://lccn.loc.gov/2019022882

ISBN: 978-1-03-295696-1 (hbk)
ISBN: 978-1-61-711986-6 (pbk)
ISBN: 978-1-00-352248-5 (ebk)

DOI: 10.4324/9781003522485

Dedication

To all of our teachers, mentors, colleagues, coworkers and friends—thank you. To all of our patients—a bigger thank you.

"We make a living but what we get, we make a life by what we give."

—Sir Winston Churchill

Contents

Acute Care Physical Therapy: A Clinician's Guide, Second Edition includes ancillary materials specifically available for faculty use. Included are PowerPoint Slides. Please visit ww.routledge.com/9781032956961 to obtain access.

ACKNOWLEDGMENTS

As noted in the preface, acute care physical therapy demands skill, resolve, and teamwork. This second edition of Acute Care Physical Therapy would never have been possible without a dedicated TEAM and I am indebted to the TEAM: My co-editor, Kathy Lee Bishop—a mentor, a colleague, and a good friend. Coworkers and colleagues who turned into coauthors and contributors—thank you for your patience and persistence. Our publisher, SLACK Incorporated—a big thank you for seeing this project through with gentle but determined prodding. Most importantly, to my wife Margie. As noted by George Bernard Shaw, "a happy family is but an earlier heaven."

—DJM

As I review my acknowledgements for the first edition, I realize how much of what I wrote still rings true. I am still so thankful for my mentors in cardiovascular and pulmonary physical therapy for the support and direction they gave me as a young clinician and as my career evolved. The passion for acute care you instilled in me is something I share with my students every day! I walked into my first intensive care unit (ICU) around 1984 and practiced as a singular entity. When I moved to Boston for graduate school and started working at Massachusetts General Hospital in 1986 the physical therapy culture around the majority of ICUs was "early intervention and mobilization." I still feel strongly that physical therapy needs to start early, be aggressive, but be part of a team that successfully progresses the patient through the acute care stay to discharge. Now I feel we need to go further. One hour of therapy by a physical or occupational therapist a day is not enough. The critically ill patient needs a coordinated team effort. What happens those other 23 hours? The persistence of ICU acquired weakness, delirium, cognitive impairments, functional limitations, and multisystem issues (eg, sleep disturbances, gastrointestinal/gastrourinary) after an ICU stay demonstrates that this aggressive team effort should not stop at 1 hour of therapy or at the ICU door when transferred to a regular floor. The care of the acute patient needs to continue after the ICU within the hospital through the time of discharge to full recovery. This textbook targets acute care, but I do not feel that is only restricted to an acute care hospital. If symptoms and impairments are persisting upwards of 5 years from a stay in the ICU, looking beyond an acute care hospital door is the right direction.

As I attend CSM each year I marvel how our profession has embraced early mobility and how ever-changing lifesaving technology and early mobilization are symbiotic. Our profession now emphasizes documentation of valid functional tools to demonstrate value added, productivity, and patient outcomes. Our documentation practices have changed over these decades since the inception of the first edition. Consider the value added if we had had validated tools and started documenting with the valid functional tools in the early 80s to demonstrate reduction in readmission rates, reduction in health care costs, percentage of return to work, and so much more.

I am in awe of my co-editor Dan Malone for all that he has accomplished as the outgoing president of the cardiovascular and pulmonary section, his many peer-reviewed publications, as well as with this second edition. Our weekly discussions, arguments, and resolutions (and sometime no resolutions) raised my critical thinking and writing. I am thankful for my dear partner Larry's support and unwavering love as the second edition goes to publication. He shows me joy, laughter, and balance each day. As for our 3 fur babies Davos, Cersie, and Riley, thank you for being so happy to see me whether I have been gone 1 hour or at the end of a long day with plenty of purrs and tail wags.

—KLB

About the Editors

Daniel J. Malone, PT, PhD, CCS, is currently an Associate Professor in the Physical Therapy Program at the University of Colorado School of Medicine and a per diem physical therapist at the University of Colorado Hospital. He earned a Master of Physical Therapy from Temple University in 1992, and a PhD in physiology from the School of Medicine at Temple University in 2008. His career as a physical therapist started at the Hospital of the University of Pennsylvania in what he thought was a 2 to 3 year trial of acute care practice. Almost 30 years later that passion and energy for working in the acute care setting has never diminished.

Over his career, Dr. Malone has had the opportunity to provide physical therapist services across the continuum of care from ICU to home, as well as rotate through all hospital service lines. Prior to transitioning to the University of Colorado, he was the Cardiopulmonary Team Leader providing direct patient care in the medical and surgical ICUs while mentoring staff and serving as an adjunct faculty member at several regional physical therapy programs. Dr. Malone is a board certified specialist in Cardiovascular and Pulmonary Physical Therapy since 1998 and an active member of the American Physical Therapy Association and the Cardiovascular & Pulmonary (CVP) Section. He served as president of the CVP Section as well the CVP Section delegate, nominating committee member, and program chair.

Although Dr. Malone is primarily a clinician educator, he continues to participate in clinical research. His research has focused on the delivery and outcomes of physical therapy services applied to the ICU population and the frail older adult in the post-acute setting. The overall goal of Dr. Malone's scholarship is to advance education, clinical practice and research related to the physical therapist's management of patients with complex medical conditions.

Kathy Lee Bishop, PT, DPT, CCS has been passionate about cardiovascular and pulmonary physical therapy for over 35 years. She received her BS in Physical Therapy from the University of Vermont and her MS and DPT from the MGH Institute of Health Professions in Boston. She is a board-certified cardiovascular and pulmonary specialist (since 1993), an advanced cardiac life support instructor, and has been teaching in the Emory Physical Therapy program since 1999. Her career has focused on acute care, early mobilization in the ICU, cardiovascular and pulmonary rehabilitation, as well as health and wellness. She completed a Master Teaching course in 2012 through Georgia State University. Her Advanced Acute Care elective offered to Emory DPT third year students focuses on using high fidelity simulation to prepare pre-professionals for the rigor of ICU practice as part of an early mobility team. She is a reviewer for the *Journal of Acute Care Physical Therapy,* and has published in that journal as well as in the *Journal of Humanities.* Dr. Bishop developed the Emory University Acute Care Physical Therapist Residency, which is in candidacy status and accepted the first resident for the Fall of 2018. Her academic interests include interprofessional simulation in acute care, particularly the ICU, and using documentation to support strategies to reduce hospital readmissions for cardiovascular and pulmonary patients. She helped design and implement the automatic referral process for cardiac rehabilitation at Emory Healthcare which resulted in an increase of referrals by nearly 60%. She was the co-director of the 2nd Interprofessional Simulation conference and is planning the 3rd conference for the fall of 2019. Presently she continues to teach at Emory University as an Assistant Professor introducing the DPT students to the challenges and critical thinking of acute care. Dr. Bishop practices as the Program Manager for the Emory St. Joseph's Hospital Cardiac Rehabilitation program where she mentors medical students, residents, and cardiology fellows about cardiac rehabilitation. She combines her love of tennis and passion for raising awareness about heart disease by hosting an annual tennis event annually to help raise monies for the American Heart Association.

Contributing Authors

Joseph Adler, PT, DPT, CCS (Chapter 8)
Acute Care Team Leader
Good Shepherd Penn Partners
Philadelphia, Pennsylvania

Heather Dillon Anderson, PT, DPT, NCS (Chapter 9)
Associate Professor, Physical Therapy
Neumann University
Aston, Pennsylvania
Physical Therapist
Good Shepherd Penn Partners
Philadelphia, Pennsylvania

Esther H. Bae, PT, DPT (Chapter 11 Appendix A)
Good Shepherd Penn Partners
Hospital of the University of Pennsylvania
Philadelphia, Pennsylvania

Colleen Chancler, PT, MHS (Chapter 9)
Assistant Professor
Widener University
Chester, Pennsylvania

Christine F. Ehlers, PT, CWS, CLWT (Chapters 10 and 15)
Adjunct Faculty
Emory University School of Physical Therapy
Atlanta, Georgia
Staff Physical Therapist
Acute Care at Self Regional Healthcare
Greenwood, SC

David Fichandler, MSPT (Chapter 12)
Director, Initiative Integration
Hartford HealthCare
Hartford, Connecticut

Zoher F. Kapasi, PT, PhD, MBA (Chapter 5)
Dean and Professor
College of Health Professions
Medical University of South Carolina
Charleston, South Carolina

Lora Packel, PT, PhD (Chapters 2 and 13)
Chair and Associate Professor
University of the Sciences
Philadelphia, Pennsylvania

Robin Stott-McNulty, MPT (Chapter 11 Appendix A)

Preface

The ability to effectively treat patients across the broad spectrum of acute care is one of the most interesting and challenging aspects of the physical therapy profession. Acute care physical therapy demands skill and resolve to focus on the impairments and functional capabilities of the individual. The physical therapist and physical therapist assistant must consider the pathophysiology of disease and the impact of medications while utilizing the benefits, but not impeding the physiologic monitoring and patient-support equipment. Therapists will often participate in patient-centered rounds that can include representatives from physician groups, nursing, nutrition, speech pathology, respiratory and occupational therapy, performance improvement, and even spiritual counseling. Often, the physical therapist is making clinical judgments that impact discharge planning after only one patient interaction. The work is demanding, challenging, and at times disheartening, but the rewards in clinical development and positive patient outcomes abound.

Acute Care Physical Therapy: A Clinician's Guide, Second Edition evolved from a bulleted list of diagnoses and procedures to a narrative text attempting to highlight the breadth and complexity of hospital-based physical therapy services. The authors understand that it is impossible to compile all diseases, disorders, diagnostic tests, and medical/surgical procedures, as well as provide a comprehensive portrayal of physical therapy examination procedures and therapeutic interventions, into one text due to the evolving nature of hospital-based practice. However, all attempts have been made to incorporate the most relevant information pertaining to this dynamic field of physical therapy practice.

Acute Care Physical Therapy: A Clinician's Guide, Second Edition is organized by organ system preceded by the common universal topics of examination and discharge planning, common medical diagnostic tests, and patient support equipment. Complications of bed rest and the ubiquitous issues of immunity and infection control are also reviewed. Each organ system chapter begins with a brief description of pertinent anatomy and physiology followed by the most common diseases and disorders associated with the described system. This should provide the reader with an understanding of the basic physiologic mechanisms underlying normal organ function contrasted with the pathophysiology of disease. Following the didactic information, the impact of these conditions on physical therapy examination and therapeutic interventions is provided and highlighted by the inclusion of real-life case studies. A section called Pharmacological Information is included at the end of each disease/disorder chapter that outlines standard medications and their respective side effects to aid in the evaluation of patient presentation and responses to therapeutic interventions. The *Guide to Physical Therapist Practice* is integrated throughout the text, and the published literature is used to support the described physical therapy practice. However, as all acute care therapists know, there is a paucity of acute care physical therapy research, and this should challenge us all to contribute to this body of evidence. *Acute Care Physical Therapy: A Clinician's Guide, Second Edition* should serve as a reference to benefit the novice practitioner and the student as well as more experienced clinicians practicing in an evolving acute care environment.

Chapter 1

Introduction to Physical Therapist Management of the Acute Care Patient

Daniel J. Malone, PT, PhD, CCS

This chapter will introduce the physical therapist's examination of the acutely ill patient. This examination process is one part of the Physical Therapist Patient/Client Management Model as noted in the *Guide to Physical Therapist Practice 3.0*.[1] As described in the *Guide*, the Physical Therapist Patient/Client Management Model includes the elements examination, evaluation, diagnosis, prognosis, intervention, and outcomes. Although patients present with diverse medical, surgical, and social histories, there are many shared elements of the examination process. These shared elements will be explored while additional examination items that typically relate to specific diagnoses, organ systems, or patient presentations can be found in the chapters that follow. A case scenario, based on a real patient, will highlight patient management at the end of this chapter and subsequent chapters. The cases use the Patient/Client Management Model from the *Guide* and the *International Classification of Functioning, Disability and Health* (ICF) (Figure 1-1).[2] The ICF model provides a framework to organize and classify functioning and disability (ie, body functions and structures, activity limitations, participation restrictions) as an interaction between the health condition (ie, disorder/disease) and the patient's individual contextual factors (eg, personal factors, environmental factors). These 2 models will provide a clinical reasoning framework for the acute care practitioner by identifying relationships between the specific tests and measures chosen by the physical therapist as part of the examination process and the interventions used to accomplish specific patient-centered goals (Figure 1-2). Finally, an examination algorithm (Figure 1-3) to guide clinical reasoning and patient safety, a table of common tests and measures, and an introduction to the discharge planning process are provided at the end of this chapter.

Malone DJ, Bishop KL, eds. *Acute Care Physical Therapy: A Clinician's Guide, Second Edition* (pp 1-50).

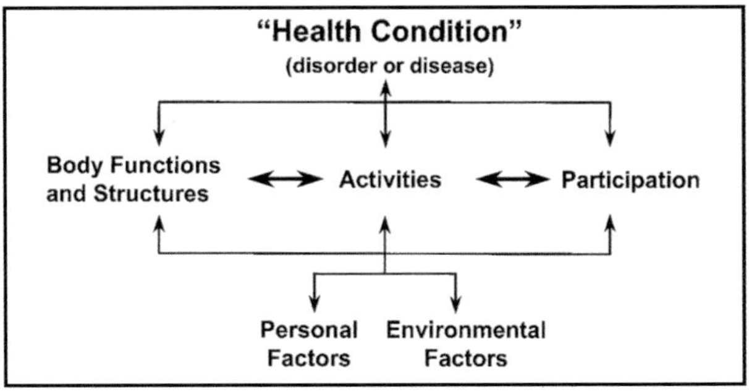

Figure 1-1. ICF model. (Reprinted with permission from *Towards a Common Language for Functioning, Disability and Health*. World Health Organization. www.who.int/classifications/icf/icfbeginnersguide.pdf. Published 2002. Accessed April 29, 2019.)

ICF Model Case Study Summary								
Health Condition								
HPI: PMHx:								
Precautions/ Contraindications								
Body Structure & Function			Activity/ Task Limitations			Participation		
Impairment/Problem	T/M	Intervention	Activity	T/M	Intervention	Participation	T/M	Intervention
Other considerations								
Personal Factors						Environmental Factors		
						Hospital Home (Discharge destination)		
Abbreviations: ICF: International Classification of Function; HPI: history of present illness; PMHx: past medical history; T/M: tests & measures								

Figure 1-2. ICF clinical reasoning tool. This tool combines the ICF[2] with the *Guide*[1] to demonstrate the relationships between tests and measures (T/M), identified examination findings, and chosen interventions to meet the patient's goals.

Examination

History

As noted in the *Guide*,[1] the elements of patient/client management include examination, evaluation, diagnosis, prognosis (including plan of care), interventions, and outcomes. This process is not a singular event but is repeated throughout the hospitalization as the patient's needs and presentation evolve. Examination of the acute care patient, as with all patients, includes 3 major categories:

1. History, including symptom investigation and review of systems
2. Systems review
3. Tests and measures

History is the systematic gathering of past and present data related to why the patient is seeking or requires physical therapy services. While reviewing the history, the patient's chief complaint or primary reasons for the hospitalization are noted. The data from the history allow the clinician to hypothesize about impairments in body structure and function, activity limitations, and participation restrictions that are commonly related to health conditions and impacted by environmental factors or personal characteristics.[1]

Review Medical History (see Chapter 1)

- Note if physical therapy is indicated based off the prior and/or current medical and surgical histories.
- Note medications that may impact mental status (MS), wakefulness, and ability to follow commands
- Note medications that may impact HR and blood pressure (BP) responses.
- Determine the prior level of function and activity tolerance (use the AHA HF Classification Scale, Borg RPE, MRC Breathlessness Scale, as indicated).

↓

Mental Status/Cognitive Decision Point

- Is the patient awake and alert (Richmond Agitation Sedation Score [RASS]: -1 to +1; Chapters 1 and 4)
- Patient follows simple commands (De Jonghe's 5 questions, Serial "A"; Chapter 4)
- Is the mental status stable? Rule out delirium (CAM-ICU, Chapter 4) or encephalopathy (encephalopathy scale; Chapter 11); or brain injury (RLAS; Chapter 9)

NO → **Patient may not be ready for physical therapy**

YES ↓

Cardiovascular Decision Point (see Chapters 4 and 6)

- Heart rate and rhythm acceptable?
  - Resting HR: >50 and <150 beats/minute
  - Heart rhythm stable? Is there an absence of a new dysrhythmia?
    - Is the atrial fibrillation ventricular response <100?
    - Are the number of premature ventricular contractions acceptable?
    - Has any recent ventricular tachycardia (VT) or non-sustained VT (NSVT) been addressed?
- Blood pressure acceptable?
  - Resting mean arterial pressure (MAP) >65 and <120 mm Hg
  - Resting Systolic BP >80 and < 200 mmHg
  - Vasopressor dose stable or decreasing with appropriate BP/MAP?
- Absence of chest pain or pressure?
- Absence of recent DVT/PE? If DVT/PE diagnosed, is anticoagulation started? Has a filter been placed?
- Surgical precautions followed?
  - Sternal precautions

NO → **Patient may not be ready for physical therapy**

YES ↓

Figure 1-3. Physical therapy examination algorithm. (PE=pulmonary embolism.) (Adapted from Adler J, Malone D. Early mobilization in the intensive care unit: a systematic review. *Cardiopulm Phys Ther J.* 2012;23[1]:5-13; Nordon-Craft A, Moss M, Quan D, Schenkman M. Intensive care unit–acquired weakness: implications for physical therapist management. *Phys Ther.* 2012;92[12]:1494-1506; and Stiller K, Phillips A. Safety aspects of mobilising acutely ill inpatients. *Physiother Theory and Pract.* 2003;19:239-257.) *(continued)*

Pulmonary Decision Point (see Chapter 7)

- Resting pulse oximetry (SpO_2) ≥88%
- Respiratory rate <35 breaths/minute at rest
- Breathing pattern acceptable? No observable respiratory distress?
- If the patient complains of shortness of breath (SOB) at rest, is it acceptable?
- Oxygen requirements and oxygen delivery device acceptable
- Mechanical ventilation parameters: PEEP < 10 cmH_20; F_iO_2 <0.7 (70% oxygen)
- Others: Arterial blood gas (ABG), PaO_2/F_iO_2 ratio acceptable?

NO → **Patient may not be ready for physical therapy**

YES ↓

Laboratory Values Decision Point (see Chapter 2)

- Are laboratory values within acceptable parameters? For example:
  - Complete blood count:
    - Hemoglobin: > 7 g/dL without cardiovascular disease and no signs of bleeding; > 8 to 10g/dL if known cardiovascular disease
    - Hematocrit: >25%
    - Platelets: >20,000 cells/mm^3
    - White blood cells: If <5,000 cells/mm^3 consider limiting patient exposure to possible infection risk; if >10,000 cells/mm^3 consider active infection (febrile versus afebrile)
  - Electrolytes:
    - Potassium (3.5 to 5.3 mEq/L)
    - Sodium (135 to 148 mEq/L
    - Calcium (8.5 to 10.5 mg/dL)
    - Magnesium (1.8 to 2.7 mg/dL)
  - Metabolic measures:
    - Glucose: >60 mg/dL and <300 mg/dL, HbA1C
    - Health condition specific testing:
      - Cardiac: Troponins, CPK, BNP
      - Renal: Creatinine
      - Hepatic: LFT
      - Is nutrition status acceptable: Albumin, pre-albmumin

NO → **Patient may not be ready for physical therapy**

YES ↓

Figure 1-3 (continued). Physical therapy examination algorithm. (Adapted from Adler J, Malone D. Early mobilization in the intensive care unit: a systematic review. *Cardiopulm Phys Ther J.* 2012;23[1]:5-13; Nordon-Craft A, Moss M, Quan D, Schenkman M. Intensive care unit–acquired weakness: implications for physical therapist management. *Phys Ther.* 2012;92[12]:1494-1506; and Stiller K, Phillips A. Safety aspects of mobilising acutely ill inpatients. *Physiother Theory and Pract.* 2003;19:239-257.) *(continued)*

Other Considerations

- Patient consent obtained?
- Patient appearance is acceptable?
- Have patient complaints been addressed?
  - Pain (Chapter 1)
  - Excessive fatigue, SOB
- Are all orthopedic considerations considered (Chapter 8)?
  - Weightbearing restrictions
  - Stable spine
- Does the patient have required orthotics/prosthetics? (Chapter 8)
- Integument considerations (Chapter 15):
  - Are skin grafts viable? Do ROM or weightbearing restrictions allow mobility?
  - Vacuum drainage system
- Is patient afebrile? (Chapter 5)
- Has life supporting equipment been reviewed?
  - Airway for mechanical ventilation (Chapters 3 and 7)
  - Vascular access placement (eg, femoral line; Chapters 3 and 6)
  - Feeding tube (Chapter 3)
  - Mechanical circulatory assist (Intra-aortic balloon pump [IABP], ventricular assist device [VAD], extracorporeal membrane oxygenation [ECMO]; Chapters 3 and 6)
  - Hemodialysis, continuous renal replacement therapy (CRRT) (Chapter 12)

NO → **Patient may not be ready for physical therapy**

YES ↓

Select appropriate physical therapy examination procedures
and
appropriate mode, intensity & duration of physical therapy interventions

Figure 1-3 (continued). Physical therapy examination algorithm. (Adapted from Adler J, Malone D. Early mobilization in the intensive care unit: a systematic review. *Cardiopulm Phys Ther J.* 2012;23[1]:5-13; Nordon-Craft A, Moss M, Quan D, Schenkman M. Intensive care unit–acquired weakness: implications for physical therapist management. *Phys Ther.* 2012;92[12]:1494-1506; and Stiller K, Phillips A. Safety aspects of mobilising acutely ill inpatients. *Physiother Theory and Pract.* 2003;19:239-257.)

Common Data Generated from a Patient History

General Demographics

Gender, ethnicity, religious beliefs, and language barriers are important considerations when working and communicating with the patient, the patient's family, and primary caregivers. Certain religious and cultural beliefs might limit a patient's acceptance of medical care by a therapist of a different sex. Language barriers may create misunderstanding of complex medical issues. Social and employment responsibilities may dictate specific goals for therapy (eg, prolonged standing for flag operator who works for the department of transportation).

Table 1-1

ACTIVITIES OF DAILY LIVING AND INSTRUMENTAL ACTIVITIES OF DAILY LIVING

Activities of Daily Living	*Instrumental Activities of Daily Living*
• Eating • Bathing • Grooming • Dressing • Bed mobility (rolling, supine↔sit) • Transfers (sit↔stand, toilet/commode, bed↔chair)	• Cooking • Shopping • Housekeeping • Balancing a checkbook • Driving a car • Ability to use public transportation

Social History

Resources and cultural beliefs of the family must be identified. Resources include family and community support and financial or insurance assets. When the current hospitalization ends, the patient may not be independent with activities of daily living (ADLs) or instrumental activities of daily living (IADLs) (Table 1-1). The clinician determines and provides recommendations regarding the minimal frequency and duration of social supports (eg, family/friends) required for safe discharge. The physical therapist and physical therapist assistant must determine if the assistance available successfully meets the needs of the patient. An individual can safely be discharged to home, although he or she may require assist for various ADLs/IADLs with an adequate support network. Clearly, the extent of social resources provides greater flexibility during the discharge planning process.

Living Environment

Therapists must understand the discharge options for the patient. Will the patient be returning to his or her primary residence or will the patient have an option of residing with a family member? Consideration of environmental factors, such as the discharge destination with special emphasis on entry/egress from the home, internal/external stairs, bathrooms, and potential space requirements for durable medical equipment (DME; eg, wheelchairs, beds, walkers, home intravenous infusion) will influence goal setting and direct the plan of care.

Additionally, the therapist must recognize that the patient's current living environment is the hospital. This environment may be overwhelming for the patient, family members, and other caregivers. It is essential that the physical therapist/physical therapist assistant is knowledgeable and understands all monitors, equipment, supplies, and alarms that are used in the care of the patient. Not understanding the indications and precautions of hospital equipment can negatively impact patient safety and undermines the therapist–patient relationship.

General Health Status

The patient's current and past capabilities and symptoms while performing the ADLs of bathing, dressing, grooming, and household and community ambulation are a guide to the general aerobic capacity of the patient. Scales such as the Borg Scale of rate of perceived exertion (RPE) or the New York Heart Association Functional Classification System (NYHA) (Table 1-2) provide objective descriptions of the prior and current level of functioning. These scales help determine the intensity of limiting

Table 1-2

COMMON SCALES FOR PERCEIVED EXERTION, ANGINA, DYSPNEA, AND CLAUDICATION

Borg Scales for Rating Perceived Exertion

6	No exertion	0	Nothing at all
7	Extremely light		
8		0.5	Very, very light
9	Very light		
10			
11	Light	2	Light
12			
13	Somewhat hard	3	Moderate
14			
15	Hard (heavy)	5	Heavy (strong)
16			
17	Very hard	7	Very heavy
18			
19	Extremely hard	9	
20	Maximal exertion	10	Very, very heavy (maximal)

New York Heart Association Functional Classification System

I: No limitations on physical activity; ordinary physical activity not resulting in symptoms

II: Slight limitation on physical activity; no symptoms at rest, but symptoms possible with ordinary physical activity

III: More severe limitations; patient usually comfortable at rest; clinical manifestations with usual physical activities

IV: Inability to carry out any physical activity without producing symptoms; symptoms often present at rest

Adapted from American College of Sports Medicine. *Guidelines for Exercise Testing and Prescription.* 9th ed. Philadelphia, PA: Lippincott Williams & Wilkins; 2014 and Borg GA. Psychophysical basis of perceived exertion. *Med Sci Sports Exerc.* 1982;14:377-387.

symptoms during functional activities and may explain participation restrictions (eg, parenting and work responsibilities).

Social/Health Habits

Social and health habits are important personal factors that may signal the need for other consults to maximize a patient's outcome. For example, smoking, alcohol, or other drug history may trigger a referral to smoking cessation or drug/alcohol rehabilitation. A social work consultation is appropriate for frequent admissions related to medical noncompliance due to financial hardship, inadequate social support, and poor living environment. A nutritionist can assist the patient with progressive weight loss or gain and provide valuable information for dietary management of many disease processes. It is never too late to consider lifestyle modifications for long-term health.

Family History

The review of a family history assists in the identification of risk for developing common health disorders, such as heart disease and hypertension (HTN), stroke, diabetes mellitus, and cancers. The increased risk is due to family members sharing common factors, such as their genes, living environment, and lifestyle. By recognizing patterns, therapists can hypothesize that individual patients may be at risk of developing a particular health disorder.

Additionally, the health status of family and primary caregivers are factors that affect the discharge plan. Does the family and primary caregiver have the ability to adequately care for the patient? Activity limitations and participation restrictions of the patient or dependence on DME, such as mechanical ventilation and negative-pressure wound therapy (ie, wound vacuum), can create a large physical and psychological burden of care that caregivers are unable to manage. Early recognition of these issues assists in appropriate discharge planning. For example, a patient with multiple medications that need to be administered at different times throughout the day may rely on the organizational skills of the caregiver to provide the correct medication at the correct dosage at the correct time.

Medical/Surgical History

The medical/surgical history represents information of critical importance that will be available in the patient's medical record; however, sometimes the medical record is incomplete and further discussion with the patient and family/caregivers is important. Of particular importance to the physical therapist are disorders or complications within the pulmonary, cardiovascular, integumentary, neuromuscular, and musculoskeletal systems. The chronicity of the medical/surgical issues and comorbid conditions will provide further information for the physical therapist regarding prognostication for outcomes and the duration of the episode of care.

Current Conditions

What is the current condition that has led to the request for physical therapy services, and is this an initial episode or a reoccurrence? Is the patient stable and is it safe for the patient to participate in therapy? What are the current treatments being provided by other health care providers? Has the patient been receiving any type of positioning, mobilization, exercise, or airway clearance? Has the patient been on bed rest? Why? How long? Are there any weightbearing, activity, or position restrictions? Are there cardiopulmonary (eg, heart rate [HR] and rhythm, BP) or pulmonary (eg, shortness of breath [SOB], dyspnea on exertion [DOE], pulse oximetry [SpO_2]) parameters that limit therapy? Do abnormal lab values warrant extra caution (see Figure 1-3)? What are the patient's and family's expectations for this episode of care and for continued care upon discharge? The answers to these questions allow the therapist to gain insight into the patient's activity patterns and tolerance preceding this episode of care. Obviously, the greater the duration of hemodynamic instability or bed rest, the more deconditioned the patient will be regardless of medical or surgical history (see Chapter 4).

Activities and Participation

As mentioned in General Health Status, determining the patient's prior level of function will provide valuable information regarding the patient's activity tolerance throughout the episode of care. For example, if the patient could only ambulate household distances secondary to DOE, community ambulation of several blocks is not a realistic goal. Comparing the current and prior functional status in relation to the duration of the hospitalization will enable the physical therapist to prognosticate on the rate and extent of functional return that will influence discharge planning.

Medications

Pharmacological interventions are a mainstay of medical and postsurgical management. Unfortunately, many medications may have significant side effects that negatively affect the patient. Side effects are symptoms that occur because of drug administration. These effects are unrelated to the intended action of the drug, and unwanted side effects do not only occur at toxic doses but may occur at therapeutic levels of the desired medication as well. Therapists should understand why medications are prescribed for specific health conditions as well as understand the medications mechanism of action. This will enable the therapist to determine the potential connection between medication side effects and a patient's mental functions, neuromuscular complaints, and hemodynamics at rest and with activity.

Following select chapters is additional information regarding common medications. Although not an exhaustive listing, the information may guide therapist practice and decision making related to patient examination and evaluation and subsequent interventions.

Other Clinical Tests

Extensive hospital derived data can be accessed, but the exact application of this data is challenging. For example, a patient who underwent a joint replacement may present with anemia and complain of SOB and increased fatigue with mobilization activities. The anemia may partially explain the decreased activity tolerance but what about the confounding opioid for pain management? Laboratory values provide information that can help in determining the patient presentation, determine the readiness for therapy, and inform the clinical responses observed during the therapy session. Laboratory data may also guide the intensity and duration of chosen interventions performed during therapy. Additional information can be found in Figure 1-3 and Chapter 2.

Systems Review

Per the *Guide*,[1] after organizing the available history information, the physical therapist begins the hands-on component of the examination. The systems review is a brief or limited examination of (1) the anatomical and physiological status of the cardiovascular/pulmonary, integumentary, musculoskeletal, and neuromuscular systems and (2) the communication ability, affect, cognition, language, and learning style of the individual. This gross examination, or quick check, provides baseline information and identifies the existence of other health problems to be considered in the diagnosis, prognosis, and plan of care. The accumulated data may trigger referral or consultation with other health care providers. The physical therapist especially notes how each of the components affects the ability to initiate, sustain, and modify purposeful movement for performance of an action, task, or activity that is pertinent to function.[1]

Cardiovascular and Pulmonary

The cardiovascular and pulmonary review should include heart/pulse rate, BP (see Table 6-11), edema (see Table 1-7), respiratory rate (RR) (see Table 7-13), and perceived level of exertion (see Tables 1-1 and 1-2) at rest and with activity. The hospitalized patient is monitored extensively and most vital signs (VS) data is available from nursing documentation. However, information documented prior to the therapist's arrival is not a substitute for current, direct monitoring of VS. The therapist should review the patient's status over the prior 12 to 24 hours to determine trends in relation to the current data. The medical record may not be up-to-date, and conferencing with the nursing staff will provide valuable and timely information.

As therapeutic exercises and progressive mobilization activities are universally prescribed for hospitalized patients, the therapist must record and understand the cardiopulmonary responses at rest and during activity to determine the presence of hemodynamic and respiratory stability and activity tolerance (Figure 1-4).

Integumentary

For the integumentary system, the assessment of pliability (ie, texture), presence of scar formation, skin color, and skin integrity is performed.[1] Patients may have fragile skin due to medications (eg, corticosteroids), poor nutrition, prolonged bed rest, and general age-related changes. Areas of skin breakdown, ecchymosis, and pressure injuries should be noted. Hospital-acquired integumentary lesions (Stage III/IV pressure injuries; see Chapter 15) are classified as **never events**, and Medicare will no longer pay the extra cost of treating these wounds while the patient is in the hospital. Skin lesions can be avoided with frequent position changes, especially out of bed (OOB) activities. Evaluation of the body habitus may elicit suggestions for beds, chairs, mattress, cushions, or mobility aids (eg, walkers, trapeze) that promote more frequent position changes and patient safety. Integumentary lesions are potential sites for infection and can negatively impact patient outcomes and prolong the length of stay. The physical therapist should examine incisions and new and old scars and determine the healing status of all wounds (see Table 15-1). Indwelling lines and tubes need to be identified and examined. Is there any evidence of infection at the insertion site? Abnormalities should be discussed with the nursing and medical team.

Musculoskeletal

For the musculoskeletal system, the assessment of gross symmetry, gross range of motion (ROM), gross strength, height, and weight is indicated.[1] Limited ROM due to soft tissue contractures occur in the hospitalized patient, particularly the bed bound patient in the intensive care unit (ICU). In addition to the extremities, consider ROM of the head, neck, and trunk. Assessment of functional strength will provide direct evidence regarding the need for further testing and the potential requirements for mobility training and ambulatory aids.

Neuromuscular

For the neuromuscular system, a general assessment of gross coordinated movement (ie, balance, gait, locomotion, transfers, transitions) and motor function (ie, motor control and learning) is completed.[1] Initial signs of neuromuscular dysfunction may not be apparent until the patient attempts to move, and the physical therapist may often be the first health care provider to mobilize or observe the patient's mobility. Abnormalities should trigger the need for a further medical consultation and more specific physical therapy examination procedures, such as deep tendon reflexes, cranial nerve testing, and myotome and dermatome testing (Tables 1-3 through 1-5; see Chapter 9).

Analysis of functional tasks (observational task analysis) comprise bed mobility, including rolling, supine to sit, and sitting at edge of the bed (ie, dangling). OOB tasks include sitting-to-standing transfers, transfers from bed to chair, wheelchair transfers, commode transfers, and ambulation on level surfaces and stairs (Table 1-6).

Communication, Affect, Cognition, Language, and Learning Style

For communication ability, affect, cognition, language, and learning style, the therapists should assess the patient's ability to make needs known, the level of consciousness, and orientation (ie, person, place, and time). The therapist should

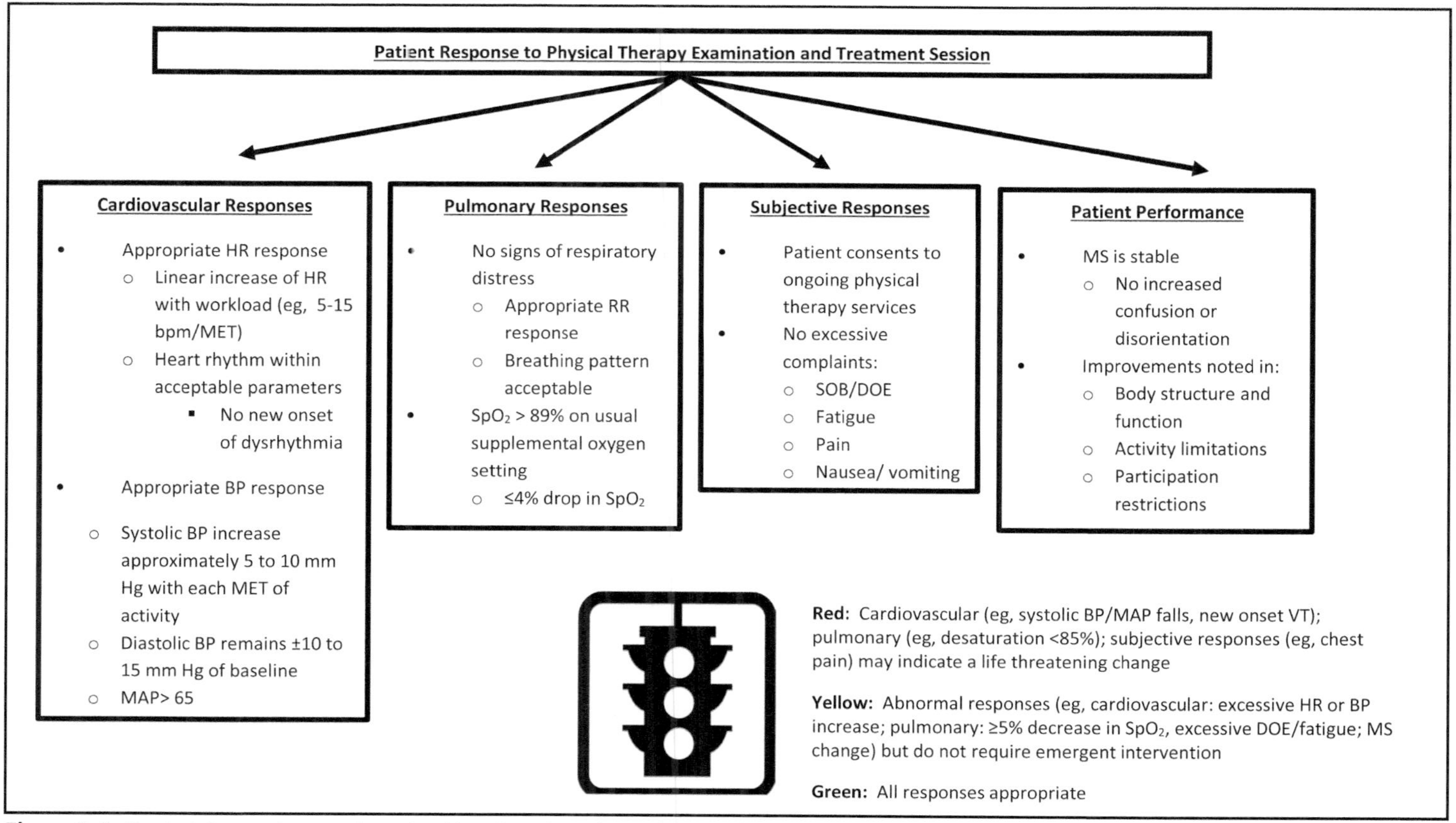

Figure 1-4. Physical therapy interventions algorithm describing the vital sign and patient responses to prescribed interventions. (Adapted from Stiller K, Phillips A. Safety aspects of mobilising acutely ill inpatients. *Physiother Theory and Pract.* 2003;19:239-257.) *(continued)*

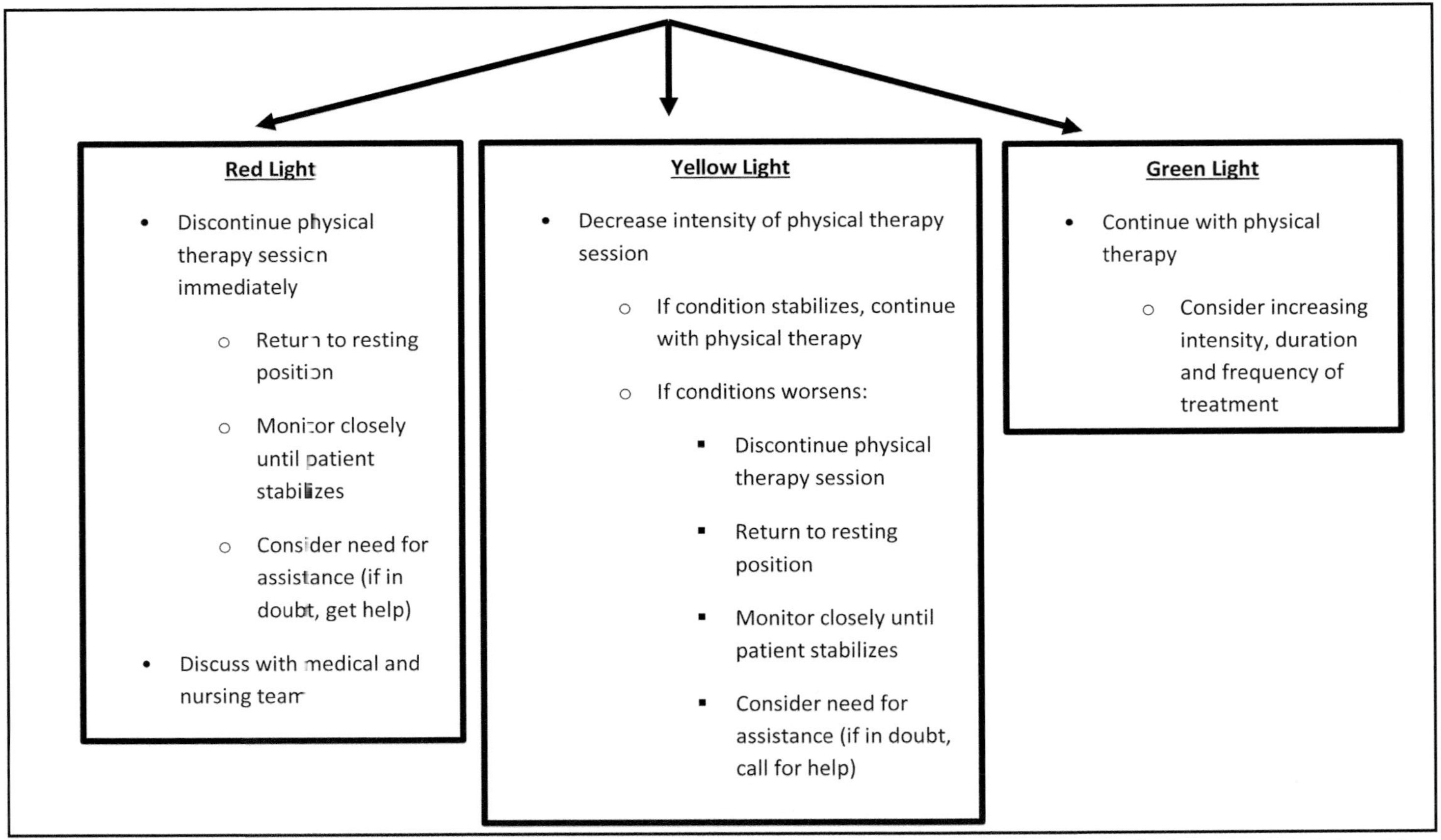

Figure 1-4 (continued). Physical therapy interventions algorithm describing the vital sign and patient responses to prescribed interventions. (Adapted from Stiller K, Phillips A. Safety aspects of mobilising acutely ill inpatients. *Physiother Theory and Pract.* 2003;19:239-257.)

Table 1-3

DEEP TENDON REFLEX TESTING

Deep Tendon	*Spinal Level*	*Grade*
Biceps	C5 and C6	0 (No response)
Brachioradial	C5 and C6	1+ (Sluggish/diminished)
Triceps	C6, C7, and C8	2+ (Active/expected/normal)
Patellar	L2, L3, and L4	3+ (More brisk than expected, slightly hyperactive)
Achilles	S1 and S2	4+ (Brisk, hyperactive, intermittent or transient clonus)

Adapted from Seidel HM, Ball JW, Dains JE, Benedict GW. *Mosby's Guide to Physical Examination.* St. Louis, MO: Mosby, Inc; 2003.

also compare the expected emotional and behavioral responses to actual responses. Identifying the patient's learning preferences (eg, learning barriers, education needs) contributes to successful patient education. It is obvious that the level of patient's consciousness and orientation will affect the delivery of physical therapy services and impact the patient's learning and ability to make needs known. Arousal and alertness can be impaired due to a variety of health conditions, as well as sleep deprivation and medications, such as sedatives, anxiolytics, and narcotics. Artificial airways, such as endotracheal or tracheostomy tubes, can alter communication and the therapist should consider alternative communication devices (eg, letter boards, electrolarynx). The therapist should consider consulting with occupational and speech therapists to manage altered communication and cognition.

Tests and Measurements

Specific tests and measures selected by the physical therapist will be determined by data gathered from the history and systems review. As stated in the *Guide,* the tests and measures performed should be only those that are necessary to (1) confirm or reject a hypothesis about the factors that contribute to making the individual's current level of function less than optimal and (2) support the physical therapist's clinical judgments about the diagnosis, prognosis, and plan of care.[1] The examination process is a dynamic and ongoing process in the acute care environment. Standardized tests and measures applied early in an episode of care establishes the baseline status of the patient and provides a means to quantify change in the patient's functioning. Common tests and measures are discussed in the following sections and included in the appendix at the end of the chapter. The appendix provides a brief description and clinical pearls of select tests and measures (Table 1-7). This table is not a comprehensive list but are the most frequently encountered by the author.

Aerobic Capacity and Endurance

The typical manner of testing aerobic capacity and endurance in adults involves some type of exercise equipment, such as bicycle or treadmill. The hospitalized patient does not usually undergo such testing; exercise testing for the patient who has recently experienced an acute myocardial infarction (MI) or electrocardiogram (ECG) abnormality may be the exception. Therapists often challenge and monitor aerobic capacity and endurance through assessment of VS responses and patient's perceived exertion with functional tasks and common ADLs, including bed mobility,

Table 1-4
Cranial Nerve Testing

Cranial Nerve #	*Name*	*Function and Description of Technique*	*Examination Findings in Common Diseases/ Disorders*
I	Olfactory	The ability to smell is tested by asking the person to identify items with very specific odors (eg, soap, coffee) placed under the nares.	**Lesion symptoms**: Loss of sense of smell *(***anosmia***)* if bilateral. May result from head injury.
II	Optic	Vision and detection of light by the pupil, the patient is tested by reading an eye chart. Detection of objects or movement from the corners of the eyes tests peripheral vision. Confrontation and extinction tests visual fields.	**Lesion symptoms**: Unilateral damage produces ipsilateral blindness; bilateral damage produces bilateral blindness.
III	Oculomotor	**Extraocular eye movements**: Eye upward, downward, and inward **Pupillary reflex**: Narrowing (constriction) or widening (dilation) of the pupil in response to light **Convergence**: Medial movements of eyes to an object at close range. The upper eyelid is observed for drooping (ptosis)	**Lesion symptoms**: Loss of medial rectus and unopposed lateral rectus muscle function results in eyeball deviation outward (**lateral strabismus**); may cause double vision (**diplopia**); involuntary back and forth motions (**nystagmus**); ipsilateral ptosis may be present.
IV	Trochlear	Extraocular movements. The ability to move each eye downward and laterally is tested by asking the person to follow a target.	**Lesion symptoms**: Loss of superior oblique muscle function results in difficulty moving eyeball down and laterally creating a **vertical, medial strabismus**; nystagmus may be present.
V	Trigeminal	Facial sensation and chewing; facial sensation is tested using a pin and cotton swab or finger. Clenching the teeth and opening the jaw against resistance tests strength and movement of jaw muscles. The **blink (corneal) reflex** is tested by touching the cornea of the eye (eg, cotton wisp).	**Lesion symptoms**: Ipsilateral loss of sensation of the head, face, and inner oral cavity; weakness of muscles of mastication make chewing difficult and jaw may deviate ipsilaterally (eg, trigeminal neuralgia). *(continued)*

Table 1-4 (continued)

Cranial Nerve Testing

Cranial Nerve #	*Name*	*Function and Description of Technique*	*Examination Findings in Common Diseases/ Disorders*
VI	Abducens	Side-to-side (lateral) eye movement.	**Lesion symptoms**: Loss of lateral rectus muscle function results in difficulty moving eyeball laterally, creating a medial strabismus; diplopia and nystagmus may be present.
VII	Facial	Facial expression (smile, open the mouth and show teeth, close eyes tightly) and taste in the front 2/3 of the tongue (eg, sweet [sugar], sour [lemon juice], salty [salt], bitter [aspirin])	**Lesion symptoms**: Decreased taste of anterior tongue; decreased corneal reflex; decreased facial movements (eg, Bell's palsy).
VIII	Vestibulo-cochlear	Hearing (tuning fork) and balance (walk a straight line, heel-toe walking, Romberg test).	**Lesion symptoms**: *Auditory*: Deafness or ear ringing (tinnitus) *Vestibular*: Decreased balance, vertigo, and/or nystagmus may be present (eg, acoustic tumor, vestibular neuritis)
IX	Glosso-pharyngeal	Swallowing, gag reflex, and speech. The patient is asked to swallow; say "ah-h-h" to check the movement of the palate and uvula (the small, soft projection that hangs down at the back of throat). A tongue blade is touched to the back of the throat to evoke the gag reflex. The person is asked to speak to check the voice for hoarseness.	**Lesion symptoms**: Loss of gag and swallowing reflex; difficulty with swallowing (dysphagia) enhancing aspiration risk.
X	Vagus	Swallowing, gag reflex, and speech; control of muscle in internal organs (including the heart). Because cranial nerves IX and X control similar functions, they are tested together.	**Lesion symptoms**: As in cranial nerve IX, tachycardia, air hunger (dyspnea), slurred speech (dysarthria), and hoarse voice (dysphonia)

(continued)

Table 1-4 (continued) **CRANIAL NERVE TESTING**			
Cranial Nerve #	*Name*	*Function and Description of Technique*	*Examination Findings in Common Diseases/ Disorders*
XI	Accessory	Neck ROM and shoulder shrugging against resistance	**Lesion symptoms**: Dysphagia; weakness for shoulder elevation ipsilateral cervical flexion/ extension and contralateral rotation.
XII	Hypoglossal	Tongue movement; stick out the tongue and observe for deviation to one side; assess symmetry of movement from side to side and observe for tongue atrophy or weakness.	**Lesion symptoms**: Ipsilateral deviation/atrophy of tongue, dysarthria, and dysphagia

Adapted from Gutman SA. *Quick Reference Neuroscience for Rehabilitation Professionals.* Thorofare, NJ: SLACK Incorporated; 2001 and Seidel HM, Ball JW, Dains JE, Benedict GW. *Mosby's Guide to Physical Examination.* St. Louis, MO: Mosby, Inc; 2003.

Table 1-5 **SIGNS OF UPPER AND LOWER MOTOR NEURON LESIONS**		
Sign	*Upper Motor Neuron Lesions*	*Lower Motor Neuron Lesions*
Weakness	Yes	Yes
Atrophy	No; however, may accompany disuse	Yes
Fasciculations	No	Yes
Reflexes	Increased	Decreased
Tone	Increased	Decreased

sit-to-stand transfers, ambulation, stair climbing, toileting, and bathing. Structured assessments can include the 6 Minute Walk Test (6MWT), shuttle tests, or step testing. The therapist should record the patient's VS prior to therapy as part of the systems review and document the physiologic responses as the therapy session proceeds. Normal exercise physiology must be kept in mind while realizing that the patient who has been admitted to the hospital can present with abnormal responses. Therefore, the therapist expectations need to be guarded. For example, a resting RR of 28 breaths per minute in a healthy person is abnormal, but this tachypnea is expected with the patient who is recovering from respiratory failure due to reduced lung compliance and decreased tidal volumes (V_T). This RR is an attempt to maintain adequate minute ventilation and is not by itself a contraindication to therapy. The work of breathing is elevated as a substantial amount of the patient's oxygen consumption is being utilized for breathing. The therapist should expect the patient to have limited

Table 1-6

FUNCTIONAL INDEPENDENCE MEASURE SCORING CRITERIA ACTIVITY MEASURE FOR POST ACUTE CARE "6 CLICKS"

Functional Independence Measure Scoring Criteria

No Helper Required	
Score	*Description*
7	Complete independence
6	Modified independence (patient requires use of a device, but no physical assistance)
Helper (Modified Dependence)	
Score	*Description*
5	Supervision or setup
4	Minimal contact assistance (patient can perform 75% or more of task)
3	Moderate assistance (patient can perform 50% to 74% of task)
Helper (Complete Dependence)	
Score	*Description*
2	Maximal assistance (patient can perform 25% to 49% of task)
1	Total assistance (patient can perform less than 25% of the task or requires more than one person to assist)
0	Activity does not occur

Activity Measure for Post Acute Care Inpatient Basic Mobility

How much difficulty does the patient currently have...	**Unable (1)**	**A lot (2)**	**A little (3)**	**None (4)**
1. Turning over in bed (including adjusting bedclothes, sheets, and blankets)?				
2. Sitting down on and standing up from a chair with arms (eg, wheelchair, bedside commode)?				
3. Moving from lying on back to sitting on the side of the bed?				
How much help from another person does the patient currently need...	**Total (1)**	**A lot (2)**	**A little (3)**	**None (4)**
1. Moving to and from a bed to a chair (including a wheelchair)?				
2. Walking in hospital room?				
3. Climbing 3 to 5 steps with a railing?				

(continued)

Table 1-6 (continued)

FUNCTIONAL INDEPENDENCE MEASURE SCORING CRITERIA ACTIVITY MEASURE FOR POST ACUTE CARE "6 CLICKS"

Activity Measure for Post Acute Care Inpatient Daily Activity				
How much help from another person does the patient currently need...	**Total (1)**	**A lot (2)**	**A little (3)**	**None (4)**
1. Putting on and taking off regular lower body clothing?				
2. Bathing (including washing, rinsing, drying)?				
3. Toileting (including using toilet, bedpan, or urinal)?				
4. Putting on and taking off regular upper body clothing?				
5. Taking care of personal grooming, such as brushing teeth?				
6. Eating meals?				
AM-PAC Scoring: Basic Mobility=XX/24; Daily Activity=XX/24				
Note: AM-PAC is a licensed tool. See https://www.onadeo.com/shop/ for licensing information.				

breathing reserve and decreased exercise capacity prompting a reduction in the intensity of therapeutic interventions.

Anthropometric Characteristics

Measures of body dimensions in adults most commonly include weight and body mass index (BMI). BMI is used to quantify tissue mass and describe the body habitus of the individual (Table 1-8). BMI is a surrogate measure of body fat and not a direct measure, although it is correlated with direct measure of body fat such as underwater weighing. BMI measures excess weight rather than excess fat and has limitations, such as overestimating body fatness in muscular individuals. Although BMI has limitations, its ease of use has allowed widespread application across populations and is an important public health measure. BMI and body weight alone do not completely define the patient's body habitus or nutrition status. Therefore, additional testing could include waist circumference to estimate visceral adiposity and review of laboratory testing data (ie, serum albumin, prealbumin, cholesterol, and C-reactive protein) provides more information regarding a patient's nutrition status and health risk (see Chapter 2).

Edema in the hospitalized adult is likely due to recent surgery, congestive heart failure, liver and/or renal dysfunction, nutritional deficits, fluid overload, and inactivity. Edema can limit joint ROM, cause pain, and impair ADL performance. Edema is often graded as noted in Table 1-9 or assessed more accurately by circumferential or volumetric measurements.

Table 1-7

COMMON TESTS AND MEASURES

The following are common tests and measures used in the acute care setting. This table is not all inclusive and is meant as a guide to assist the clinician in choosing an outcome measure. Standardized tests and measures early in an episode of care establish the baseline status of the patient, direct and provide focus for interventions, provide a means to quantify change throughout the hospitalization, may serve as a patient motivation tool, provides quantifiable outcomes for caregivers and third party payers, and assist with discharge planning. The clinician is referred to the bibliography for further descriptions, access to the tools themselves, psychometric properties, and normative data.

Test and Measures Category	*Description/Procedure*	*Clinical Pearl*
Mobility (Including Locomotion) and Activities of Daily Living		
AM-PAC 2 versions of "6 Clicks": • Basic Mobility • Daily Activities	• Designed as a functional outcomes system that can be used across settings • Basic Mobility includes rolling, sit-to-stand transfer, supine-to-sit transfer, bed-to-chair transfer, walking in room, and stair climbing. • Daily Activities includes upper and lower body dressing, bathing, toileting, personal hygiene, and eating.	• Validated, reliable, demonstrates responsiveness, has been used to predict discharge destination
Acute Care Index of Function (ACIF)	• 20 items divided into 4 subscales: 1. Mental status 2. Bed mobility 3. Transfers 4. Mobility	• Validated, reliable, demonstrates responsiveness, and has been used to predict discharge destination • Primarily developed for use with neurological population
Barthel Index	• Assesses the ability of a patient to perform ADLs • Includes 10 ADL/mobility items	• Self-report or direct observation • Surrogate (eg, family member) can be used to provide information if patient is unreliable

(continued)

Table 1-7 (continued)

Common Tests and Measures

Test and Measures Category	*Description/Procedure*	*Clinical Pearl*
Functional Independence Measure (FIM)	• 18 items (13 motor and ADL tasks, 5 cognitive tasks) • Uses a well-defined 7-point scale • Designed to measure functional status of people in inpatient rehabilitation facilities (IRFs) • Provides a uniform measure of disability; how much assistance is required for the individual to carry out ADLs	• Maximum score: 126 • Operationally defined FIM provides a common language for all rehabilitation team members • Team approach (eg, physical therapist, occupational therapist, speech-language pathologist, nurse) • Not designed for use in the acute care setting • AlphaFIM developed for use in the acute care setting
Functional Status Score for the Intensive Care Unit (FSS-ICU)	• 5 items (rolling, supine-to-sit transfers, unsupported sitting, sit-to-stand transfers, ambulation) • Uses the 7-point scoring system from the FIM	• Maximum score: 35 • Used to identify functional improvements of patients in the ICU and long-term acute care hospital (LTACH) settings. ¤ Could be useful for additional settings
Physical Function in the ICU Test-scored (PFIT-s)	• A 4-item test battery that includes the patient's upper and lower extremity strength; the ability of the patient to stand from a chair and march on the spot	• Can be used with patients in the ICU, including patients who require mechanical ventilation • Valid, reliable, responsive to change
Walking Speed; 10 Meter Walk Test (10MWT)	• Examines walking speed in meters/second (m/s) • Time is measured while the individual walks the set distance • The patient is given extra space to accelerate to his or her self-selected walking speed • If needed, an assistive device should be used.	• Complete 1 practice and then 2 timed trials. ¤ Best time is recorded ¤ Normal walking speed is 1.2 to 1.4 m/s ¤ Minimally clinically important difference ~ 0.05 to 0.1 m/s • Walking speed is considered a functional vital sign. • ± at least 0.1 m/s is a predictor for future well-being

(continued)

Table 1-7 (continued)

Common Tests and Measures

Test and Measures Category	*Description/Procedure*	*Clinical Pearl*
Aerobic Capacity/Endurance		
6MWT	• Open hallway (30 meter or 100 foot walkway) • If needed, an assistive device should be used. • Patient is instructed to walk as far as possible for 6 minutes.	• 2 tests increase reliability because of a practice effect. • Consistency with encouragement is important because this influences total walk distance • Calculate miles per hour (MPH): ¤ Walk distance/6 x 0.0136 = mph • Minimally clinically important difference ~ 50 meters (164 feet)
2-Minute Walk Test (2MWT)	• Open hallway • If needed, an assistive device should be used. • Patient is instructed to walk as far as possible for 2 minutes	• Highly correlated with 6MWT in select population (eg, chronic obstructive pulmonary disease [COPD], cerebrovascular accident [CVA], multiple sclerosis [MS], geriatric populations)
Muscle Performance (Including Strength, Power, Endurance, and Length)		
Grip Strength (Hand Held Dynamometry [HHD])	• Assessment of muscle strength using a HHD	• Grip strength is a simple test to identify ICU-acquired weakness ¤ Males, < 11 kg-force; females, < 7 kg-force
5 Times Sit to Stand	• A measure of lower extremity muscle strength • Patient sits in a standard chair with arms folded across chest. • Time starts with "go" and ends when buttocks touches chair after fifth repetition.	• Use of arm rests is a modification. • Also used as fall risk assessment ¤ Generally, scores > 12 to 15 seconds associated with increased fall risk.

(continued)

Table 1-7 (continued)

COMMON TESTS AND MEASURES

Test and Measures Category	*Description/Procedure*	*Clinical Pearl*
Manual Muscle Test (MMT)/ Medical Research Council (MRC) Strength Examination	• MMT evaluates the patient's ability to generate muscle force; can be used to isolate specific muscles and/or myotomes; each movement is graded from 0 to 5 • MRC evaluates 6 muscles (3 upper extremity [UE], 3 lower extremity [LE]) on both sides; each movement is graded from 0 to 5.	• MRC scores of 60 is normal. • MRC score <48 indicate ICU-acquired weakness.
30 Second Chair Stand	• Examines functional LE strength. • Patient is seated in chair with his or her arms folded across chest. • Patient rapidly rises to fully erect stand and returns to sitting. This is repeated for 30 seconds.	• If patient uses UEs, he or she is scored 0 and test is stopped. • Do not count incomplete stand, but more than halfway up at the end of 30 seconds counts as a full stand.
Balance		
Function in Sitting Test (FIST)	• 14-item bedside examination of sitting balance	• Performed using a standard hospital bed but without an air mattress.
Functional Reach Test (FRT) and Modified Functional Reach Test (mFRT)	• Examines a patient's stability in standing (FRT) or sitting (mFRT).	• Reach <6 inches associated with high risk of falling
Berg Balance Scale (BBS)	• 14-item fall risk measure that examines static and dynamic balance.	• Maximum score: 56 • Increased fall risk: ¤ Score <42 if no fall history ¤ Score <51 if history of falls • Norms available
Dynamic Gait Index (DGI)	• 8 items that examine gait, balance, and fall risk. • Combines walking with head turns, changing directions, managing obstacles, and stairs.	• Maximum score: 24 ¤ Generally, scores ≤19 associated with increased fall risk

(continued)

Table 1-7 (continued)

Common Tests and Measures

Test and Measures Category	*Description/Procedure*	*Clinical Pearl*
Timed Up and Go (TUG) Test	• Assesses transfers, gait and fall risk. • Patient should sit in a standard armchair, placing his or her back against the chair and arms on the chair's arms. • Patient walks 3 meters (9.8 feet), turns around, walks back to chair, sits down • A stopwatch is used to time the test. • If needed, an assistive device can be used.	• Often used as a mobility outcome measure. • Generally, scores >14 seconds associated with increased fall risk.
Integumentary Integrity		
Braden Scale	• Assesses the likelihood of developing pressure ulcers • 6 items are examined: 1. Sensory perception 2. Moisture 3. Activity 4. Mobility 5. Nutrition 6. Friction/shear	• Total scores range from 6 to 23 points. ¤ Scores <12 lower scores indicate a higher risk.
Pressure Ulcer Scale for Healing (PUSH)	• Examines and categorizes the ulcer with respect to surface area, exudate, and type of wound tissue.	• A comparison of total scores measured over time provides an indication of the improvement or deterioration in pressure ulcer healing. ¤ Decreasing scores indicate healing.

Adapted from ATS Committee on Proficiency Standards for Clinical Pulmonary Function Laboratories[11]; Fritz and Lusardi[12]; Jette et al[13]; Rehabilitation Measures Database[14]; and Thrush et al.[15]

Obesity is associated with multiple disorders, including diabetes, coronary artery disease, obstructive sleep apnea, and hypothyroidism to name a few (see Chapter 11, *Surgical Information*, and Table 11-21). Obesity can independently limit the patient's mobility and is a leading risk factor for integumentary and cardiopulmonary disorders. Appropriate bariatric equipment is required to successfully initiate OOB activities (see Tables 11-24 through 11-27). Conversely cachexia is also prominent in long-standing disease, and impaired nutrition status is associated with poor outcomes. Acute illness is associated with hypermetabolism and hypercatabolism, resulting

Table 1-8

BODY MASS INDEX (KG/M^2)

18.5 or less	Underweight
18.5 to 24.9	Normal
25.0 to 29.9	Overweight
30.0 to 34.9	Obesity Class I
35.0 to 39.9	Obesity Class II
40 or greater	Obesity Class III/Severe Obesity

Table 1-9

GRADING EDEMA

Scale	*Depression (cm)*	*Description*
1+ (Trace)	Slight	Barely perceptible
2+ (Mild)	0.0 to 0.6	Skin rebounds <15 seconds
3+ (Moderate)	0.6 to 1.3	Skin rebounds in 15 to 30 seconds
4+ (Severe)	1.3 to 2.5	Skin rebounds in >30 seconds

Adapted from Perloff JK. *Physical Examination of the Heart and Circulation.* 3rd ed. Philadelphia, PA: WB Saunders; 2000 and Seidel HM, Ball JW, Dains JE, Benedict GW. *Mosby's Guide to Physical Examination.* St. Louis, MO: Mosby, Inc; 2003.

in increased energy expenditure and excessive metabolic breakdown of body tissues, leading to unintentional weight loss. Malnutrition promotes muscle wasting, reduced respiratory and peripheral muscle strength and endurance, increased rates of infection, increased mortality, and reduced pulmonary function.

Assistive and Adaptive Devices

Assistive technology is any item, piece of equipment, or product system—acquired commercially off the shelf, modified, or customized—that is used to increase, maintain, or improve the functional capabilities of a person with a disability. Discrete types of assistive technology include aids for locomotion, orthotic devices, prosthetic requirements, seating and positioning technology, and other assistive technology to improve function.[1] Assistive technologies are applied in the acute care setting to aid patients in performing tasks (eg, long-handled reachers, splints) or promote safe movement (eg, walkers, canes, wheelchairs [see Table 8-15]). Some equipment may be necessary due to medical or surgical management (eg, orthotic, splints [see Tables 8-10 through 8-14 and 9-20]), and the therapist's job is to optimize mobility within the constraints of the prescribed device.

Orthotics devices are externally applied equipment used to support or protect weak or ineffective joints/muscles or other part of the body and may serve to enhance performance.[1] Common orthotic devices include braces, casts, shoe inserts, and splints. Protective devices include braces, cushions, and helmets, as well as compression garments, abdominal binders, neck collars, serial casts, and slings. Common orthotics and protective and supportive devices are described in Chapter 8 (see Tables 8-10 through 8-14) and Chapter 9 (see Table 9-20). Physiologic support devices include mechanical ventilation and supplemental oxygen (Chapter 3), mechanical circulatory assist devices (Chapters 3 and 6) and renal replacement therapy (Chapter 12).

A prosthesis is an artificial device used to replace a missing body part.[1] Patients are rarely prescribed a final version of their prosthesis in the acute care setting; however, the physical therapist may need to evaluate a previously prescribed prosthetic device for a patient who is admitted to the hospital. In all cases, the therapist provides valuable patient and family education; objective measurement and training regarding the successful care, alignment, and fit of all equipment; and the benefits, safety, and potential modifications of existing equipment to optimize patient outcomes.

Seating and positioning technology includes individually selected, configured, or custom-designed technology for one or more of the following purposes: (1) to provide support to a person's body in a desired sitting position, (2) to provide support in positions other than a sitting position (eg, standing, side-lying, supine), (3) to provide support in a way that will assist in maintaining or restoring skin integrity, or (4) to provide a mechanical method to change position relative to gravity (eg, tilt, recline, elevate, stand).[1] Therapists may also need to evaluate previously prescribed and possibly outdated seating technologies and provide recommendations. More commonly, positioning to optimize pressure relief and pressure distribution is an important and often daily aspect of acute care physical therapy. Chapter 15 provides a more detailed discussion.

Other assistive technology to improve function includes 3 categories of technology: (1) transfer technologies, including gait belts, sliding boards, sliding sheets, and manual or electric lifts designed to move a person from one surface to another; (2) assistive devices used in a bathroom setting, including raised toilet seats, adaptive commodes, shower commodes, shower chairs, benches, and sliders; and (3) electronic aids to daily living (EADLs), including environmental controls and access methods to electronic technologies (eg, sip-and-puff switch to control a power wheelchair, adapted switch to control an automatic door opener or hospital bed movement). The therapist provides valuable patient and family education and training for safe mobility in both the hospital and the home. Overall, the physical therapist assesses the patient's safety and determines if the device enables or disables task completion. Determining the patient's prior, present, and future utilization of assistive technologies can prevent ordering duplicate or unnecessary equipment. Therapists need to be fiscally aware of the costs associated with assistive and adaptive devices and realize that many patients may not have adequate insurance coverage for DME. Therapists will need to investigate ways to provide necessary equipment for those with limited insurance or financial resources (eg, contact DME companies, consult social work).

Balance

Balance is defined in the *Guide* as the ability to maintain the body in equilibrium with gravity both statically (ie, while stationary) and dynamically (ie, while moving), and while upright (ie, standing, ambulating) and while sitting (ie, supported, unsupported).[1] This definition highlights the importance of assessing balance in multiple postures and while at rest and with activity. Common structured balance assessments used in the acute care setting include the FIST, FRT, BBS, DGI and the TUG test (see Table 1-7).

Balance disorders are common in older adults and falls can lead to injury and loss of independence with negative consequences on quality of life. The identification of balance disorders obviously influences the physical therapist's plan of care and discharge planning. Falls in the hospital are an important public health issue. Injurious falls are viewed as **never events** and typical fall prevention strategies promote immobility and may exacerbate gait and balance problems. It has been proposed that promoting mobility in the hospital may actually help to prevent injurious falls.[3] Physical therapists/physical therapist assistants will play a crucial role in these types

Table 1-10

GRADING PULSES

Upper Extremity: Carotid artery (medial and inferior to angle of the jaw)/brachial artery (medial to biceps tendon)/radial artery (medial and ventral side of wrist)
Lower Extremity: Femoral artery/popliteal artery (popliteal fossa with knee bent and patient in prone)/dorsalis pedis artery (medial side of dorsum of foot)/posterior/tibial artery (inferior to medial malleoli)

Scale	*Description*
4+	Bounding
3+	Full, increased
2+	Normal
1+	Weak, thready
0	Absent

Adapted from Perloff JK. *Physical Examination of the Heart and Circulation.* 3rd ed. Philadelphia, PA: WB Saunders; 2000 and Seidel HM, Ball JW, Dains JE, Benedict GW. *Mosby's Guide to Physical Examination.* St. Louis, MO: Mosby, Inc; 2003.

of initiatives to identify patients at risk of falls and assist with progressive mobilization and rehabilitation.

Circulation (Arterial, Venous, Lymphatic)

Circulation is the movement of blood through organs and tissues to deliver oxygen and nutrients while removing waste products. Cardiac and integumentary disorders should trigger a more thorough examination of the circulatory system. As noted during the system review, measurements of HR/pulse rate, BP, and the description of edema are standard elements. The physical therapist should also include rate of perceived exertion, descriptions of pulse quality (Table 1-10), activity tolerance and cardiovascular symptoms, such as angina, claudication, and dyspnea, as noted in Table 1-2. Further examination procedures would include interpretation of heart rhythm if the patient is attached to a cardiac monitoring system (see Chapter 6, Monitoring Information). Additional cardiovascular examination techniques are found in Chapter 6 (see Table 6-6 and Monitoring Information) and Chapter 15 (see Table 15-2). The examination of circulation and ventilation and respiration are often performed concurrently (see Tables 1-2 and 1-7) because cardiovascular and pulmonary health conditions present with similar signs and symptoms.

Cranial and Peripheral Nerve Integrity and Reflex Integrity

The cranial nerves are 12 pairs of nerves exiting directly from the brain to various parts of the head, neck, and viscera. The peripheral nerves include the spinal nerves and their efferent and afferent components. Reflex integrity is the soundness of the neural path involved in a reflex. A reflex is a stereotypic, involuntary reaction to sensory stimuli.[1]

Muscular weakness, abnormal movement patterns, or altered sensation and proprioception identified during the system review (musculoskeletal and neuromuscular systems) or diagnosed neuromuscular disorders should lead to further testing. Common measurements of nerve integrity include manual muscle testing, deep tendon reflexes (see Table 1-3), and cranial nerve testing (see Table 1-4). Sensory testing includes light touch (eg, cotton swab or finger), sharp vs dull (eg, safety pin), and joint position sense. Sensory testing should be performed bilaterally. Classification of ascending and descending spinal tract and UE and lower extremity motor and sensory nerve root distributions (eg, dermatome/myotome) are found in Chapter 9.

Environmental Factors

Environmental factors make up the physical, social, and attitudinal environment in which people live and conduct their lives. Environmental factors may be facilitators or barriers.[1] Environmental factors to consider include the physical features of the home (eg, stairs, width of doorways, bedroom/bathroom locations) as well as the health status of the primary caregiver. The therapist can hypothesize on caregiver burden based off the patient status as determined by specific tests and measures (eg, aerobic capacity/endurance, assistive technology, balance, gait, mental function, mobility [including locomotion]). Caregiver mental function, safety awareness, and physical capabilities are important factors affecting the discharge plan. Social support networks increase flexibility for safe and effective discharge planning and ease the caregiver's burden of care. Therapists typically provide patient/family education on modification to the discharge environment (eg, grab bars, shower chair, removal of throw rugs, lighting) that will enhance safety and mobility. Goals to overcome environmental barriers may warrant the referral to another level of care post-discharge. A simple tool used to predict discharge disposition after joint replacement that includes environmental factors is the Risk Assessment Predication Tool (RAPT).

Gait

Gait is the manner in which a person walks and may be characterized by rhythm, cadence, step, stride, and speed.[1] Additional descriptors include difficulty initiating or stopping the gait cycle, distance, posture, trunk and arm movements, stability, and observation of involuntary movements during walking (eg, spasticity/genu recurvatum). Ideally, therapists typically observe the gait pattern with the patient walking toward and away from the observer; however, safety and guarding of the patient, especially with changes of direction and turns, may necessitate standing next to the patient. Tests of gait (see Table 1-7) may include the TUG test, walking speed/10MWT, 2MWT or 6MWT, or observational gait analysis. Tests used to assess gait provide the physical therapist with objective information regarding fall risk and the abilities to independently perform ADLs and IADLs. This information provides evidence for the prescription of specific assistive and adaptive devices and is critical when determining the discharge plan.

Integumentary Integrity

Integumentary integrity refers to the intactness of the skin and the ability of the skin to serve as a barrier to environmental threats, such as bacteria, pressure, shear, friction, and moisture.[1] The skin is important for immune defense, provides sensory feedback, protects the internal organs, maintains fluid status and thermoregulation (ie, conservation and dissipation of heat), and synthesizes Vitamin D. As a component of the systems review, examination of the integument is standard practice in the acute care setting. Examination of sensation, incisions, scar tissue, bony prominences and pressure points, feet/shoes, and indwelling lines are critical in reducing infection risk and wound development. Chapter 15 (see Table 15-1) provides a more detailed description of the wound care examination.

Joint Integrity and Mobility and Range of Motion

Joint integrity and mobility represent the structure and function of the joint and are classified in biomechanical terms as **arthrokinematic motion**. Joint mobility is the capacity of the joint to be moved passively, evaluating the structure and integrity of the joint surface in addition to periarticular soft tissue characteristics.[1] ROM is the arc through which active and passive movement occurs at a joint or a series of joints and the angles created during this limb or trunk movement. Muscle length (ie, the maximum extensibility of a muscle-tendon unit), in conjunction with joint and soft tissue extensibility, determines flexibility. ROM in biomechanical terms is classified as **osteokinematic motion.** Evaluating ROM abnormalities includes consideration of arthrokinematics (ie, accessory movement at joint surfaces); tissue extensibility, such as muscle-tendon length and movement; and muscle tone, including spasticity.[1]

As mentioned previously, ROM examination is an important consideration for the acute care therapist. LE ROM is necessary for the patient to successfully transfer and initiate gait activities while UE ROM impacts ADL performance. The therapist must also consider chest wall and spine asymmetries that may be associated with surgical incisions, pain, neuromuscular disease, prior thoracic trauma, or orthopedic conditions (eg, scoliosis). Chest wall and spine asymmetries can affect the patient's breathing pattern and contribute to trunk pain. Joint integrity and mobility should be examined in more than the orthopedic or bed bound patient populations.

Mental Functions

The degree of patient arousal, attention, and cognition greatly influences the mobility status, independence with ADLs and IADLs, and the discharge plan. **Cognition** is defined as the act or processing of knowing, including awareness, memory, and judgment. Cognition, including the ability to process commands, is frequently assessed through a structured mental status examination. Specific instruments used include the Glasgow Coma Scale (GCS) (see Table 9-5), Montreal Cognitive Assessment (MoCA), Mini-Mental State Examination (MMSE), and the Confusion Assessment Method for the Intensive Care Unit (CAM-ICU) (see Table 4-2 and Figure 4-2).

Arousal is defined as a state of responsiveness to stimulation or physiologic readiness for activity and the patient's level of arousal and cognition is assessed throughout the episode of care. Frequent descriptors are provided in Table 1-11. Arousal, agitation and sedation can be quantified using the Richmond Agitation Sedation Scale (RASS). The RASS is a 10-point scale, with 4 levels of anxiety or agitation, 1 level to denote a calm and alert state (0), and 5 levels of sedation (see Table 4-2). Orientation is assessed by asking the patient his or her name, current location, month, day, year, and reason for admission (oriented x4). Asking patients to repeat your name and discipline, provided at the beginning of the interaction, challenges short-term memory. Having the patient repeat number sequences assesses immediate recall. Asking patients to recall past personal or historical events assesses long-term memory. Attention, an important aspect of task completion while performing ADLs, is the selective awareness of the environment or selective responsiveness to stimuli. Spelling "world" backward or counting by 2s to 20 determines attention.

As noted previously, mental status function might fluctuate throughout a hospitalization due to medication side effects, sleep deprivation, sensory deprivation secondary to bed rest, or a prior history of mental illness. Screening tools provide valuable data that can assist with determining alterations in status as well as determining appropriate therapeutic interventions and discharge recommendations.

Mobility (Including Locomotion), Self-Care, and Domestic Life

Mobility (including locomotion) is an individual moving by changing body positions or locations or by transferring from one place to another. This includes ambulation and wheeled mobility.[1] Self-care is caring for oneself, washing and drying oneself, caring for one's body parts, dressing, eating and drinking, and looking after one's health. Domestic life management is carrying out everyday actions and tasks associated with home life, such as acquiring and maintaining a living space, shopping, performing household tasks, caring for dependents, and performing yard work.[1] Although mobility and self-care are separate constructs in the *Guide,* these 2

Table 1-11

DESCRIPTORS OF LEVELS OF ALTERED CONSCIOUSNESS OR COGNITIVE FUNCTION

Disorientation: Beginning loss of consciousness (LOC); disorientation to time, place; impaired memory; loss of self-recognition.
Lethargy: Limited spontaneous movement or speech; easy arousal with normal speech or touch; may or may not be oriented to time, place, or person.
Obtundation: Mild to moderate reduction in arousal with limited response to the environment; falls asleep unless stimulated verbally or tacitly; answers questions with minimal responses.
Somnolence: Roused by various stimuli; makes appropriate motor and verbal responses.
Stupor: A condition of deep sleep or unresponsiveness from which the person may be aroused or caused to make a motor or verbal response only by vigorous and repeated stimulation; response is often withdrawal, grabbing at stimulus, or patient may be combative.
Coma: No motor or verbal response to the external environment or to any stimuli; even noxious stimuli, such as deep pain or suctioning; no arousal to any stimulus.
Semicoma: The organized withdrawal to painful stimuli or similar responses to persistent tactile stimuli.
Confusion: Loss of ability to think rapidly and clearly; impaired judgment and decision making.
Delusion: A false belief brought about without appropriate external stimulation and inconsistent with the individual's own knowledge and experience.
Psychosis: A mental disorder where alterations in personality and emotional state, and irrational behaviors and thinking are of psychogenic origins (ie, without clearly defined physical cause or structural alteration in the brain). Hallucinations and delusions are often present.
Illusions: The misinterpretation of sensory input, shadows, noises, odors, bodily sensations, etc.
Hallucination: Subjective sensory perceptions that may occur in any of the sensations (ie, auditory, visual, gustatory [taste], olfactory [smell], tactile).
Compulsion: Repetitive acts that a person feels driven to do.
Obsession: Repetitive thoughts that enter the patient's mind that the patient is unable to control (eg, thoughts of aggression, sexual thoughts).
Ruminations: Repetitive or continuous speculations; often circular and abstract.
Indecision: The inability to make up one's own mind.

Adapted from Huether SE, McCance KL. *Understanding Pathophysiology*. St. Louis, MO: Mosby-Year Book Inc; 1996.

categories are often examined together. Initiated during the neuromuscular portion of the systems review, functional task analysis is the most common examination test and measure. Functional tasks typically include bed mobility, transfers from bed to out of bed, and ambulation. Additional functional tasks include bathtub transfers, wheelchair use, and ADLs. Distances and use of mobility aides are included in functional task analysis. Beyond general observation, therapist will often grade patient performance of these functional tasks using portions of the FIM. Another measure used in hospital settings include the AM-PAC. The AM-PAC "6 Clicks" are short forms measuring the functional domains of basic mobility and daily activities. Each item is scored on 1 of 4 levels based on the amount of difficulty a patient has or how much help is needed from another person in completing the task (see Table 1-3). The PFIT-s, FSS-ICU, and ICU Mobility Scale (IMS) are other measures commonly used in the ICU but can be used in other settings as well. These tools are outlined in Chapter 4. Additional measures of function may include the Katz Index of Independence in Activities of Daily Living, Barthel Index, ACIF, and AlphaFIM to name a few (see Table 1-7).

Motor Function

Motor function is the ability to learn or demonstrate the skillful and efficient assumption, maintenance, modification, and control of voluntary postures and movement patterns.[1] Examination procedures include tests of dexterity and coordination, including rapid rhythmic alternating movements (eg, turning palms over and back, touch thumb to each finger in sequence, foot tapping) and accuracy of movements (eg, finger-nose, heel up/down alternate LE shin [heel-shin test]). Functional tests may include buttoning a shirt, tying shoes, or performance tests such as the TUG. Additional measures may include the 9-Hole Peg Test and the patient reported Disabilities of the Arm, Shoulder and Hand (DASH)/QuickDASH. Motor function provides valuable information regarding ADL/IADL performance and patient safety.

Muscle Performance

Muscle performance is the capacity of a muscle or a group of muscles to generate forces to produce, maintain, sustain, and modify postures and movements that are the prerequisite to functional activity. Strength is the muscle force exerted by a muscle or a group of muscles to overcome a resistance under a specific set of circumstances. Power is the work produced per unit of time or the product of strength and speed. Endurance is the ability for a muscle to sustain forces repeatedly or to generate forces over a period of time. Length refers to the maximum extensibility of a muscle-tendon unit. Recruitment of motor units, fuel storage, and fuel delivery, in addition to balance, timing, and sequencing of contraction, mediate integrated muscle performance.[1]

The most common strength tests are manual muscle testing, HHD, and the MRC Strength Examination (see Table 4-3). The MRC Strength Examination is a common screening tool used in the ICU for detection of ICU-acquired neuromuscular dysfunction but can also be applied throughout the hospital. Additional examination tools include functional tests, such as repeated transfers (eg, 5 Times Sit To Stand, 30 Second Chair Stand) (see Table 1-7). Functional tasks, such as repeated transfers, stair climbing, and self-care activities (eg, grooming, dressing, bathing), challenge not only strength but also endurance, motor planning, and motor control. Timed activity tests (eg, 2- or 6 Minute Walk Test) are helpful to examine cardiopulmonary and muscular endurance. While performing specific tests of muscle performance, keep in mind signs of an upper or lower motor neuron lesion as noted in Table 1-5, the potential negative impact of bed rest (see Chapter 4), and medication side effects. Newly discovered focal weakness or weakness patterns (eg, hemiplegia) discovered during the examination should lead to consultation with the medical team.

Pain

Pain is a disturbed sensation that causes disability, suffering, or distress. Pain can be viewed as adaptive and maladaptive. **Adaptive pain** refers to pain that is mainly a protective mechanism for the body where the individual reacts to remove the pain stimulus (eg, flexor withdrawal to nail bed pressure). Maladaptive pain is pain that interferes with normal physiologic processes leading to further activity limitations and restricted participation (eg, chronic pain leading to prolonged bed rest and loss of employment). The peripheral mechanisms of pain define pain as arising from stimulation of free nerve endings, the nociceptors, by mechanical (ie, pressure, deformation), chemical (ie, histamine, potassium, bradykinin), or thermal (ie, cold/heat) stimuli. Somatic pain includes superficial and deep pain. Superficial pain is defined as pain at the body surface, while deep pain arises from muscles, joints, bones, and connective tissues. Visceral pain originates from internal organs and is typically related to ischemia, deformation, infection, and inflammation. Therapists will frequently encounter patients with peripheral, somatic, and visceral pain in the acute care setting. Therapists will also encounter patients with chronic pain. Chronic pain is associated with multiple common conditions, such as back injury, osteoarthritis, diabetic neuropathy, rheumatic disease, and cancer. Chronic pain results not just from a physical insult but also from a combination of physical, emotional, psychological, and social factors. Pain science continues to evolve, and it is now recognized that pain is multidimensional. Mechanistically, the International Association for the Study of Pain (IASP) defines painful conditions as[4,5]:

- Nociceptive pain arises from actual or threatened damage to non-neural tissue and is due to activation of nociceptors
- Neuropathic pain is caused by a lesion or disease of the somatosensory nervous system
- Pain of unknown origin persists in the absence of tissue injury or is out of proportion to the initial insult and is thought to have enhanced central excitability, loss of central inhibition, or both.

Therapists should assess the intensity, quality, location, and duration of all pain. Pain scales provide an objective measurement of pain intensity and may guide therapeutic interventions (Figure 1-5). The impact of pain on the patient's participation restrictions (eg, quality of life [Short Form-36]) and activity limitations (eg, 6MWT) should also be investigated.[4] Effective pain management is essential to maximize patient interactions and involves coordinated multidisciplinary management. In addition to pain medications, the therapist can employ patient education, including education on pain physiology, manual therapy, peripheral desensitization techniques, relaxation techniques, and pain-relieving modalities.[5,6]

Posture

As noted in the *Guide*, posture is the alignment, positioning of the body in relation to gravity, center of mass, or base of support and optimal posture is a state of musculoskeletal balance and skeletal alignment that may protect the individual against injury or progressive deformity.[1] Therapists will assess posture through observation but may also use posture grids, plumb lines, tape measures, and video-assisted technology.[1]

Skeletal Integrity

Skeletal integrity is the optimal alignment, density, and soundness of the bony structures of the body. [1] Related to posture, skeletal integrity is assessed by observation and palpation and bone mineral density is most often noted during the history. However, signs and symptoms of interrupted bony integrity (eg, erythema, pain, edema, point tenderness at mid-sections of long bones)[1] may warrant further investigation and discussion with the medical team.

Ventilation and Respiration

The *Guide* defines ventilation as the movement of a volume of gas into and out of the lungs and respiration is the exchange of oxygen and carbon dioxide across a membrane either in the lungs or at the cellular level.[1] Examination of ventilation and respiration is performed at rest and repeated following activity (see Aerobic Capacity/Endurance; Mobility [Including Locomotion]). Observation of the breathing pattern and use of perceived exertion scales (see Table 1-2) supplement the measurement of respiratory rate. Pulse oximetry is indicated if the patient presents with supplemental

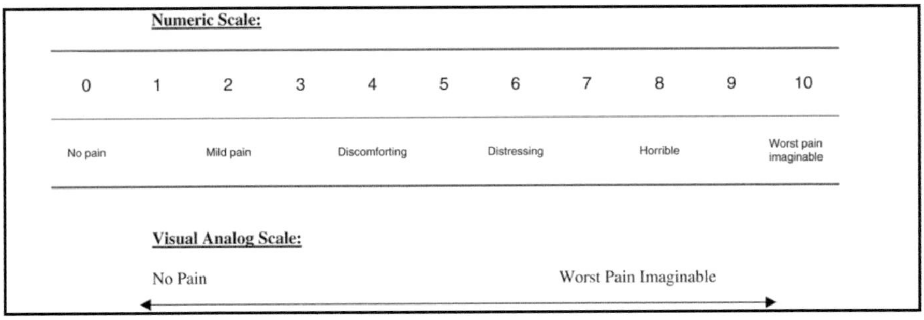

Figure 1-5. Pain scales.

oxygen, cyanosis, history of hypoxemia and prior/current need for oxygen therapy, complaints of SOB, or is diagnosed with cardiac or pulmonary disease. Capnography, the noninvasive measurement of the partial pressure of carbon dioxide (CO_2) in exhaled breath, is becoming more common in the hospital. Additional examination items include the review of pulmonary function testing during the history and assessment of cough, chest wall mobility, and breath sounds. Chapter 7 provides a more detailed description of the pulmonary examination.

Interventions

As stated in the *Guide*, intervention is the purposeful interaction of the physical therapist with an individual, and, when appropriate, with other people involved in that individual's care, to produce changes in the conditions that are consistent with the diagnosis and prognosis.[1] Obviously, the physical therapist's examination findings direct the therapist to prescribe and apply the most beneficial interventions (Table 1-12). For example, the need to prescribe strengthening, balance activities, and/or assistive technology can be determined from the findings of the tests and measures during the motor function, muscle performance, and/or mobility (including locomotion) examination. The need for airway clearance will be determined from the findings of ventilation and respiration. The dynamic nature of acute care practice requires the therapist to constantly reexamine the patient in real time as interventions are performed as noted in Figure 1-4. It is beyond the scope of this chapter to discuss each intervention category; however, specific interventions will be highlighted in the chapters and the case studies in the proceeding chapters to provide guidance and context.

Summary

This chapter introduced the physical therapist's examination of the patient in the acute care setting using the *Guide* as the foundation. As stated previously, this chapter is not all inconclusive but provides a rational approach to patient care. The physical therapist's examination is an ongoing process that is continuously applied throughout the hospitalization because the patient's status can change daily, if not minute-by-minute. The application of objective tests and measures provides concrete data to help drive care planning and decision making for discharge. Shorter lengths of stay in the hospital has limited the duration of the acute episode of care and the physical therapist has a greater role as a discharge planner and case manager. The appendix that follows this chapter on the discharge planning process provides an overview of the complex decisions that go into the transition from the hospital to the next appropriate level of care. Physical therapists/physical therapist assistants play a pivotal role in these decisions and are an integral part of the acute care health care team.

Table 1-12

INTERVENTION OVERVIEW

Intervention	*Description*	*Clinical Suggestions*
Patient or client instruction (used with every patient and client)	• Process of informing, educating, or training patients, families, significant others, and caregivers with intent to promote and optimize physical therapist episode of care. • Topics may be related to: ¤ Current condition (eg, specific impairments in body functions or structures, activity limitations, participation restrictions) ¤ Plan of care ¤ Transition to different role or setting ¤ Risk factors for developing impairments in body functions or structures, activity limitations, or participation restrictions ¤ Need for health, wellness, and fitness programs • Patient instruction engages patients in own health care and recovery	• Identify patient's needs: Topics should focus on "needs to know" not "nice to know." • Identify patient's concerns, readiness to learn, preferences for learning, support, and possible barriers to learning. ¤ Examples of learning preferences include verbal, visual, demonstration, written brochures/handout, models/props, or video. • Well-recognized barrier (patient and caregiver's) is **health literacy** ¤ Degree to which individuals have capacity to obtain, process, and understand basic health information and services needed to make appropriate health decisions[1] • Education plan: Frequently adjusted based on patient's health status and environmental factors • Examples of goals to achieve may include improved or increased: ¤ Understanding of health conditions and impairments in body structures/function and activity limitations or participation restrictions ¤ Behaviors fostering healthy habits, wellness, and prevention, including modifiable risk factors ¤ Self-advocacy for own health decisions combined with improved collaboration with health care team ¤ Awareness and use of community resources ¤ Adherence with prescribed medications, weightbearing restrictions, home or bedside exercise programs, etc. ¤ Patient and caregiver safety

(continued)

Table 1-12 (continued)

INTERVENTION OVERVIEW

Intervention	*Description*	*Clinical Suggestions*
Airway clearance techniques (ACTs)	• Therapeutic activities intended to manage or prevent consequences of impaired mucociliary transport or inability to protect airway (eg, impaired cough). • May include breathing strategies for airway clearance and symptom control, manual/mechanical techniques for airway clearance, positioning, and postural drainage • Breathing strategies: ¤ Huff cough ¤ Active cycle of breathing (ACB); autogenic drainage ¤ Deep breathing, incentive spirometry, staircase breathing ¤ Pursed-lip breathing (PLB) ¤ Pacing of ADLs and energy conservation • Manual/mechanical techniques: ¤ Chest wall percussion and vibration ¤ Assisted cough ¤ Bracing of incisions ¤ Airway suctioning • Positioning: ¤ Bronchial drainage ¤ Head of bed elevation or sitting upright to improve cough effectiveness ¤ Positioning to maximize ventilation and perfusion relationship • Techniques to maximize ventilation: ¤ Inspiratory hold maneuver, staircase breathing, manual hyperinflation, incentive spirometry	• Postoperative pulmonary complications increase patient morbidity, mortality, and health care costs. • ACT may benefit more than pulmonary patients • Data from history and pulmonary examination will guide prescription and performance of ACT. ¤ Patient with atelectasis, collapse of part of lung, ACT emphasis on deep breathing (eg, incentive spirometry, stacked breathing, diaphragm breathing) • Identify patient's concerns, readiness to learn, preferences and ability to participate. For example: ¤ Patient has reduced arousal (cannot actively participate); ACT of choice: chest wall percussion and vibration combined with positioning or high frequency chest wall oscillation (ie, the Vest [Hill-Rom]) ¤ Patient with cystic fibrosis effectively performs autogenic drainage at home, continue in hospital. Autogenic drainage as brand new technique in hospital, overwhelming and ineffective • Outcomes after performance of ACT demonstrates improvements in patient's status. ¤ Coarse crackles and diminished breath sounds prior to ACT. After ACT breath sounds louder and reduction in crackles due to mucus removal and increased ventilation

(continued)

Table 1-12 (continued)

Intervention Overview

Intervention	*Description*	*Clinical Suggestions*
	¤ Extension of trunk combined with flexion/abduction of UE for inspiration; flexion of trunk combined with extension/adduction of UE for expiration • Supplemental oxygen (O_2) therapy: ¤ Know/discuss variables of O_2 prescription including: ° Lowest acceptable SpO_2 value ° O_2 flow (2 to 6 liters per minute and F_IO_2 (percentage [eg, 21%, 50%] of O_2 delivered) ° Delivery device (eg, nasal cannula, face mask)	• Examples of goals to achieve may include increased or improved: ¤ Breath sounds ¤ Volume of mucus expectoration ¤ Independence with ACT regimen ¤ Incentive spirometry volumes ¤ Exercise/activity tolerance (eg, endurance, walk distance) ¤ Decreased symptoms (eg, SOB, DOE, chest wall pain) with exercise/activity
Assistive technology	• Includes prescription, application, and, fabrication or modification of: ¤ Aids for locomotion (eg, crutches, canes, walkers, wheelchairs) ¤ Seating and positioning technologies (eg, molded seating, lateral trunk support, support trays for wheelchair, prone cart) ¤ Orthotic devices (eg, ankle-foot orthoses [AFOs], knee-ankle-foot orthoses [KAFOs], wrist cock-up splints, shoe inserts)	• Used to reduce level of physical disability and/or pain. • Promote activities and participation. • Be aware of financial implications. • Examples of goals to achieve may include increased or improved: ¤ Quality and quantity of movement between and across body segments ¤ Balance ¤ Endurance ¤ Weightbearing status ¤ Pressure on specific body segment reduced and protection of body parts

(continued)

Table 1-12 (continued)

INTERVENTION OVERVIEW

Intervention	*Description*	*Clinical Suggestions*
	¤ Prosthetic devices (transtibial and transfemoral prostheses) ¤ Other assistive technologies to improve functioning (eg, transfer boards, mechanical lifts, raised toilet seat, commode)	• Decreased or reduced: ¤ Level of supervision required for task performance ¤ Edema and joint swelling ¤ Pain
Biophysical agents	• Broad group of agents that use various forms of energy and intended to: ¤ Assist muscle force generation and contraction (electrical muscle and nerve stimulation) ¤ Maintain strength after injury or surgery (electrical muscle and nerve stimulation) • Increase or improve: ¤ Joint mobility, muscle performance, and neuromuscular performance (eg, electrical stimulation, standing frames, tilt table) ¤ Rate of healing of open wounds and soft tissue (eg, hydrotherapy[pulsed lavage]) ¤ Tissue perfusion (eg, thermotherapy [hot packs]) • Modulate or decrease pain (eg, compression bandaging/garments, taping, cryotherapy [ice packs], thermotherapy) • Reduce or eliminate edema (eg, compression therapies [wrappings, garments, taping], electrical stimulation)	• Use in acute care environment vary widely based on practitioner preference and patient need. • Consider waxing/waning of communication abilities (ie, can patient make needs known) and mental functions (eg, arousal, cognition) when prescribing and applying. • Consider permanent and temporary physiological support equipment (eg, indwelling catheters, pacemakers, orthopedic hardware) prior to prescribing or applying. • Examples of goals to achieve may include increased or improved: ¤ Muscle performance (eg, activation, strength, power, endurance) ¤ Quality and quantity of movement between and across body segments ¤ Ability to perform functional tasks or activities related to self-care with and without devices and equipment ¤ Performance of and independence in ADLs and IADLs with or without devices and equipment ¤ Weightbearing status ¤ ROM ¤ Postural alignment ¤ Wound healing

(continued)

Table 1-12 (continued)

Intervention Overview

Intervention	*Description*	*Clinical Suggestions*
	• Decrease inflammation, connective tissue extensibility, or restriction associated with musculoskeletal injury or circulatory dysfunction (eg, mechanical devices [continuous passive motion], standing frames, tilt table) • Remodel scar tissue (compression therapies including wrappings and garments)	• Decreased or reduced: ¤ Pain ¤ Joint and soft tissue swelling, inflammation, or restriction ¤ Nonviable tissue in wound
Functional training in self-care and domestic, work, community, social, and civic life	• Functional training in self-care and domestic life integration and reintegration is the education and training of individuals to improve their ability to perform physical actions, tasks, or activities in an efficient, typically expected, or competent manner. ¤ Self-care includes ADLs, such as bed mobility, transfers, dressing, grooming, bathing, eating, and toileting ¤ Domestic life includes more complex ADLs and IADLs, with training in activities such as caring for dependents, maintaining a home, performing household chores and yard work, and shopping ¤ Education and training may include accommodation to or modification of environmental and home barriers, guidance and instruction in injury prevention or reduction, functional training programs, training in use of assistive technology during self-care and domestic life activities, task simulation and adaptation, and travel training.	• Essential part of most acute physical therapy episodes of care. ¤ Combine interventions with test and measures to identify beneficial outcome of physical therapy services. For example, if working on bed mobility, transfers, dressing, grooming, bathing, eating, and toileting, these tasks can be measured with FIM, AM-PAC, Katz, and Barthel. • Examples of goals to achieve may include increased or improved: ¤ Balance ¤ Endurance ¤ Motor function (motor control and motor learning) ¤ Muscle performance (strength, power, and endurance) ¤ Postural alignment and control ¤ Performance of and independence in ADLs and IADLs with or without devices and equipment • Decreased or reduced: ¤ Level of supervision required for task performance

(continued)

Table 1-12 (continued)

INTERVENTION OVERVIEW

Intervention	*Description*	*Clinical Suggestions*
Integumentary repair and protection techniques	• Application of therapeutic methods and techniques to enhance wound perfusion and establish optimal environment for wound healing by any of these mechanisms: ¤ Facilitation of cellular changes needed for wound healing ¤ Removal of nonviable tissue ¤ Removal of wound exudate ¤ Elimination of peripheral edema ¤ Management of scar tissue. • Methods and techniques may include: ¤ Debridement ¤ Dressing selection ¤ Orthotic selection ¤ Protective and supportive device recommendations and modifications ¤ Biophysical and topical agents	• Include functional and motor training as part of the wound management plan of care as many wounds may develop from impaired body structures/function (eg, tone, weakness, ROM) and activity limitations • Integumentary repair • Examples of goals to achieve may include decreased or reduced: ¤ Peripheral edema ¤ Pain levels ¤ Risk of recurrence of wound • Wound size decreases: ¤ Wound tissue is healthy (eg, granulation, new epithelium) ¤ Clinical infection signs are not present ¤ Inflammation signs are not present ¤ Necrotic tissue debrided ¤ Wound exudate minimized ¤ Wound healing advances to next phase
Manual therapy techniques	• Skilled hand movements and skilled passive movements of joints and soft tissue; are intended to improve tissue extensibility; increase ROM; induce relaxation; mobilize or manipulate soft tissue and joints; modulate pain; and reduce soft tissue swelling, inflammation, or restriction	• Examples of goals to achieve may include increased or improved: ¤ Quality and quantity of movement between and across body segment ¤ Integumentary integrity ¤ Weightbearing status

(continued)

Table 1-12 (continued)

INTERVENTION OVERVIEW

Intervention	*Description*	*Clinical Suggestions*
	• Techniques may include: ¤ Manual lymphatic drainage ¤ Manual traction ¤ Massage ¤ Mobilization/manipulation ¤ Passive ROM	¤ Improved ability to perform movement tasks ¤ Ability to perform physical actions, tasks, or activities related to self-care and domestic, education, work, community, social, and civic life with and without devices and equipment • Decreased or reduced: ¤ Pain ¤ Edema, lymphedema, or effusion ¤ Joint swelling, inflammation, or restriction ¤ Soft tissue swelling, inflammation, or restriction
Motor function training	• Systematic performance or execution of planned physical movements, postures, or activities • May include: ¤ Balance training, both static and dynamic ¤ Gait and locomotor training ¤ Perceptual training ¤ Postural stabilization and training	• Essential part of most acute physical therapy episodes of care • Self-care and domestic life integration and reintegration should be combined with motor function training (ie, gait and locomotor training). ¤ Combine interventions with tests and measures to identify beneficial outcomes. For example, if working on balance and gait, can be measured with TUG, BBS, AM-PAC, 2MWT, 6MWT, gait speed. • Examples of goals to achieve may include increased or improved: ¤ Balance ¤ Endurance ¤ Muscle performance (strength, power, and endurance) ¤ Postural alignment and control ¤ Level of supervision required for gait/locomotion ¤ Ability to perform tasks or activities related to self-care and domestic, education, work, community, social, and civic life with or without devices and equipment

(continued)

Table 1–12 (continued)

INTERVENTION OVERVIEW

Intervention	*Description*	*Clinical Suggestions*
Therapeutic exercise	• Systematic performance or execution of planned physical movements or activities intended to enable patient or client to remediate or prevent impairments of body functions and structures, enhance activities and participation, reduce risk, optimize overall health, and enhance fitness and well-being • May include: ¤ Aerobic/endurance, conditioning/reconditioning, increased workload over time ¤ Training (gait and locomotor, agility, body mechanics, developmental activities, movement pattern, neurodevelopment activities, perceptual) ¤ Breathing exercises ¤ Coordination exercises ¤ Muscle lengthening ¤ Neuromuscular education or reeducation ¤ ROM exercises and soft tissue stretching ¤ Relaxation exercises ¤ Strength, power, and endurance exercises	• Combine with tests and measures to identify beneficial outcome of physical therapy services. For example: ¤ If working on aerobic/endurance conditioning, can be measured with 2- or 6MWT. ¤ If working on strength, power and endurance exercises, tasks measured with 5 Times Sit to Stand, MMT, HHD, MRC sum score, PFIT-s or Borg RPE during functional or motor function training. • Examples of goals to achieve may include increased or improved: ¤ Aerobic capacity/endurance ¤ Airway clearance and/or breathlessness ¤ Ability to perform physical actions, tasks, or activities related to self-care ¤ Performance of and independence in ADLs and IADLs with or without devices and equipment ¤ Tolerance of positions and activities • Decreased or reduced: ¤ Level of supervision required for task performance

Adapted from American Physical Therapy Association. *Guide to Physical Therapist Practice*. 3rd ed. http://www.apta.org/Guide. Updated October 21, 2015. Accessed October 5, 2018.

Case Study

A 78-year-old female, Mrs. Carter, was admitted from the emergency department after her daughter found her on the floor of her apartment. Mrs. Carter was on the floor for approximately 15 hours. After evaluation in the emergency department, she is admitted to the hospital for medical management of dehydration, presumed syncope, ECG changes, and diabetes mellitus. On the day of admission, a physical therapy consult is ordered because of her fall.

Patient/Client History

General Demographics, Social History, and Living Environment

The patient lives alone in a third-floor apartment with a working elevator. She has 2 daughters who visit approximately every other day. She reports that her apartment is on 1 level and there are 4 steps to enter the apartment building and a handrail on both sides.

General Health Status, Social/Health Habits, and Family History

Patient appears overweight and denies smoking or alcohol use. She does not consider herself active but states "I get along all right by myself." Her hobbies include being active in her church, playing bridge with some friends, and knitting. Her family history is unrelated to the current condition.

Systems Review

Cardiovascular and Pulmonary

Resting BP is 108/78, HR 108 (atrial fibrillation per telemetry), respiratory rate is 16 breaths/minute and there is no observable edema.

Integumentary

Mrs. Carter appears overweight and there are no observed sores or skin lesions. She has been wearing pneumatic compression stockings on both LEs.

Musculoskeletal

Gross examination of bilateral upper extremities (BUEs)/bilateral lower extremities (BLEs) reveals no specific deficits. Strength is 5/5 and active range of motion (AROM) appears within normal limits (WNL).

Neuromuscular

Sensation to light touch and gross proprioception are intact throughout. Patient reports "tingling" sensation of her distal BLEs. She reports this is "the way it's been for several years."

Communication, Affect, Cognition, Language, and Learning Style

Mrs. Carter is awake, alert, and oriented to person, place, and time. She reports feeling anxious about moving because of the fear of falling again. Her primary language is English.

Tests and Measures

Aerobic Capacity and Endurance

The patient demonstrated a substantial increase in HR when standing at the bedside with minimal change in BP or SpO_2 (see Circulation [Arterial, Venous, Lymphatic] section).

Assistive and Adaptive Device

The patient was assisted into a standing position with use of a rolling walker. The physical therapist was not going to use a walker initially, but Mrs. Carter requested a mobility aid because she was afraid. The patient was able to assist with bed mobility by grabbing the bed rails. The nursing staff has ordered a bedside commode.

Balance, Gait, and Mobility (Including Locomotion)

The patient required minimal assistance to transition from supine to sit at the edge of the bed and minimal assistance to complete the sit-to-stand transfer and maintained abbreviated standing with a rolling walker and supervision. A gait assessment was not performed at this time due to the dramatic HR increase and blunted BP response with standing.

Circulation (Arterial, Venous, Lymphatic) and Ventilation/Respiration

The pulse is weak/thready (1+) and irregularly irregular due to the atrial fibrillation. SpO_2 is 97% on 2 liters per minute (lpm). Breath sounds are diminished bilateral bases, and otherwise clear to auscultation (CTA). After sitting at the edge of the bed, standing, and transferring to a bedside chair, her VS are BP 100/68, HR 146, SpO_2 94%. Patient reports feeling fatigued but denies lightheadedness. VS return to baseline after 3 minutes.

Pain

Mrs. Carter complains of discomfort along her left flank and using a visual analogue scale she reports the pain is 3/10 pain (aching) at rest and 4/10 (sharp) with moving. Subjectively, she states it's "not too bad" and the pain diminishes with rest.

Evaluation

The patient is an elderly female currently hospitalized secondary to a fall at home. The etiology of the fall appears multifactorial. She has been admitted with a medical history including dehydration, atrial fibrillation, and diabetes. These disorders can increase her fall risk due to reduced blood volume and a decreased cardiac output with resultant hypotension. Additionally, subjective sensory changes are noted in BLE probably due to diabetes. She denies fainting or a LOC but did report feeling "funny" for several hours prior to the fall.

Diagnosis

The patient presents with activity limitations related to atrial fibrillation with a rapid ventricular response (RVR) and a blunted BP response. She reports moderate pain with movement. Her laboratory values confirm the renal insufficiency, resolving dehydration, and diabetes (now insulin dependent). Her neuromuscular, musculoskeletal, and integumentary examination is unremarkable except for the subjective report of "tingling" in the LE.

Prognosis

The patient will most likely return to independent mobility status with improved rate control of her atrial fibrillation and correction of the dehydration and abnormal electrolytes. This should improve her BP responses with activity. Per nursing, she requires supervision for her medications. Social work has initiated nursing home placement while the family decides on discharge options. The patient will receive physical therapy 2 to 3 times/week with short-term goals of increasing OOB tolerance and decreasing level of assistance required for bedside mobilization, transfers, and ambulation. Interventions included ADL training (eg, bed mobility, transfers, toilet and gait training, wheelchair management), assistive and adaptive device training (eg, walker, reacher), therapeutic exercise (eg, UE/LE AROM and resistive exercises), education on use of blood sugar monitoring, bedside AROM exercise program, fall precautions, and review of prescribed medications.

Intervention

The plan of care primarily focused on progressive functional training in self-care and motor function training with the use of assistive technology. The therapists performed transfers and gait training with a walker and balance exercises. Patient instruction included education on fall prevention, importance of blood glucose monitoring, and safe use of the walker. Promoting increasing time spent OOB was discussed with nursing.

Outcomes

Mrs. Carter received a fluid bolus and she was encouraged to increase her free water consumption after the first physical therapy session secondary to mild orthostasis and readjustment of her cardiac medications. Reexamination the following day revealed a supervision level of assistance for OOB activities and ambulating 75 feet with an appropriate VS response, including an elevation in HR, BP, and stable SpO_2 without complaint of dizziness or excessive fatigue.

Mrs. Carter was treated for 3 days, including the initial physical therapy examination. At this point she was independent with a rolling walker walking 120 feet, a TUG was performed (16 seconds) and she was discharged to her elder daughter's home. Home care physical therapy was recommended.

ICF Clinical Reasoning Tool Case Study Summary								
Health Condition								
HPI: S/p fall, severe dehydration, presumed syncope, flank hematoma, and atrial fibrillation PMHx: NIDDM, HTN, ARF, and overweight								
Precautions/Contraindications								
Pain, atrial fibrillation with RVR, dehydration, lab values show elevated hct, sodium, creatinine, fasting blood glucose and leukocytosis; fatigue, deconditioning, syncope, and universal precautions Risk factors: CAD, depression, diabetes, atrial fibrillation, HTN, obesity, sedentary lifestyle								
Body Structure and Function			*Activity/Task Limitations*			*Participation*		
Impairment/ Problem	*Tests and Measures*	*Intervention*	*Activity*	*Tests and Measures*	*Intervention*	*Participation*	*Tests and Measures*	*Intervention*
• Excessive HR response • Flat BP response • Diminished breath sounds • Abnormal lab values • Decreased endurance • Left flank pain • Decreased balance • RF for cardiovascular disease • Weight exceeds IBW	• VS including ECG • Breath sounds • Review lab values • ROM/MMT • Balance • Pain scale • Risk factor assessment • BMI	• Breathing exercises • Bedside ROM • Progressive resistance training • Education on breathing exercises and safety/fall prevention • Consult registered dietician	• ADLs • Bed mobility • Transfers • Gait	• Functional task analysis • VS including ECG • TUG	• Progressive functional retraining • Balance retraining • Education on safety with transfers/gait	• Unable to return to independent living • Unable to play bridge	• QoL measure • Interview patient and family	• Continue physical therapy services • Consult social worker and family regarding discharge plans

(continued)

ICF Clinical Reasoning Tool Case Study Summary (continued)

Personal Factors	*Other Considerations*	*Environmental Factors*
• Age: 78 y/o female • A & O • Primary language: English • Lives alone • Self-management of diabetes • Self-management of nutrition and hydration • Anxiety about moving and fear of repeat falls		Home: • 4 entrance steps to apartment building • Emergency access to portable phone • Relies on elevator once in building and family for shopping/ groceries/cleaning/ financial management Hospital: • Urinary catheter, ECG monitor, NP oxygen, IV

A & O = alert and oriented; ARF = acute renal failure; CAD = coronary artery disease; ECG = electrocardiogram; hct = hematocrit; HPI = history of present illness; IBW = ideal body weight; IV = intravenous; NIDDM = non–insulin dependent diabetes mellitus; NP = nasal prongs; PMHx = past medical history; QoL = quality of life; RF = risk factors; RVR = rapid ventricular rate; s/p = status post; y/o = years old.

Adapted from American Physical Therapy Association. *Guide to Physical Therapist Practice*. 3rd ed. http://www.apta.org/Guide/. Updated October 21, 2015. Accessed October 5, 2018 and *Towards a Common Language for Functioning, Disability and Health*. World Health Organization. www.who.int/classifications/icf/icfbeginnersguide.pdf. Published 2002. Accessed April 29, 2019.

Chapter Review Questions

1. What are the key elements of the patient/client management as outlined in the *Guide to Physical Therapist Practice*?
   a. Examination, evaluation, diagnosis, prognosis
   b. Systems review, medications, chief complaints, current conditions
   c. Family history, consultation, coordination, collaboration
   d. Medical and surgical history, functional status, communication
2. What impact does previous function, current medical and functional status, and future discharge destination have on physical therapy examination?
   a. Helps determine number of outpatient encounters on follow-up
   b. Key information for comparison to current examination findings and potential discharge destination during examination
   c. Helpful to determine number of anticipated encounters in acute care
   d. Previous functional status is beneficial to use for the determining FIM value
3. What is the benefit of knowing the social and health habits of the patient when formulating the treatment plan?
   a. Prior social and health habits have no impact on the treatment plan.
   b. Prior social and health habits only benefit the communication and coordination of care.
   c. Prior social and health habits influence admission status but have no impact on discharge planning.
   d. Prior social and health habits are beneficial to determine goals, prognosis, and plan of care.
4. Which of the following components will best assist a therapist in the discharge decision-making process?
   a. Good home support 24 hours/day following hospital discharge
   b. Will patient achieve pre-hospital work status?
   c. Can the patient tolerate greater than 2 hours of skilled therapy per day?
   d. Will the patient qualify for disability?
5. Which of the following would most impact the decision to safely discharge a patient to home?
   a. Was the patient safe at home following hospitalization and able to return to full time work status?
   b. Does the patient have access to an elevator and was the patient an independent driver prior to hospital admission?
   c. Does the patient have access to a van service for transportation because he or she cannot drive?
   d. Can the patient ambulate safely on all surfaces and is the patient cognitively intact?

Answers: 1a, 2b, 3d, 4a, 5d

References

1. American Physical Therapy Association. *Guide to Physical Therapist Practice*. 3rd ed. http://www.apta.org/Guide/. Updated October 21, 2015. Accessed October 5, 2018.
2. *Towards a Common Language for Functioning, Disability and Health*. World Health Organization. www.who.int/classifications/icf/icfbeginnersguide.pdf. Published 2002. Accessed April 29, 2019.
3. Kosek E. Medical management of pain. In: Sluka KA, ed. *Mechanisms and Management of Pain for the Physical Therapist*. Seattle, WA: IASP Press; 2009:231-255.
4. Hoeger Bement MK, St. Marie BJ, Nordstrom TM, et al. An interprofessional consensus of core competencies for prelicensure education in pain management: curriculum application for physical therapy. *Phys Ther*. 2014;94(4):451-465.
5. Kumar SP, Saha S. Mechanism-based classification of pain for physical therapy management in palliative care: a clinical commentary. *Indian J Palliat Care*. 2011;17(1):80-86.
6. Growdon ME, Shorr RI, Inouye SK. The tension between promoting mobility and preventing falls in the hospital. *JAMA Intern Med*. 2017;177(6):759-760. doi: 10.1001/jamainternmed.2017.0840
7. Shepperd S, Lannin NA, Clemson LM, McCluskey A, Cameron ID, Barras SL. Discharge planning from hospital to home. *Cochrane Database Syst Rev*. 2013;1:CD000313. doi: 10.1002/14651858.CD000313.pub4
8. Smith BA, Fields CJ, Fernandez N. Physical therapists make accurate and appropriate discharge recommendations for patients who are acutely ill. *Phys Ther*. 2010;90(5):693-703.
9. Jette DU, Grover L, Keck CP. A qualitative study of clinical decision making in recommending discharge placement from the acute care setting. *Phys Ther*. 2003;83(3):224-236.
10. Agency for Healthcare Research and Quality. *Strategy 4: care transitions from hospital to home: IDEAL discharge planning*. http://www.ahrq.gov/professionals/systems/hospital/engagingfamilies/strategy4/index.html. Published June 2013. Accessed October 5, 2018.
11. ATS Committee on Proficiency Standards for Clinical Pulmonary Function Laboratories. ATS statement: guidelines for the Six-Minute Walk Test. *Am J Respir Crit Care Med*. 2002;166(1):111-117.
12. Fritz S, Lusardi M. White paper: walking speed: the sixth vital sign. *J Geriatr Phys Ther*. 2009;32(2)2-5.
13. Jette DU, Stilphen M, Ranganathan VK, Passek SD, Frost FS, Jette AM. AM-PAC "6-Clicks" functional assessment scores predict acute care hospital discharge destination. *Phys Ther*. 2014;94(9):1252-1261.
14. Rehabilitation Measures Database. http://www.rehabmeasures.org. Accessed January 15, 2016.
15. Thrush A, Rozek M, Dekerlegand JL. The clinical utility of the functional status score for the intensive care unit (FSS-ICU) at a long-term acute care hospital: a prospective cohort study. *Phys Ther*. 2012;92(12):1536-1545.

Bibliography

Huether SE, McCance KL. *Understanding Pathophysiology*. St. Louis, MO: Year Book Inc; 1996.

Jette AM. Physical disablement concepts for physical therapy research and practice. *Phys Ther*. 1994;74:380-386.

Rothstein JM, Echternach JL, Riddle DL. The Hypothesis-Oriented Algorithm for Clinician II (HOACII): a guide for patient management. *Phys Ther*. 2003;83:455-470.

Seidel HM, Ball JW, Dains JE, Benedict GW. *Mosby's Guide to Physical Examination*. 5th ed. St. Louis, MO: 2003.

Appendix

The Discharge Planning Process

Discharge planning is the development of an individualized discharge plan for the patient prior to leaving the hospital. The discharge plan should determine the most appropriate post-acute care destination, determine the need for follow-up services, contain medical costs and improve patient outcomes. A structured discharge plan tailored to the individual probably brings about small reductions in hospital length of stay and readmission rates.[7] Many factors go into the discharge plan including cognitive, physical, social, and financial status, environmental factors, and access to formal and informal care. Many health care disciplines will contribute to the discharge plan, including formal discharge planning coordinators, nurses, social workers, physical and occupational therapists, and physicians.[8]

Specific to physical therapy, data from the initial and repeated examinations allow the clinician to create an efficacious plan of care with goal-directed interventions. The intervention chosen attempts to improve and prevent impairments in body structure and function while negating activity limitations and participation restrictions to transition the patient to the next level of care. Therapists must make decisions on assistive technology, appropriate intensity, levels of continued rehabilitation, and whether or not the patient is safe to go home. These recommendations are sought not only by patients and their families, but also the physician, nursing, social work, and case management teams. Discharge planning can be a daunting and often confusing process. Figure 1-6 provides a conceptual model for discharge decision making and Figure 1-7 provides a practical approach to determining the discharge destination. These 2 models are not mutually exclusive but interact and influence each other. The conceptual model establishes that discharge recommendations requires a multi-step process where the therapist examines the patient and collects information about the structural impairments, activity limitations, and participation restrictions, determines the patient's ability to participate (eg, activity tolerance >3 hours/day) and the patient's and family's wants and needs and considers contextual factors such as home set up (eg, stairs) and social and family support. This information is further influenced by the patient's prognosis (eg, trajectory of recovery; expected length of stay; ongoing medical, surgical, nursing needs), insurance constraints, and ultimately by the therapist's experience.[9] The discharge decision-making process is changeable because the patient's medical needs, functional status, and other factors can change rapidly within the acute care setting. Figure 1-7 provides a practical model to determine the discharge destination. It is worth repeating that Figure 1-6 and 1-7 are linked. Unfortunately, no simple formula exists to accurately determine the most appropriate discharge decision. However, studies have demonstrated that therapists are able to integrate multiple factors contributing to the discharge needs of the patient to make accurate and appropriate discharge recommendations.[9,10] In fact, when therapist discharge recommendations are implemented and recommended follow-up services were received by the patient, the patient and the hospital had an increased likelihood of positive outcomes, including reduced readmission rates. As hospitals attempt to balance efficiency and quality of health care, the ability of physical therapists to provide accurate and appropriate discharge recommendations becomes even more important.[8]

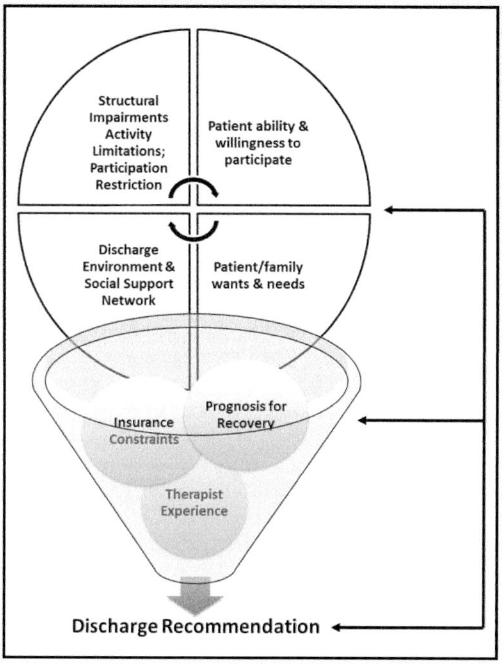

Figure 1-6. Discharge decision-making model. (Adapted from Jette DU, Grover L, Keck CP. A qualitative study of clinical decision making in recommending discharge placement from the acute care setting. *Phys Ther.* 2003;83[3]:224-236.)

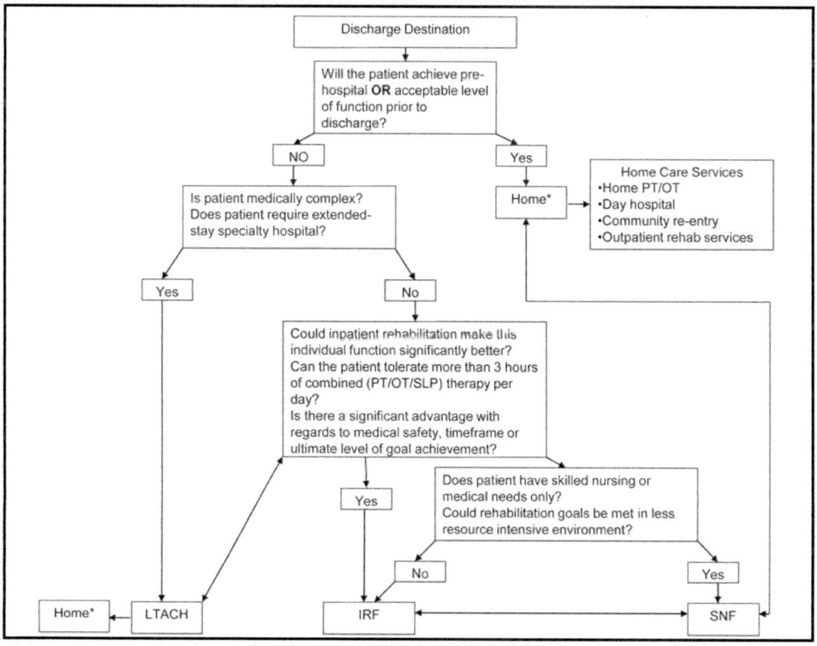

Figure 1-7. Discharge destination. (OT = occupational therapy; PT = physical therapy; SLP = speech-language pathology; SNF = skilled nursing facility.)

The Agency for Healthcare Research and Quality (AHRQ) developed the *Guide to Patient and Family Engagement in Hospital Quality and Safety*, a tested, evidence-based resource to help hospitals work as partners with patients and families to improve quality and safety. With the goals of reducing adverse events and preventing readmissions, it has been noted that discharge from hospital to home requires the successful transfer of information from clinicians to the patient and family. This requires active engagement of patients and families in the discharge planning process to make the transition in care safe and effective. With these goals in mind, the AHRQ created the IDEAL strategy highlighting the key elements of engaging the patient and family in discharge planning[10]:

I: Include the patient and family as full partners in the discharge planning process.

D: Discuss with the patient and family 5 key areas to prevent problems at home:

1. Describe what life at home will be like
2. Review medications
3. Highlight warning signs and problems
4. Explain test results
5. Make follow-up appointments

E: Educate the patient and family in plain language about the patient's condition, the discharge process, and next steps throughout the hospital stay.

A: Assess how well doctors, nurses, and other health care providers explain the diagnosis, condition, and next steps in the patient's care to the patient and family and use teach back.

L: Listen to and honor the patient's and family's goals, preferences, observations, and concerns.

Physical therapists and physical therapist assistants have unique opportunities to impact and participate in the IDEAL strategy. Although patients are "discharged sicker and quicker," it is not uncommon for the rehabilitation team to have repeated and prolonged interactions with patients and families. This should allow for open communication and multiple patient/family education sessions to incorporate many of the key elements of IDEAL. Finally, the acute care therapist should appreciate the pressure under which hospital-based medical care functions. Physicians are required, by their daily documentation, to justify why the patient requires ongoing hospital-based care. When that care is completed, the patient is generally considered medically stable and ready for discharge regardless of functional independence. One of the great rewards of being an acute care therapist is assisting a patient with seemingly insurmountable activity limitations become more independent through accurate diagnosis and interventions that facilitate a mutually advantageous discharge plan. It is essential that the physical therapist participate in the discharge planning process to transition the patient to the next level of appropriate care whether that is home, inpatient rehabilitation, or some other suitable post-acute setting.

Chapter 2

Clinical Laboratory Values and Diagnostic Testing

Daniel J. Malone, PT, PhD, CCS and Lora Packel, PT, PhD

Laboratory testing provides physical therapists with key information that can be used to make clinical decisions. Although physical therapists rarely order specific diagnostic tests, the results will influence therapeutic interventions and the prognosis of our patients. The goal of this chapter is to present the most common laboratory testing encountered by the acute care therapist and provide a background on the normal homeostatic mechanisms that form a part of the foundation of clinical decision making. Common abnormalities will be described and how these perturbations influence physical therapy services will be discussed.

Although a complete description of laboratory testing is beyond the scope of this text, additional information regarding organ- and disease-specific laboratory and diagnostic testing is included in the proceeding chapters. Additionally, the reader should utilize many of the listed references for expanded descriptions and supplementary information.

Laboratory Tests and Measures

The survival of cells in the body is contingent upon tight regulation of electrolyte concentration and pH. Alterations in electrolytes, acid-base status, and fluid balance disrupt cellular functioning, impair organ function, and can potentially lead to death.[1] The physical therapist must understand the mechanisms for maintenance of homeostasis, as well as the pathophysiologic consequences associated with alterations of this dynamic environment. Fluid, electrolyte, and acid-base status are constantly disrupted, but the human body has extensive mechanisms to preserve homeostasis. Blood chemistry testing identifies many chemical blood constituents, and repeated testing is used to establish patterns. Tests are diverse and can be grouped into **profiles**, or tests that screen for certain conditions. Routine tests that screen the integrative organ systems of the body, termed **standard panels**, are listed in Table 2-1.

Malone DJ, Bishop KL, eds. *Acute Care Physical Therapy: A Clinician's Guide, Second Edition* (pp 51-91).

Table 2-1

COMMON SCREENING PROFILES

Group Heading	Routine Tests
Electrolyte panel (lytes)	Sodium (Na^+), potassium (K^+), chloride (Cl^-), carbon dioxide (CO_2), pH
Metabolic panel	Na^+, K^+, Cl^-, CO_2, glucose, blood urea nitrogen (BUN), creatinine
Kidney function	BUN, creatinine, creatinine clearance, glucose, calcium (Ca^{++}), CO_2
Liver function/hepatic panel	Total bilirubin, alkaline phosphatase, aspartate aminotransferase (AST), gamma glutamyl transferase (GGT), lactate dehydrogenase (LDH), prothrombin (PT), total protein, albumin (ALB)
Cardiac markers (myocardial infarction/congestive heart failure) (see Table 2-17)	Chemistry panel, cardiac troponins, creatine kinase MB (CK-MB), B-type natriuretic peptide (BNP), C-reactive protein (CRP), homocysteines
Lipid panel (see Table 2-19)	Cholesterol, high-density lipoprotein (HDL), low-density lipoprotein (LDL), very low-density liproprotein (VLDL), triglycerides
Complete blood count (CBC) (see Tables 2-12 and 2-13)	Red blood cells (RBC), hemoglobin (Hb), hematocrit (hct), platelet count, white blood cells (WBC) and WBC differential

Adapted from Fischbach FT, Dunning MB. *A Manual of Laboratory and Diagnostic Tests*. Philadelphia, PA: Lippincott Williams & Wilkins; 2004.

Fluid Balance/Body Water

The adult body is composed of approximately 60% water that is distributed between the intracellular (40%) and extracellular (20%) compartments. The extracellular fluid compartment is further divided into 2 spaces: one within the vessels (intravascular) and the other in the interstitial space.[2] Interstitial fluid surrounds the cells of the tissues and organs of the body (Figure 2-1).

Osmosis and hydrostatic pressures govern the movement of fluid between the body compartments. Osmosis is the movement of fluids across a semipermeable membrane from an area of high concentration to low concentration (ie, concentration gradient). Osmotic pressures are derived from the concentrations of ions of the body. The major ions of the body are potassium, sodium, bicarbonate, chloride, calcium, magnesium, phosphate, and bicarbonate (Table 2-2). The intracellular fluid compartment is maintained by the function of the sodium–potassium pumps embedded in the cell membrane. The action of these pump results in high concentrations of potassium intracellularly and high concentrations of sodium extracellularly. The extracellular compartment is primarily a function of the concentrations of sodium , bicarbonate, and **chloride** and is regulated by kidney function.[2] Hydrostatic pressure is the pressure that a fluid exerts on a vessel wall. The movement of water across cell membranes due to hydrostatic pressures is termed **filtration**. Fluid movement across capillary membranes is essential for the delivery of gasses (oxygen and carbon dioxide) and nutrients. Fluid movement is summarized by the Starling equation:

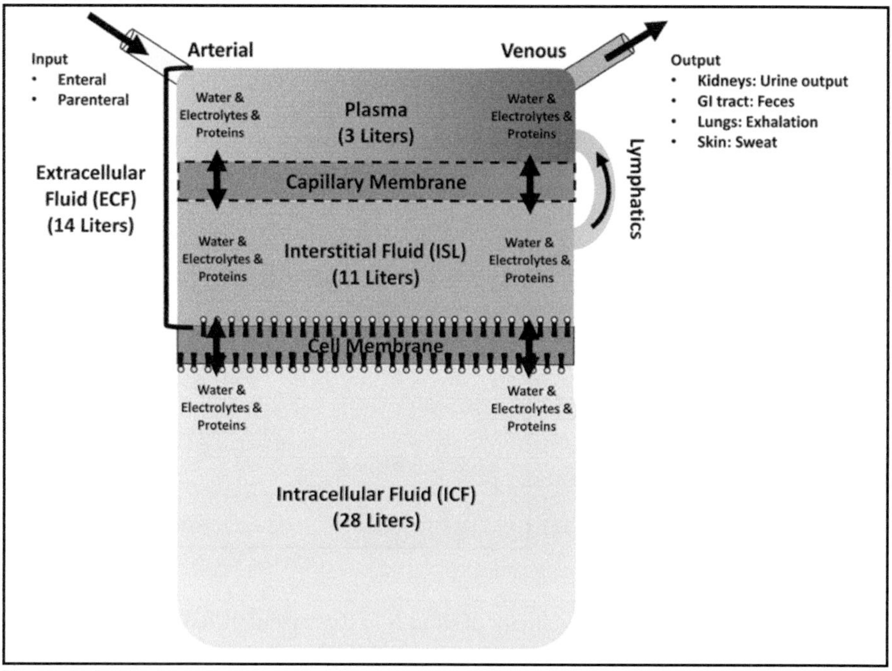

Figure 2-1. Fluid compartments.

Table 2-2

MAJOR CATIONS AND ANIONS

	Extracellular	*Intracellular*
Cations	Na^+: 135 to 148 mEq/L K^+: 3.5 to 5.3 mEq/L Ca^{++}: 8.5 to 10.5 mg/dL; 4.5 to 5.5 mEq/L Magnesium (Mg): 1.8 to 2.7 mg/dL	Na^+: 10 to 14 mEq/L K^+: 140 to 150 mEq/L Ca^{++}: <1 mEq/L Mg: 40 mEq/L
Anions	Bicarbonate ($HCO3^-$): 23 to 27 mEq/L Cl^-: 98 to 106 mEq/L Phosphate: 2.5 to 4.5 mg/dL Proteins: 16 mEq/L ALB: 3.5 to 5.5 mg/dL	$HCO3^-$: 7 to 10 mEq/L Cl^-: 3 to 4 mEq/L Phosphate: 40 to 85 mEq/L Proteins: 54 mEq/L

Adapted from Baumberger-Henry M. *Quick Look Nursing: Fluids and Electrolytes*. Thorofare, NJ: SLACK Incorporated; 2004.

$$\text{fluid movement} = Kf[(Pc - Pi) - (\pi_c - \pi_i)]$$

Forces that promote the movement of fluid out of the vasculature and into the interstitial space include vascular hydrostatic pressure (P_c) and interstitial osmotic pressures (π_i).

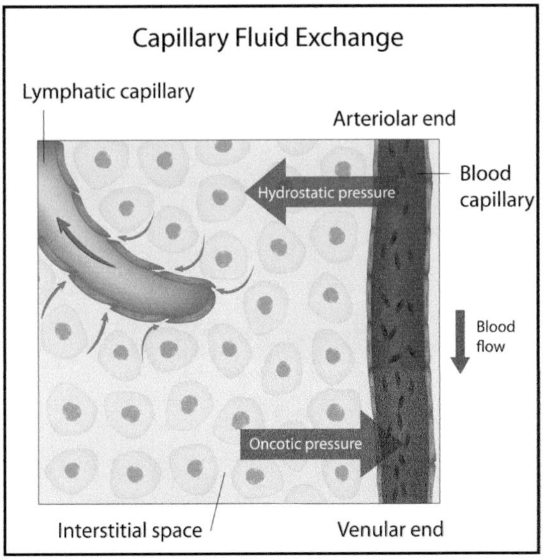

Figure 2-2. Fluid homeostasis. (Alila Medical Media/Shutterstock.com)

Forces that promote the movement of fluid into the vasculature include interstitial hydrostatic pressures (P_i) and intravascular osmotic pressures (π_c). Normally, the forces promoting fluid efflux from the vasculature is greater at the arterial end of a capillary bed, while the forces promoting influx of fluid into the vasculature are higher at the venous end of the capillary (Figure 2-2). Alteration in these forces result in many pathologic sequelae of various disorders as outlined in Table 2-3. Examples include pulmonary edema in congestive heart failure (CHF) (increased vascular hydrostatic pressure promoting fluid efflux), ascites in liver failure (increased vascular hydrostatic pressure [portal hypertension], decreased production of plasma proteins decreased production of plasma proteins [albumin] decreasing intravascular osmotic pressures), or dehydration related to burns (increased capillary permeability [increased K_f]).[1]

Electrolyte Balance

Electrolyte balance is important for nerve conduction, muscle contraction, cardiac rhythm, bone health, blood coagulation, and fluid balance. The balance of electrolytes and water is primarily under the control of the renal system but influenced by the neurologic, endocrine, gastrointestinal (GI), and musculoskeletal systems. Electrolyte disorders are among the most frequent and challenging problems facing acute care practitioners, resulting in significant morbidity and mortality.[3]

Sodium is the principal positively charged electrolyte of the extracellular fluid and is the primary determinant of the extracellular fluid volume.[4]

The balance between body water and sodium are closely linked due to their osmotic relationships. Kidney function determines sodium concentrations, adrenal handling of sodium and water is influenced by the sympathetic nervous system, hormones such as aldosterone (increased renal water absorption), antidiuretic hormone (ADH or vasopressin; increased renal water excretion), and atrial natriuretic factor (ANF; increased renal water excretion) and medications, most notably diuretics (increased renal water excretion).[3]

The common manifestations of sodium imbalance are neurologic symptoms as noted in Table 2-4. **Hyponatremia**, low sodium (<135 mEq/L), is more common in

Table 2-3

Fluid Status

Fluid Overload/Hypervolemia	
Common Causes	**Manifestations**
• Excess intake: ¤ Excess intravenous (IV) fluids ¤ Hypertonic fluids • Inadequate output: ¤ CHF ¤ Cirrhosis ¤ Renal insufficiency and failure/nephrotic syndrome ¤ Hyperaldosteronism ¤ Low dietary protein ¤ Steroid use	• Pitting peripheral edema • Shortness of breath (SOB) • Anasarca • Bounding pulse/jugular venous distension (JVD) • Hypertension (HTN) • Tachycardia • Moist crackles in the lungs
Fluid Deficit/Dehydration/Hypovolemia	
Common Causes	**Manifestations**
• Limited oral intake: ¤ Cerebrovascular accident (CVA) ¤ Dementia ¤ Neglect • Excess loss: ¤ Vomiting, diarrhea, nasogastric suction ¤ Diabetes mellitus, diabetes insipidus ¤ Burns ¤ Excessive sweating	• Dry mucus membranes • Poor skin turgor • Postural hypotension/hypotension • Tachycardia • Tachypnea • Oliguria • Altered mental status

hospitalized elderly and is often related to the patient's fluid status.[1,4,5] Common manifestations of hyponatremia include muscle weakness and twitching, confusion, headache, nausea, malaise, and fatigue.[1] **Hypernatremia**, excess sodium ($>$147 mEq/L), may result from dehydration, increased sodium intake with normal fluid volumes, and is also associated with surgery and febrile illnesses.[4] Elevated sodium concentrations draw water out of cells resulting in intracellular dehydration. Patients with normal fluid intake may have symptoms of **hypervolemia** (excess fluid in the extracellular spaces), including elevated blood pressure (BP), weight gain, venous distention, edema, and muscle weakness. Hypernatremia resulting from decreased water intake leads to **hypovolemia** leading to postural hypotension, tachycardia, weak pulses, and confusion.

Potassium is the most abundant cation within the intracellular fluid compartment. Potassium leakage out of the cell contributes to the normal negative resting membrane potential, but potassium concentration remains high inside the cell due to cell membrane sodium–potassium (Na^+–K^+) pumps.[2,6] These pumps requires energy in the form of adenosine triphosphate (ATP) to remove intracellular sodium and promote the influx of potassium against their respective concentration gradients.

Potassium balance is important for normal functioning of multiple organ systems as noted in Table 2-5. Similar to sodium, long-term regulation of potassium balance is under direct control of the kidneys.

Table 2-4

Electrolytes: Sodium

Hypernatremia ($Na^+ > 147$ mEq/L)	
Common Causes	**Manifestations**
• Hypovolemia/poor water intake • Excess Na^+ intake/hypertonic IV solutions • Severe vomiting • CHF • Renal insufficiency and failure • Cushing syndrome • Diabetes insipidus	• Irritability/agitation • Seizure, coma • Hypotension • Tachycardia • Weak, thready pulse • Decreased urine output
Hyponatremia ($Na^+ < 135$ mEq/L)	
Common Causes	**Manifestations**
• Hypovolemia: ¤ Diuretic use ¤ GI loss ¤ Burns/wound drainage ¤ Adrenal insufficiency • Hypervolemia: ¤ Hypotonic IV fluids ¤ CHF ¤ Cirrhosis ¤ Renal failure ¤ Syndrome of inappropriate antidiuretic hormone (SIADH)	• Headache • Lethargy, confusion • Absent/diminished reflexes • Seizures, coma • Nausea/vomiting • Diarrhea • Hypovolemic hyponatremia: ¤ Poor skin turgor ¤ Dry mucus membranes ¤ Orthostatic hypotension, tachycardia, weak pulse • Hypervolemic hyponatremia: ¤ HTN, tachycardia ¤ Pitting edema

Hypokalemia, low potassium (<3.5 mEq/L), or potassium deficiency, usually occurs due to loss of body potassium (eg, diarrhea, vomiting), reduced intake (ie, malnutrition), or increased cellular uptake. Hormones that promote a shift of potassium from the extracellular fluid into the intracellular fluid are insulin and the catecholamines, norepinephrine and epinephrine. Aldosterone increases renal excretion of potassium in the urine.[1] Hypokalemia hyperpolarizes cells, making the cell membrane potential more negative. This decreases the excitability of cells, necessitating greater stimuli for formation of action potentials. The clinical manifestations of hypokalemia include muscle weakness and conduction abnormalities (see Table 2-5).[1]

Hyperkalemia, elevated potassium (>5.5 mEq/L), is rare due to efficient renal excretion and cellular uptake. Causes of hyperkalemia include increased potassium intake combined with renal insufficiency and shifts of potassium from the intracellular fluid to the extracellular fluid due to cellular damage (eg, hypoxia, acidosis, muscle damage, burns) and insulin deficiency (type 1 diabetes). Medications, including heparin, potassium sparing diuretics, nonsteroidal anti-inflammatory drugs (NSAIDs), angiotensin converting enzyme (ACE) inhibitors, and beta blockers, can lead to hyperkalemia.[3-5]

Table 2-5
Electrolytes: Potassium

Hyperkalemia (K^+ >5.5 mEq/L)	
Common Causes	**Manifestations**
• Impaired excretion: ¤ Renal failure ¤ Metabolic acidosis, diabetic ketoacidosis (DKA) ¤ Addison's disease ¤ Potassium-sparing diuretics, NSAIDs, ACE inhibitors • Excess intake: ¤ Oral K^+ supplements ¤ Blood transfusions ¤ Excessive IV administration	• Muscle weakness, flaccid paralysis • Paresthesias • Bradycardia, heart block, ventricular fibrillation • Cardiac arrest
Hypokalemia (K^+ <3.5 mEq/L)	
Common Causes	**Manifestations**
• Excess loss: ¤ Diarrhea, vomiting ¤ GI losses/nasogastric suction ¤ Diuretics ¤ Cushing syndrome ¤ Steroid use • Inadequate intake: ¤ Malnutrition/restrictive diets ¤ Alcoholism ¤ Inadequate IV replacement	• Extremity weakness • Hyporeflexia • Paresthesias • Leg cramps • Electrocardiogram (ECG) changes (ST depression, T wave inversion, U waves), dysrhythmias, cardiac arrest • Hypotension • Diminished bowel function, constipation, abdominal distension, paralytic ileus

Hyperkalemia produces partial depolarization (hypopolarization) of cell membranes leading to increased excitability as well as decreasing the amplitude of the action potential. This leads to muscle weakness and cardiac conduction abnormalities, including sinus bradycardia and, potentially, ventricular fibrillation and cardiac arrest.[1,5]

Calcium ions play major roles in bone formation, cell division and growth, blood coagulation, muscle contraction, and release of neurotransmitters.[2] The majority of calcium (99%) is stored in bone and teeth, while the remainder is found in 2 forms: ionized calcium, also called free calcium, and calcium bound to albumin. Normal serum levels of free calcium are 4.5 to 5.5 mEq/L and total calcium levels are 8.5 to 10 mg/dL.[7,8] The amount of calcium absorbed by the GI tract, excreted by the kidneys, and mobilized from bone determines total body calcium. Total body calcium is influenced by the interactions of 3 hormones: parathyroid hormone (PTH) (increased extracellular fluid calcium), calcitonin (decreased extracellular fluid calcium), and calcitriol/Vitamin D (increased extracellular fluid calcium)[7] (see Chapter 10).

Hypercalcemia (>10 mg/dL of total calcium or >5.5 mEq/L of free calcium) often results from hyperparathyroidism and malignancy (Table 2-6). Hypercalcemia may present as fatigue, weakness, confusion, nausea, and constipation.

Table 2-6

ELECTROLYTES: CALCIUM

Common Causes	Manifestations
Hypercalcemia (Ca^{++} > 10.5 mg/dL or > 5.5 mEq/L)	
• Excess intake or release: ¤ Ca^{++} antacids/supplements ¤ Bone destruction (eg, tumor, immobilization, bed rest, trauma, multiple fractures) ¤ Excess Vitamin D ¤ Cancer (eg, lung, breast, ovary, prostate, GI, leukemia) • Inadequate excretion: ¤ Renal failure ¤ Thiazide diuretics ¤ Increased PTH ¤ Hypophosphatemia	• Ventricular dysrhythmias, bradyarrythmias, heart block, asystole • Stupor/coma • Lethargy • Muscle weakness • Diminished reflexes • Constipation • Nausea/vomiting • Renal calculi
Hypocalcemia (Ca^{++} < 8.5 mg/dL or < 4.5 mEq/L)	
Common Causes	**Manifestations**
• Inadequate intake: ¤ Alcoholism ¤ Poor dietary intake ¤ Limited GI absorption/chronic diarrhea • Excess loss: ¤ Hypoparathryoidism ¤ Renal failure ¤ Hyperphosphatemia ¤ Pancreatitis ¤ Laxatives	• Anxiety, confusion, irritability • Seizures • Cardiac dysrhythmias (eg, prolonged QT interval) • Fatigue • Numbness/tingling • Hyperreflexia • Muscle cramps/tetany

Hypocalcemia (<8.5 mg/dL of total calcium or <4.5 mEq/L of free calcium) is loss of serum calcium and is associated with hypoparathyroidism and disorders that impair GI absorption of calcium, including Vitamin D deficiency and pancreatitis. Additional causes include rhabdomyolysis, chronic renal insufficiency, malignancy, and limited calcium intake (see Table 2-6).[1,7] Patients show signs of enhanced neuromuscular excitability resulting in tetany, muscular twitching, hyperreflexia, and, potentially, convulsions. Common symptoms include numbness, tingling, fatigue and muscle cramps.[7] ECG abnormalities include a prolonged QT interval increasing the risk of developing ventricular tachycardia/fibrillation.[1]

Phosphate, 2.4 to 4.5 mg/dL, is necessary for bone formation, and 85% of the body's stores are within the skeleton. Phosphate is necessary for acid-base balance and cellular energy production (eg, ATP). Abnormalities in serum phosphate are often inversely related to calcium levels because both electrolytes are regulated by PTH and Vitamin D. **Hyperphosphatemia** is associated with hypocalcemia, but most commonly with renal failure. **Hypophosphatemia** is associated with hypercalcemia,

Table 2-7

ELECTROLYTES: PHOSPHATE (2.4 TO 4.5 MG/DL)

Common Causes	Manifestations
Hyperphosphatemia (>4.5 mg/dL) (see Hypocalcemia [Table 2-6])	
• Excess intake: ¤ Phosphate containing medications (eg, laxatives, fosphenytoin) • Inadequate excretion: ¤ Renal failure • Increased renal reabsorption: ¤ Acromegaly ¤ Hypoparathyroidism • Cell lysis (eg, chemotherapy/tumor lysis syndrome, rhabdomyolysis) • Bisphosphonates • Diabetic ketoacidosis	• Mild; often asymptomatic • Altered mental status (eg, delirium, obtundation, coma) • Muscle weakness • Muscle cramping • Paresthesias • Subcutaneous nodules
Hypophosphatemia (<2.4 mg/dL) (see Hypercalcemia [Table 2-6])	
Common Causes	**Manifestations**
• Inadequate intake: ¤ Alcoholism ¤ Chronic malnutrition (refeeding syndrome) • Excess loss: ¤ Vitamin D deficiency ¤ Hyperparathyroidism • Excessive use of antacids • Kidney transplantation • Severe burns	• Mild; often asymptomatic • Disorientation • Bone and muscle pain • Osteopenia • Muscle weakness • Fatigue • Seizures

hyperparathyroidism, diabetic ketoacidosis, and alcoholism. Symptoms of phosphate disorders are noted in Table 2-7.[7]

Chloride, 104 to 110 mEq/L, is the major serum anion and its movements between the extracellular fluid and intracellular fluid is tied to sodium maintaining electroneutrality but also contributes to fluid and acid-base balance. **Hypochloremia** (chloride concentrations <104 mEq/L) is often due to GI loss (ie, vomiting, nasogastric suction, diarrhea) combined with metabolic alkalosis. Additional causes include massive diuresis, fluid overload with resultant hyponatremia, or compensated respiratory acidosis.[1,5] **Hyperchloremia** (elevated chloride >110 mEq/L) is associated with hypernatremia, dehydration, hyperventilation, and anemia (Table 2-8).[1,5]

Magnesium, 1.8 to 2.7 mEq/L, is the fourth most abundant cation in the body and is concentrated in bone and muscle (Table 2-9). It is essential for the use of ATP for energy and is necessary for carbohydrate metabolism, protein synthesis, and muscular contraction. **Hypomagnesemia** (<1.8 mEq/L; symptoms <1.0 mEq/L) resembles hypocalcemia with patients presenting with increased neuromuscular excitability, hyperreflexia, and tetany.[5] Hypomagnesemia is observed in chronic alcoholism, eating disorders, and may be associated with increased urinary excretion as seen with diabetic crisis. **Hypermagnesemia** (>2.7 mEq/L) is relatively rare but occurs in the

Table 2-8

Electrolytes: Chloride (104 to 110 mEq/L)

Hyperchloremia ($Cl^- > 110$ mEq/L)	
Common Causes	**Manifestations**
• Increased intake/exchange: ¤ High salt diet without water ¤ Hypertonic IV solutions ¤ Metabolic acidosis • Decreased loss: ¤ Hyperparathyroidism ¤ Hyperaldosteronism ¤ Renal failure	• Lethargy, reduced level of consciousness • Weakness • Edema • Tachypnea, dyspnea • HTN, tachycardia
Hyperchloremia ($Cl^- < 104$ mEq/L)	
Common Causes	**Manifestations**
• Decreased intake: ¤ Low salt diet ¤ Water intoxication • Increased loss: ¤ Diuresis ¤ Excessive vomiting, nasogastric suction, ileostomy, diarrhea	• Agitation/irritability • Hypertonicity/hyperreflexia • Cramping/twitching/tetany

aged and critically ill patients and is frequently encountered in patients with renal insufficiency.[4,5] Patients may present with lethargy, dysarthria, hypoactive deep tendon reflexes, and hypotension.

Acid-Base Balance

Acid-base balance describes the equilibrium in extracellular fluid between substances that release hydrogen (H^+) ions (ie, acids) and those capable of accepting hydrogen (ie, alkalines or bases). The concentration of hydrogen is described by pH in an inverse relationship; the greater the pH, the less hydrogen in the extracellular fluid.[2,9] Virtually all cells, tissues, and organs of the body are sensitive to pH, and life cannot exist outside a pH range from 6.8 to 7.8.[2] Acids and bases are ingested in the diet or produced by cellular processes continuously; however, the body has developed multiple buffering mechanisms that maintain pH in a narrow range. Buffers act like a sponge and absorb excess acids (hydrogen ions or base [OH]) without significant changes in pH. Common buffers include bicarbonate, hemoglobin, phosphate, and plasma proteins. Ultimately, the respiratory and renal systems maintain the acid-base status of the body. For example, impaired ventilation as seen in lung disease (ie, hypoventilation) will increase arterial carbon dioxide, which decreases the pH, creating respiratory acidosis.

Acid-base imbalance, acidosis or alkalosis, may be of respiratory, metabolic, or mixed origin (Tables 2-10 and 2-11).[1,5] **Acidosis** is either a loss of base or excess acid, while **alkalosis** is either excess base or loss of acid. Respiratory-initiated imbalances are compensated by the kidneys by producing more acidic or basic urine, and metabolic abnormalities are compensated by the respiratory system by varying the rate and depth of breathing.[1] Normal arterial **carbon dioxide** is 35 to 45 mm Hg and is

Table 2-9

ELECTROLYTES: MAGNESIUM (1.8 TO 2.7 MEQ/L)

Hypermagnesemia (Mg > 2.7 mEq/L)	
Common Causes	**Manifestations**
• Increased intake: ¤ Medications: Antacids, lithium, magnesium sulfate medications • Decreased loss: ¤ Renal failure ¤ Adrenal insufficiency ¤ Leukemia ¤ Hyperparathryoidism ¤ Dehydration	• Diaphoresis/warm, flushed appearance • Nausea/vomiting • Drowsiness/lethargy • Weakness/flaccidity • Diminished deep tendon reflexes • Hypotension, bradycardia, heart block
Hypomagnesemia (Mg < 1.8 mEq/L; symptoms, Mg < 1.0 mEq/L)	
Common Causes	**Manifestations**
• Decreased intake: ¤ Alcoholism ¤ Eating disorders (eg, bulimia,anorexia) ¤ Hyperalimentation • Increased loss: ¤ Diuresis ¤ Primary aldosteronism ¤ DKA ¤ Medications: Aminoglycosides, amphotericin, cisplatin	• Neuromuscular irritability, hyperreflexia, tremors, twitching, spasticity • Seizures • Nystagmus • ECG changes: ¤ Prolonged PR/QT intervals and QRS complex, flattened T waves ¤ Ventricular dysrhythmias (eg, premature ventricular contraction, ventricular tachycardia, ventricular fibrillation), supraventricular tachycardia (SVT) • Emotional lability

Table 2-10

ACID-BASE/ARTERIAL BLOOD GAS ANALYSIS

Acid-base balance (pH)	7.35 to 7.45
Partial pressure of oxygen (PaO_2)	80 to 100 mm Hg
Partial pressure of carbon dioxide ($PaCO_2$)	35 to 45 mm Hg
HCO_3^-	22 to 28 mEq

the primary regulator of ventilation. A rise in carbon dioxide stimulates the central chemoreceptors of the medullary respiratory center resulting in an increase in ventilation and subsequent reductions in the **partial pressure of arterial carbon dioxide** ($PaCO_2$). **Hyperventilation**, an arterial carbon dioxide less than 35 mm Hg, is due to increased alveolar ventilation and leads to **respiratory alkalosis**. Hyperventilation is associated with nervousness and anxiety, pain, pregnancy, and pulmonary emboli. Patients may present with dizziness, confusion, and paresthesias.[1,9] **Hypoventilation**,

Table 2-11

ACID-BASE DISORDERS

Respiratory Acidosis (pH <7.35, $PaCO_2$ >45 mm Hg, HCO_3^- normal or >27 mEq/L)	
Common Causes	**Manifestations**
• Obstructive airways disease • Thoracic trauma/incision pain • Medication/drug overdose	• Irritability, lethargy • Headache • Tremors, muscle twitching • Vertigo • Tachycardia • Peripheral vasodilation
Respiratory Alkalosis (pH >7.45, $PaCO_2$ <35 mm Hg, HCO_3^- normal or >27 mEq/L)	
Common Causes	**Manifestations**
• Pain • Fever • Hyperthyroidism • Meningitis • Brain tumor • Psychogenic	• Convulsions • Coma • Numbness/tingling • Lightheadedness/dizziness • Sweating • Palpitations
Metabolic Acidosis (pH <7.35, $PaCO_2$ normal or low, HCO_3^- <23 mEq/L)	
Common Causes	**Manifestations**
• Chronic diarrhea • Shock, sepsis • Trauma • DKA • Renal failure/uremia	• Stupor/coma • Headache • Malaise/fatigue, weakness • Decreased cardiac contractility/ decreased cardiac output • Dysrhythmias • Hyperkalemia
Metabolic Alkalosis (pH >7.45, $PaCO_2$ normal or high, HCO_3^- >27 mEq/L)	
Common Causes	**Manifestations**
• Severe vomiting, nasogastric suction • Excessive use of antacids • Diuretics • Hypokalemia • Hyperaldosteronism	• Seizures • Confusion • Neuromuscular irritability, hyperreflexia, tingling • Tetany • Respiratory insufficiency

an arterial carbon dioxide greater than 45 mm Hg, is due to reduced alveolar ventilation and leads to **respiratory acidosis**. Common causes of elevated carbon dioxide and hypoventilation are chronic obstructive pulmonary diseases (eg, emphysema, chronic bronchitis, asthma), thoracic or abdominal surgery, kyphoscoliosis, sleep apnea, head trauma, and depression of the respiratory drive to breath due to oversedation, pain medications, and alcohol or drug abuse. Manifestations of respiratory acidosis include restlessness followed by lethargy, muscle twitching, and tremors.[1,9]

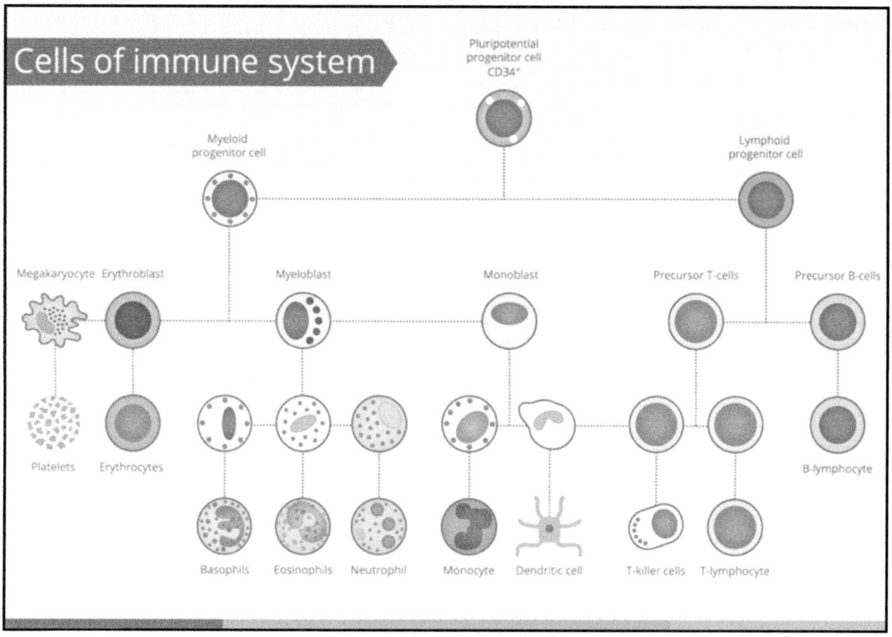

Figure 2-3. Origin of cells of the immune system, RBCs and platelets. (Marina Mandarina/ Shutterstock.com)

Bicarbonate is the primary metabolic buffer and its serum concentration is determined by renal function. **Metabolic acidosis**, a deficit of bicarbonate, is associated with renal failure, DKA, lactic acidosis, diarrhea, and hypoxia. **Metabolic alkalosis** is due to loss of normal metabolic acids, specifically gastric acids induced by severe vomiting, or excess base due to hyperaldosteronism or diuretic use. Patients may present with weakness and muscle cramps, hyperreflexia, tetany, confusion, and dysrhythmias, including atrial tachycardia.

Hematology Studies

Blood is a specialized connective tissue consisting of cells and plasma. The plasma, the fluid component of blood, contains the plasma proteins, lipids, vitamins, amino acids, and hormones.[10] The **CBC** evaluates RBCs, WBCs, and platelets (PLTs) and is obtained from a simple blood draw from a peripheral vein. A CBC with differentials breaks down these cells to look more closely at their component parts. Erythrocyte indices include the mean corpuscular volume (MCV) and mean corpuscular hemoglobin concentration (MCHC). WBC differential includes the 5 types of WBCs: neutrophils, eosinophils, basophils, lymphocytes, and monocytes.

To understand the CBC, one must first start with an overview of hematopoiesis, or the formation of the blood cells. In adults, hematopoiesis begins in the bone marrow, and certain components mature in the thymus gland. All blood cells develop from a pluripotent stem cell (Figure 2-3). This stem cell, as it matures, differentiates and is committed to one of 3 cell types: RBC, WBC, or PLT.

The erythrocyte or RBC's primary functions are the delivery of O_2 to tissues, the uptake of cellular metabolic byproducts (carbon dioxide and hydrogen), and maintenance of acid-base balance. Normal RBC values (Table 2-12) vary depending on the type of sample, age, and sex. Generally, the RBC count, or erythrocyte count, is

Table 2-12

Common Hematology Studies

Blood Component and Indices	*Normal Values*	*Common Abnormalities/Diseases/Disorders*
RBCs • MCV • MCH • MCHC	• Men: 4.2 to 5.4 x 106/mm3 • Women: 3.6 to 5.0 x 106/mm3 • 84 to 99 μm3 • 5 to 25 pg/cell • 20 to 30 g/dL	Anemia: ↓ RBCs, Hb, and/or hct • Normal MCV: Hemolytic anemia, posthemorrhagic anemia, aplastic anemia • ↓ MCV: Microcytic anemia (eg, iron deficiency, chronic disease) • ↑ MCV: Macrocytic anemia (eg, Vitamin B_{12} deficiency, intrinsic factor deficiency, ileal resection, pancreatic disease, neoplastic disease, hyperthyroidism, alcoholism)
Hematocrit	• Men: 42% to 52% • Women: 36% to 48%	Polycythemia (↑ RBC): Renal cancer, hepatocellular cancers, lung disease, altitude
Hemoglobin	• Men: 14 to 17.4 g/dL • Women: 12 to 16 g/dL	↑ Hb: Chronic obstructive pulmonary disease (COPD), CHF, polycythemia, altitude
WBCs • Neutrophil • Basophil • Eosinophil • Monocyte • Lymphocyte	• 4 to 10,000/mm3 • ~50% of WBCs; 3000 to 7000/mm3 • 0% to 1% of total WBCs; 15 to 50/mm3 • 0% to 3% of total WBCs; 0 to 0.7 x 109/L • 3% to 7% of total WBCs; 100 to 500/mm3 • 25% to 40% of total WBCs; 1500 to 4000 cells/mm3	Leukocytosis: WBCs >11,000/mm3 • Infection, leukemia/myeloproliferative disorders, malignant neoplasms, trauma/surgery Leukopenia: WBCs <4000/mm3 • Viral infections, chemotherapy, aplastic anemia Neutropenia: <40% or <1800/mm3 • Stem cell disorders, overwhelming bacterial or viral infections, ionizing radiation, hypersensitivity reactions
Platelets	• 140 to 400 x 103/mm3	Thrombocytopenia: <140 x 103/mm3 • Idiopathic thrombocytopenia purpura, anemias, CHF, renal insufficiency, sepsis, prosthetic heart valve, hemorrhage, acute/chronic myelogenous leukemia, drug interaction Thrombocytosis: >400 x 103/mm3

performed to calculate indices, the MCV (RBC size) and MCH (Hb content) for further classification of specific anemias.[11] The **hematocrit** (hct) is a percentage of whole blood occupied by cells. A single RBC contains 4 Hb molecules and, when fully saturated, can carry 4 molecules of O_2 for a total O_2 content of approximately 20 mL/dL of blood.[12] RBCs last 120 days in the bloodstream and are removed by macrophages in the liver and spleen. Hypoxia due to pulmonary disease, heart failure, severe anemia, chronic smoking, or altitude may upregulate RBC production in response to the production of the hormone **erythropoietin** made by the kidneys. Erythropoietin signals the stem cells to produce more RBCs, thus increasing the body's capabilities of delivering oxygen. Elevated levels of RBCs is termed **polycythemia**. Polycythemia may not be directly due to an increase in RBC production, but the concentration of RBC is increased when the plasma volume is low. Plasma volume may be low in people who are dehydrated, those with severe diarrhea or vomiting, or due to extensive burns.[11] Polycythemia is usually well-tolerated, but therapists should consider the associated increased viscosity of blood increasing myocardial oxygen demand in those patients with cardiac disease and the potential reduced peripheral blood flow in patients with vascular disease.

Anemia, a decrease in the number of erythrocytes, low hemoglobin concentrations, or both is demonstrated by a reduced hct, Hb concentration, and erythrocyte count. Anemia is generally classified as:

- Hypoproliferative anemia due to defective RBC production (eg, deficiencies in iron [microcytic/hypochromic anemia], folate, Vitamins B_{12} [pernicious anemia] or B_6, bone marrow failure [aplastic anemia])
- Anemia due to loss of RBC (eg, trauma, hemorrhage, GI bleeding)
- Hemolytic anemia resulting from excessive RBC destruction (hemolysis)[13]

As the primary function of RBCs is to deliver oxygen to tissues, low levels can impact a person's ability to participate in therapy. It is common practice for therapists to reduce the intensity and duration of exercise and mobilization programs to accommodate for lower levels of hemoglobin as noted in Table 2-12. However, the evidence supporting cessation of physical therapy services with Hb values less than 8 g/dL is lacking and may be tied to transfusion recommendations. Medical practice previously followed the **10/30 rule** where transfusion was advised to maintain Hb concentration above 10 g/dL and a hematocrit above 30%; however, recent evidence has challenged this standard. Physicians must balance the benefit of treating anemia while avoiding unnecessary transfusion with its associated costs and potential harm (eg, infection risk [HIV, hepatitis], transfusion-associated circulatory overload [TRACO], transfusion-related acute lung injury [TRALI]). The following are proposed guidelines for hemodynamically stable patients without active bleeding:

- Hb <6 g/dL: Transfusion recommended except in exceptional circumstances
- Hb 6 to 7 g/dL: Transfusion generally likely to be indicated
- Hb 7 to 8 g/dL: Transfusion should be considered in postoperative surgical patients, including those with stable cardiovascular disease, after evaluating the patient's clinical status
- Hb 8 to 10 g/dL: Transfusion generally not indicated, but should be considered for some populations (eg, those with symptomatic anemia, ongoing bleeding, acute coronary syndrome with ischemia)
- Hb >10 g/dL: Transfusion generally not indicated except in exceptional circumstances

These recommendations are more restrictive with regards to administering blood products than those presented in Table 2-13. Therapists should also note the more

Table 2-13

HEMATOLOGY: BLOOD VALUES AND COMMON PHYSICAL THERAPY CONSIDERATIONS

Component	*Values and Considerations*
Hemoglobin	Normal: • Men: 14 to 17.4 g/dL • Women: 12 to 16 g/dL Subnormal values: Anemias • >10 g/dL: Therapy as indicated; no distinct precautions 8 to 10 g/dL: ¤ Anticipate poor cardiopulmonary reserve/limited endurance ¤ Monitor vital signs closely ¤ Patient symptoms: Exercise intolerance, DOE, tachycardia, pallor • <8: g/dL: Therapy may be contraindicated, blood transfusion probable ¤ <5 g/dL: Leads to heart failure and death Elevated values: • 20 g/dL: Increased blood viscosity leading to capillary blockage and tissue ischemia
Platelets	Normal • 140 to 400 x 103/mm^3 Subnormal values: Thrombocytopenia: <10 x 103/mm^3 • 50 to 140 x 103/mm^3: ¤ Low-intensity progressive resistive exercise (PRE) and aerobic exercise (no to minimal grade/elevations) • 30 to 50 x 103/mm^3 (50 x 103/mm^3 typically not associated with spontaneous bleeding) ¤ Active range of motion (AROM) exercise, walking ad lib • <20 x 103/mm^3: ¤ Risk of spontaneous bleeding, petechia, ecchymosis, and prolonged bleeding time ¤ Therapy may be contraindicated/minimal AROM ¤ No brushing of teeth Elevated values: Thrombocytosis: >400 x 103/mm^3 • No distinct recommendation; note paradoxical increased risk of bleeding
WBCs	Normal WBC. 5,000 to 10,000 cells/mm^3
Leukopenia	WBC <4,000/mm^3 • Infection risk; patient is immunocompromised
Leukocytosis	WBC >11,000/mm^3 • Infection present
Neutropenia	<40% or <1800/mm^3 • ↑ infection risk; patient should wear mask outside room • Physical therapist/physical therapist assistant should wear mask if respiratory infection • No fresh fruit/flowers

liberal transfusion recommendation for patients with acute coronary syndrome (<10 g/dL) or those with stable preexisting cardiovascular disease (<8 g/dL).[14]

For patients with anemia, therapists should monitor for signs and symptoms of hypoxia, low oxygen in tissues, such as:

- Chest pain/pressure
- Dizziness
    - Orthostatic hypotension
    - Tachycardia
- SOB or dyspnea on exertion (DOE)
- Fatigue

Therapists must be aware that many of these symptoms are vague complaints and may also reflect recovery from anesthesia or medication side effects.

WBCs, or **leukocytes**, are important components of the immune system and primarily fight infection. If a CBC with differential is ordered, information on the 5 types of WBCs, neutrophils, eosinophils, basophils, monocytes, and lymphocytes, is provided as outlined in Table 2-12.

Granulocytes

- **Neutrophils:** Kill bacteria by phagocytosis and make up 58% of WBC.
- **Eosinophils:** Kill parasites and play a role in allergic disorders. Eosinophils comprise 2% of WBCs.
- **Basophils:** Play a role in some allergies, are responsible for the release of histamine and heparin, and are approximately 1% of WBCs.

Agranulocytes

- **Monocytes:** Differentiate into **macrophages** and ingest bacteria by phagocytosis. Monocytes are found primarily in the liver, spleen, lungs, and lymph nodes and are responsible for destroying old or damaged cells. Monocytes make up 4% of WBCs.
- **Lymphocytes:** Consist of T lymphocytes and B lymphocytes.
    - **T lymphocytes** are responsible for cell-mediated immunity. They begin their maturation in the bone marrow and complete differentiation in the thymus gland.
    - **Helper T** cells orchestrate the immune response via the use of cytokine messengers. These cells stimulate B cells to form antibodies, stimulate production of cytotoxic T cells, and activate macrophages.
    - **Cytotoxic T** cells release toxins that kill infected or dysfunctional cells and invading organisms.
    - **Memory T** cells preserve a memory of previous antigens. When the antigen is reintroduced into the body, memory T cells accelerate the immune response and direct antibodies specific to the offending pathogen.
    - **Suppressor T** cells modulate the intensity of the immune response .
    - **B lymphocytes** are responsible for humoral immunity by producing antibodies. B cells make up 33% of WBCs.

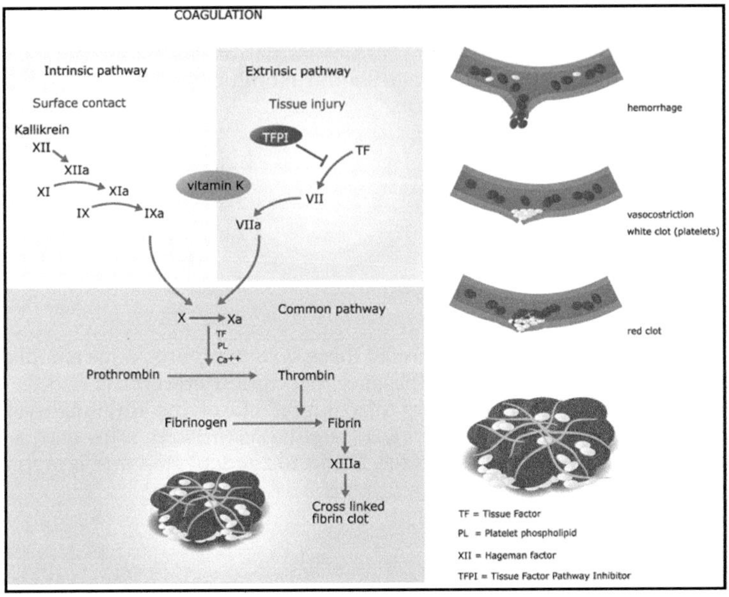

Figure 2-4. Hemostasis (blood clotting): sequence of activated factors of coagulation of human blood. (ellepigrafica/Shutterstock.com)

Leukocytosis, a high WBC count, can indicate infection, inflammation, or rapid abnormal proliferation of WBCs (eg, leukemia). **Leukopenia**, a low WBC count, indicates a compromised immune system as a result of chemotherapy, radiation, medications, or hematologic disorders. Exercise intensity and duration may need to be modified or withheld during fever depending on the clinical stability of the patient. If a patient has a low WBC count, take caution to avoid infectious exposures. Handwashing, wearing masks, and cleaning exercise equipment will help prevent infections.

Platelets, Blood Coagulation, and Venous Thromboembolism

Under normal conditions, the body maintains a finely-tuned balance of blood coagulation, hemostasis, and clot breakdown, or fibrinolysis. **Platelets** (PLT) are an essential component of hemostasis, initiating the clotting mechanism to arrest bleeding (Figure 2-4).[10] PLTs adhere to disruptions of the endothelial lining of a wound and to each other and release multiple vasoactive substances that promote the aggregation and activation of other PLTs to form a platelet plug. Coagulation factors from the blood plasma, PLT, and damaged blood vessels promote the sequential activation of approximately 13 plasma proteins, giving rise to fibrin, a polymer that forms a network of fibers trapping RBCs, leukocytes, and PLT to form a blood clot, or thrombus.[10,12] Many of these coagulation factors require calcium for activation. The blood clotting cascade is composed of an intrinsic and an extrinsic pathway, which both converge to produce fibrin as outlined in Figure 2-3.

Normal platelet values in adults are 150 to 450,000/mm^3 (see Table 2-12). **Thrombocytopenia,** or platelet count below 150,000/mm^3 of blood, can result from:

- Decreased production of PLT (eg, bone marrow depression/leukemia, cytoxic drugs)
- Increased destruction of PLT (eg, **idiopathic thrombocytopenic purpura** [ITP]), disseminated intravascular coagulation, drug reaction (eg, penicillin, digoxin, sulfonamides)

- Aggregation of PLT in the microvasculature (eg, **thrombotic thrombocytopenic purpura** [TTP])[1,10]

Patients with thrombocytopenia are at an increased risk for bleeding and may present with petechia, epistaxis, purpura, and menorrhagia.[1] Common precautions include avoidance of activities that might cause bruising or loss of balance and falls. Caution should be taken when prescribing resistive exercise or weight training in the person with low PLT to avoid intramuscular bleeding. Therapists should consider avoidance of weights when platelets drop below 50,000/mm^3. Finally, avoidance of valsalva is important, as small blood vessels in the eyes and nose may burst causing bleeding.

Thrombocytosis, defined as a platelet count greater than 450,000/mm^3, may be a response to stress, infection and inflammation, trauma, exercise, and ovulation. Thrombocytosis may also be a consequence of splenectomy, rheumatoid arthritis, and cancer.[1] Thrombocytosis may be associated with increased thrombus formation and, paradoxically, an increased risk of bleeding.[11]

Blood tests are used to determine efficacy of the clotting cascade and to pinpoint specific deficiencies for a targeted treatment as noted in Table 2-14. **Bleeding time** measures platelet functioning by determining the time it takes for a blood clot to form from a punctured capillary. The duration of bleeding depends on the quantity and quality of PLT and the ability of the vessel to constrict. Normal bleeding time is 3 to 10 minutes and bleeding after 15 minutes is highly significant. **Prothrombin time** tests the functioning of the extrinsic system of the clotting cascade. Specifically, it evaluates the efficacy of Factors I (fibrinogen), V, VII, and X.[6] The PT is measured by taking venous blood and adding substances to initiate the extrinsic pathway of the clotting cascade, and the time to form a clot is usually measured in seconds. Normal PT is 11 to 13.5 seconds. The **International Normalization Ratio** (INR) is used to correct for differences in the laboratory substances used to test the PT. The PT/INR are used to monitor the dosage of Coumadin (warfarin). The **partial thromboplastin time** (PTT) evaluates the clotting factors found in the intrinsic (surface contact activation pathway) and common pathways.[6] The PTT evaluates the functioning of Factors I, II, V, VIII, IX, X, XI, and XII. PTT is drawn from venous blood similar to the PT. This blood is then separated into plasma and cells. Substances are added to the vial that activate the intrinsic pathway of the clotting cascade. Normal PTT values are 30 to 45 seconds. This test may also be done by adding a substance to shorten the clotting time, an **activated partial thromboplastin time** (APTT). Normal APTT is between 25 to 40 seconds. The PTT are used to monitor the dosage of heparin. Low molecular weight heparins (LMWH) (ie, Lovenox [enoxaparin], Arixtra [fondaparinux]) may be monitored by monitoring factor Xa in the blood. Newer anticoagulants, such as the **direct acting oral anticoagulants** (DOAC), also termed **novel oral anticoagulants** (NOACs), do not require laboratory monitoring (eg, Pradaxa [dabigatran], Xarelto [rivaroxaban], Eliquis [apixaban]). Anticoagulants are prescribed to treat and prevent blood clot formation from mechanical valves, dysrhythmias, and DVT. Therapists should consider bleeding risk when treating patients with prolonged clotting times and the risk of embolic events for patients with shortened clotting times. It is important to review institutional guidelines regarding specific policies and procedures outlining activity restrictions. **D-dimers** are produced by the action of plasmin on cross-linked fibrin and their presence in the blood confirms that clotting has occurred. Blood tests for D-dimers are used to screen for DVT, pulmonary emboli, and disseminated intravascular coagulation (DIC).

Venous thromboembolism (VTE) is blood clotting in a vein and is most often defined as **DVT,** a thrombus typically found in the deep veins of the lower extremity but sometimes may form in the arm or other veins, or a **pulmonary embolism**, a DVT that has broken free (ie, embolized) and traveled to the lung and lodged within the pulmonary arterial circulation. Estimates suggest that at least 350,000, and as many as 600,000, Americans each year have DVT/pulmonary emboli, and at least 100,000

Table 2-14

HEMOSTASIS AND COAGULATION

Normal Values	*Common Abnormalities/Diseases/Disorders*
Platelet count: 140 to 400 x 103/mm^3 **Clotting time**: 3 to 10 minutes **PT**: 11 to 13.5 seconds **INR**: <1.1 **PTT**: 30 to 45 seconds **APTT**: 25 to 40 seconds **D-dimer**: 0.5 µg/mL fibrinogen-equivalent units (FEU)	↑ **PT/INR**: • Malabsorption • Vitamin K deficiency • Patient is on Coumadin (disrupts Vitamin K, which is essential for the activity of Factors VII, IX, X) • Deficiencies in Factors V, VII, X, fibrinogen, or PT • Hepatitis, cirrhosis, hepatic dysfunction (liver produces many of the clotting factors) • DIC ↑ **PTT/APTT**: • Malabsorption • Hemophilia A (Factor VIII deficiency) • Hemophilia B (Factor IX deficiency) • Cirrhosis • von Willebrand's disease • Heparin therapy (increases action of Antithrombin III, which inhibits multiple clotting factors) • Therapy contraindicated if PT/PTT values >2.5 reference range due to bleeding risk; need to check institution guidelines ↑ **D-dimer**: • Activation of clotting • May trigger further workup of VTE (DVT, pulmonary emboli) • Inflammation • DIC ↓ **D-dimer**: • May rule out VTE (DVT, pulmonary emboli) if low pretest probability (unlikely; see Wells Criteria, see Figure 2-6)

deaths are thought to be related to VTE each year. It should be noted that recurrence is common and impacts men greater than women. Survivors of VTE have long-term complications, such as post-thrombotic syndrome leading to varicose veins, skin breakdown, venous stasis ulcers, and chronic pain and burning impacting walking and quality of life.[15] Risk factors for VTE are diverse and the development of thrombosis is classically define by 3 broad categories (ie, Virchow's Triad): blood stasis, hypercoagulability, and endothelial injury/dysfunction (Table 2-15). Not surprisingly, most patients in the hospital have 3 or more risk factors for VTE.

If the there is concern that a patient is at risk for VTE (DVT/pulmonary emboli), the therapist should apply a clinical prediction rules to ascertain the potential risk. A validated clinical prediction rule, the Wells Criteria for DVT or pulmonary emboli, risk stratifies patients for clotting and has been validated in multiple settings and patient populations (Figure 2-5). As noted in the flow chart in Figure 2-6, the Wells Criteria is used to determine the clinical probability of DVT and is followed by diagnostic testing, including D-Dimer, duplex ultrasound, and computed tomography (CT) scan,

Table 2-15

Risk Factors and Signs and Symptoms for Venous Thromboembolism

Risk Factors

Stasis	Hypercoagulability	Endothelial Damage
• Older age • Major surgery (eg, abdominal or thoracic operations that require general anesthesia lasting ≥30 minutes, orthopedic surgery) • Fracture of the pelvis, hip, or long bones • Inactivity and immobility • Long air travel • Stroke, paralysis, spinal cord injury • COPD • Polycythemia, dehydration • Obesity	• Cancer, chemotherapy • Sepsis • Inflammatory disease (eg, inflammatory bowel disease, rheumatological disease) • Nephrotic syndrome • Antiphospholipid antibody syndrome • Pregnancy, postpartum • Oral contraceptives and hormone replacement therapy • Smoking	• Surgery • IV access, central lines • Trauma • Previous history of VTE (DVT, pulmonary embolism)

Signs/Symptoms

Pulmonary Embolism	Deep Vein Thrombus
• Unexplained SOB • Chest pain, pain with deep breathing • Coughing up blood (hemoptysis) • Tachypnea • Tachycardia • New onset dysrhythmia • Feelings of anxiety or dread, light-headedness or fainting, sweating	• Pain • Swelling of the leg or along a vein in the leg • Pain or tenderness in the leg • Increased warmth in the leg that is swollen or painful • Red or discolored skin on the leg • Can often be asymptomatic

Adapted from Anderson FA, Spencer FA. Risk factors for venous thromboembolism. *Circulation*. 2003;107(23 suppl 1):19-26; Kesieme E, Kesieme C, Jebbin N, Irekpita E, & Dongo A. Deep vein thrombosis: a clinical review. *J Blood Med*. 2011;2:59-69; and Zierler BK. Ultrasonography and diagnosis of venous thromboembolism. *Circulation*. 2004;109(12 suppl 1):19-14.

DVT Criteria	Points
Active cancer (treatment ongoing, within 6 months, or palliative	1
Bedridden recently >3 days or major surgery within 4 weeks	1
Calf swelling >3 cm compared to the other leg (measured 10 cm below tibial tuberosity)	1
Collateral (nonvaricose) superficial veins present	1
Entire leg swollen	1
Localized tenderness along deep venous system	1
Pitting edema, greater in symptomatic leg	1
Paralysis, paresis, or recent plaster immobilization of the lower extremity	1
Previously documented DVT	1
Alternative diagnosis to DVT as likely or more likely	-2

Probability for DVT	
DVT unlikely	< 2
DVT likely	≥ 2

PE Criteria	Points
Previous PE or DVT	1.5
Heart > 100 beats/minute	1.5
Recent surgery within past 4 weeks or immobilization (≥ 3 days)	1.5
Clinical signs of DVT	3
Alternative diagnosis less likely than PE	3
Hemoptysis	1
Malignancy/ Cancer (treated within last 6 months) or palliative	1

Probability of PE	
PE unlikely	≤ 4
PE likely	> 4

Figure 2-5. Wells Prediction Rule for deep vein thrombosis (DVT) and pulmonary embolism. (Adapted from Wells PS, Anderson DR, Rodger M, et al. Derivation of a simple clinical model to categorize patients probability of pulmonary embolism: increasing the models utility with the SimpliRED D-dimer. *Thromb Haemost.* 2000;83[3]:416-420 and van Belle A, Büller HR, Huisman MV, et al; Christopher Study Investigators. Effectiveness of managing suspected pulmonary embolism using an algorithm combining clinical probability, D-dimer testing, and computed tomography. *JAMA.* 2006;295[2]:172-179.)

magnetic resonance imaging (MRI), or other testing (not shown) based upon the predicted risk. The therapist should discuss the clinical findings and concerns with the medical team. Because of the seriousness of VTE, the frequency that therapists encounter patients with a suspected or confirmed VTE, and the need to prevent future VTE, a clinical practice guideline (CPG) has been developed that can guide therapists in their clinical decision making.[16] Specific recommendations from this CPG include:

- Therapists should screen for VTE risk prior to mobilization and always screen for fall risk if a patient requires anticoagulation.
- Therapists should advocate for a culture of mobility and physical activity unless medical contraindications for mobility exist.
- Therapists should initiate mobilization when therapeutic threshold levels of anticoagulants have been reached. This requires therapists to understand the target (ie, INR/PT, PTT), mechanism, and onset of action of multiple anticoagulants (eg, LMWH, heparin sulfate, warfarin, NOAC/DOAC), and antiplatelet medications (eg, aspirin, clopidogrel, prasugrel). If a patient has known VTE and has not received anticoagulation or an inferior vena cava filter, the medical team should be consulted prior to mobilization.
- Therapists should provide preventive measures for patients who are identified as high risk for lower extremity (LE) DVT. These measures should include education regarding signs and symptoms of LE DVT, activity, hydration, mechanical compression, and referral for medication. Mechanical compression (eg, intermittent pneumatic compression) is indicated not only as a preventative measure but also if a DVT is present and beneficial to help post-thrombotic syndrome.[16]

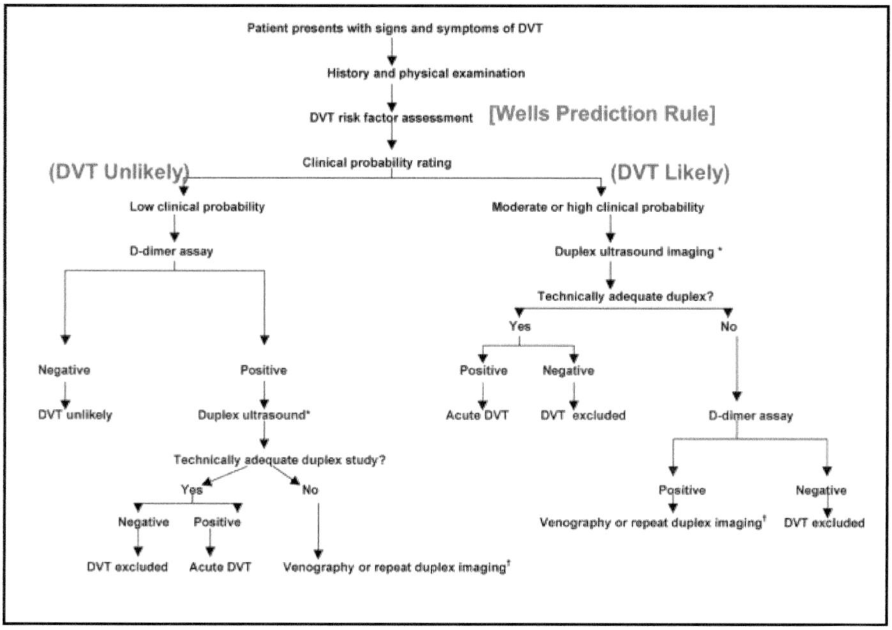

Figure 2-6. Algorithm for diagnosing DVT using clinical assessment, clinical prediction rule, duplex ultrasound, and D-dimer testing. (Adapted from Zierler BK. Ultrasonography and diagnosis of venous thromboembolism. *Circulation.* 2004;109[12 suppl 1]:19-14.)

As noted previously, hemostasis and fibrinolysis are usually balanced. This balance is disrupted in **DIC**. DIC results in exaggerated clotting, while simultaneously activating fibrinolysis and increasing bleeding. The result is ischemia and multiorgan failure with complicating hemorrhage. DIC is often a complicating factor from another underlying condition, usually in those with a critical illness such as sepsis and severe infections. DIC may also be associated with cancer, trauma, and extensive burns.

Proteins, Protein Metabolites, Enzymes, and Pigments

Amino acids are the building blocks of **proteins**. Proteins function as enzymes, detoxifying agents, antibodies, hormones, buffers, and energy sources. Serum proteins include albumin, globulins (alpha$_1$ alpha$_2$, beta, and gamma), and fibrinogen, and the remainder consists of hormones, enzymes, complements, and lipid transporters. Protein metabolites are the byproducts of protein degradation. **Enzymes** are proteins that facilitate chemical reactions in cells, with unique enzymes needed for different biochemical processes. The **bile pigments** are waste products of heme degradation, initiated by the breakdown of RBCs. Detection of organ- and tissue-specific enzymes, protein, protein metabolites, and pigments allows for precise diagnosis and monitoring of therapeutic interventions. Standard values and common abnormalities are presented in Tables 2-16 and 2-17.

Cardiac and Skeletal Muscle Enzymes and Proteins

Creatine kinase, also termed **creatine phosphokinase** (CPK), is found in high concentration in skeletal and cardiac muscle and in smaller concentration in brain tissue. CK is used as a specific index of injury to myocardial and skeletal muscle.

Table 2-16

Proteins, Protein Metabolites, and Trace Elements

Component	*Normal Values*	*Common Abnormalities*
Ammonia (NH_3)	15 to 56 μg/dL	↑ NH_3: Liver disease/cirrhosis, renal disease, GI infections/hemorrhage, total parenteral nutrition (TPN)
BUN	6 to 20 mg/dL	↑ BUN: CHF, diabetes, myocardial infarction, urinary tract obstruction, burns, cancer ↓ BUN: Liver failure, malnutrition, SIADH
Creatinine (Cr)	0.9 to 1.3 mg/dL	↑ Cr: Renal dysfunction, nephritis, urinary tract obstruction, muscular dystrophy, myasthenia gravis, rhabdomyolysis, hyperthyroidism, CHF, acromegaly, dehydration
Bilirubin	0.3 to 1.0 mg/dL	↑ Bilirubin: Liver disease (eg, cirrhosis, hepatitis), bile or hepatic duct obstruction (obstructive jaundice), pernicious anemia, sickle cell disease, CHF
ALB and Prealbumin (PAB)	3.5 to 4.8 g/dL 19 to 38 mg/dL	↓ ALB: Acute/chronic infections and inflammation, cirrhosis/liver disease, nephrotic syndrome, Crohn's disease, burns, starvation/malnutrition, thyroid disease
Iron (Fe^{3+})	Men: 65 to 175 μg/dL Women: 50 to 170 μg/dL	↓ Fe^{3+}: Iron deficiency/malabsorption, blood loss/hemorrhage, systemic lupus erythematosus, rheumatoid arthritis, chronic infections

When skeletal or cardiac muscle are damaged or die, they leak CK into the plasma, which can be detected with a laboratory test. These values are used in the diagnosis of myocardial infarction, myocarditis, inflammatory muscle disorders, rhabdomyolysis, muscular dystrophies, and trauma. CK occurs in multiple forms and can be subdivided into 3 isoenzymes to increase testing specificity. **CK-BB** is found in brain and neural tissue, **CK-MB** is found in heart muscle, and **CK-MM** is found in skeletal muscle.

Troponins are proteins associated with the contractile apparatus of muscle. Cardiac troponins are highly specific to heart tissue and are released into the serum following myocardial injury and infarction (see Table 2-17).

Lactate dehydrogenase (LDH) catalyzes the conversion of lactic acid to pyruvic acid, which then enters the Krebs's or tricarboxylic acid (TCA) cycle resulting in energy (ATP) formation. LDH is found in most cells of the body, limiting its specificity to detect tissue abnormalities. However, LDH is present in 5 tissue-specific isoenzymes enhancing diagnostic accuracy.

BNP and **atrial natriuretic peptide** (ANP) are hormones secreted by the heart due to pressure or volume overload. BNP is a marker of heart failure severity.

CRP is a protein produced by the liver and is a nonspecific marker of inflammation. CRP is elevated in a variety of disorders, including cancer, bacterial or

Table 2-17

Cardiac and Skeletal Muscle Enzymes and Hormones

Component	*Normal Values*	*Peak*	*Release*	*Decline*	*Common Abnormalities*
Myoglobin	<55 ng/mL				↑ CK/DC-MB: Acute myocardial infraction, perisurgical myocardial infraction, unstable angina, myocarditis
CPK • CK-MB	0 to 120 ng/mL • 3 ng/mL; 0 to 3%	3 to 6 hours	1 to 2 days	3 to 4 days	
Troponin • Cardiac troponin I • Cardiac troponin T	<0.4 ng/mL • <0.35 ng/mL • <0.2 ng/mL	3 hours	7 to 10 days 10 to 14 days		↑ Troponin: Acute myocardial infraction, unstable angina, myocarditis
LDH	140 to 280 U/L	1 to 2 days	8 to 14 days		
AST/SGOT	Men: 14 to 20 U/L Women: 10 to 36 U/L	8 to 12 hours	3 to 4 days		↑ AST: Myocardial infraction, hepatitis, cirrhosis, dermatomyositis, polymyositis, cerebral infarction, trauma, pulmonary embolism, gangrene, hemolytic anemia
ANF and BNP	20 to 77 pg/dL <100 pg/dL				↑ ANP/BNP: CHF, heart disease with elevated filling pressures, volume overload, paroxysmal atrial tachycardia
CRP	<8 mg/L				↑ CRP: Elevated cardiac risk/atherosclerosis (coronary artery disease [CAD])
Homocysteine	4 to 17 µmol/L				↑ Homocysteine: Elevated cardiac risk/atherosclerosis (CAD) ↓ Homocysteine: Folic acid/folate deficiency, homocystinuria

fungal infections, inflammatory disorders (eg, inflammatory bowel disease, Crohn's disease, ulcerative colitis), autoimmune disorders (eg, systemic lupus erythematosus [SLE]), and rheumatoid arthritis. Elevated CRP values are used to screen for cardiovascular risk as well as predict future cardiovascular events, such as CVA or myocardial infarction.

Homocysteine is an amino acid that is an intermediate of the metabolic pathway to synthesize cysteine from methionine. Homocysteine measurements are used to assess risk for coronary artery disease (CAD) and thromboses, anemia and abnormalities in folate, methionine, and Vitamins B_6 and B_{12}.

Hepatic Enzymes

Aspartate aminotransferase (AST), also termed **serum glutamic-oxaloacetic transaminase** (SGOT), is an enzyme present in tissues of high metabolic activity, including the liver, skeletal, and cardiac muscle. AST is released into the circulation following cellular damage or death (see Table 2-17).

Alanine aminotransferase (ALT) and **gamma glutamyl transferase** (GGT) are found primarily in the liver. The major amino acid precursor to produce glucose is alanine, and ALT catalyzes the chemical reaction that creates pyruvate from alanine for gluconeogenesis. GGT is important in the transport of amino acids into the cells of the intestines and kidneys. These enzymes are commonly monitored in hepatitis, cirrhosis, and drug therapy to determine the extent of liver damage.

Alpha-1 antitrypsin (AAT) is produced in the liver and functions to neutralize elastase, which breaks down elastic fibers. Elastic fibers are an important component of many organs, especially the bronchioles and alveoli of the lungs. AAT deficiency is associated with enhanced elastase activity leading to damaged elastic fibers, loss of lung recoil, and the development of early onset emphysema.

Pancreatic Enzymes

Amylase/Lipase

Amylase is a digestive enzyme that converts starch into glucose and is produced primarily in the salivary (parotid) glands and pancreas. **Lipase**, also produced in the pancreas, is vital for fat digestion and absorption, especially of triglyceride. Amylase and lipase from the pancreas are secreted into the small intestine. Laboratory testing is performed to determine the presence and management of pancreatitis. Normal serum amylase is 25 to 125 U/L and lipase is 10 to 140 U/L.

Proteins and Protein Metabolites

Transferrin/Ferritin

Transferrin, a glycoprotein formed in the liver and functions as a transporter of serum iron. Iron comes from the diet or the breakdown of RBCs, and transferrin transports iron to the bone marrow for hemoglobin synthesis or to the spleen, liver, and bone marrow for storage as **ferritin**. Transferrin and iron concentrations are used in the assessment of iron-deficiency anemia, thalassemias, and hemochromatosis (see Table 2-16).

Ammonia

Nitrogen from amino acids forms **ammonia** that is converted to **urea** and is excreted in the urine. Ammonia is toxic to the body, impacting acid-base balance and neurologic functioning and is usually excreted rapidly. Serum levels of ammonia may rise due to renal disease, parenteral nutrition, and liver disease leading to hepatic encephalopathy (see Table 2-16).

Creatinine

Creatinine is a breakdown product of CPK and its production is fairly constant. Creatinine is readily excreted by the kidneys, keeping serum values low. The serum concentration of creatinine is the most useful indicator of renal function, specifically the glomerular filtration rate (GFR). A rise in serum creatinine is assumed to result from decreased GFR and the extent of the rise is directly related to the severity of kidney dysfunction.

Blood Urea Nitrogen

Urea forms in the liver from the breakdown of proteins and amino acids, and urea excretion varies with dietary protein intake, metabolic state of the body, and the presence of disease. **BUN** is used to measure renal excretory capacity and estimate protein catabolism and/or tissue necrosis.

Albumin/Prealbumin

Albumin (ALB) and **prealbumin** (PAB) are values used to analyze nutrition status. ALB is the primary protein for maintaining the osmotic pressure in the vascular and extravascular spaces and is vital to fluid distribution. Decreased serum ALB leads to peripheral edema and potentially hypotension. Serum levels of ALB and transferrin may indicate the degree of protein malnutrition; however, ALB has a half-life of approximately 21 days and does not provide an accurate estimate of recent nutrition status. PAB is the preferred marker of nutrition status due to its short half-life, approximately 2 days, while ALB is slower to respond to a patient's recent change in nutrition status.

Carbohydrates and Ketone Bodies

Carbohydrates (CHOs) are the largest source of dietary calories in the typical diet. The primary CHOs consist of starch, a polysaccharide of multiple glucose molecules; lactose, a disaccharide of glucose and galactose; and sucrose, a disaccharide composed of glucose and fructose. Polysaccharides and disaccharides are converted to monosaccharides by digestive enzymes and absorbed via specific cell membrane transporters in the GI tract. **Glucose**, the body's major energy source, is principally obtained from the diet but can also be synthesized from amino acids. CHOs, stored in limited quantities in the liver and muscle as **glycogen**, provide a major source of energy via ATP production for the majority of metabolic processes, sparing protein breakdown. CHOs also function as a primer for fat metabolism. It should be noted that the use of any one fuel source at rest or during exercise does not occur in isolation. Rather, multiple fuel sources are simultaneously being used at a given time depending on the body's metabolic needs and substrate availability. For example, both CHOs and fat are oxidized at rest to provide the energy required for basal metabolic processes in skeletal muscle, and there is a reciprocal relationship between the utilization of CHOs and fat during exercise. It should also be noted that CHOs are a necessary fuel for the central nervous system and are the only energy source utilized by the brain.

Glucose metabolism is governed by the inverse actions of the pancreatic hormones, insulin, and glucagon (see Chapter 10). **Insulin** promotes the cellular absorption of glucose, production of hepatic and skeletal muscle glycogen, muscle protein synthesis and amino acid storage, and synthesis of triglycerides in adipose tissues. **Glucagon**, which is secreted during periods of fasting or low blood glucose, stimulates glycogen breakdown (ie, **glycogenolysis**) and glucose formation from protein and fat (ie, **gluconeogenesis**). Glucagon also stimulates lipolysis of adipose tissue resulting in the formation of fatty acids and glycerol. Monitoring of blood glucose is one of the most commonly performed laboratory tests in the acute care setting.

Fasting plasma glucose test is the measurement of plasma glucose after a 12-hour fast and is performed using a small blood sample and glucometer. The **oral glucose tolerance test** (OGTT) is used to diagnose borderline cases of diabetes, as well as gestational diabetes. In this test, the patient fasts overnight and then gets a fasting plasma glucose test. The patient then drinks a solution that is high in glucose and returns a few hours later for another blood draw. If gestational diabetes is a concern, the patient may have their blood drawn at 2 hours after ingestion of the glucose solution and again 3 hours after ingestion. The OGTT is based on the fact that the insulin response to a large oral glucose dose is almost immediate with a return to normal levels within 3 hours.

The OGTT and fasting glucose test provide information regarding the immediate plasma levels of glucose but provide limited information regarding the long-term management of blood glucose. The **glycosylated hemoglobin test** or **hemoglobin A1C** (HbA1C) is used to monitor the effectiveness of diabetes therapy. Hemoglobin, like other proteins, may be chemically modified by the addition of CHOs in a chemical reaction termed **glycosylation**. The addition of glucose to heme occurs spontaneously over the lifespan of RBCs (90 to 120 days) in proportion to the blood glucose concentration. Therefore, HbA1C is an indicator of blood glucose levels over the preceding 3 to 4 months.

Ketones consist of acetone, beta-hydroxybutyric acid, and acetoacetic acid synthesized in the liver resulting from the metabolism of fatty acids. Ketones are formed when fatty acid levels are elevated in the blood, as seen in fasting, starvation, high fat–low carbohydrate diets, and lack of insulin function. Normally, ketones are completely metabolized by extrahepatic tissues so that negligible amounts enter the urine. However, when carbohydrate metabolism is disturbed, fats and proteins become the predominate fuel sources, resulting in enhanced ketone formation. Excess ketones in the blood (ie, **ketonemia**), may result in **ketoacidosis**, a potentially lethal metabolic state due to ketones lowering blood pH. Ketones can be measured in the urine (ie, **ketonuria**) and can be used to monitor control of diabetes, alcoholism, malnutrition, and metabolic acidosis. Ketoacidosis is more common in type 1 diabetes compared to type 2, due to the absolute absence of insulin. Table 2-18 lists normal values for plasma glucose, insulin, and glucagon and diagnostic criteria for diabetes.

Bilirubin, a breakdown product of hemoglobin, is transported to the liver and primarily excreted in the bile. Bilirubin is found in the serum, and small amounts are present in the urine as **urobilinogen** (see Table 2-16). **Hyperbilirubinemia**, elevated bilirubin levels, usually indicates hepatic damage, biliary obstruction, or hemolytic anemia. The deposition of bilirubin in tissues produces the yellow appearance of **jaundice**.

Lipids and Lipoproteins

Lipids can be categorized into simple, compound, and derived forms. The simple lipids consist primarily of triglycerides, the major fat of the diet and the major storage form of fat in tissues. Compound lipids include the phospholipids and glycolipids, which are components of cell membranes, and the lipoproteins such as VLDL, LDL, and HDL. The lipoproteins, the combination of plasma proteins with triglycerides, allow the transport of fat in the blood. Specifically, HDL transports cholesterol in the periphery to the liver, while LDL and its precursor VLDL, carry cholesterol synthesized in the liver to the peripheral cells of the body. The apolipoproteins A and B are specific surface proteins on the lipoprotein molecules. HDL and LDL maintain cellular cholesterol balance and are important markers of cardiovascular risk assessment (Table 2-19). Derived lipids include the fatty acids used for energy production and steroids that are components of hormones, bile acids, and Vitamin D.

Table 2-18

CARBOHYDRATES AND KETONE BODIES—INSULIN AND GLUCAGON: DIABETES CRITERIA

Component	*Normal Values*	*Prediabetes*	*Diabetes*
Insulin	0 to 35 μIU/mL		
Glucagon	20 to 100 pg/mL		
Blood glucose	70 to 110 mg/dL		
Urine glucose	1 to 15 mg/dL/24 hours		
Fasting glucose test	<110 mg/dL	110 to 200 mg/dL	>126 mg/dL
OGTT	<140 mg/dL	140 to 200 mg/dL	>200 mg/dL
HbA1C	4% to 6.7% of total Hb		>8.1% of total Hb
Blood ketones			
Acetone	<2 mg/dL		
Beta-hydroxybutyric acid	0.21 to 2.81 mg/dL		
Acetoacetic acid	<1 mg/dL		
Urine ketones	Negative		

Cholesterol and lipid testing are measures that evaluate the risk for cardiac disease including atherosclerosis and CAD. Additionally, cholesterol and lipid measurements are used in the assessment of thyroid, renal, and liver function and diabetes.

COMMON DIAGNOSTIC TESTS

The following section will describe the mechanistic principles behind several common diagnostic tests. These descriptions are a general overview to provide the therapist with an understanding of how these devices and procedures promote an accurate diagnosis or promote safe and competent patient care. Additional procedures are described in the chapters that follow.

Ultrasonagraphy

Ultrasonagraphy, **sonogram**, or **ultrasound** is a noninvasive procedure for visualizing soft tissue structures of the body. High-frequency sound waves from a transducer are directed at a structure or organ. The sound waves are reflected back to the transducer producing a structural image on a monitor, providing information characterizing the position, size, and shape of the organ. Ultrasound is also used to determine the presence of fluid collections around organs. The **Doppler effect** is used during sonography to provide information about the presence, quality, and changing nature of the circulation. Sound waves strike moving RBCs and reflect back allowing

Table 2-19

Common Lipids and Cardiovascular Risk

The present clinical philosophy is to drive down total cholesterol as low as possible if the person has known atherosclerotic cardiovascular disease (ASCVD), specifically targeting LDL. Target goals for total cholesterol are less important than the targets for cholesterol components and triglycerides.

Lipid	*Targets for Primary and Secondary Prevention*	*Associations*
Total cholesterol		• High cholesterol: High cholesterol diet, hypothyroidism, chronic renal disease, alcoholism, obesity • Low cholesterol: Myeloproliferative diseases, malabsorption syndromes, malnutrition, severe burns, chronic anemias, hyperthyroidism
LDL	• If high risk for ASCVD optimal LDL is 70 mg/dL • If LDL is elevated, heart healthy lifestyle changes, pharmacological therapy (statins/non-statin)	• High LDL: High cholesterol/high fat diet, diabetes, chronic renal disease, nephrotic syndrome, hepatic obstruction, multiple myeloma • Low LDL: Hyperthyroidism, chronic anemias, acute stress (eg, burns, illness)
HDL	• Normal: 35 to 65 mg/dL • Target: >60 mg/dL • Elevated risk: ¤ Males: <40 mg/dL ¤ Females: <50 mg/dL	• Low HDL: Diabetes, chronic renal failure, nephrotic syndrome
Triglycerides (Tg)	• High: >175 mg/dL • Target: <150 mg/dL	• High Tg: Liver disease, alcoholism, pancreatitis, renal disease, myocardial infarction • Low Tg: Malnutrition,malabsorption, hyperthyroidism, hyperparathyroidism, COPD.

ASCVD Risk Estimator available at http://tools.acc.org/ASCVD-Risk-Estimator-Plus/#!/calculate/estimate/

Risk Estimator includes the following variable to assign risk:

- Age, sex, race
- Blood pressure
- Total cholesterol, HDL cholesterol, LDL cholesterol
- Medical history including diabetes, HTN
- Smoking

Adapted from Grundy SM, Stone NJ, Bailey AL, et al. 2018 AHA/ACC/AACVPR/AAPA/ABC/ACPM/ADA/AGS/APhA/ASPC/NLA/PCNA Guideline on the Management of Blood Cholesterol: Executive Summary: A report of the American College of Cardiology/American Heart Association Task Force on Clinical Practice Guidelines. *J Am Coll Cardiol*. 2019;73(24):3168-3209. doi: 10.1016/j.jacc.2018.11.002

direct listening and recording of blood flow patterns, including direction, velocity, and magnitude of flow. For example, narrowed blood vessels produce high velocities, indicating possible stenosis or vasospasm or potential arteriovenous malformations. **Duplex scans** are the combination of anatomic imaging of blood vessels and hemodynamic information provided by Doppler ultrasound. Duplex scans provide information regarding the direction, pulsatile nature, and resistance of blood flow.

Common sonographic and duplex procedures include:

- Echocardiography/transesophageal echocardiography (TEE)/Doppler echocardiography to evaluate the cardiac structures and blood flow through the chambers and valves
- Upper extremity (UE)/LE duplex scans to evaluate arterial and venous blood flow to identify clot (eg, DVT)
- Abdominal sonograms to evaluate soft tissue organs (eg, hepatobiliary, pancreas, kidneys, spleen, aorta/other large abdominal vessels, lymph nodes)
- Head and neck sonograms to evaluate pathologies of the thyroid/PTH glands, assess carotid and vertebral arteries, and cerebral blood flow

Endoscopy

Endoscopy is an invasive procedure that provides direct visualization of internal body structures by means of a lighted lens system, or fiberoptic, attached to either a rigid or flexible tube. Separate ports allow the administration of drugs, suction, and insertion of lasers, brushes, forceps, or other instruments for excision or tissue sampling. Examples of common endoscopic procedures include the following:

- Arthroscopy to examine the interior of a joint
- Bronchoscopy to examine the airways
- Laparoscopy to examine the intra-abdominal and pelvic cavities
- Cystoscopy to examine the lower urinary tract

Radiography

Radiographs (x-rays) are short-wavelength electromagnetic vibrations that are absorbed or deflected as they pass through tissue. The density of the tissue will determine the degree of absorption allowing the differentiation of various body structures. Dense tissues will appear white, while air-filled regions will appear black. X-ray studies are usually used for more dense structures, but the additions of **contrast agents** of varying densities are used to further differentiate tissue, especially hollow viscera. Contrast agents are generally described as radiopaque, or high absorption, resulting in no transmission of x-rays onto the film, or radiolucent, which allow partial transmission of the x-rays. Contrast agents may by injected or administered orally or rectally. Contrast agents are not benign, and the risk of allergic reactions can range from simple nausea to severe anaphylaxis. Radiographs produce a 2-dimensional image in grayscale and superimposed structures may create odd appearing lines, shadows, or apparent structural abnormalities. X-rays are termed by the radiographic view that describes the direction of the beam entry and exit. For example, an anterior-posterior (A-P) view implies the beam entered the patient anteriorly and exited posteriorly, a lateral view is from the side, while an oblique view is on an angle.

Fluoroscopy

Fluoroscopy uses a continuous stream of x-rays and the direct viewing of the image on a fluorescent screen to view real-time movement of anatomic structures or contrast material through anatomic structures. The image clarity is limited, but fluoroscopy is often used for central line placement and assessment of diaphragm function, digestive tract motility, or swallowing dysfunction.

Angiography

Angiography involves the injection of a contrast medium into the vasculature to allow radiographic examination. Angiography is used to detect aneurysms, arteriovenous malformation (AVM), thrombosis, vasospasm, and narrowing or occlusion of suspect vessels. Angiography is a diagnostic tool commonly used to assess the coronary circulation, the carotid and vertebral vessels, and cerebral circulation.

Digital subtraction angiography (DSA) uses fluoroscopic imaging before and after injection of contrast material to remove, or subtract, common features from the 2 images. Common features subtracted include bone and soft tissue, providing an enhanced image of the vasculature. DSA is used to visualize the intracranial and carotid vessels, aorta, visceral organ vessels, and other peripheral vessels.

Computed Tomography

CT scan or **computerized axial tomography** (CAT) **scan** combines multiple x-ray beams and computer-based calculations to determine the different absorption patterns of soft tissues providing delineation of minor differences in tissue densities. The image is displayed in cross-section, or slices, without superimposing structures. A **spiral CT** employs a continuous corkscrew scan pattern that allows the reconstruction of a 3-dimensional image. Use of contrast media can further accentuate differences in tissue densities, providing a more accurate description of the anatomy.

Magnetic Resonance Imaging

MRI uses a superconducting magnet to polarize protons, the positively charged nucleus of hydrogen atoms, and a radio-frequency signal that is pulsed through the hydrogen atoms causing them to become energized or knocked out of alignment and resonate. The hydrogen atoms will eventually reestablish the previous equilibrium and the decay of the resonation signal is monitored by sensors and recorded and processed by computer. The greater the concentration of protons in a tissue, the greater the resonance and longer decay time, allowing the computer to construct an image. For example, tissues that contain a lot of water, and therefore, a high concentration of hydrogen, have high signal strength and are detected more readily than tissues with little water, such as adipose tissue. MRI allows multiplanar scanning and contrast-free 3-dimensional imaging.

Nuclear Medicine Imaging

Nuclear medicine imaging includes **single photon emission computed tomography** (SPECT) and **positron emission tomography** (PET). These diagnostic modalities study the function of organs of the body through the use of a radiopharmaceutical that incorporates a radioactive label (radioisotope), and a pharmaceutical (the substrate) that is specified for the organ or tissue of interest. The radiopharmaceutical chosen are biologically active and will remain in the organ to be studied long enough to produce a usable image but with relatively short half-lives to minimize radiation exposure to the patient's tissues. The radiopharmaceutical is inhaled, ingested, or injected, and the target tissue takes up the radiolabeled substrate. The radioisotope emits gamma rays, allowing the target organ to be scanned by a camera providing quantitative and qualitative physiologic data.

Electrodiagnostic Studies

Electrophysiology studies are invasive tests for the diagnosis and treatment of supraventricular and ventricular dysrhythmias, syncope, and sick sinus syndrome. The EP studies measure cardiac electrical conduction system activity through solid electrode catheters that are guided via fluoroscopy through the venous system to the right atrium and ventricle. In addition to measuring baseline electrical activity, the EP catheters may be used to pace the heart in an attempt to induce the suspected dysrhythmia.

Electromyography and Nerve Conduction Studies

Electromyography (EMG) and **nerve conduction studies** (NCV) measure the functional state and structural integrity of the lower motor neurons to discriminate between myopathy and neuropathy. Conventional EMG uses concentric or monopolar electrodes, while needle EMG involves the percutaneous insertion of a needle electrode into the desired muscle. EMG records the electrical activity of selected muscle fibers at rest, during voluntary contraction, or in combination with electrical stimulation.

NCV studies involve the application of an electrical stimulus to a nerve of interest with the recording of the action potentials a known distance from the point of stimulation, allowing computation of the conduction velocity.

Tests of repetitive motor nerve stimulation are intended to distinguish disorders of neuromuscular junction transmission, presynaptic, or postsynaptic failure as the cause of muscle weakness.

Electroencephalogram and Evoked Potentials

Electroencephalograms (EEGs) measure and record the electrical impulses from the brain cortex. Electrodes are attached to areas of the patient's scalp and brain waves are recorded. Common waveforms include the following:

- Alpha waves: Frequency of 8 to 11 Hz; occur in the wakened state
- Beta waves: 13 to 30 Hz; associated with anxiety, depression, and sedatives
- Theta waves: 4 to 7 Hz; common in frontal and temporal regions of children and young adults
- Delta waves: 0.5 to 3.5 Hz; common in children and sleep

Waveforms are evaluated for symmetry, amplitude, distinct patterns, and observation for transient discharges and responses to stimulation. Common indications for an EEG include epilepsy and seizure activity, focal brain abnormalities, including tumor, abscess, or hemorrhage, as well as various diseases including Parkinson's and Alzheimer's.

Evoked potentials evaluate the integrity of visual, somatosensory, and auditory nerve pathways by measuring the brain's electrical responses to specific stimulation.

Case Study

Mrs. Gloria Bennet is a 74-year-old female diagnosed with a right fibula fracture following a fall at home. Her past medical history is significant for hypertension (HTN), obesity, and rheumatoid arthritis. The fracture is aligned, stabilized with a short leg cast, and physical therapy is consulted.

Patient/Client History

General Demographics, Social History, and Living Environment

Mrs. Bennet is married, and lives in a 2-story home with 4 steps to enter and a handrail. There is a bedroom and bathroom on the second floor and a bathroom on the first floor. Her husband is also 74 years old and is reportedly in good health.

General Health Status, Social/Health Habits, and Family History

Mrs. Bennet is overweight with a body mass index (BMI) of 32. She denies smoking or drug use but does "enjoy my nightly glass of white wine". She does not consider herself active and has no regular exercise routine. Hobbies include watching movies and knitting. Her family history is unremarkable and unrelated to the current condition.

Medical/Surgical History

Mrs. Bennet has HTN, obesity, and rheumatoid arthritis. Surgical history includes a caesarean section. Knee replacement surgery was recommended approximately 2 months ago but she does not wish to do this prior to the current fall and hospitalization. She states that she was fearful of the recovery following knee replacement surgery. Upon further questioning, her fear is primarily related to infection risk.

Current Conditions

Mrs. Bennet is status-post (s/p) right lower extremity (RLE) fibula fracture repair by cast immobilization. She is weightbearing as tolerated (WBAT). She states her pain is "okay," but she is fearful to use pain medications because of a prior experience of severe constipation.

Activities and Participation

Prior to admission, the patient was independent with all aspects of mobility and activities of daily living (ADLs)/instrumental activities of daily living (IADLs) and occasionally used a straight cane for walking outside and stairs. She reports "walking very little" over the last 2 weeks because of increased knee pain. Currently, the patient is WBAT on the RLE, allowed out of bed ad lib, and requires assistance for all mobility secondary to pain and the WBAT status.

Medications

Her usual medications include metoprolol (a beta blocker) and furosemide (a diuretic) for HTN, leflunomide (a disease-modifying antirheumatic drug [DMARD]) and an NSAID for "aches and pains" as needed. She was receiving DVT prophylaxis with Lovenox (enoxaparin sodium; a LMWH).

Other Clinical Tests

Abnormal Laboratory Findings

CBC revealed Hb = 9.4 g/dL, WBCs 13,500/mm3, and electrolytes were sodium < 130 mEq/L and K^+ of 3.1 mEq/L.

Systems Review

Cardiovascular and Pulmonary

Resting heart rate (HR) 84 beats per minute (bpm), blood pressure (BP) is 136/78 mm Hg, and respiratory rate (RR) is 20 breath per minute. Her toes are visible and swollen on the RLE and her left lower extremity (LLE) also presents with pitting edema below the knee. Mrs. Bennet reports that this is new.

Integumentary

Her RLE is casted and has been placed on a pressure relieving, low air loss mattress based on body habitus and lack of mobility. There are pneumatic compression stockings hanging from the bed, but she has not worn them stating "it's uncomfortable on my leg."

Musculoskeletal

Gross myotome assessment and AROM of bilateral upper extremities (BLEs) and LLE appears normal except RLE strength limited by pain and weight of the cast.

Neuromuscular

Sensation to light touch and gross proprioception are intact throughout.

Communication, Affect, Cognition, Language, and Learning Style

Mrs. Bennet is awake, alert, and oriented to person, place, time, and situation. She reports feeling anxious about moving because of the pain. Her primary language is English. She reports that she likes to plan ahead so "please let me know what is going to happen next."

Tests and Measures

Aerobic Capacity and Endurance

As noted in the Mobility assessment that follows, the patient demonstrated tachycardia and complained of chest discomfort with standing at the bedside.

Assistive and Adaptive Devices

Mrs. Bennet was assisted into a standing position with use of a standard walker. The patient could assist with bed mobility but might benefit from an overhead trapeze bar and reacher. A bedside commode has been ordered. There is a RLE cast.

Balance, Gait, and Mobility (Including Locomotion)

Mrs. Bennet required moderate assistance to transition from supine↔sitting at the edge of the bed (Functional Independence Measure [FIM] definitions FIM 3) and maximal assistance to complete the sit↔stand transfer (FIM 2) and maintain abbreviated standing with a standard walker. Mrs. Bennet required maximal assistance (FIM 2) to take 10 steps with a standard walker. She complained of an expected RLE and unexpected LLE ache while reporting a sudden discomfort in her right flank. Her Activity Measure for Post Acute Care (AM-PAC) "6 Clicks" basic mobility score is 8/24.

Circulation (Arterial, Venous, Lymphatic) and Ventilation/Respiration

After sitting at the edge of the bed and standing to a walker, her vital signs are BP 136/78-156/80 mm Hg, HR 84-115 bpm, SpO_2 94%-90% on 2 liters/minute (l/m). Patient reports feeling chest discomfort in the right lateral thorax during gait training and is returned to bed. The nursing and medical staff is notified. RLE/toes demonstrate brisk capillary refill.

The SpO_2 is 94% on 2 lpm at rest and decreased to 90% during gait assessment. Auscultation of breath sounds at rest reveals decreased breath sounds being clear to auscultation (CTA). Incentive spirometry averages 450 mL.

Mental Function

The patient was alert, cooperative and could follow commands easily. She appears anxious.

Muscle Performance

Muscle strength was 4/5 in all major muscle groups of bilateral upper extremities (BUEs)/BLEs with the exception of the RLE, which was not formally assessed secondary to pain with motion.

Pain

Using a numeric pain rating scale, the patient reports RLE 3/10 pain at rest (aching) and 8/10 (sharp) while moving. Rest and RLE elevation relieve the pain.

Evaluation

Mrs. Bennet is an older female currently hospitalized secondary to a fall and RLE fibula fracture. Past medical history is remarkable for HTN, rheumatoid arthritis, and obesity. The complaint of right chest wall discomfort is concerning for pulmonary embolism and per the Wells Criteria she scores a 6 (HR >100 bpm), recent surgery and clinical signs of DVT (immobilization, RLE and LLE swelling). The desaturation on SpO_2 is also an abnormal response. Her laboratory reveals anemia, hyponatremia, and hypokalemia. Each of these may contribute to feelings of weakness and fatigue. The electrocardiogram (ECG) should be consistently reviewed because hypokalemia may result in ECG abnormalities. Although uncommon at the current serum concentrations, hypokalemia can result in atrial and ventricular tachycardia and potentially ventricular fibrillation.

Diagnosis

Mrs. Bennet presents with activity limitations including deficits with transfers and gait primarily related to pain with movement and weakness. The right flank discomfort combined with tachycardia, tachypnea, and a Wells score that indicates a pulmonary emboli is likely requires immediate consultation with the nursing and medical staff. She will require ongoing physical therapy services to facilitate safe discharge, but the immediate concern is potential pulmonary emboli.

Prognosis

Complete fibula fracture healing should allow return to the prior level of function, but an assistive device may be required for a prolonged time. The immediate concern is the potential for pulmonary emboli. It is important to recognize that patients can still develop VTE even in the presence of anticoagulation and this patient was at great risk due to the immobility and her history of RA and obesity. A CT scan was performed and ruled out the pulmonary emboli. The patient will require ongoing episodes of physical therapy, including outpatient services, to facilitate a complete return to the prior level of function. She has already been recommended to undergo a total knee arthroplasty so pre-rehabilitation could be very beneficial.

Intervention

The orthopedic service agreed that the patient's presentation (vital sign response, patient complaint, Wells criteria) was very serious and ordered a CT scan and modified the dosage of anticoagulation. The CT scan was negative for pulmonary emboli. It appears that the patient experienced a muscle strain while trying to mobilize into standing and attempt walking. Although the CT was negative, the therapist was correct in determining that this was a potential life-altering situation and immediate action was required.

Daily physical therapy intervention with short-term goals of increasing out of bed tolerance and decreasing level of assistance required for bedside mobilization, transfers, and gait training was emphasized. Interventions included functional training (eg, bed mobility, transfers, toilet and gait training), assistive technology training included use of walker, trapeze, and reacher. The trapeze will be used intermittently until the patient can independently perform bed mobility tasks. Therapeutic exercises (eg, UE/LE AROM and resistive exercises) and patient instruction (eg, pain control, skin integrity, incentive spirometry, WBAT progression, bedside ROM exercise program) were initiated and progressed throughout this episode of care.

Outcomes

As noted previously, the CT scan was negative, but the physical therapist made the correct decision to alert the medical and nursing teams. The patient presented with multiple risk factors for VTE including immobility, recent orthopedic surgery, obesity, and RA. Additionally, the Wells Criteria was positive with the sudden onset of chest discomfort combined with tachycardia and tachypnea and BLE swelling being significant.

The patient was treated for 5 additional sessions at which point she was discharged to home. The patient was independent transferring from supine to sit (FIM 7), supervision for sit to stand (FIM 5), and was ambulating 75 feet x 2 with a rolling walker independently (FIM 6). She could ascend/descend 10 steps with minimal assist using a railing and straight cane (FIM 4). Her AM-PAC "6 Click" basic mobility score increased from 8 to 21/24. It was recommended that she continue with outpatient physical therapy to return to her prior level of function emphasizing gait training, stair climbing, and potentially progressing to a less restrictive assist device. This ongoing physical therapy care may also help if she decides to pursue knee replacement surgery.

ICF Clinical Reasoning Tool Case Study Summary								
Health Condition								
HPI: Fall in the home, RLE fibula fracture s/p cast immobilization PMHx: Rheumatoid arthritis, HTN, obesity and increasingly sedentary lifestyle. Potential need for bilateral knee arthroplasty at later date								
Precautions/Contraindications								
WBAT; initial concern for pulmonary emboli with Wells Criteria indicating a "likely" probability for pulmonary emboli; safety/fall risk; pain; universal precautions								
Body Structure and Function			*Activity/Task Limitations*			*Participation*		
Impairment/ Problem	*Tests and Measures*	*Intervention*	*Activity*	*Tests and Measures*	*Intervention*	*Participation*	*Tests and Measures*	*Intervention*
• Impaired endurance • Bilateral knee pain • Chest wall discomfort • Abnormal lab values • Obesity	• ROM/MMT • VS including SpO_2 and ECG • NPRS • BMI • Lab values	• Breathing exercises (incentive spirometry, deep breathing) • Pain management • Education for risk for falls/ safety • Consult registered dietician	• ADLs • IADLs • Bed mobility • Transfers • Gait	• Functional task analysis • FIM • AM-PAC Basic Mobility ("6 Clicks") • RPE • Pain scale • PSFS	• Progressive functional retraining • Careful monitoring of VS due to hypokalemia	• Unable to return home and perform regular ADLs/ IADLs as homemaker	• PSFS	• Continue physical therapy services • Consult social worker • Family meeting to discuss discharge plans

(continued)

ICF Clinical Reasoning Tool Case Study Summary (continued)

Personal Factors	*Other Considerations*	*Environmental Factors*
• Age: 74 y/o female • AAO x 3 • Primary language: English • Full time homemaker • Married • 1 grown son lives nearby and can assist intermittently as care provider • Independent prior to fall and fracture but reports recent sedentary lifestyle due to knee pain • Anxious and fearful of pain with movement		Home: • 2 story home; doesn't wish to stay on 1st floor but will consider if necessary (and temporary); 3 steps to enter with handrail, bedroom/bathroom on 2nd floor and bathroom on 1st floor Hospital: • 2 L NP, urinary catheter, RLE cast, bedside commode, OOB and WBAT RLE

AAO = awake, alert, oriented; BMI = body mass index; HPI = history of present illness; NP = nasal prongs; OOB = out of bed; PMHx = past medical history; PSFS = Patient Specific Functional Scale; ROM = range of motion; RPE = rate of perceived exertion; y/o = year old.

Adapted from American Physical Therapy Association. *Guide to Physical Therapist Practice*. 3rd ed. http://www.apta.org/Guide/. Updated October 21, 2015. Accessed October 5, 2018 and *Towards a Common Language for Functioning, Disability and Health*. World Health Organization. www.who.int/classifications/icf/icfbeginnersguide.pdf. Published 2002. Accessed April 29, 2019.

CHAPTER REVIEW QUESTIONS

1. What are the benefits of laboratory testing, sonography, radiology, and nuclear imaging for the physical therapist in the acute care setting?
   a. This information allows the therapist to better understand the medical diagnosis and how well major organs are functioning.
   b. This information is only considered adjunct information and has no impact on examination or evaluation of the patient.
   c. This information is beneficial to discuss and review with the patient and family.
   d. This information is helpful in planning discharge destination especially if skilled nursing facility recommended.
2. What is the best test to monitor the effectiveness of long-term diabetes management?
   a. Oral glucose tolerance test
   b. Urine ketone test
   c. Fasting blood glucose test
   d. HbA1c
3. Which of the following signs and symptoms would lead to altering the intensity and duration of an exercise program due to anemia?
   a. Increased dysrhythmias, hemoptysis, decreased resting HR, and pallor
   b. Increased tachycardia with transfers, nausea with position change, and paroxysmal nocturnal dyspnea
   c. Increased DOE, muscle cramping, dizziness, and chest pressure
   d. Increased crackles in lower lobes, decreased chest expansion, +S3, and pain with inhalation
4. What are clinical manifestations that a therapist may observe if a patient has hypernatremia?
   a. Seizure, hypotension, tachycardia, and a weak, thready pulse
   b. Headache, lethargy, diarrhea, and dry mucus membranes
   c. Pitting edema, HTN, absent reflexes, and decreased urine output
   d. Agitation, vomiting, orthostatic hypotension, and bradycardia
5. The clinical symptoms associated with a decreased extracellular potassium concentration (hypokalemia include:
   a. Heart block and positive Homan's sign
   b. HTN and hyperreflexia
   c. Diarrhea and leg cramps
   d. Paresthesia and dysrhythmias

Answers: 1a, 2d, 3c, 4a, 5d

References

1. Huether SE, McCance. *Understanding Pathophysiology.* St. Louis, MO: Mosby; 1996.
2. Koeppen BM, Stanton BA. *Renal Physiology.* St. Louis, MO: Mosby; 2001.
3. Ackril P, France MW. Common electrolyte problems. *Clin Med.* 2002;2:205-208.
4. Luckey AE, Parsa CJ. Fluid and electrolytes in the aged. *Arch Surg.* 2003;138:1055-1060.
5. Crutchlow EM, Dudac PJ, MacAvoy S, et al. *Pathophysiology.* Sudbury, MA: Jones and Bartlett; 2002.
6. Ravel R. *Clinical Laboratory Medicine.* 6th ed. St. Louis, MO: Mosby; 2004:86-88.
7. Bushinsky DA, Monk RD. Electrolyte quintet: calcium. *Lancet.* 1998;352:305-311.
8. Bove LA. Restoring electrolyte balance: calcium & phosphorus. *RN.* 1996;59:47-52.
9. Horne C, Derrico D. Mastering ABGs: the art of arterial blood gas measurement. *Am J Nurse.* 1999;99:26-32.
10. Kierszenbaum AL. *Histology and Cell Biology.* St. Louis, MO: Mosby; 2002.
11. Abramo L, Alexander IM, Bastien D, et al. *Professional Guide to Diagnostic Tests.* Philadelphia, PA: Lippincott Williams & Wilkins; 2005.
12. Junqueira LC, Carneiro J. *Basic Histology Text and Atlas.* 10th ed. New York, NY: McGraw-Hill; 2003.
13. Hand H. Blood and the classification of anaemia. *Nursing Standard.* 2001;15:45-55.
14. Carson JL, Grossman BJ, Kleinman S, et al. Clinical Transfusion Medicine Committee of the AABB. Red blood cell transfusion: a clinical practice guideline from the AABB. *Ann Intern Med.* 2012;157(1):49-58.
15. Office of the Surgeon General, National Heart, Lung, and Blood Institute. *The Surgeon General's Call to Action to Prevent Deep Vein Thrombosis and Pulmonary Embolism.* Rockville, MD: Office of the Surgeon General. https://www.ncbi.nlm.nih.gov/books/NBK44178. Published 2008. Accessed October 15, 2018.
16. Hillegass E, Puthoff M, Frese EM, Thigpen M, Sobush DC, Auten D, for the Guideline Development Group. Role of physical therapists in the management of individuals at risk for or diagnosed with venous thromboembolism: evidence-based clinical practice guideline. *Phys Ther.* 2016;96(2):143-166.

Bibliography

Chen MY, Pope ML, Ott DJ. *Basic Radiology.* New York, NY: McGraw-Hill; 1996.

Fischbach FT, Dunning MB. *A Manual of Laboratory and Diagnostic Tests.* Philadelphia, PA: Lippincott Williams & Wilkins; 2004.

Halperin ML, Kamel KS. Electrolyte quintet: potassium. *Lancet.* 1998;352:135-140.

Johnson EW, Pease WS. *Practical Electromyography.* Baltimore, MD: Lippincott Williams & Wilkins; 1997.

Marks DB, Marks AD, Smith CM. *Basic Medical Biochemistry.* Philadelphia, PA: Lippincott Williams & Wilkins; 1996.

McArdle WD, Katch FI, Katch VL. *Exercise Physiology: Energy, Nutrition, and Human Performance.* Philadelphia, PA: Lippincott Williams & Wilkins; 2001.

Mettler RA, Guibereau MJ. *Essentials of Nuclear Imaging.* Philadelphia, PA: WB Saunders; 1991.

Chapter 3

Physiologic Monitors and Patient Support Equipment

Daniel J. Malone, PT, PhD, CCS

Providing physical therapy services in the acute care and critical care settings continues to evolve.[1] Physical therapists may be intimidated to provide care in the intensive care unit (ICU) due to the tenuous pathophysiologic state of the patient and the overwhelming nature of the monitors and equipment attached to the patient. The use of life support and monitoring equipment; the prescription of sedative and paralytic agents; and the presence of pain, malnutrition, and sleep deprivation further complicate the patient's functional status.[2] The information that needs to be processed can be daunting; however, the monitoring equipment provides immediate data regarding the patient's physiologic responses to therapeutic interventions, and appropriate measures can be undertaken to avoid untoward events. In addition, the other health professionals who work in the ICU are skilled in providing emergency services in the unlikely event that the patient does not tolerate the therapy session. The physical therapist plays a pivotal role in providing and guiding care throughout the entire acute care continuum with the introduction of patient care often taking place in the ICU. It is the physical therapist's responsibility to integrate the patient's pathophysiologic status; the surgical, medical, and pharmacologic interventions; and the physiologic monitors and support equipment.

The goal of this chapter is to provide the physical therapist/physical therapist assistant with a working knowledge of the diverse equipment present within the ICU and to provide guidelines that will enable the practitioner to provide safe and effective care.

Central Venous and Pulmonary Artery Catheter (Swan-Ganz Catheter) Monitoring

The pulmonary artery catheter (PAC) was first introduced by Swan and colleagues[3] in 1970 and has become a widely used tool to measure central hemodynamics and modify medical therapy in the critically ill. Although controversy exists regarding

Malone DJ, Bishop KL, eds. *Acute Care Physical Therapy: A Clinician's Guide, Second Edition* (pp 93-117).

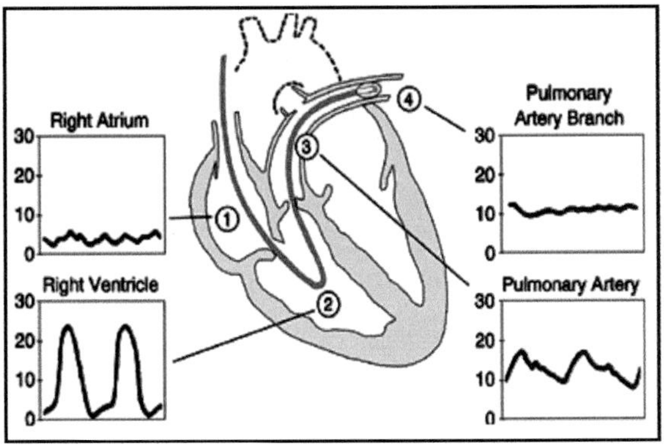

Figure 3-1. PAC for hemodynamic monitoring. The catheter passes through the right atrium and ventricle into the pulmonary artery. Note the pressure differences in the different chambers of the heart and pulmonary artery. (Reprinted with permission from Marino PL. *The ICU Book*. Baltimore, MD: Lippincott Williams & Wilkins; 1998.)

the use of these devices in septic shock, acute respiratory distress syndrome, and acute decompensated heart failure, the PAC is extensively used for hemodynamic monitoring in pulmonary hypertension, cardiogenic shock, mixed shock states, cardiac tamponade, and complicated myocardial infarction.[4,5] The PAC is a flexible, balloon-tipped, flow-directed catheter that is inserted in a large peripheral vein, usually the subclavian or internal jugular veins, and guided through the right side of the heart into the pulmonary artery (Figure 3-1).[6,7] The catheter's balloon is inflated upon insertion and rapidly migrates into the heart and pulmonary vasculature as it is carried by the force of blood flow against the inflated balloon until it impacts upon a medium-sized pulmonary artery whose internal diameter is the same or less than that of the balloon.[6] The PAC is commonly a triple lumen catheter with a proximal port for measuring right atrial pressure (RAP), a distal port for measuring pulmonary artery pressure (PAP), and a thermistor that allows calculation of the cardiac output.[8] The left atrial pressure (LAP), an estimate of left ventricular preload, can be obtained with the PAC by determining the pulmonary capillary wedge pressure (PCWP; sometimes called the **pulmonary artery occlusion pressure**). The PCWP is measured with the balloon inflated, preventing flow of blood in the occluded pulmonary artery. This creates a static column of fluid. The static column of fluid transmits LAP and, therefore, the left ventricular end diastolic pressure (LVEDP), which is the estimate of preload.[4,5,7] Segmental lung infarction may occur if the catheter balloon is left inflated for long periods of time; therefore, PCWP is only measured intermittently. PCWP should be determined at end expiration because respiratory variation of the waveform occurs due to changes in intrathoracic pressures.[9] Other hemodynamic variables can be derived from these basic measures as outlined in Table 3-1.

As the therapist begins to review the data generated from the PAC, it is important to consider that there are assumptions that must be met for the values to be valid. For example, pressure may be used as a surrogate for blood volume; however, pressure may not directly reflect volume due to vascular and cardiac chamber compliance and the degree of vasodilation and constriction. For example, reduced right ventricular compliance combined with pulmonary artery vasoconstriction would increase right ventricular and right atrial pressures without a change in blood volume.

RAP, also termed **central venous pressure** (CVP), is recorded from the proximal port of the PAC situated in the superior vena cava or right atrium. The RAP should be equivalent to right ventricular end diastolic pressure when there is no obstruction or tricuspid valve abnormality between the right atrium and ventricle. CVP represents the blood volume that is returned to the right heart creating the **filling pressure** or **preload**. The left heart's filling pressure is provided by the PCWP and represents the volume of blood across the pulmonary circulation to the left atria. The LAP should

Table 3-1

Common Measured and Calculated Hemodynamic Values

Parameter	*Normal Value (Mean)*	*Equation*
Indicator of preload • RAP/CVP • PAWP/LVEDP	 • 2 to 8 mm Hg • 8 to 15 mm Hg	
Indicators of afterload • PVR • SVR	 • <250 dynes–s/cm[5] • 800 to 1200 dynes–s/cm[5]	 PVR = (mean PAP-PAWP/CO) x 80 SVR = (mean BP-CVP/ CO) x 80
PAP • Systolic • Diastolic • Mean	 • 20 to 30 mm Hg • 5 to 10 mm Hg • 10 to 20 mm Hg	
Cardiac output (CO)	• 5.2 to 7.4 (L/min) (6)	CO = HR x SV
Cardiac index (CI)	• 2.6 to 4.2 ($L/min\text{-}m^2$) (3.2)	Thermodilution: CO = amount of indicator injected/area under curve Fick equation: $CO = VO_2/(CaO_2 - CvO_2)$ CI = CO/BSA
Arterial BP (see Table 6-3)	• <130/85	
Mean arterial pressure (MAP)	• 70 to 110 mm Hg	MAP = DBP + 1/3 PP PP = SBP – DBP

Pressure (mm Hg) = pressure (cm H_2O) x 1.36

DBP = diastolic blood pressure; PP = pulse pressure; SBP = systolic blood pressure.

Adapted from Hillegass EA. *Essentials of Cardiopulmonary Physical Therapy*. 3rd ed. St. Louis, MO: Elsevier: WB Saunders Co; 2011 and Tibby SM, Murdoch IA. Monitoring cardiac function in intensive care. *Arch Dis Child*. 2003;88:46-52.

also be equivalent to the LVEDP when there is no obstruction or mitral valve abnormality between the left atrium and ventricle (PCWP = LAP = LVEDP).[8-10]

Cardiac output is measured by the thermodilution technique (also called **indicator washout method**). Thermodilution is a computer-assisted measurement of cardiac output that uses the injection of a known volume of cold saline. The cold saline mixes with the blood in the right atrium and as this cooled blood flows over the thermistor in the pulmonary artery, the cardiac output is calculated based off the changes in blood temperature. The calculation is founded on the premise that when a known concentration of an indicator solution is added to circulating blood, the rate of blood flow is proportional to the change in concentration of the indicator over time (ie, washout).[4,9,11] Delayed washout is indicative of decreased cardiac output, while rapid washout is associated with good cardiac output. This technique provides an estimate of the cardiac output as long as there is no shunting of blood (eg, ventricular septal defect) and the tricuspid valve is normal.[4,8,11] Continuous measurement of **cardiac output** is a derivation of the thermodilution method using a catheter equipped with a thermal filament. The filament generates low-energy heat pulses that are transmitted to the surrounding blood. The resulting change in blood temperature is then used to generate a thermodilution curve for determining cardiac output.[9] Cardiac output can be corrected to body size by indexing the values to the body surface area (BSA) and is expressed as the **cardiac index**.

Mixed venous oxygen saturation (S_VO_2) is the saturation of hemoglobin in the pulmonary artery. Blood is sampled and analyzed through one of the ports of the PAC. $\mathbf{S_VO_2}$ reflects the balance between oxygen delivery and the amount consumed. Values of 60% to 80% are normal.[10] A low S_VO_2 is associated with a decrease in the cardiac output or anemia, or may indicate pulmonary dysfunction and poor gas exchange.[8] If the S_VO_2 changes ±10% from the baseline value, confirm that the change reflects a change in the patient's condition and alert the medical team.[10]

For patients who present with a central indwelling catheter, the most common complication is a transient dysrhythmia as the catheter passes through the tricuspid and pulmonary valves during insertion. Dysrhythmias are usually self-limiting and cause no harm.[8] Other complications include infection of the insertion site, line-related sepsis, thrombus, and, rarely, pulmonary infarction, pulmonary artery rupture, and death.[8]

Interpretation of the data obtained from a PAC is complicated. The absolute values of the measured variables are often difficult to decipher, and it is the trend in values that is most relevant.[8] Although patients with a PAC and other central indwelling catheters can participate in all positioning, airway clearance, and mobilization, it is critical that the physical therapist determines patient stability prior to initiating physical therapy interventions.[12,13] The physical therapist must continuously determine the hemodynamic, respiratory, and electrophysiological stability of the patient before, during, and after patient interactions.

Arterial Blood Pressure Monitoring

Invasive arterial blood pressure (BP) monitoring is accomplished by an indwelling catheter inserted into a peripheral artery and connected to a transducer and a pressurized flush device (Figure 3-2). The transducer is set at a reference point, usually the level of the atrium (phlebostatic axis: fourth intercostal space, mid axillary line in supine), and the transducer is zeroed to atmospheric pressure. BP is represented by the height of a column of blood that would rise above the reference point. The systolic BP can increase as much as 20 mm Hg from the proximal aorta to the radial or femoral arteries due to the reflection of the pressure waves back from the periphery (Figure 3-3). This increase in peak systolic pressure is offset by the narrowing of the systolic pressure wave, so that the **MAP** remains unchanged. Therefore, the MAP is a more accurate measure of central aortic pressure and reflects the tissue perfusion pressure.[4,9,12] MAP is the true driving pressure for peripheral blood flow. The electronic measurement of MAP is preferred to the estimated mean pressure, which is derived as the diastolic pressure plus one-third of the pulse pressure (MAP = diastolic BP + 1/3 pulse pressure). This formula is based on the assumption that diastole represents 2/3 of the cardiac cycle, which corresponds to a heart rate (HR) of 60 beats per minute (bpm). Therefore, HRs faster than 60 bpm, which are common in critically ill patients, lead to errors in the estimated MAP.[9]

Arterial BP monitoring using indwelling catheters is the gold standard for monitoring BP and is also used to sample arterial blood to monitor arterial blood gases (ABG). The ABG is monitored in some patients with pulmonary disorders and those patients who may also require mechanical ventilation. Common sites for insertion include the radial, femoral, and dorsalis pedis arteries. Weightbearing and repeated

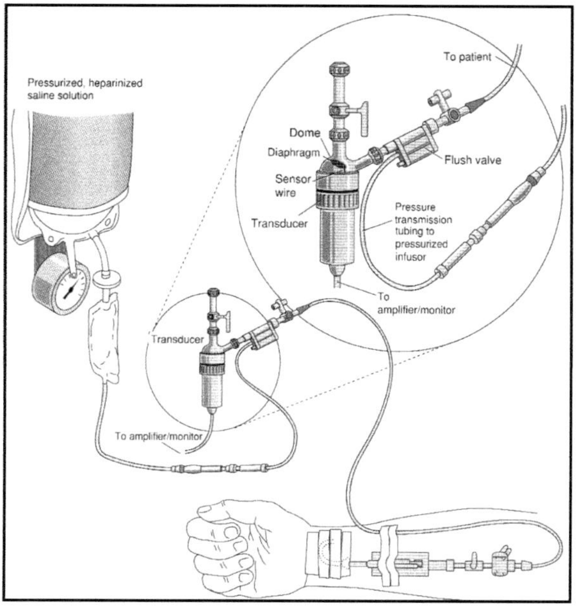

Figure 3-2. Arterial line showing catheter, transducer and pressure bag. (Reprinted with permission from Hillegass E, Sadowsky S. *Essentials of Cardiopulmonary Physical Therapy*. 2nd ed. Philadelphia, PA: WB Saunders; 2001.)

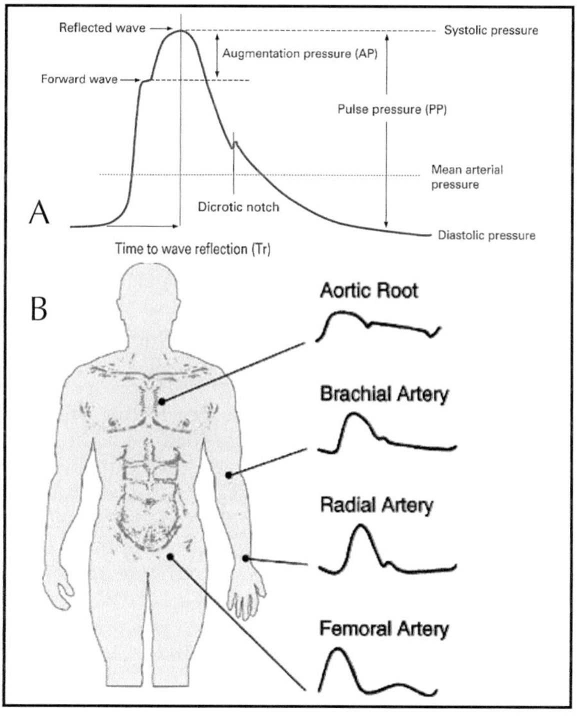

Figure 3-3. Arterial waveforms. Note the systolic pressure, diastolic pressure, mean arterial pressure, pulse pressure, and the dicrotic notch in the upper panel. The pulse pressure is systolic pressure – diastolic pressure. The lower panel highlights the changes in the arterial waveforms throughout the body. (B reprinted with permission from Marino PL. *The ICU Book*. 2nd ed. Baltimore, MD: Lippincott, Williams & Wilkins; 1998.)

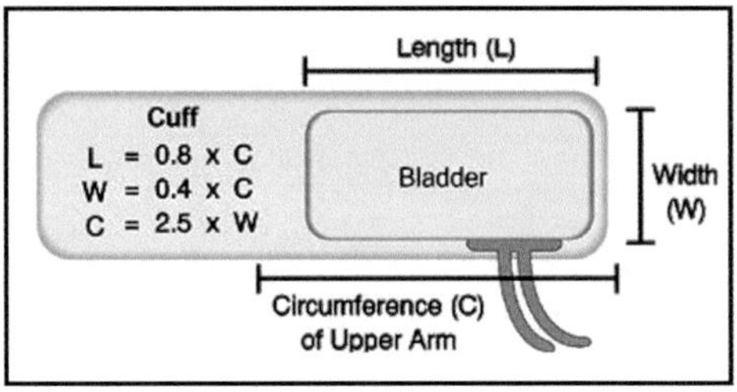

Figure 3-4. BP cuff dimensions for accurate measurements. (Reprinted with permission from Marino PL. *The ICU Book*. Baltimore, MD: Lippincott Williams & Wilkins; 1998.)

joint movement near the sites of insertion should be limited to prevent vascular damage or accidental line removal. The physical therapist should note the position of the transducer and the arterial pressure waveform to determine the accuracy of the numerical readings prior to initiating a therapy session.[11,13] The arterial pressure waveform consists of 3 distinct components as shown in Figure 3-3:

1. Peak systolic pressure
2. The dicrotic notch indicating closure of the aortic valve due to retrograde blood flow
3. The diastolic pressure point

Similar to the PAC and other central indwelling catheters, patients with invasive arterial BP monitoring can participate in all aspects of physical therapy, including positioning, airway clearance, and mobilization, providing that the patient is hemodynamically stable and the arterial line is secure.[12,13] The physical therapist should always monitor the waveform to determine if any interventions result in damping of the arterial waveform. If the catheter becomes dislodged, immediately apply direct pressure and call for assistance. While mobilizing the patient, the transducer must be aligned with the heart (ie, phlebostatic axis) to maintain an accurate reading. If the transducer height is below the heart, the displayed BP will be falsely high, while a higher transducer height will result in a falsely low BP reading.

The more common approach to BP measurement uses a sphygmomanometer and stethoscope. Cuff size is important, as noted in Figure 3-4. An oversized cuff will provide a falsely low reading and an undersized cuff will result in a falsely high reading (see Table 6-8).[14,15] Brachial artery pressure can be accurately performed in an obese patient using the forearm provided that the forearm is cylindrical and not conical in shape, and an appropriately sized cuff allows even distribution of pressure.[14] BP should be taken in both arms because the systolic pressure tends to be somewhat higher(as much as 15 mm Hg in adults) in the right upper extremity.[14] Lower extremity BP tends to be higher than upper extremity measurements due to the reflection of the pressure wave and the influence of gravity. Finally, it is worth repeating that accuracy is critical. Accuracy includes not just an appropriately sized cuff but also the positioning (ie, sitting with back supported, legs uncrossed) and relaxed state of the of the patient (eg, sitting quietly for 5 minutes, arm fully relaxed, bared with no constrictive clothing, and fully supported) and the positioning of the arm (ie, heart level). Documentation should reflect the procedures performed and note any deviations. As already mentioned, an inappropriately sized cuff can impact the BP reading. Other common variations include:

- If the upper arm is below the level of the heart, the readings will be higher; if the upper arm is above heart level, the readings will be lower.
- If the arm is unsupported, the pressure will be higher.
- Talking during the procedure can cause errors in the measurement.
- Supine measurements are often higher than sitting.

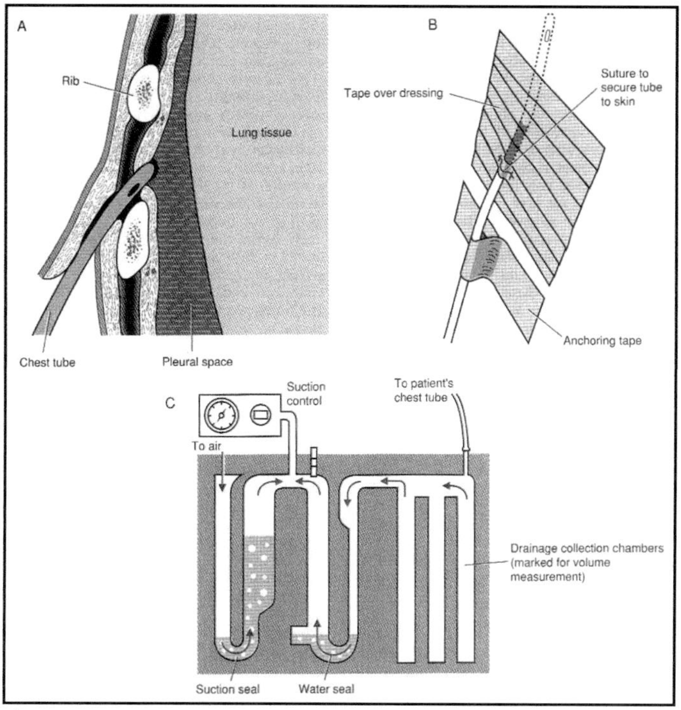

Figure 3-5. Chest tube/intrapleural drainage tube. (Reprinted with permission from Hillegass E, Sadowsky S. *Essentials of Cardiopulmonary Physical Therapy.* 2nd ed. Philadelphia, PA: WB Saunders; 2001.)

- Standing measurements tend to be the lowest.
- Recognize subject factors, such as pain or anxiety, can impact the reading.

Chest Drains

Injury, disease, or surgical procedures that result in the accumulation of air or fluid in the pleural cavity will result in loss of lung volume due to compression. The accumulation of fluid within the mediastinum or pericardium can compress the heart, resulting in reduced ventricular filling and reduced cardiac output; this is termed **cardiac tamponade**. A chest drain is a large catheter placed within the pleural space, mediastinum, or pericardium to evacuate fluid or air (Figure 3-5). Mediastinal/pericardial tubes are often placed after open-heart surgery. Common indications requiring intrapleural drainage include pneumothorax, hemothorax, pleural effusion, and empyema.[16,17] Chest drainage systems consist of 3 chambers:

1. Collection chamber
2. Water seal chamber
3. Suction chamber

The collection chamber allows measurement and analysis of the evacuated fluid. The water seal chamber acts as a one-way valve, allowing escape of fluid and air from the body while preventing retrograde flow into the pleural or mediastinal space. The suction chamber allows the application of negative pressure (ie, vacuum) through the drainage system, promoting removal of fluid and air. Goals of drainage systems include the removal of intrapleural and mediastinal collections and lung re-expansion.[17-19]

Drain insertion sites can vary but the thoracic cavity is usually accessed through the fourth or fifth intercostal space in the mid or anterior axillary line with the site of entry posterior to the lateral border of the pectoralis major muscle. If the intention is to remove air from a pneumothorax, the drain is directed to the apex of the lung. If the goal is to drain a fluid collection, the drain is directed toward the base or dependent portion of the lung. Drainage of loculated fluid collections are often performed using radiologic or ultrasound guidance.[17]

The patient's pain level and vital signs should be monitored with special emphasis on respiratory status (eg, respiratory rate [RR], breathing pattern, breath sounds, oxygen saturation [see Table 7-13]). The therapist should note any bubbling within the water seal chamber indicating an air leak. Bubbling is typically more pronounced during expiration and coughing. If bubbling is noted continuously, either the patient has a significant air leak from the lung or there is a leak in the drainage system. If this is a new occurrence, the medical/surgical team should be notified. **Swinging** refers to the usual 5- to 10-cm fluctuation in the underwater seal chamber associated with the respiratory cycle (ie, inspiration/expiration). If swinging is not observed, reposition the patient and check to determine that the drainage tube is not blocked or kinked. Patients are allowed to participate fully in therapeutic interventions as long as the drainage system is maintained lower than the insertion site and the prescribed level of suction is maintained. The patient should be encouraged to perform frequent position changes and deep breathing exercises to facilitate drainage. If the drainage tube becomes disconnected or falls out, an occlusive dressing should be placed at the insertion site or the remaining tube should be clamped to prevent air entry into the pleural space. If the collection chamber falls over, immediately return the chambers to upright to reestablish the underwater seal and alert the medical/surgical team.[12,13,16]

Pulse Oximetry

Pulse oximetry provides a noninvasive, continuous assessment of pulse rate and oxyhemoglobin saturation, a key determinant of oxygen delivery to systemic tissues (Figure 3-6).[17] The principles of pulse oximetry are based on the different light-absorbing characteristics of oxyhemoglobin and deoxyhemoglobin and the pulsatile nature of arterial blood flow.[20] The pulse oximeter consists of a probe that emits 2 wavelengths of light and a photodetector that measures the differences between light absorbances during and between arterial pulsations (ie, systole and diastole), providing an estimate of arterial oxygen saturation of available hemoglobin (% SpO_2).[17,20] Confirming the accuracy of the reading is important, especially with values below 90%.[17] Common sources of error include poor peripheral perfusion (ie, low cardiac output or vasoconstriction), anemia, skin pigmentation and nail polish, presence of carboxyhemoglobin (smokers), methemoglobin, and motion artifact. Accuracy of readings is enhanced if the therapist pays careful attention to signal strength and pulse rate.

The interpretation of pulse oximetry readings is based off knowledge of the oxyhemoglobin dissociation curve (see Figure 3-6). The flat portion of the curve illustrates the loading of oxygen onto hemoglobin. This portion of the curve shows that with large increases in the amount of oxygen dissolved in the arterial blood, the PaO_2, there is little change in %SpO_2; however, the steep portion of the curve illustrates the unloading of oxygen. This portion of the curve demonstrates that large changes in %SpO_2 are associated with small but critical changes in PaO_2. SpO_2 values <90%, indicate that the patient is becoming increasingly hypoxemic and

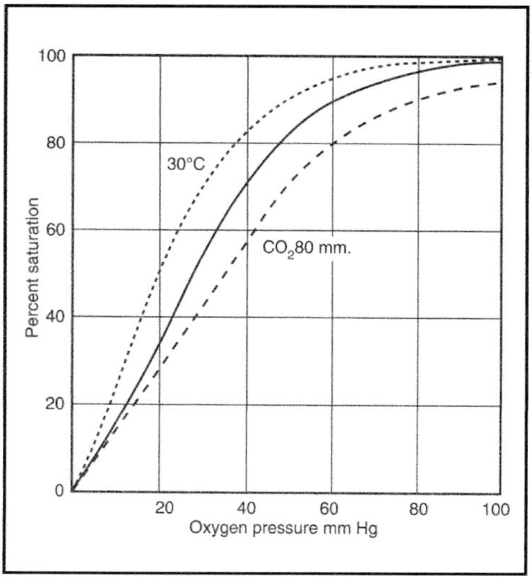

Figure 3-6. Oxyhemoglobin dissociation curve. (Reprinted with permission from Sheldon LK. *Oxygenation*. Sudbury, MA: Jones and Bartlett; 2001.)

tissue damage may result. **Hypoxemia** is defined as abnormally low concentration of oxygen in the blood, a low PaO_2. Supplemental oxygen is often provided to boost the PaO_2 to increase SpO_2 and correct the hypoxemia. The therapist must also consider the factors that shift the oxyhemoglobin dissociation curve. A rightward shift occurs with increased $PaCO_2$, acidosis, temperature, and increased 2,3-diphosphoglycerate (2,3-DPG is created by glycolysis in red blood cells). A rightward shift signifies a reduced affinity of hemoglobin for oxygen and results in reduced $\%SpO_2$ for a given PaO_2. This may result in inadequate oxygen delivery to peripheral tissues because the majority of oxygen is carried by red blood cells. A leftward shift results from decreased pH, temperature or 2.3 DPG. A leftward shift signifies an increase in the binding of hemoglobin for oxygen and reduced unloading of oxygen at low PaO_2 values. This may limit oxygen delivery to the peripheral tissues due to decreased unloading of oxygen.

Oxygen Delivery Devices

Oxygen is a medication that is prescribed in specific dosages and delivery modes. Oxygen is administered to raise the PaO_2 and reverse hypoxemia.[4] Once hemoglobin is saturated with oxygen, additional oxygen administration will not raise the oxygen content of the blood (ie, flat portion of the oxyhemoglobin dissociation curve) and may result in toxicity. The physical therapist requires a physician prescription to modify either the mode or dose of oxygen provided to the patient. Common delivery devices include low- and high-flow devices as listed in Table 3-2 and Figures 3-7 and 3-8. **Low flow** refers to a delivery system that does not meet the inspiratory flow demands of the patient resulting in the entrainment of ambient (room) air. The fraction of inspired oxygen (F_IO_2) is the percentage of oxygen being administered to the patient. Room air is a F_IO_2 of 0.21 or 21% oxygen. As the patient receives oxygen-enriched air, this means the patient is provided a higher-than-atmospheric F_IO_2. The actual F_IO_2 delivered to the patient depends on the patient's respiratory drive and breathing pattern.[4] **Nasal prongs** or **nasal cannula** are inserted into the patient's nose and oxygen is delivered from 0.5 to 6 lpm. Typically flow rates >6 lpm do not further increase tracheal F_IO_2. High-flow systems minimize the variability

Table 3-2
Oxygen Delivery Devices

Low-Flow Devices		*High-Flow Devices*	
Dose	**F_IO_2**	**Dose**	**F_IO_2**
Nasal Cannula		*Venturi Mask*	
1 L/minute	0.24	4 L/minute	0.24 to 0.28
2 L/minute	0.28	6 to 8 L/minute	0.32 to 0.36
3 L/minute	0.32	10 to 12 L/minute	0.40 to 0.50
4 L/minute	0.36	*Non-Rebreather Face Mask*	
5 L/minute	0.40	10 to 15 L/minute	1.0
6 L/minute	0.44		

Adapted from Hillegass EA. *Essentials of Cardiopulmonary Physical Therapy.* 3rd ed. St. Louis, MO. Elsevier: WB Saunders Co; 2011 and Sheldon LK. *Nursing Concepts: Oxygenation.* Thorofare, NJ: SLACK Incorporated; 2001.

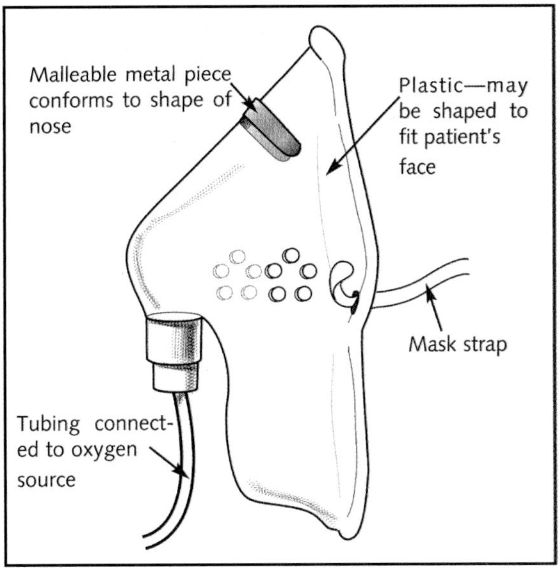

Figure 3-7. Example of oxygen delivery devices: simple face mask. Oxygen flow rates are 5 to 8 L/minute providing an oxygen concentration between 40% and 60%. The F_IO_2 will be diluted by room air and expired air and will vary depending on the fit of the mask and the patient's RR and breathing pattern. (Reprinted with permission from Sheldon LK. *Oxygenation.* Sudbury, MA: Jones and Bartlett; 2001.)

in F_IO_2 and usually consist of **face masks** that deliver oxygen at any F_IO_2 up to 1.00. The exact F_IO_2 provided to the patient will depend upon the fit of the mask, oxygen flow rate, and the patient's breathing pattern.[21] **Non-rebreather masks** have one-way valves that prevent the rebreathing of exhaled gas and the inspiration of ambient air. **Venturi masks** rely on air entrainment around a jet of oxygen to deliver a precise F_IO_2. The oxygen flow rate and the jet orifice opening determine the precise F_IO_2.[4,21] A **transtracheal catheter** provides oxygen directly into the trachea and requires a small incision (mini-trach) for the catheter. This device provides higher oxygen flows and must be cleaned daily to prevent mucus plugging of the catheter tip.[21]

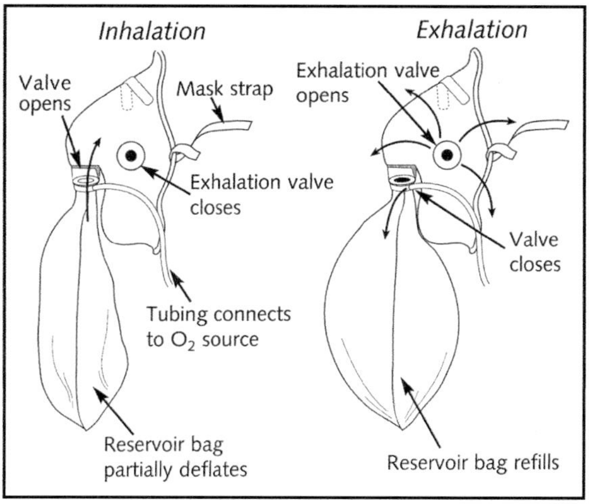

Figure 3-8. Example of oxygen delivery devices: non-rebreather face mask. Note oxygen flowing into a reservoir bag and one-way valves limiting the rebreathing of expired air. This type of face mask will deliver the highest oxygen concentration. (Reprinted with permission from Sheldon LK. *Oxygenation*. Sudbury, MA: Jones and Bartlett; 2001:125.)

Oxygen therapy is well-tolerated with few complications. Potential complications include mucosal membrane dryness, oxygen toxicity (especially in children), and elevations in $PaCO_2$. Patients with severe lung disease may demonstrate an increase in the $PaCO_2$ due to changes in the ventilation/perfusion (V/Q) relationship and the decreased ability of hemoglobin to carry carbon dioxide if hyperoxia is present (PaO_2>100 mm Hg); this is called the **Haldane Effect**. Ventilation/perfusion mismatch may result from correction of hypoxemia, which reduces hypoxic pulmonary vasoconstriction. This can increase the perfusion to poorly ventilated alveoli resulting in worsening gas exchange (decreased PaO_2; increased $PaCO_2$). Complications are avoided by providing humidification and administering oxygen at the lowest flow rate, or F_IO_2, that provides an acceptable arterial oxygen level.[16,21] The exact target for pulse oximetry readings is currently undetermined and titrating oxygen to keep the $SpO_2 \geq 88\%$ seems reasonable, while normalization of the PaO_2 (80 to 100 mm Hg) or pulse oximetry readings ($SpO_2 > 95\%$) does not appear to add extra benefit.[22,23] Therapists should consider these values in relationship to sleep, resting posture, and with ambulation and activities of daily living. If abnormal readings are noted, the therapist should discuss this with the medical team, and provide recommendations regarding the oxygen prescription based off the pulse oximeter, patient's vital sign responses, and subjective symptoms, such as dyspnea. An algorithm to guide clinical decision making and communication with the medical team is presented in Figure 3-9. Criteria for the prescription of home supplemental oxygen include $PaO_2 \leq 55$ mm Hg or $SpO_2 \leq 88\%$ and/or in the presence of cor pulmonale, a PaO_2 55 to 59 mm Hg or $SpO_2 \leq 89\%$.

Mechanical Ventilation

Mechanical ventilation is a cornerstone of intensive respiratory medicine and is lifesaving in acute respiratory failure, severe hypoxemia, and worsening respiratory acidosis.[16,20,21] Mechanical ventilation is provided either noninvasively or invasively. Invasive mechanical ventilation requires an artificial airway, such as an endotracheal tube (ETT) or tracheostomy tube. Noninvasive ventilation is applied through a variety of interfaces, such as a mouth piece or mask covering the nose or face. Mechanical ventilation decreases the work of breathing and improves alveolar gas exchange. Although there are multiple indications and modes of mechanical ventilation, there

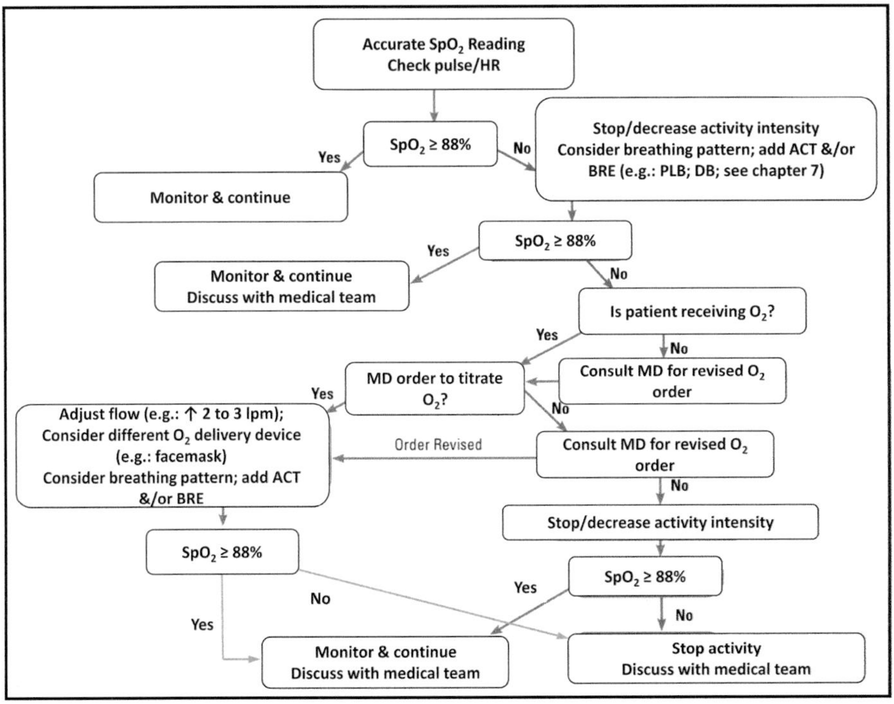

Figure 3-9. Algorithm to guide decision making regarding monitoring, application of supplemental oxygen and communication with the medical team. (ACT = airway clearance techniques; BRE = breathing retraining exercises; DB = diaphragm breathing; PLB = pursed-lip breathing.) (Adapted from Hillegass E, Fick A, Pawlik A, et al. Supplemental oxygen utilization during physical therapy interventions. *Cardiopulm Phys Ther J*. 2014;2[25]:38-49.)

Table 3-3
Mechanical Ventilation

Indications	*Goals (Measure)*
• Inadequate alveolar ventilation • Inadequate lung expansion • Inadequate respiratory muscle strength • Excessive work of breathing • Insufficient or unstable respiratory drive • Severe hypoxemia	• Improve alveolar ventilation and gas exchange • Decrease elevated $PaCO_2$, thereby increasing pH • Improve oxygenation by increasing PaO_2 and SpO_2 • Decrease work of breathing

Adapted from Albert RK, Spiro SG, Jett JR. *Comprehensive Respiratory Medicine*. Philadelphia, PA: Mosby; 1999.

are common objectives as listed in Table 3-3. Mechanical ventilation has historically been accomplished by the application of negative pressure to the thorax (eg, iron lung) or through the application of positive pressure to the airways and lungs. Currently, mechanical ventilation is almost always applied through positive pressure ventilators and there are 2 primary types: volume ventilators and pressure ventilators.

Volume ventilators provide a stable minute ventilation (mVE) with known tidal volumes (V_T) and RRs (mVE = RR x V_T). However, the tidal volume is delivered at the expense of peak airway pressure. Pressure ventilators prevent sudden changes in inspiratory pressures as lung and chest wall compliance change; however, tidal volume may be variable. For example, if compliance falls due to increased stiffness of the lung, the patient will quickly reach the predetermined peak airway pressure and the mechanical ventilation will stop the inspiration, resulting in an inadequate tidal volume. Mechanical ventilators provide 3 basic modes of ventilation:

1. A/C mode
2. Pressure support/pressure control mode
3. Synchronized intermittent mandatory ventilation (SIMV) mode

Current mechanical ventilator technology allows these modes to be used in isolation or hybrid modes that combine features of volume- and pressure-targeted ventilation.[4,17,21] A description of the common and alternative modes of positive pressure ventilation are provided in Table 3-4. The mechanical ventilation modes include additional settings that can be controlled, such as the trigger, limit, and cycle variables. The trigger variable determines what initiates inspiration—a preset pressure (pressure triggering), a preset volume, a designated flow, or an elapsed time. The limit variable is the pressure, volume, or flow that cannot be exceeded during inspiration. The cycle variable refers to the factor (ie, pressure, volume, flow, time) that terminates the inspiration. The physician and respiratory therapist will determine the appropriate setting for the mechanical ventilation.

To date, there is no firm evidence that the alternative modes of mechanical ventilation have improved adult patient outcomes.[24] However, the therapist may encounter these modes depending on the physician's and respiratory therapist's experience, preference, and patient presentation. The dangers of ventilator-induced lung and diaphragm injury have led to many changes in the prescription and monitoring of ventilator settings. Patients are often placed on lung protective ventilation strategies consisting of low tidal volume ventilation to avoid high inflation pressures and alveolar distension.[25] As a result of this protocol, patients may present with acceptable abnormal blood gasses, including permissive hypercapnia (reduced pH, elevated $PaCO_2$) or mild hypoxemia.[25,26]

Positive end expiratory pressure (PEEP) is a mechanical means of increasing the end-expiratory volume of the lungs, the **functional residual capacity**. Pressure is deliberately raised above atmospheric pressure and all inspiratory and expiratory breaths begin and end at this elevated pressure. PEEP improves oxygenation by keeping alveoli open and reinflates collapsed alveoli (atelectasis). The result is an increased lung volume that better matches ventilation and perfusion (V/Q ratio), reduces right to left (intrapulmonary) shunt, and ultimately improves oxygenation.[4,17,21,24] PEEP increases lung volume and pressures and this may lead to pulmonary vascular compression. Pulmonary vascular compression can diminish venous return and increase pulmonary vascular resistance. The result is decreased cardiac output and possible reduced oxygen delivery to the peripheral tissues.[9,17] **Continuous positive airway pressure** (CPAP) is analogous to PEEP during spontaneous breathing. Inspiration and expiration are pressurized to a preset level throughout the respiratory cycle. **Bilevel positive airway pressure** (BiPAP) is similar to CPAP in that the patient is breathing spontaneously but the machine delivers a preset inspiratory positive airway pressure and a reduced expiratory positive airway pressure. BiPAP is commonly prescribed for patients with chronic obstructive pulmonary disease who retain CO_2. As CPAP and BiPAP require spontaneous breaths, the patient must have an intact respiratory drive and adequate tidal volume. CPAP and BiPAP can be provided invasively but may also be provided noninvasively (eg, a patient with obstructive sleep apnea).

Table 3-4

MODES OF MECHANICAL VENTILATION

Conventional Modes of Mechanical Ventilation

Mode	Description
Controlled mechanical ventilation	• All mechanical ventilation breaths are delivered at a fixed RR and tidal volume ensuring a preset mVE. • Variables cannot be changed by patient.
Assist/control (A/C)	• Combination mode of mechanical ventilation • Assist: Mechanical ventilation delivers fixed tidal volume in response to patient's efforts (ie, assist mode); patient determines the RR but mechanical ventilation determines tidal volume. • Control: If patient fails to initiate breath within specific time period (ie, patient fails to trigger), mechanical ventilation automatically delivers fixed tidal volume.
SIMV	• Combination mode of mechanical ventilation • Mechanical ventilation delivers a fixed number of assisted breaths guaranteeing a preset tidal volume. Mechanical ventilation delivered breaths are synchronized with the patient's effort (ie, assist mode). • Patient can breathe spontaneously between assisted mechanical ventilation breaths.
Pressure support ventilation	• Patient breathes spontaneously and determines RR and inspiratory time; during each patient breath, the mechanical ventilation delivers a preset inspiratory pressure. • Tidal volume is determined by inspiration pressure and patient's lung and chest wall compliance; the mVE may vary. • Pressure support ventilation can be added to spontaneous breaths in SIMV. *(continued)*

Although mechanical ventilation is necessary lifesaving technology for patients with respiratory failure, it may cause lung and diaphragm damage. **Ventilator-induced lung injury** (VILI) results from the cyclic opening/closing (atelectotrauma) and overdistension of alveoli due to excessive pressure (barotrauma) or excessive tidal volumes (volutrauma). VILI results in pulmonary edema, alveolar hemorrhage, and surfactant dysfunction.[27] Mechanical ventilation may also lead to structural changes in the muscles of breathing, termed **ventilator-induced diaphragm dysfunction** (VIDD). Diaphragm atrophy and contractile dysfunction lead to weakness and poor endurance and is more often related to mechanical ventilation modes that are designed to have patients perform little or no work of breathing (eg, controlled mechanical ventilation, A/C).[28] The mechanical ventilation settings can be changed to minimize VILI (eg, small tidal volumes; higher PEEP) and prevent VIDD by allowing the patient to assume a greater proportion of the work of breathing.

Table 3-4 (continued) **MODES OF MECHANICAL VENTILATION**	
Alternative Modes of Mechanical Ventilation	
Mode	**Description**
Pressure-controlled ventilation	• Mechanical ventilation is set to provide a fixed inflation pressure, inspiratory time, and RR. • Tidal volume and mVE are determined by patient's lung and chest wall compliance.
High-frequency oscillatory ventilation and high-frequency jet ventilation	• Mechanical ventilation is set to deliver high breathing frequencies (typically 3 to 15 Hz; 180 to 900 breaths/minute) coupled with very small tidal volume. • High-frequency oscillatory ventilation: Inspiration and expiration are actively performed by mechanical ventilation. • High-frequency jet ventilation: Combined with conventional mechanical ventilation;, inspiration is active, expiration is passive. • More common in neonatal and pediatric patients.
Airway pressure release ventilation; also called bilevel (different than BiPAP)	• Combination mode where the mechanical ventilation provides CPAP (pressure control) for a set time interval and then releases the applied pressure. The pressure is applied with an inverse ratio (prolonged inspiratory time; shorter expiratory time). • Mechanical ventilation can provide mandatory breaths interspersed with the patient's spontaneous breathing.
Pressure-regulated volume control	• Similar to A/C where breaths are mechanical ventilation initiated (control) and patient initiated (assist) where inspiratory pressures are controlled to provide a preset tidal volume. • Mechanical ventilation adjusts inspiratory pressure breath-to-breath to deliver predetermined tidal volume
Proportional assist ventilation	• Mechanical ventilation performs a predetermined percentage of the total work of breathing. • Inspiratory pressure and air flow are augmented by the mechanical ventilation in proportion to the patient's effort.
Adaptive support ventilation	• Mechanical ventilation automatically adjusts the RR and tidal volume to achieve a predetermined mVE. • Mechanical ventilation alters the inspiratory pressure and inspiratory time or airflow according to the patient's respiratory mechanics.
Neurally adjusted ventilatory assist	• Mechanical ventilation uses electromyogram (EMG) sensors to determine diaphragm activity. • EMG activity triggers the mechanical ventilation to deliver assistance in proportion to and in synchrony with the patient's respiratory efforts.
Adapted from Lanken P. *The Intensive Care Unit Manual.* 2nd ed. Philadelphia, PA: Elsevier Saunders; 2014.	

Table 3-5

SIGNS AND SYMPTOMS OF WEANING INTOLERANCE

• Increased RR (>35 bpm) • Decreased tidal volumes • Change in HR, heart rhythm, or BP • Altered level of consciousness • Altered breathing pattern: ¤ Rapid, shallow pattern ¤ Paradoxical pattern (abdominal paradox)	• ABG analysis: ¤ Hypercarbia/hypoxemia (respiratory acidosis) • Decreasing pulse oximetry • Patient complaint of shortness of breath (eg, SOB, dyspnea)

Weaning From Mechanical Ventilation

Weaning is an individualized process involving a change in the interaction between the patient and the ventilator. Throughout the weaning process, the level of support provided by the ventilator is decreased requiring the patient to assume a greater proportion of the workload.[4,26] Weaning may be accomplished in multiple ways: a step wise reduction of the mechanical ventilation settings (eg, reduction in the preset inspiratory pressure [pressure support wean]); decrease in the number of machine-assisted breaths [SIMV wean]); increasing the time spent with less mechanical ventilation support; or the patient may proceed to a spontaneous breathing trial where he or she is provided minimal pressure support and PEEP, CPAP alone, or use of a T-piece. The physical therapist needs to consider the physiologic demands associated with a weaning trial and needs to estimate the patient's pulmonary reserve. Providing physical therapy during a weaning trial is acceptable but routine daily ICU activities including bathing, range of motion, and chest physical therapy can significantly increase the metabolic rate. Daily ICU activities can increase HR, BP, and oxygen consumption by 20% to 35% greater than resting.[29,30] In addition, the patient with advanced lung disease may be utilizing upwards of 25% of his or her oxygen consumption simply to breathe due to increases in the work of breathing. The therapist should be familiar with the signs of weaning intolerance (Table 3-5). Therapists should coordinate with the medical team to determine appropriate times to provide physical therapy services. Coordination of medications, airway clearance, mobilization activities, and weaning helps to ensure a positive outcome. Successful therapy sessions during weaning trials may provide feedback that the patient can be weaned more aggressively, while evidence of limited pulmonary reserve during therapy may lead to a slower, more deliberate weaning schedule. For patients who are undergoing a prolonged wean, it may be beneficial to schedule therapy during the rest period or recommend placing the patient on the rest settings during therapy with a return to the weaning setting post-therapy. Finally, therapists must also be familiar with common alarms that may sound on the mechanical ventilator as noted in Table 3-6. The therapist should not silence these alarms unless a rationale is determined for the alarm trigger.

Table 3-6 COMMON ALARMS AND MECHANICAL VENTILATION
Ventilator Alarms
High/low pressure: Indicates the need for elevated/decreased pressure to deliver the desired volume of air. • High pressure: Mucus plug/bronchospasm • Low pressure: Disconnection/tube leak High/low RR: Patient's RR has exceeded/declined below a preset limit. • High RR: Pain, discomfort, agitation, exercise, fatigue • Low RR: Fatigue, sedation

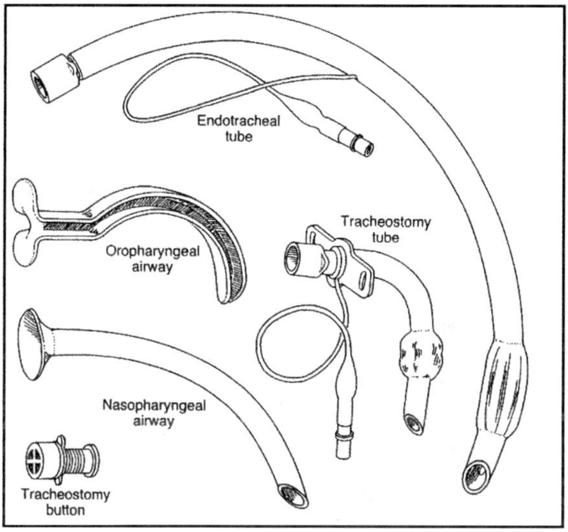

Figure 3-10. Common airways. (Reprinted with permission from Luce JM, Pierson DJ, Tyler ML. *Intensive Respiratory Care*. 2nd ed. Philadelphia, PA: WB Saunders; 1993:16.)

ARTIFICIAL AIRWAYS

Artificial airways are indicated whenever airway protection is compromised or the gas-exchanging function of the lungs is abnormal.[17,21] Airways can be divided into those that occupy the nose or mouth, cross the larynx, are placed directly into the trachea (Figure 3-10). The common advantages and disadvantages of artificial airways are listed in Table 3-7.

An **oropharyngeal airway** prevents obstruction of the upper airway by moving the tongue anteriorly. These airways limit biting and compression of the tongue and ETT and are most common in the unconscious patient. The **nasopharyngeal airway** provides a direct connection between the nose and the upper airway and is often used for nasotracheal suctioning. Patients may require nasotracheal suctioning if they present with retained secretions, a poor cough, and do not have an ETT. An **ETT** or a **tracheostomy tube** provides a sealed, closed system for mechanical ventilation. These airways have an internal balloon that surrounds the outer cannula or distal ETT. When inflated, the internal balloon fills the trachea promoting the one-way flow of delivered air into the lungs. The ETT and tracheostomy tube may also be

Table 3-7

ARTIFICIAL AIRWAYS

Advantages	*Disadvantages*
• Provide a sealed, closed system for mechanical ventilation • Prevent/relieve upper airway obstruction • Facilitate tracheal suctioning/ airway clearance	• Decreased cough effectiveness • Reduced ciliary motion • Interference with communication and nutrition • Bypasses respiratory defense mechanisms • Increased risk of infection • Loss of dignity • Tracheal stenosis

used to relieve upper airway obstruction and facilitate tracheal suctioning.[21] The ETT is a shorter duration airway as compared to the tracheostomy tube. Tracheostomy tubes are usually inserted between the second or third cartilaginous ring, inferior to the vocal cords, and fixated initially with a stitch and later by knotted string ties or Velcro strapping around the neck. The typical tracheostomy tube consists of an outer cannula that is stabilized at the neck and a removable inner cannula that can be cleaned and replaced.[13] Both ETT and tracheostomy tubes terminate above the carina to allow airflow to both lungs. Tracheostomy tubes allow patient communication by mouthing words and patients may be fed orally if appropriate. A **fenestrated tracheostomy** tube has an opening in the superior aspect of the outer cannula that allows airflow to enter the upper airway when the inner cannula of the tracheostomy tube is removed. **Tracheostomy buttons** extend from the anterior surface of the trachea to the skin. These airways maintain an open stoma and allow direct tracheal suctioning.

Speaking valves or caps may be placed over the tracheostomy tube or tracheostomy button to promote use of the upper airway, assess the patient's ability to clear secretions, and allow for speaking (phonation). The balloon must be deflated with tracheostomy tubes and the patient must be able to adequately clear his or her own airway or asphyxiation may occur.

Patients with artificial airways can participate in all aspects of physical therapy and may require airway clearance. The insertion of an artificial airway results in loss of the normal upper airway functions of humidification, warming, and filtration of inspired air. As a result, these patients are at risk for impaired mucociliary transport, retained secretions, and an increased risk of infections and pneumonia. The physical therapist must determine the stability of the airway. Breath sounds should be assessed to determine the degree of aeration and presence of adventitious sounds. ETT are usually marked in standard increments along the length of the tube allowing the therapist to check the relative position before, during, and after the therapy session. ETT should be monitored by checking the position of the tube in relationship to the lip, teeth, or gum line. Excessive movements of all airways, but especially ETT and tracheostomy tubes, should be avoided due to tracheal irritation, accidental extubation, or accidental intubation of a single mainstem bronchi with an ETT. Patients may produce grunting noises due to air leaking around the balloon. Air leaks are common during mobilization and are typically a harmless nuisance. An air leak may be hazardous if a large volume of air escapes through the upper airway decreasing alveolar ventilation. The respiratory therapist should be notified to check the airway stability and balloon inflation pressure (usually <30 cm H_20).

Extubation, the removal of an airway, is considered when the patient demonstrates adequate ventilatory drive, respiratory muscle strength and gas exchange, a satisfactory breathing pattern, a patent airway with intact protective reflexes (eg, gag and cough reflexes), and is hemodynamically stable.[27] The therapist should note that a patient who has been extubated from mechanical ventilation is vulnerable and may require reintubation due to bronchospasm, laryngospasm, aspiration, inadequate airway patency, impaired ventilatory drive, or mucus plugging.[29] The physical therapist needs to examine the patient at rest and with activity by assessing vital signs to determine hemodynamic stability and determine the patient's pulmonary reserve by assessing RR, cough, breath sounds, breathing pattern, SOB/dyspnea on exertion and pulse oximetry (see Chapter 7).

Suctioning

The goals of suctioning are to clear the airway, normalize breath sounds and breathing pattern, reduce dyspnea, and improve oxygenation.[31] Suctioning can be an extremely unpleasant experience for the patient, and complications including bronchial epithelial damage, transient hypoxemia, bronchospasm, and vasovagal events (eg, bradycardia, hypotension) can occur.[32] Due to the risks and potential complications, suctioning should be applied judiciously. Noninvasive techniques, such as optimizing positioning, applying assisted coughing and chest wall exercises, splinting of incisions, and instruction in directed coughing or huffing, should be considered first.[12,32] The procedure for suction is outlined in Table 7-17.

Intra-Aortic Balloon Pump/ Intra-Aortic Balloon Counterpulsation

An intra-aortic balloon pump (IABP) is used for patients with cardiac pump dysfunction associated with myocardial infarction, unstable angina, cardiogenic shock, and after cardiac surgery. IABP increases coronary blood flow while also increasing cardiac output and improving peripheral perfusion.[4,33] The device consists of a balloon mounted on a catheter that is attached to a console (Figure 3-11). The catheter is frequently inserted into the femoral artery and advanced to the descending thoracic aorta. Alternate insertion sites may also be used, including the axillary-subclavian artery, that allow greater mobilization. The balloon inflates during diastole, which increases diastolic pressure promoting increased coronary artery perfusion. Balloon deflation occurs prior to systole, which reduces afterload pressures in the aorta, promoting enhanced cardiac output and reduced myocardial oxygen demand. If physical therapy services are indicated, the physical therapist must ensure hemodynamic stability, review HR and BP, and maintain patency of the insertion catheter at all times.

Extracorporeal Membranous Oxygenation and Extracorporeal Carbon Dioxide Removal

Extracorporeal membranous oxygenation (ECMO) and extracorporeal carbon dioxide removal are methods of replacing the gas exchange functions of the lung via a modified heart–lung bypass machine. Blood is removed from the venous system, and oxygen is added and carbon dioxide removed by a membrane oxygenator outside

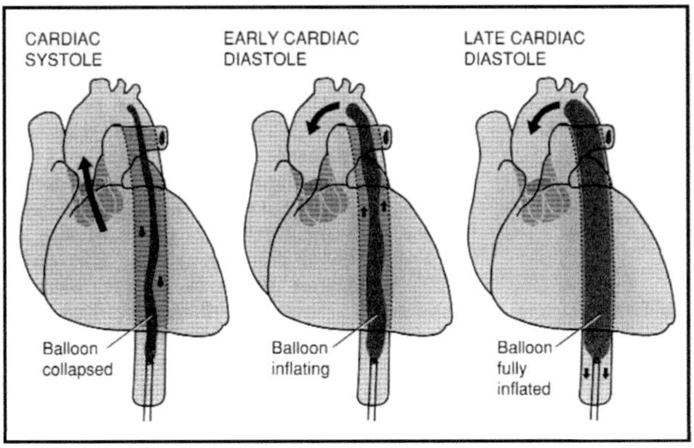

Figure 3-11. IABP. Note deflation of the balloon during cardiac systole (ejection) and inflation during cardiac diastole (filling). (Reprinted with permission from Hillegass E, Sadowsky S. *Essentials of Cardiopulmonary Physical Therapy*. 2nd ed. Philadelphia, PA: WB Saunders.)

the body and returned to the arterial or venous circulation.[10] These highly technical devices are reserved for critically ill patients and provide a means of limiting lung damage resulting from mechanical ventilation.[32] These devices may require the administration of paralytic agents and sedation if the patient's condition is life threatening; however, similar to IABP, ambulatory ECMO has been initiated as a bridge to transplant or recovery. The physical therapist must remember that patients are critically ill and avoid cannula dislodgement due to the risk of immediate hemorrhage. The cannula must be secured and visible while diligent continuous cardiopulmonary monitoring is performed before, during, and after therapy.[10] Hemodynamic stability must be assessed by determining HR and rhythm and BP. Respiratory stability is assessed by measuring the RR, observing the breathing pattern, assessing pulse oximetry, and measuring the patient's complaints of SOB and dyspnea on exertion. A team approach is recommended for mobilization. The physical therapist manages the patient, the perfusionist manages ECMO circuit and cannula, the nurse manages lines, and the physician is available in case of emergency. Pre-planning is necessary for successful mobilization.

Nutrition Support/Feeding Tubes

Nutrition support plays a vital role in the management of acutely ill patients. Delivery is accomplished through the parenteral route through central venous access, or the enteral route using the gastrointestinal (GI) tract. Enteral nutrition is preferred due to the ease of administration, decreased cost, decreased prevalence of infection, no need for central venous access, and improved GI function. **Total parenteral nutrition** is reserved for those patients who cannot use their GI tract due to dysmotility, ischemia, GI obstruction, or for those who demonstrate an intolerance to tube feedings and cannot meet their nutritional requirements.[4,34] Total parenteral nutrition is the delivery of food and nutrients intravenously, bypassing the GI tract, allowing the intestines to rest or heal, or if there are absorption deficiencies, it provides missing nutritional elements to the patient. The formula is customized for each patient and is based on basic nutritional elements as well as height, weight, and desired nutritional needs. The patient's clinical status will determine the specific contents (eg, carbohydrates, proteins, fats, electrolytes, vitamins, trace elements) of the formula. Special formulations include pulmonary formulas that are designed to be high in fat and low in carbohydrates to reduce carbon dioxide production. Hepatic formulas contain large amounts of branch chain amino acids to improve the nitrogen balance and limit encephalopathy. Renal formulas are usually calorically dense, low in protein, and contain variable amounts of branch chain amino acids.[35]

The **nasogastric tube** is a tube inserted through a nostril that terminates in the stomach. The nasogastric tube is usually short term. Complications may include gastroesophageal reflux and aspiration, rhinitis, pharyngitis, esophagitis and stricture, and upper GI bleeding. **Nasoduodenal** and **nasojejunal** feeding may reduce the risk for aspiration. **Percutaneous endoscopic gastrostomy** (PEG) and **percutaneous endoscopic jejunostomy** (PEJ) tubes are surgically inserted directly into the GI tract through the abdominal wall and are usually a longer-term solution for nutrition support. PEG and PEJ tubes eliminate nasal and esophageal irritation and reduce potential aspiration. Complications include skin breakdown and wound dehiscence associated with gastric content leak through the incision site and GI bleeding.[36-38]

Patients receiving nutrition support can participate in all aspects of physical therapy. Risk of aspiration should be minimized by maintaining the head in an upright position (bed >30 degrees to 45 degrees during feeding and for 1 hour after) and limiting Trendelenburg or other head-down positions. If appropriate, temporarily suspend nutrition support during the session; however, the therapist needs to first consider the feeding schedule (ie, bolus feeding [intermittent feeding most similar to eating a periodic meal] or continuous feeding) and if the patient has recently received insulin because of the hypoglycemia risk. The therapist must confirm that the feeding tube is properly secured to prevent leakage and accidental removal. Changes in bowel habits or other GI complaints may provide evidence of poor tolerance to the nutritional support, and this information should be passed on to the medical and nursing teams (see Tables 11-18 and 11-19).

Additional Drains and Catheters

Following surgery or trauma, patients may have devices that drain excess blood or fluids from the wound, either mechanically or manually. These drains can be categorized as either active or passive drains.

Active Drains

These drains typically use suction to create a vacuum that pulls excess fluid from the surgical site or anatomic region. Active drains are closed systems and are not gravity dependent. A chest drainage tube connected to suction would be an example of an active drain. Additional examples of active drains include:

- **Jackson-Pratt drains** and **Hemovac**: **Jackson-Pratt drains** are small, bulbous drains while a **Hemovac** is a collapsible chamber that resembles an accordion. The drains are surgically placed into the wound, and as they expand a small negative pressure (ie, vacuum) draws fluid into the receptacle.
- **Sump drains**: These larger drains are surgically placed into the wound and are then connected to a suction device to mechanically remove the contents from the wound. These drains are common in the management of fistulas and nonhealing open wounds.

Passive Drains

Passive drains are gravity dependent so patient positioning must be considered. A chest tube that is to underwater gravity seal (ie, not connected to suction) would be an example of a passive drain. Additional examples of passive drains include:

- **Penrose drains**: These drains consists of soft, pliable rubber tubing that is placed at the site of injury or surgery to prevent fluid accumulation. The tubing length is variable, but part of the tubing is typically externalized and exits the skin. Penrose drains are a type of passive drain and are gravity dependent.
- **Pigtail catheters**: This catheter consists of tubing with a coiled end that is connected to a collection bag. The coiled end holds the catheter in place. A pig tail catheter is typically used to drain bile, pancreatic, or pleural fluids.
- **T tube**: This T-shaped tube is typically used in bile duct surgery. The unique shape allows some bile to flow down the bile duct through the cross piece while excess fluid is removed into a drainage bag flowing through the tail piece that exits the abdomen.
- **Foley catheter**: This flexible balloon-tipped catheter is placed directly into the bladder through the urethra allowing direct elimination of urine providing skin protection and assessment of urine output to determine fluid balance.
- **Rectal catheter**: A large indwelling balloon catheter (similar to Foley catheter) that is connected to a drainage bag to collect liquid stool. The balloon provides a seal and directs stool into the collection bag while limiting leakage.
- **Rectal tube**: A short piece of flexible tubing that is inserted into the rectum.

The Foley catheter, rectal catheter, and rectal tube attempt to minimize caregiver's contact with body fluids and minimize exposure of the patient's skin in the perineal region from urine and liquid stool that can promote skin breakdown and infection.

Chapter Review Questions

1. Which of the following best describes how pulmonary artery wedge pressure is measured?
   a. Inflate balloon in the left atrium allowing a pressure measurement of cardiac output
   b. Inflate balloon in the pulmonary artery creating a dynamic column of fluid to measure cardiac index
   c. Inflate balloon in the pulmonary artery creating a static column of fluid to measure LVEDP
   d. Inflate balloon in the pulmonary vein thereby allowing a pressure measurement of LVEDP
2. The clinical findings that are associated a low S_VO_2 include:
   a. Cardiac output and end diastolic volume
   b. Oxygen consumption and ventricular filling
   c. Anemia and blood volume
   d. Oxygen delivery and amount consumed

3. The MAP represents:
   a. Central aortic pressure and tissue perfusion pressure
   b. Systemic vascular pressure and oxygen consumption
   c. Peripheral resistance and myocardial oxygen consumption
   d. Diastolic pressure plus half of pulse pressure
4. What is the most common complication with central venous and pulmonary artery monitoring?
   a. Infection and transient dysrhythmias
   b. Central line occlusion and pneumothorax
   c. Empyema and line-related sepsis
   d. Thrombocytopenia and deep vein thrombosis
5. The following are some common sources of error when interpreting oxygen saturation?
   a. Coronary artery disease and ectopy
   b. Anemia and nail polish
   c. Vasodilation and skin pigmentation
   d. Carboxyhemoglobin and elevated cardiac output

Answers: 1c, 2d, 3a, 4a, 5b

References

1. Stiller K. Physiotherapy in intensive care: towards an evidence-based practice. *Crit Care Review.* 2000;118:1801-1813.
2. Sciaky AJ. Mobilizing the intensive care unit patient: pathophysiology and treatment. *Phys Ther Pract.* 1994;3:69-80.
3. Swan HJ, Ganz W, Forrester J, et al. Catheterization of the heart in man with the use of a flow-directed balloon tipped catheter. *N Engl J Med.* 1970;283:447-551.
4. Lanken P. *The Intensive Care Unit Manual.* 2nd Edition. Philadelphia, PA: Elsevier Saunders; 2014.
5. Kelly CR, Rabbani LE. Pulmonary-artery catheterization. *N Engl J Med.* 2013;369(25):e35
6. Pinsky MR. Pulmonary artery occlusion pressure. *Intens Care Med.* 2003;29:19-22.
7. Dulak SB. A PA catheter refresher course. *RN.* 2003;66:28-35.
8. Manikon M, Grounds M, Rhodes A. The pulmonary artery catheter. *Clin Med.* 2002;2:101-104.
9. Marino PL. The ICU Book. Baltimore, MD. Lippincott Williams & Wilkins; 1998.
10. Nettina SM. *The Lippincott Manual of Nursing Practice.* Philadelphia, PA: Lippincott Williams & Wilkins; 2001.
11. Tibby SM, Murdoch IS. Monitoring cardiac function in intensive care. *Arch Dis Child.* 2003;88:46-62.
12. Hillegass E. *Essentials of Cardiopulmonary Physical Therapy.* 3rd Edition. Philadelphia, PA: Elsevier Saunders; 2011.

13. Ciesla ND, Murdock KR. Lines, tubes, catheters, and physiologic monitoring in the ICU. *Cardiopulmonary Phys Ther.* 2000;11:10-25.
14. Perloff JK. *Physical Examination of the Heart and Circulation.* Philadelphia, PA: WB Saunders; 2000.
15. Manning DM, Kuchira C, Kaminski J. Miscuffing: inappropriate blood pressure cuff application. *Circulation.* 1983;68(4):763-766.
16. Allibone L. Nursing management of chest drains. *Nursing Standard.* 2003;17:45-56.
17. Albert RK, Spiro SG, Jett JR. *Comprehensive Respiratory Medicine.* Philadelphia, PA: Mosby; 1999.
18. Baumann MH, Strange C, Heffner JE, et al. Management of spontaneous pneumothorax: an American College of Chest Physicians Delphi consensus statement. *Chest.* 2001;119:590-602.
19. Baumann MH, Strange C. Treatment of spontaneous pneumothorax: a more aggressive approach? *Chest.* 1997;112:789-804.
20. Mengelkock LJ, Martin D, Lawler J. A review of the principles of pulse oximetry and accuracy of pulse oximeter estimates during exercise. *Phys Ther.* 1994;74:40-49.
21. Luce JM, Pierson DJ, Tyler ML. *Intensive Respiratory Care.* 2nd ed. Philadelphia, PA: WB Saunders; 1993.
22. Ekström M. Clinical usefulness of long-term oxygen therapy in adults. *N Engl J Med.* 2016;375(17):1683-1684.
23. The Long-Term Oxygen Treatment Trial Research Group. A randomized trial of long-term oxygen for COPD with moderate desaturation. *N Engl J Med.* 2016;375:1617-1627.
24. Tobin MJ. Current concepts: mechanical ventilation. *N Engl J Med.* 1994;330:1056-1061.
25. Acute Respiratory Distress Network. Ventilation with lower tidal volumes as compared with traditional tidal volumes for acute lung injury and the acute respiratory distress syndrome. *N Engl J Med.* 2000;342:1301-1308.
26. Tobin MJ. Medical progress: advances in mechanical ventilation. *N Engl J Med.* 2001;344:1986-1996.
27. Slutsky AS, Ranieri MV. Ventilator-induced lung injury. *N Engl J Med.* 2013;369:2126-2136
28. Petrof BJ, Jaber S, Matecki S. Ventilator-induced diaphragmatic dysfunction. *Curr Opin Crit Care.* 2010;16(1):19-25.
29. Weissman C, Kemper M, Damask MC, et al. Effect of routine intensive care interactions on metabolic rate. *Chest.* 1984;86:815-818.
30. Verderber A, Gallagher KF. Effects of bathing, passive range of motion exercises, and turning on oxygen consumption in healthy men and women. *Am J Crit Care.* 1994;3:374-381.
31. Griggs A. Tracheostomy: suctioning and humidification. *Nurs Stand.* 1998;13:49-53, 55-56.
32. Bach JR. *Pulmonary Rehabilitation: The Obstructive and Paralytic Conditions.* Philadelphia, PA: Hanley E. Belfus; 1996.
33. Bavin TK, Self MA. Weaning from intra-aortic balloon pump support. *Am J Nurs.* 1991;10:54-59.
34. Smith HG, Orlando R. Enteral nutrition: should we feed the stomach? *Crit Care Med.* 1999;27:1652-1653.
35. Chan S, McGowen KC, Blackburn GL. Nutrition management in the ICU. *Chest.* 1999;115:145S-148S.

36. Barrera R, Schattner M, Nygard S, et al. Outcome of direct percutaneous endoscopic jejunostomy tube placement for nutritional support in critically ill, mechanically ventilated patients. *J Crit Care*. 2001;16:178-181.
37. Kennedy JF. Enteral feeding for the critically ill patient. *Nurs Stand*. 1997;11:39-43.
38. Marik PE, Zaloga GP. Early enteral nutrition in acutely ill patients: a systematic review. *Crit Care Med*. 2001;29:2264-2270.

Chapter 4

Bed Rest, Deconditioning, Hospital-Acquired Neuromuscular Disorders, and Evidenced-Based Early Mobilization

Daniel J. Malone, PT, PhD, CCS

"Teach us to live that we may dread unnecessary time in bed. Get people up and we may save our patients from an early grave."[1]

The profound impact of bed rest is well-documented, and confinement to bed is, unfortunately, a common treatment for patients with acute and chronic disease and injury. Functional status and maintenance of activity levels in hospitalized patients are often overshadowed by patient care requirements for comfort and pain management, fluid and electrolyte maintenance, medication administration, hemodynamic monitoring, nutrition, wound care, and emotional and psychological support.[2] Patients are often confined to bed due to the severity of their illness, simply feeling poor, multiple lines and tubes, medication side effects, depression and anxiety, or a lack of personnel to assist with mobility. Hospitalization is a major risk for older persons and is often followed by an irreversible decline in functional status and a change in quality of life.[3,4] The spectrum of immobilization ranges from a minimal reduction of usual activity levels to the extreme immobilization of spinal cord injury (SCI).[5] This chapter will use information derived from imposed and simulated bed rest, as well as research using microgravity, to draw many correlations of bed rest in hospitalized patients. This chapter will illustrate the sequelae of immobility and bed rest and provide evidence that many of these complications can be prevented and improved through the provision of physical therapy services.

Bed Rest and Deconditioning Overview

Deconditioning is defined as the loss of physiologic and performance adaptations, and occurs rapidly when a person terminates regular participation in activities of daily living (ADLs) and exercise.

Malone DJ, Bishop KL, eds. *Acute Care Physical Therapy: A Clinician's Guide, Second Edition* (pp 119-147).

Only 1 week of bed rest or inactivity can significantly reduce exercise capacity.[6] It should be remembered that almost all hospitalized patients have a reduction in usual activity. Even a patient who gets up and walks 5 times/day is still not performing his or her usual routine and is subject to deconditioning. The older adult is especially vulnerable. It is well known that hospitalization, even as short as 2 days, contributes to the functional decline and the inability to perform basic ADLs and often leads to nursing home placement.[7,8] The causes of functional decline are multifactorial and include a variety of physiological adaptations, including changes in cardiovascular, pulmonary, hematologic, musculoskeletal, metabolic, thermoregulatory, immune, neuroendocrine, and psychological functions as noted in Table 4-1.[9-13]

Cardiovascular

The performance of short-duration, all-out tasks requires skill, motivation, and the ability to generate mechanical power. Mechanical power is related to muscular strength and the ability to produce energy via anaerobic metabolic pathways. Many tasks that make up ADLs (eg, toileting, grooming) may challenge the anaerobic power of bed-bound patients. Activities of longer duration, such as walking household distances, challenge the aerobic pathways of energy production. Additionally, many ADLs, such as cleaning the house, may include both aerobic and anaerobic components, challenging both metabolic pathways. Most ADLs are submaximal activities related to total possible energy production. However, many hospitalized patients may be functioning near their peak aerobic and anaerobic levels during routine ADL performance.

Cardiovascular Adaptations

Prolonged bed rest results in a reduction in aerobic (VO_{2max}) and muscular power that is dependent on the duration of bed rest.[12-15] The longer the duration, the greater the loss. Heart rate (HR) will be elevated at all submaximal workloads in an attempt to maintain cardiac output and the delivery of blood to exercising muscles. CO and VO_{2max} are initially reduced due to a decrease in blood volume that limits cardiac filling (end-diastolic volume) and the stroke volume.[16,17] The reduction in circulating blood volume (hypovolemia) occurs most rapidly during the first few days of bed rest due to renal excretion of sodium (natriuresis) and diuresis.[18] Venous compliance also increases, promoting venous pooling, which may be exacerbated with upright postures. Venous pooling further compromises venous return and cardiac filling contributing to orthostatic intolerance.[16,19] Additional factors that contribute to resting tachycardia include reduced cardiac vagal tone, greater plasma norepinephrine, and enhanced beta-adrenergic receptor sensitivity.[16,20,21]

Orthostatic hypotension is a common risk after prolonged bed rest. Bed rest reduces a person's habitual exposure to the upright posture, which deprives the cardiovascular system of stimulation to maintain blood pressure (BP) regulation.[18] Initially, orthostasis is related to hypovolemia and resultant decrease in cardiac filling and stroke volume. However, past 1 week, the contribution of autonomic reflex function, impaired carotid-cardiac baroreflex responses, and impaired peripheral vascular vasoconstriction contribute to hypotension.[18,22]

Hematologic

Bed rest reduces red blood cell (RBC) mass by 5% to 25%, resulting in anemia and a diminished oxygen carrying capacity that may limit oxygen delivery to exercising muscle. The reduced RBCs combined with the reduced blood volume may

Table 4-1

Consequences of Bed Rest and Immobility

Cardiovascular	*Metabolic/Endocrine/Electrolytes*
• ↓ exercise tolerance/↓ VO_{2max} • ↓ cardiac output • ↓ resting HR • ↓ resting and maximum stroke volume • ↑ venous compliance • ↓ orthostatic tolerance • Venous pooling	• ↑ insulin resistance • ↑ urinary excretion of sodium, potassium, calcium, and phosphorus • Hypercalcemia/renal stone formation
Hematologic	*Psychiatric*
• ↓ blood volume • ↓ RBCs • ↑ DVT risk	• ↑ anxiety • ↑ agitation • ↑ delirium • ↑ depression
Musculoskeletal	*Nutrition*
• Muscle atrophy (disuse atrophy) • ↓ mitochondria density and aerobic enzymes • Bone demineralization, osteopenia, osteoporosis	• Cachexia/malnutrition • Obesity
Pulmonary	
• ↓ lung volumes and capacities • ↓ respiratory muscle strength • ↑ risk for pneumonia/pulmonary emboli	

be represented by a normal or slightly elevated hematocrit. An elevated hematocrit increases the resistance to blood flow that may stress a compromised cardiovascular system as well as increase the risk of deep vein thrombosis (DVT). Further exacerbating limited blood flow is reduced capillary network of peripheral muscle, which impairs blood flow to exercising muscle.

Musculoskeletal

Muscle and bone are dynamic structures with an extraordinary adaptive potential. In hospitalized patients, muscle damage can occur during prolonged immobility and from external sources, such as mechanical injury (eg, trauma, surgery), or as a medication side effect (eg, corticosteroids).[23] Multiple factors interact to influence skeletal muscle structure including genetics, neural activation, mechanical loading, and hormones.[24] Key elements of bed rest contributing to changes in the musculoskeletal system include:

- The lack of usual weightbearing forces acting on bones of the lower limb in the vertical position
- The decrease in number and magnitude of muscle contractions, especially in the postural musculature[5]

Muscle starts adapting to decreased loading within a matter of hours, with the predominant response being atrophy.[25] Atrophy is the process where muscle size is reduced, almost exclusively because of reduction in the contractile proteins actin and myosin.[25] This increased protein degradation results in a negative nitrogen balance, which is a diagnostic marker for muscle atrophy.[5] The amount of muscle atrophy a patient will experience depends on the usage prior to bed rest and the function of the muscle.

Muscular weakness tends to favor decrements in muscle force of the antigravity muscles. For example, antigravity muscles, such as the quadriceps, will have greater atrophy than the antagonist muscles, the hamstrings.[5,23,26] Strength loss in the upper extremity (UE) muscle groups is somewhat spared in relation to lower extremity (LE) disuse.[11] The magnitude of loss of muscle mass and strength, as well as the decrease in bone mineral density (BMD), is roughly proportional to the duration of the immobilization period.[27] Atrophy accounts for most, but not all, of the decrease in force production, suggesting that the ability to activate muscle by neuromuscular transmission and electrical contraction coupling is also compromised.[25,28]

Atrophy involves all muscle fibers but Type IIB (fast twitch fibers) are impacted to a greater extent than Type I (slow twitch fibers) and Type IIA (intermediate fibers).[25,29,30] Skeletal muscle fibers also undergo a slow to fast transition with Type IIA transitioning to Type IIX and Type IIB.[30] It is possible that the fiber type transition can further exacerbate endurance impairments.

Interestingly, patient positioning may influence disuse atrophy associated with bed rest. Studies demonstrate that immobilization in shortened positions increases atrophy while immobilization in lengthened and stretched positions may slow the loss of muscle fiber proteins.[31] This has important clinical considerations for patients who are diagnosed with an orthopedic or neuromuscular condition limiting active movements of the extremities or patients who are medically paralyzed, or who require excessive sedation.

Muscle metabolism is greatly affected by disuse and bed rest. Aerobic enzymes associated with the Krebs cycle and beta-oxidation pathway (ie, fatty acid metabolism) decrease while enzymes associated with anaerobic metabolic pathways, glycolysis, appear to be spared. These changes, loss of aerobic capability, and sparing of glycolytic pathways, contribute to the early fatigue observed after disuse and immobility.[27] Fiber atrophy results in decreased total mitochondria content, also contributing to reductions in muscle endurance. However, the mitochondria-to-fiber ratio may not change significantly, but due to fiber atrophy and mitochondria loss, the remaining muscle and contractile proteins must work against greater absolute workloads. Long-term unloading, as seen in SCI, is associated with fewer mitochondria per muscle fiber.[25]

Skeletal Adaptations

Bed rest contributes to loss of BMD and is termed **disuse osteopenia**. This loss of BMD is delayed compared to the loss of muscle strength, but the combined loss of muscle and bone mass increases a patient's risk of bone fracture with even minor falls. Normal homeostasis of the skeletal system involves a balance among bone formation by osteoblasts and bone resorption due to osteoclastic function. Bone homeostasis is a balance of normal mechanical forces acting on bones and the interaction of several endocrine hormones. For example, parathyroid hormone increases bone resorption by stimulating osteoclasts and calcitonin promotes bone formation by stimulating osteoblasts, and calcitriol (also called 1, 25 dihydroxyvitamin D), which promotes absorption of calcium via the intestines (see Chapter 10). Evidence for disuse osteopenia includes the increased excretion of calcium in the urine and feces that may be observed within 1 week of bed rest.[5] This increased calcium excretion increases the risk of stones forming in the kidneys and urinary tract.

The LEs appear to be the most susceptible to disuse osteopenia. Loss of BMD at the calcaneus is greatest followed by the femoral neck and spine with minimal changes in the UEs.[25] Interestingly, the BMD of the spine of SCI patients is maintained within normal limits, possibly reflecting the ongoing mechanical loads associated with wheelchair mobility and transfers.[27] This provides further evidence for the common use of closed chain exercise and the facilitation of weightbearing upright activities for all hospitalized patients.

Respiratory Function

Pulmonary complications are a leading cause of hospital morbidity resulting in prolonged lengths of stay and admission into the intensive care unit (ICU).[30] Common abnormalities following bed rest include reduced lung volumes and expiratory airflow rates, loss of respiratory muscle strength, decreased lung and chest wall compliance, and impaired gas exchange.[32-34] Overall, these factors increase the patient's work of breathing and increase the patient's risk for pneumonia and atelectasis. This increased risk is potentially exacerbated by thoracic and abdominal surgery as well as advancing age.[3,35] Abnormalities in respiratory muscle strength and limited tidal volume may impair the cough mechanism, further increasing the risk for pulmonary infections during a prolonged hospitalization. Finally, the increased work of breathing combined with impaired gas exchange may increase complaints of dyspnea on exertion and increased desaturation with activity.

Metabolic Alterations

Insulin resistance increases as a result of bed rest, and physical inactivity has been implicated in type 2 diabetes, obesity, and metabolic syndrome. Glucose transport into skeletal muscle is primarily a function of the glucose transporter protein 4 (Glut4). In the absence of insulin, Glut4 resides predominantly within intracellular vesicles within the cytoplasm of cells decreasing the transport of blood glucose into the cell. Insulin stimulation of cells translocates the Glut4 protein to the cell surface leading to the uptake of blood glucose.[36] Muscle activity is of paramount importance for the expression of Glut4 proteins in muscle. Detraining and immobilization have been shown to decrease the expression of Glut4 in skeletal muscle, and glucose intolerance has been demonstrated after only 3 days of bed rest.[36,37]

Bed rest can also elicit marked changes in plasma and urinary electrolyte concentrations. Enforced bed rest of 7 days results in increased urinary excretion of sodium, potassium, calcium, and phosphorus (see Chapter 2 for clinical manifestations of these electrolyte abnormalities).[38] Bed rest can also lead to alterations in endocrine function, such as the parathyroid, as noted previously. Another example is decreased erythropoietin concentrations in the blood. Erythropoietin is a hormone produced by the kidneys to stimulate RBC production. Reduced erythropoietin may partially explain the reduced RBC number and anemia associated with prolonged bed rest.[39]

Thermoregulatory Changes

Thermoregulatory responses are altered secondary to bed rest and physical inactivity. The primary source of heat gain is internal heat generated by energy metabolism. Patients in the hospital may have elevated metabolic rates due to infections, fever, or stress, leading to elevations in body temperature. The primary responses to elevated body temperatures is to increase HR to promote elevations in cardiac output, vasodilate cutaneous blood vessels to promote convective and radiant heat loss, and initiate sweating to promote evaporation.[27] Deconditioning and bed rest alters

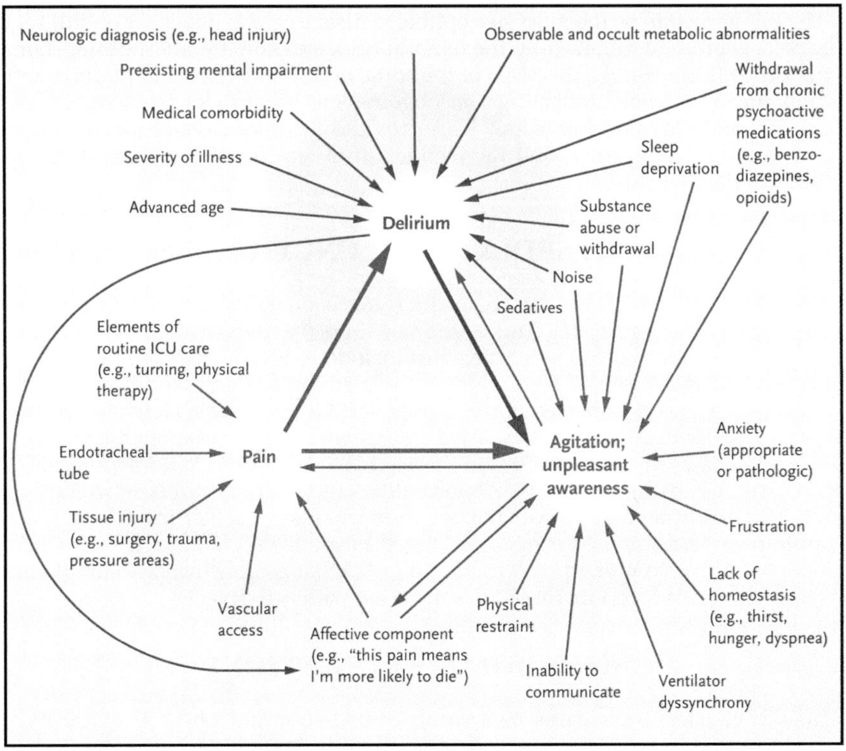

Figure 4-1. ICU triad. (Reprinted with permission from Reade MC, Finfer S. Sedation and delirium in the intensive care unit. *N Engl J Med.* 2014;370:444-454.)

thermoregulation resulting in increases in internal core temperatures with exercise. The threshold for cutaneous vasodilation and sweating to promote heat dissipation is shifted to a higher core temperature.[40] Impaired regulation of body heat limits exercise performance, resulting in increased complaints of fatigue and can increase the risk of heat-related abnormalities including cramping in fatigued muscles and, in extreme circumstances, syncope and heat stroke.[27]

Psychiatric

Alterations in psychological functioning often accompany acute illness and may promote functional decline, increasing morbidity and mortality of hospitalized adults.[39] Pain, anxiety, agitation, delirium, and depression are common findings affecting more than 50% of all patients.[41,42] Pain, agitation, and delirium are common in the ICU and have overlapping etiologies and management. The linking of pain, agitation and delirium is termed the **ICU triad** (Figure 4-1).[43] Altered sleep patterns, presence of noxious stimuli (eg, surgical incisions, vascular access, endotracheal tube suctioning), noise, loss of circadian light patterns, sedative medications, and communication deficits are several factors contributing to the ICU triad. The physical therapist needs to recognize these factors and perform accurate mental status examinations to identify psychiatric disorders and alert the medical team so appropriate interventions can be initiated. Table 4-2 and Figure 4-2 provide common examination items that should be routinely performed by the physical therapist.

Delirium is disturbances in consciousness, orientation, memory, thought, perception, and behavior. Delirium is typically abrupt in onset and fluctuating in its course. The prevalence of delirium in the ICU has varied from 20% to 80% and is recognized as a frequent and serious event in critically ill patients. Delirium is associated with self-extubation and removal of catheters, failed extubation and prolonged hospitalization. Delirium is classified into hyperactive, hypoactive, and mixed forms. Hyperactive delirium is characterized by agitation, diaphoresis, tachycardia, and tremor. Patients with hypoactive delirium are often passive and present with decreased responsiveness, withdrawal, and apathy and are at risk for dehydration, pressure sores, and nutrition abnormalities.[41] The majority of patients with delirium will have a mixed presentation. Importantly, delirium is frequently unrecognized and underdiagnosed by bedside clinicians. However, standard examination tools, such as the Confusion Assessment Method for the Intensive Care Unit (CAM-ICU), are available and should be used routinely by therapists (see Figure 4-2).[43-45]

Anxiety is a condition characterized by apprehension and increased motor activity with autonomic arousal.[41] Anxiety is associated with hyperreactivity, tremor, shaking, and avoidance behaviors. Agitation is represented by excessive motor activity leading to inappropriate verbal behavior and physical aggression. Agitation is driven by internal factors such as pain, anxiety, and delirium. Agitation can be deleterious, resulting in removal of catheters and vascular access, self-extubation, and increased energy expenditure, oxygen consumption, and ventilator dysynchrony.[46,47]

Depression is the persistence of a low mood or loss of interest in most activities for at least 2 weeks. Depression is associated with weight change, altered sleep patterns, lack of energy, agitation, poor self-esteem, and suicidal ideations.[45,46] Patients with symptoms of depression are more likely to be dependent and require assistance with basic ADLs or instrumental ADLs independent of comorbidities or illness severity.[46]

Nutrition Issues

Cachexia and malnutrition are prominent in prolonged hospitalization. Critical illness results in hypermetabolism, an increase in energy expenditure, and hypercatabolism, increased destruction of existing tissues.[43] These effects promote rapid depletion of body tissue stores and critical protein elements leading to reduced protein synthesis, enhanced protein breakdown, and malnutrition.[48,49] Malnutrition results in muscle wasting, reduced respiratory and peripheral muscle strength and endurance, increased rates of infection, reduced pulmonary function, and increased mortality. Cachexia is associated with a spectrum of clinical diseases including HIV/AIDS, cancers, rheumatologic diseases, chronic heart failure, chronic obstructive pulmonary disease (COPD), end-stage renal disease, inflammatory bowel disease, and hepatitis. Cachexia is also frequently found in the elderly.[49]

Intensive Care Unit–Acquired Weakness and Acute Neuromuscular Disorders

Severe weakness with respiratory failure is a complication of critical illness. Neuromuscular weakness occurs in critically ill patients with an incidence approaching 70% to 80% of patients hospitalized with sepsis or multiorgan failure.[50,51] The most common acquired neuromuscular disorders include **acute myopathy**

Table 4-2
Mental Status Examination

Orientation

Awake, alert, oriented x4 (person, place, time, situation):
Does the patient know:
1. What their name is (person)?
2. Where they are (place)?
3. What date it is (time)?
4. What is the cause or circumstances of their hospitalization (situation)?

Following Simple Commands

Sometimes called De Jonghe's 5 orders.

Procedure for 5 orders:
1. "Open (close) your eyes."
2. "Look at me."
3. "Open your mouth and put out your tongue."
4. "Nod your head."
5. "Raise your eyebrows when I have counted up to 5."

Patient must follow ≥3/5 to be able to "follow simple commands."

Level of Consciousness: Arousal, Agitation, and Sedation

Richmond Agitation-Sedation Scale (RASS):

Points	*Classification*	*Description*
+4	Combative	Overtly combative or violent; immediate danger to staff
+3	Very agitated	Pulls on or removes tubes or catheters or has aggressive behavior toward staff
+2	Agitated	Frequent nonpurposeful movement or patient-ventilator dyssynchrony
+1	Restless	Anxious or apprehensive but movements not aggressive or vigorous
0	Alert and calm	
-1	Drowsy	Not fully alert, but has sustained (more than 10 seconds) awakening, with eye contact, to voice
-2	Light sedation	Briefly (less than 10 seconds) awakens with eye contact to voice
-3	Moderate sedation	Any movement (but no eye contact) to voice
-4	Deep sedation	No response to voice, but any movement to physical stimulation
-5	Unarousable	No response to voice or physical stimulation

(continued)

Table 4-2 (continued)

Mental Status Examination

Procedure for RASS:

1. Observe patient. Is patient alert and calm (score 0)? Does patient have behavior that is consistent with restlessness or agitation (score +1 to +4 using the criteria listed previously, under Description)?
2. If patient is not alert, in a loud speaking voice state patient's name and direct patient to open eyes and look at speaker. Repeat once if necessary. Patient has eye opening and eye contact, which is sustained for more than 10 seconds (score -1). Patient has eye opening and eye contact, but this is not sustained for 10 seconds (score -2). Patient has any movement in response to voice, excluding eye contact (score -3).
3. If patient does not respond to voice, physically stimulate patient by shaking shoulder and then rubbing sternum if there is no response to shaking shoulder. Patient has any movement to physical stimulation (score -4). Patient has no response to voice or physical stimulation (score -5).

Attention Span

Procedure for Letters Attention Test

1. Say to the patient, "I am going to read you a series of 10 letters. Whenever you hear the letter A, indicate by squeezing my hand."
2. Read letters from the following letter list in a normal tone 3 seconds apart.

S A V E A H A A R T or C A S A B L A N C A or A B A D B A D A A Y

3. Errors are counted when patient fails to squeeze on the letter A and when the patient squeezes on any letter other than A.
4. If patient has ≥2 errors this is classified as "inattentive."

Adapted from De Jonghe B, Sharshar T, Lefaucheur JP, et al; Groupe de Réflexion et d'Etude des Neuromyopathies en Réanimation. Paresis acquired in the intensive care unit: a prospective multicenter study. *JAMA*. 2002;288(22):2859-2867 and Sessler CN, Gosnell MS, Grap MJ, et al. The Richmond Agitation–Sedation Scale. *Am J Respir Crit Care Med*. 2002;166(10):1338-1344.

syndrome (AMS) and **critical illness polyneuropathy** (CIP). Patients develop acute, diffuse, flaccid weakness often first identified due to the failure to wean from mechanical ventilation.[52] AMS, also known as **critical care myopathy** or **acute necrotizing myopathy**, is associated with neuromuscular blocking agents, intravenous corticosteroids, and aminoglycosides.[52-54] Other predisposing conditions include liver and lung transplantation, hepatic failure, and acidosis.[54] AMS results in preferential necrosis of the Type II (myosin heavy chain) muscle fibers. Sensory function is typically spared. CIP is defined as an axonal neuropathy associated with intense inflammation accompanying sepsis and multiorgan failure. Features of CIP include flaccid tetraplegia, hyporeflexia, muscle atrophy, and distal sensory disturbances.[55-57] AMS and CIP are conclusively diagnosed by electrophysiological testing (eg, electromyography, nerve conduction velocity) and muscle biopsy but these tests are difficult to perform and may be unreliable in the ICU. AMS and CIP often overlap and a clinical diagnosis, intensive care unit–acquired weakness (ICU-AW), is an overarching term used to define neuromuscular disease in the critically ill. ICU-AW can result in profound paralysis requiring months of rehabilitation. An ICU-AW

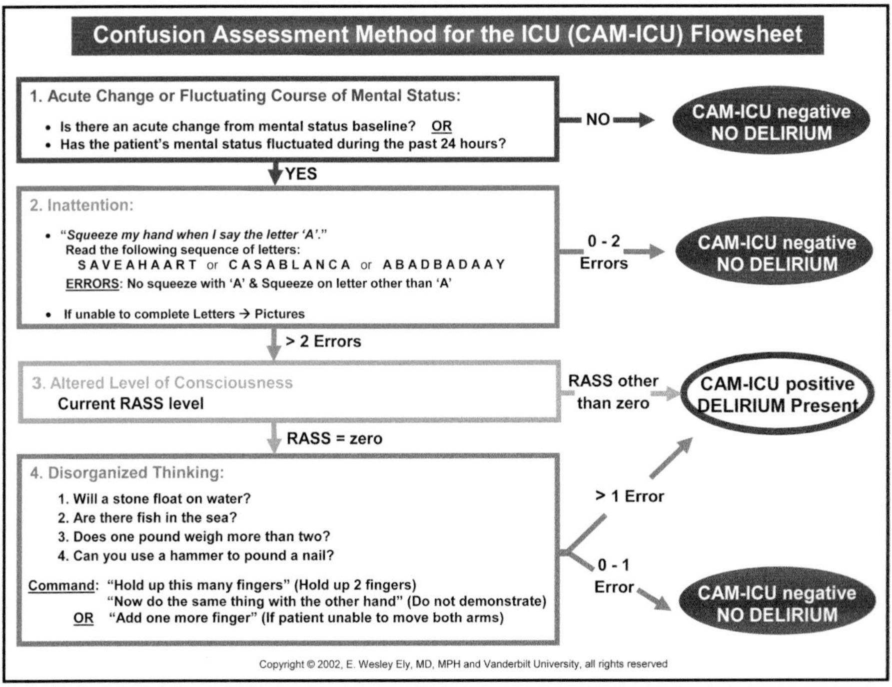

Figure 4-2. CAM-ICU. (Reprinted with permission from Critical Illness, Brain Dysfunction, and Survivorship Center. *Confusion Assessment Method for the ICU (CAM-ICU): The Complete Training Manual.* Revised ed. http://www.icudelirium.org/docs/CAM_ICU_training.pdf. Published 2014. Accessed October 17, 2018.)

diagnostic algorithm is presented in Figure 4-3 and additional diagnostic considerations are provided in Figure 4-4. The Medical Research Council (MRC) examination is provided in Table 4-3. It is important to remember that transient causes of acute muscle weakness often accompany acute changes in endocrine function, medication side effects, and electrolyte disturbances as seen in Figure 4-4.[57-59] (see Chapter 2 for further details).

Steroid-induced myopathy is the most common drug-induced myopathy and can occur acutely or may be associated with chronic glucocorticoid therapy. Steroid-induced myopathy is often associated with fluorinated glucocorticoids (eg, triamcinolone, betamethasone, dexamethasone) and is dose dependent. Risk is increased in the elderly, those who are inactive, those with cancer, and those who are nutritionally depleted.[54] Steroids alter muscle lipids, carbohydrates, and protein metabolism; however, the main effect of glucocorticoids is to induce muscle protein catabolism and myocyte apoptosis leading to the preferential atrophy of type 2 muscle fibers.[54,55] The hospitalized patient is at increased risk because malnutrition and inactivity worsen the course of steroid-induced myopathy. Weakness is primarily proximal, with the legs more severely involved than the arms; cranial nerves and sphincters are spared. Myalgias and electrolyte abnormalities (eg, hypokalemia) occur frequently.[60,61] Weakness typically improves with reduction of the steroid dose, but full recovery may require extensive rehabilitation.

Rhabdomyolysis is a syndrome characterized by muscle necrosis and the release of cellular contents into the circulation due to disruption of the sarcolemma and influx of extracellular calcium into the muscle cell. The elevated intracellular calcium

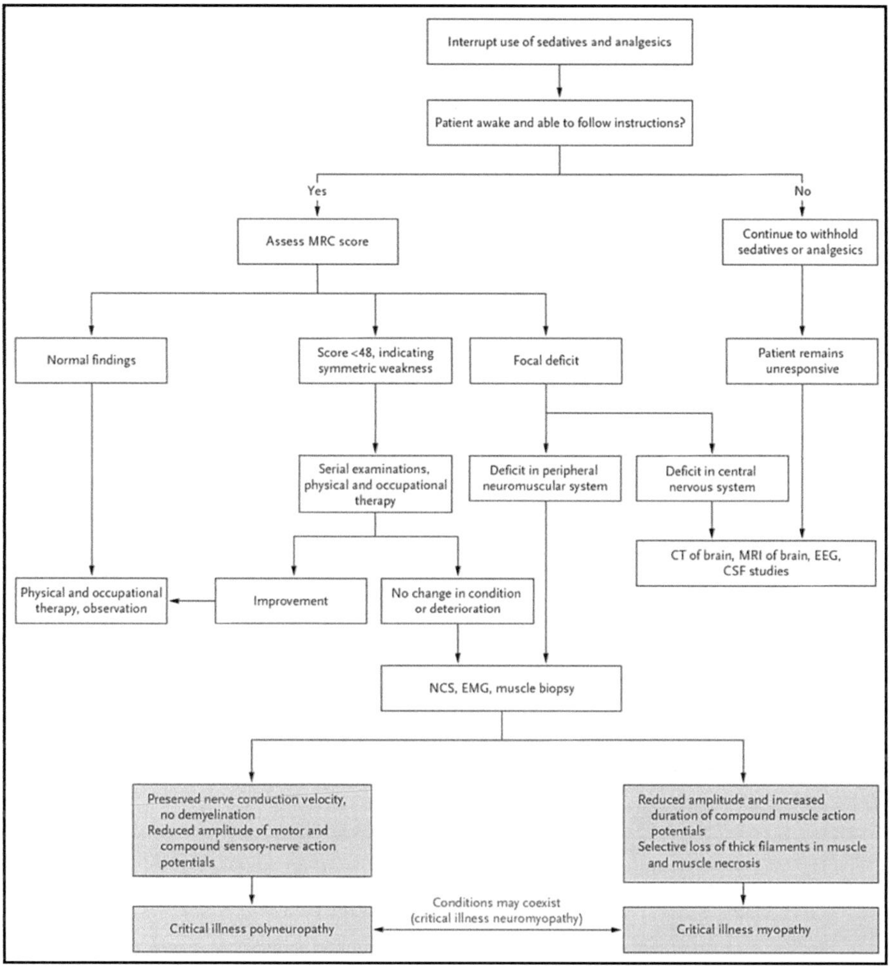

Figure 4-3. Diagnostic algorithm for ICU-AW. (CT = computed tomography; CSF = cerebrospinal fluid; EEG = electroencephalogram; EMG = electromyogram; MRC score = Medical Research Council Examination [see Table 4-3]; MRI = magnetic resonance imaging; NCS = nerve conduction study.)

causes a pathologic interaction of actin and myosin resulting in muscle destruction and fiber necrosis.[62,63] Risk factors for rhabdomyolysis include:

- Trauma and crush injuries
- Prolonged muscle compression and ischemia, static positioning due to excessive alcohol ingestion, operative positioning, or coma/paralysis
- Seizures and agitation
- Heat stress and extreme exertion
- Alcohol, amphetamine, cocaine, and heroin overdose
- Electrolyte disturbances, including hypokalemia, hypophosphatemia, hypocalcemia, hypernatremia, and hyponatremia

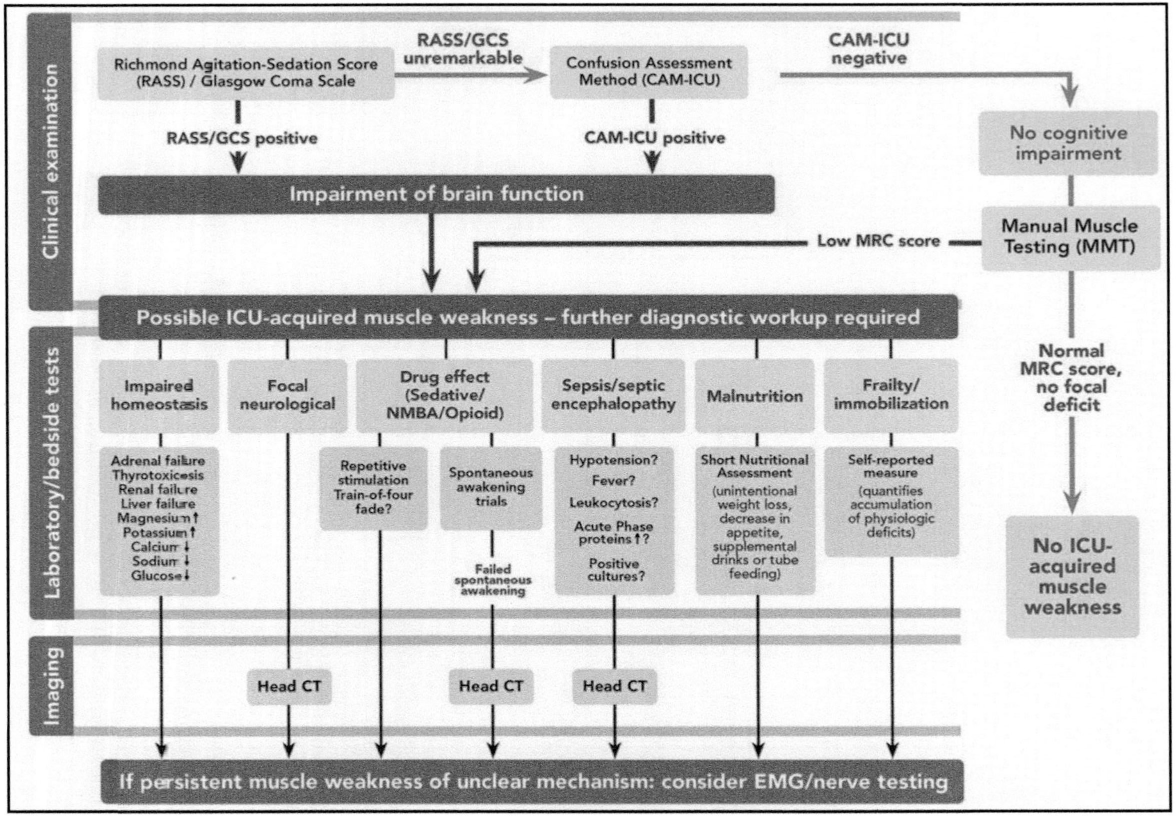

Figure 4-4. Differential diagnosis of ICU-AW. (NMBA=neuromuscular-blocking agent.) (Reprinted with permission from Farhan H, Moreno-Duarte I, Zafonte R, Eikermann M. Acquired muscle weakness in the surgical intensive care unit: nosology, epidemiology, diagnosis, and prevention. *Anesthesiology*. 2016;124[1]:207-34.)

Table 4-3

MEDICAL RESEARCH COUNCIL EXAMINATION

Score	*Description*	*Upper Extremity Movements Assessed*	*Lower Extremity Movements Assessed*
0	No visible contraction		
1	Visible muscle contraction, but no limb movement		
2	Active movement, but not against gravity	Shoulder abduction	Hip flexion
3	Active movement against gravity	Elbow flexion	Knee extension
4	Active movement against gravity and resistance	Wrist extension	Dorsiflexion
5	Active movement against full resistance		

Maximum score: 60 (4 limbs; 3 movements per extremity with maximum score of 15 points per limb)
Minimum score: 0 (quadriplegia); ICU-AW <48.

Adapted from Schweickert WD, Pohlman MC, Pohlman AS. Early physical and occupational therapy in mechanically ventilated, critically ill patients: a randomized controlled. *Lancet.* 2009;373:1874-1882.

Patients present with acute muscle necrosis resulting in myalgias, elevated serum creatine kinase levels, myoglobinuria (ie, brown discoloration of urine) and acute renal failure. Muscle weakness is in proportion to the severity of muscle damage.

INFLAMMATORY MYOPATHIES

The inflammatory myopathies are autoimmune diseases including **dermatomyositis, polymyositis**, and **inclusion body myositis**. These disorders often overlap with connective tissue diseases (eg, scleroderma, mixed connective-tissue disease) and cancers (eg, gastrointestinal, lung, breast, ovarian, non-Hodgkin's lymphoma). Patients with dermatomyositis and polymyositis may also have cardiac involvement leading to dysrhythmias and heart failure (see Chapter 6). Common to these disorders are moderate to severe weakness and muscle inflammation. Symptoms typically develop over weeks to months, but acute cases have been noted.[64] Symmetric proximal muscle weakness, including trunk muscle weakness, is common to dermatomyositis and polymyositis, but inclusion body myositis may be asymmetric and present with distal to proximal weakness. Patients with dermatomyositis present with characteristic rashes on the extremities and trunk. Diagnosis is confirmed by muscle biopsy and patients present with elevations in serum CK. Facial muscles and cranial nerves are typically spared, and myalgias are noted early in disease course.[64,65]

Examination and Interventions for the Weak Patient: Early and Progressive Rehabilitation

Examination of neuromuscular status is important for all patients but is especially important for patients who have remained on prolonged bed rest and all patients in the ICU. Neuromuscular dysfunction may be suggested when patients have difficulty weaning from mechanical ventilation or may be discovered by the physical therapist during the initial mobilization attempts. Movement patterns and observation of bed mobility and transfers (observational task analysis) may provide insight into the neuromuscular integrity of the patient. Tone, motor control, strength and sensation should be noted to further evaluate the patient's condition and may trigger the need for a further referral. Figure 4-3 provides a diagnostic algorithm for patients suspected of having ICU-AW. The clinical diagnosis of ICU-AW relies on a specific Manual Muscle Test (MMT) procedure, the MRC scale for grading the strength (see Table 4-3). Patients who score <48 on the MRC exam are diagnosed with ICU-AW. Confounding the diagnosis of ICU-AW is that some duration of bed rest is common, and the pre-admission neuromuscular status is typically unknown. Patients can have ICU-AW with superimposed deconditioning. Patients with bed rest–induced weakness will often present with a specific weakness pattern. Weakness is typically symmetric; LE weakness is greater than UE and antigravity muscle groups will be most affected. Weakness will be in proportion to the duration of the bed rest. Deep tendon reflexes (DTRs), sensation, and proprioception should be intact. Patients with ICU-AW will also present with symmetric extremity weakness as well as respiratory muscle weakness. The weakness is disproportionate to the duration of bed rest. Critical illness myopathy (CIM) occurs more frequently than CIP, and CIM is associated with a more favorable trajectory of recovery.[66] However, CIM and CIP seldom occur in isolation, so patients often present with muscle weakness, diminished DTRs and sensory changes (ie, pain, temperature, vibratory sense). Electrophysiological testing will show axonal damage (ie, reduction in sensory nerve action potential amplitudes and compound muscle action potential amplitudes).[66,67] Additional examination items include the Physical Function in Intensive Care Test–scored (PFIT-s), the Functional Status Score for the Intensive Care Unit (FSS-ICU), and the ICU Mobility Scale (IMS). The PFIT-s was designed as a measure of function for prescribing exercise and evaluating rehabilitation outcomes in the critically ill population. The PFIT-s includes 4 items (Table 4-4) designed to assess endurance, muscle strength, cardiovascular capacity and functional ability.[68,69] The IMS (Table 4-5) uses an 11-point ordinal scale, ranging from nothing (ie, lying/passive exercises in bed; score of 0) to independent ambulation (score of 10).[70] The FSS-ICU (Table 4-6) consists of 3 pre-ambulation categories (ie, rolling, supine-to-sit transfers, unsupported sitting) and 2 ambulation categories (ie, sit-to-stand transfers, ambulation). Each functional category is rated similar to the Functional Independence Measure (FIM) using a scale of 1 to 7, with a score of 1 corresponding to total dependent assistance and score of 7 corresponding to complete independence.[71,72]

No specific interventions can be recommended at this time, although progressive mobilization is the most common chosen intervention in the literature. Figure 4-5 is a protocol adapted from clinical research on early mobilization in the ICU. This protocol starts with a brief screen of cardiopulmonary and neurological stability, and the physical therapists should see Figure 1-3 for greater detail. Once the patient is deemed ready for physical therapy, progressive mobilization is initiated based off the patient's response and tolerance of the activity. As the patient is mobilized, orthostatic hypotension should be expected until proven otherwise and the therapist should monitor the cardiopulmonary and neurological responses as well as patient symptoms. Gait and transfer training can be performed with patients who require

Table 4-4

Physical Function in Intensive Care Test Scored

Component	*Definition*
Assist for sit to stand	0, 1, or 2 person assistance
Marching on the spot (cadence)	Number of steps/time in seconds
UE strength (shoulder flexion)	Greatest of left or right using 0 to 5 MRC scale (see Table 4-3)
LE strength (knee extension)	Greatest of left or right using 0 to 5 MRC scale (see Table 4-3)

Physical Function in Intensive Care Test Score	*0*	*1*	*2*	*3*	*Ordinal Score Total*
Assistance	Unable	Assist x2	Assist x1	No assist	
Cadence (steps/min)	Unable	>0 to 49	50 to <80	80+	
Shoulder (grade)	0, 1, or 2	3	4	5	
Knee (grade)	0, 1, or 2	3	4	5	

The PFIT-s (interval score) is then obtained from the Rasch analysis algorithm

Ordinal score /12	0	1	2	3	4	5	6	7	8	9	10	11	12
Interval PFIT score /10	0	2.0	3.2	3.9	4.4	4.9	5.4	5.9	6.4	7.1	7.9	8.8	10

Adapted from Denehy L, de Morton NA, Skinner EH, et al. A physical function test for use in the intensive care unit: validity, responsiveness, and predictive utility of the physical function ICU test (scored). *Phys Ther.* 2013;93(12):1636-1645. doi: 10.2522/ptj.20120310

mechanical ventilation using a self-inflating anesthesia bag or portable ventilators with an attached oxygen source. This task is cumbersome, especially if the patient has difficulty ambulating because of weakness and balance dysfunction. Careful preparation and planning may include premedication for anxiety, airway clearance techniques, including suctioning, a portable oxygen source, monitoring equipment (eg, electrocardiogram, pulse oximetry), assistive devices, including a wheelchair, gait belt, portable suction unit for chest tubes, and extra staff for guarding and transporting equipment. The assistance of nursing, respiratory therapists, or an additional therapist will promote safety and task completion. Few interventions provide more positive feedback to the patient and medical team as walking the mechanically ventilated patient.

Additional interventions may include the use of equipment to perform in-bed cycling, body weight support devices to allow assisted transfers, standing, and ambulation, treadmills and bicycles, as well as neuromuscular electrical stimulation.[73] Maintenance of aerobic work capacity, strength, and endurance may best be accomplished by an interval training approach rather than longer duration submaximal exercise as reported in ambulatory subjects.[74] The majority of the bed rest literature use healthy men and women as subjects, and the typical exercise workloads are

Table 4-5

ICU Mobility Scale

Classification		Definition
0	Nothing (lying in bed)	Passively rolled or passively exercised by staff, but not actively moving
1	Sitting in bed, exercises in bed	Any activity in bed, including rolling, bridging, active exercises, cycle ergometry and active assisted exercises; not moving out of bed or over the edge of the bed
2	Passively moved to chair (no standing)	Hoist, passive lift or slide transfer to the chair, with no standing or sitting on the edge of the bed
3	Sitting over edge of bed	May be assisted by staff, but involves actively sitting over the side of the bed with some trunk control
4	Standing	Weightbearing through the feet in the standing position, with or without assistance. This may include use of a standing lifter device or tilt table.
5	Transferring bed to chair	Able to step or shuffle through standing to the chair. This involves actively transferring weight from one leg to another to move to the chair. If the patient has been stood with the assistance of a medical device, they must step to the chair (not included if the patient is wheeled in a standing lifter device.)
6	Marching on spot (at bedside)	Able to walk on the spot by lifting alternate feet (must be able to step at least 4 times, twice on each foot), with or without assistance
7	Walking with assistance of 2 or more people	Walking away from the bed/chair by at least 5 meters (5 yards) assisted by 2 or more people
8	Walking with assistance of 1 person	Walking away from the bed/chair by at least 5 meters (5 yards) assisted by 1 person
9	Walking independently with a gait aid	Walking away from the bed/chair by at least 5 meters (5 yards) with a gait aid, but no assistance from another person. In a wheelchair-bound person, this activity level includes wheeling the chair independently 5 meters (5 years) away from the bed/chair
10	Walking independently without a gait aid	Walking away from the bed/chair by at least 5 meters (5 yards) without a gait aid or assistance from another person.

Reprinted with permission of American Thoracic Society. Copyright © 2019 American Thoracic Society. Tipping CJ, Bailey MJ, Bellomo R, et al. The ICU Mobility Scale has construct and predictive validity and is responsive. A multicenter observational study. *Ann Am Thorac Soc*. 2016;13(6):887-893. doi: 10.1513/AnnalsATS.201510-717OC. The *American Journal of Respiratory and Critical Care Medicine* is an official journal of the American Thoracic Society.

Table 4-6

Functional Status Score for the Intensive Care Unit

FSS-ICU Categories	*FSS-ICU (FIM) Scoring (0-7)*
Pre-Ambulation Categories	
Rolling	
Supine to sit transfer	
Unsupported sitting	
Ambulation Categories	
Sit to stand transfer	
Ambulation	
Total FSS-ICU Score (xx/35)	

FSS-ICU scoring categories are rated using the FIM rating scale of 0 to 7: 0 = unable to perform; 1 = total assistance; 2 = maximum assistance; 3 = moderate assistance; 4 = minimal assistance; 5 = supervision; 6 = moderate independence; 7 = complete independence.
The maximum score is 35/35.

Reprinted with permission from Zanni JM, Korupolu R, Fan E, et al. Rehabilitation therapy and outcomes in acute respiratory failure: an observational pilot project. *J Crit Care*. 2010;25:254-262.

over 50% the one repetition maximum for resistive exercise prescriptions or over 50% of VO_{2max} for aerobic work. Few studies outside of the ICU mobilization literature include hospitalized patients with multiple comorbid medical conditions, limiting generalizations to the acute care setting; however, the premise that deconditioning can be partly explained independent of disease underscores the importance of physical activity, resistive exercise, early intermittent transfers, standing, and ambulation.[11] Although passive range of motion (PROM) is routinely used to prevent pressure ulcers and contractures and stimulate circulation, PROM cannot prevent atrophy of affected muscles.[21] Muscle contraction of certain minimal force and frequency are necessary to maintain strength. Additionally, the continued performance of ADLs supports the cardiovascular system and improves muscle strength alleviating many of the hazards of bed rest and inactivity.[13,23] Overall, exercise can diminish and potentially alleviate the muscle atrophy in an exercise-specific manner. This specificity of training is demonstrated in studies addressing LE strengthening. For example, cycling and leg press type exercises promote improvements in quadriceps and hamstring force production with minimal changes in plantar and dorsiflexion strength,[75-78] whereas specific programs aimed at the plantar flexor muscle group can attenuate the deconditioning of this muscle group.[76] Specificity of training is important considering that bed rest promotes the greatest loss of strength in the postural and LE muscles. Specificity is also related to orthostatic intolerance. Reduction of carotid vagal baroreflex activity after bed rest was dependent on chronic supine positioning. Supine exercise does not correct orthostatic intolerance even with correction of blood volumes.[74,77] This provides further evidence of the importance of facilitating out of bed activities and maximizing upright positioning, including head of bed elevation and sitting. Joint ROM for the prevention of contractures is important for all patients who are mobility challenged, especially those patients who require mechanical ventilation. Joint contractures and muscle tightness interfere with functional

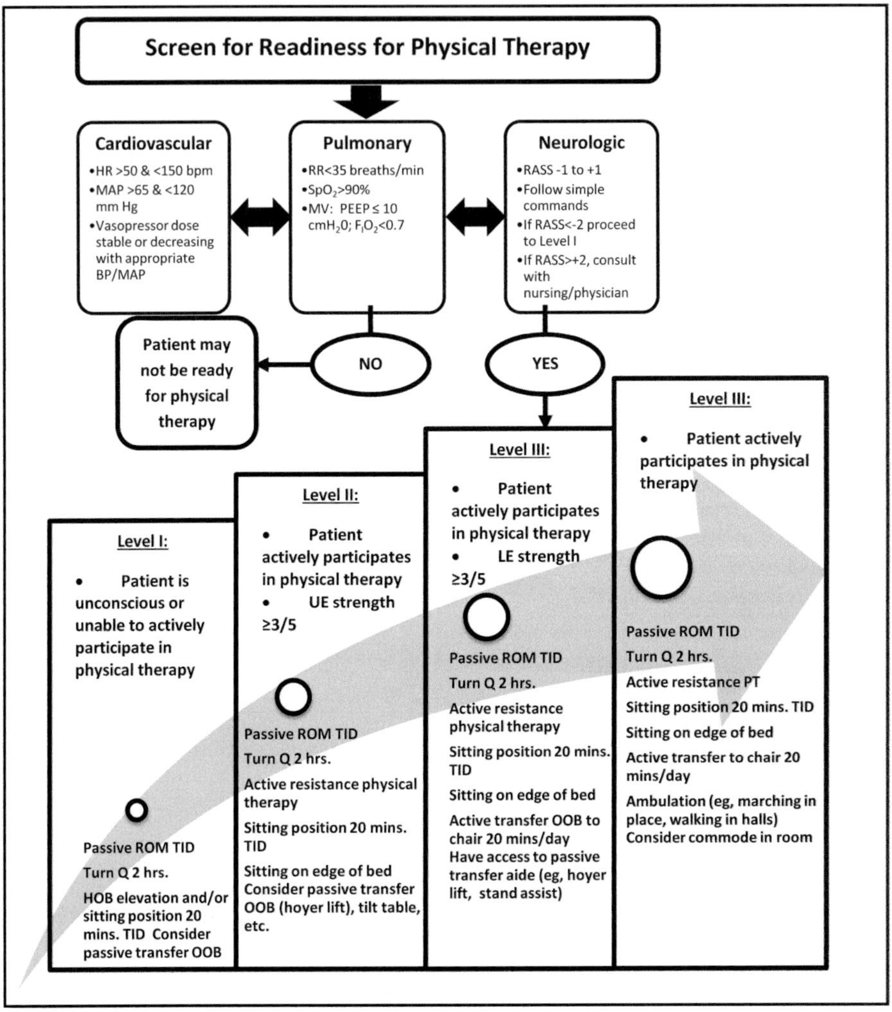

Figure 4-5. Sample mobility protocol. (HOB = head of bed; OOB = out of bed; ROM = range of motion; TID = three times per day.) (Adapted from Morris PE, Goad A, Thompson C, et al. Early intensive care unit mobility therapy in the treatment of acute respiratory failure. *Crit Care Med.* 2008;36[8]:2238-2243.)

mobility and proper bed positioning. Frequent turning and repositioning, use of splints and footboards, and encouragement of self-care activities supplement ROM exercises in preventing contractures. Physical constraints imposed by monitoring or life support equipment can restrict the patient from carrying out ROM exercises and changing positions. Positioning in functional or lengthened/stretched positions and frequent ROM needs to be considered for those who are unable to move, pharmacologically sedated, or paralyzed. Positioning in shortened positions should be avoided and active assisted and active muscular activity and upright positioning should be promoted as much as possible.

Additional benefits of exercise training during prolonged bed rest include increased fluid intake and maintenance of a positive fluid balance and RBC volume.[74,76,77] Hospital guidelines emphasizing frequent mobilization and activity decrease the incidences of DVT, pulmonary embolism, pneumonia, and urinary tract infections.[2] Exercise tends to maintain quality of sleep and leads to improvements in depression symptoms.[74,76,77] Exercise may also lead to maintenance or improvements in proprioception, further reducing fall and fracture risk.[61]

Finally, it has been shown that physical therapy, including deep breathing exercises, huffing, coughing, and early mobilization, can improve oxygen saturation and reduce the incidence of postoperative pulmonary complications.[79-82] All hospitalized patients should be involved in an airway clearance and/or mobility regimen.

Case Study

Mrs. Morton is a 60-year-old female transferred from a local community hospital per the family's request for further treatment of a severe exacerbation of COPD and possible evaluation for lung transplantation. She was transferred to the medical intensive care unit, intubated, and sedated. Physical therapy is consulted for evaluation and treatment as part of the early mobilization protocol.

Patient/Client History

General Demographics, Social History, and Living Environment

Her husband states that they live in a split-level with 4 steps to enter from the outside, 2 steps from the garage, and a bathroom on each level of the house. On clarification, the bathrooms are either up or down 6 steps in the house. Mrs. Morton is a retired pharmacist, but still manages a chain of pharmacies.

General Health Status, Social/Health Habits, and Family History

Chart review reveals that Mrs. Morton had been a 100 pack/year smoker who quit smoking 5 years ago. Her weight on admission to the outside hospital was 205 pounds at a height of 70 inches (body mass index [BMI] = 29.4). Mrs. Morton's father died of a heart attack at age 55, and she lost a brother to a heart attack last year.

Medical/Surgical History

Mrs. Morton has successfully quit smoking. She was dependent on 15 mg of prednisone for the past 6 months to manage her COPD symptoms. She has a past medical history (PMHx) that includes hypertension (HTN) that has been well-controlled with medication and diet. Her surgical history is significant for an anterior cruciate ligament (ACL) repair on the right 15 years ago due to a skiing accident.

Current Conditions

Mrs. Morton was admitted to the community hospital 3 weeks ago for an exacerbation of her COPD. She has not responded to intravenous (IV) antibiotics and corticosteroids, bronchodilators, supplemental oxygen therapy, or noninvasive and mechanical ventilation. She currently requires mechanical ventilation because of acute on chronic respiratory failure. The mechanical ventilation settings are synchronized intermittent mandatory ventilation (SIMV) of 12 breaths/minute, a F_IO_2 of 0.40 (40%), and positive end expiratory pressure (PEEP) of 10 cm H_2O. The chest x-ray demonstrates hyperinflation, flattened diaphragms, and some patchy haziness at the right base.

She is not awake or responsive, most likely due to sedation to lessen her "fighting" the ventilator. The medical staff has noticed minimal active muscle activity during examination and her DTRs are diminished.

Activities and Participation

Mrs. Morton was independent with all ADLs, enjoyed getting together with her children and grandchildren, and played golf with friends 2 times/week prior to hospital admission. Her husband states she could walk 2 blocks before getting "winded."

Medications

Mrs. Morton is receiving IV steroids (methylprednisolone), antibiotics (doxycycline), proton pump inhibitor (pantoprazole), sedatives (dexmedetomidine), and inhaled bronchodilators (albuterol, Atrovent [ipratropium bromide]) related to the COPD and respiratory failure. She is also receiving heparin for DVT prophylaxis and Norvasc (amlodipine) for the HTN.

Other Clinical Tests

Laboratory results of the complete blood count (CBC) revealed white blood cell (WBC) elevation of 22,500 cells/µL, hemoglobin of 9.4 g/dL, and hematocrit (hct) 33%. The electrolyte panel results were sodium 131 mEq/L, creatinine 1.7 mg/dL, albumin 2.8 g/dL. Arterial blood gas values were pH 7.34/PCO_2 48/PO2 70/HCO_3^- 26.

Systems Review

Cardiovascular and Pulmonary

The patient has resting vital signs (VS) of HR 94 bpm, sinus rhythm, respiratory rate (RR) 12 breaths/minute, BP 130/90 mm Hg, and SpO_2 93% on SIMV 12, F_IO_2 0.40 (40%), and PEEP of 10.

Integumentary

Mrs. Morton has a radial arterial line in her right forearm with a supportive board, an IV line in her left antecubital space, and a central venous line in the right subclavian. She also has a Foley catheter in place. Her skin appears dry and fragile with purplish marks on the forearms. Her legs have pneumatic boots on, but upon removal the skin is also very dry and fragile, but there are no pressure sores on elbows, heels, or buttock region. Slight pitting edema (+2) noted in the low back and buttock area and distal extremities.

Musculoskeletal

Mrs. Morton is able to move bilateral upper extremities UEs and LEs to command but she is weak. ROM is limited at the shoulders, hips, and ankles.

Neuromuscular

Gross sensation appeared intact for light touch and although she was weak, there are no observed abnormal movement patterns or tone.

Communication, Affect, Cognition, Language, and Learning Style

Mrs. Morton primarily speaks English per her husband. She is somnolent and easily aroused and became more alert during the examination. Mrs. Morton did follow simple direction and could squeeze eyelids with yes/no questions. Presently she is orally intubated and did not attempt to mouth words.

Tests and Measures

Aerobic Capacity and Endurance

Poor endurance is demonstrated during supine evaluation of MMT, ROM, and bed mobility. Mrs. Morton had a significant change in HR, BP, RR, drop in SpO_2, and complaint of shortness of breath (SOB) with a minimal intensity challenge. Five minutes were required for VS to return to baseline. Laboratory results are indicative of hypoxemia along with borderline nutritional, pulmonary, and kidney function. Anemia is noted on the CBC. Partial thrombinplastin time should be monitored because she is anticoagulated (heparin) due to her risk for DVT.

Assistive and Adaptive Devices

Recommend resting ankle/foot orthosis to prevent breakdown and prevent worsening of distal LE ROM deficits. Recommend elevation of distal UE/LE in supine position and placing patient on a pressure relief mattress for wound prevention.

Balance, Gait, and Mobility (Including Locomotion)

Currently, bed mobility (rolling and supine to sit) is moderate assistance (FSS-ICU=3) and sitting at edge of the bed was accomplished with moderate assistance (FSS-ICU=3) for 2 minutes. Mrs. Morton was significantly fatigued following the supine examination and bed mobility tasks. Further mobility testing was postponed at this time due to fatigue as demonstrated by subjective complaints and vital sign changes with minimal exertion. Her IMS classification was 3 (sitting over edge of bed). Her total FSS-ICU score was 9/35 and the Activity Measure for Post Acute Care (AM-PAC) 6 clicks basic mobility score was 8/24.

Circulation (Arterial, Venous, Lymphatic) and Ventilation/Respiration

MMT, ROM, and bed mobility were evaluated with a vital sign response of HR 94-128 bpm, RR 12-28 breaths/minute, BP 130/90-166/96 mm Hg, and SpO_2 93%-87%.

Mrs. Morton desaturated during bed mobility (SpO_2 93%-87%) and complained of severe SOB. Breath sounds on the ventilator are coarse anteriorly and laterally but diminished posteriorly at the lung bases. A weak cough was elicited with moving side to side while assessing bed mobility.

Mental Function

Mrs. Morton is CAM-ICU negative and her RASS score is -1.

Muscle Performance

MMT reveals 1/5 shoulder flexion and abduction, 3/5 UE elbow and wrist flexion/extension and grasp. She has 2/5 for hip flexion and knee extension and 1/5 dorsiflexion bilaterally. The MRC strength examination is 24/60. ROM is limited to <100 degrees at bilateral shoulders, hip flexion is limited to <50 degrees bilaterally, knee extension is within normal limits, but flexion is limited to 40 degrees, and dorsiflexion is -10 bilaterally.

Pain

The patient was unable to quantify her pain, but pain is confirmed by nonverbal communication when Mrs. Morton squeezed her eyelids tight with end ROM at the ankles, knees, hips, and shoulders.

Reflex Integrity

Reflexes are diminished (1+).

Sensory Integrity

Light touch, pressure, and proprioception are intact.

Evaluation

Mrs. Morton presents with profound motor weakness with intact sensation. The therapist cannot distinguish between disuse atrophy or a myopathic process, but an acquired neuromuscular disorder would be consistent with the history and an MRC score of 24. Additionally, the cardiopulmonary reserve is diminished as evidenced by the VS responses during bed mobility activities.

Diagnosis

Mrs. Morton demonstrates severe quadriparesis consistent with ICU-AW. The weakness may be a myopathy related to her critical illness, prolonged bed rest, and chronic corticosteroids use.

Prognosis

Mrs. Morton will benefit from daily physical therapy services for progression of functional level and to assist with weaning from mechanical ventilation. It is anticipated that she will need prolonged rehabilitation services that will span acute care through inpatient rehabilitation or other post-acute care settings.

Intervention

Mrs. Morton will receive daily physical therapy consisting of airway clearance and breathing exercises, therapeutic exercise, and progressive mobility training. She will also benefit from occupational and speech therapy as well as a nutrition consult for weight loss of >25 pounds and a decreased albumin since outside hospital admission. The nursing staff and the patient's family are instructed in ROM exercises to be performed daily.

ICF Clinical Reasoning Tool Case Study Summary

Health Condition								
HPI: Severe exacerbation of COPD and possible evaluation for lung transplant. Low hct, Hb (anemia) and albumin, Na^+ (hyponatremia), patchy haziness right base, elevated WBC, creatinine, and universal precautions PMHx: COPD, HTN, obesity, and distant surgical repair of ACL, family history of heart disease.								
Precautions/Contraindications								
Intubated and sedated on MV, prolonged bed rest, challenge to wean and universal precautions Risks: Delirium/depression, skin breakdown, and ICU-AW; VS parameters								
Body Structure and Function			*Activity/Task Limitations*			*Participation*		
Impairment/ Problem	*Tests and Measures*	*Intervention*	*Activity*	*Tests and Measures*	*Intervention*	*Participation*	*Tests and Measures*	*Intervention*
• Impaired ventilation • Limited ROM • Muscle weakness • Decreased endurance • Edema • Diminished reflexes • Impaired communication • Abnormal lab values • Weight exceeds IBW	• VS including ECG/SpO_2 • Breath sounds • ROM • MMT/MRC • Grade pitting edema • CAM-ICU • DTRs • Lab values • BMI	• Breathing exercises and airway clearance • Bedside ROM and progressive resistance exercise • Consider NMES • Maintain HOB >30 degrees • Consult registered dietician, occupational therapist, and speech pathologist • Education: Bedside team and family for positioning and AAROM	• ADLs • Bed mobility including rolling, supine to sit, and sitting at edge of bed (dangling) • Sitting balance • Standing transfers	• Functional task analysis • FSS-ICU (FIM) • PFIT when able • FIST • IMS	• Early mobilization program	• Unable to work • Unable to golf • Unable to play with grandchildren	• MMSE • SGRQ • SF-36	• Continue physical therapy services • Consult social work and family regarding discharge plan • Consult occupational therapy • Discuss findings with transplant team

(continued)

ICF Clinical Reasoning Tool Case Study Summary (continued)

Personal Factors	*Other Considerations*	*Environmental Factors*
• Age: 60 y/o female • Not awake or responsive • Primary language: English • Married, pharmacist manages chain of pharmacies • Prior to admission independent with all ADLs • Active with children/grandchildren • Played golf with friends twice/week • Former 100 pk/yr smoker • Fear, anxiety, unable to verbally communicate		Home: • Lives in split-level • 4 steps to enter from outside; 2 from garage • Bathrooms up or down steps Hospital: • Multiple IVs, arterial line, ETT, urinary catheter, sedation, limited communication, medications, access and timing for interventions, HOB ≥30 degrees VAP prevention protocol

AAROM = active assistive range of motion; ECG = electrocardiogram; ETT = endotracheal tube; FIST = Function in Sitting Test; Hb = hemoglobin; HOB = head of bed; HPI = history of present illness; IBW = ideal body weight; IMS = ICU Mobility Scale; MMSE = Mini-Mental State Examination; MV = mechanical ventilator; Na^+ = sodium; NMES = neuromuscular electric stimulation; pk/yr = packs per year; PMHx = past medical history; SF = Short Form; SGRQ = Saint George's Respiratory Questionnaire; VAP = ventilator-associated pneumonia; y/o = year old.

Adapted from American Physical Therapy Association. *Guide to Physical Therapist Practice*. 3rd ed. http://www.apta.org/Guide/. Updated October 21, 2015. Accessed October 5, 2018 and *Towards a Common Language for Functioning, Disability and Health*. World Health Organization. www.who.int/classifications/icf/icfbeginnersguide.pdf. Published 2002. Accessed April 29, 2019.

Outcomes

Mrs. Morton was transferred to the intermediate medical care unit and underwent a tracheostomy and gastric tube insertion for supplemental feeding 5 days post-admission. Her arterial line was removed, but the Foley catheter was continued. Mrs. Morton is OOB in a chair for at least 1 hour twice/day. Her ventilator settings have been decreased to SIMV 8, PEEP 6, F_IO_2 30%, and she has started short trach collar trials (1 to 3 hours). Her UE strength has increased to 2/5 at the shoulder, and 3/5 at the elbow, wrist, and hand. Her LE strength has increased to 3/5 at the hip, knee, and ankle. The MRC strength score has increased from 24 to 34/48. She is able to roll side-to-side in bed with the head of the bed flat with minimal assistance of 1 (FSS-ICU = 4), transfer to dangling at edge of bed with moderate assist of one (FSS-ICU = 3) and tolerates this unsupported sitting for 5 minutes times 2. Standing is attempted, and she requires maximal assistance of 2 people (FSS-ICU = 1). Her total FSS-ICU score increased from 9 to 13/35 and the AM-PAC 6 clicks basic mobility score increased from 8 to 12/24. The IMS increased from 3 to 4.

Mrs. Morton needs to continue with the present therapy services and will remain in the acute care setting for another 2 weeks. Her activity limitations continue to be an inability to perform bed mobility, transfers, or ADLs without assistance. She is being evaluated for discharge to a skilled nursing unit.

Chapter Review Questions

1. How does prolonged bed rest impact the patient?
   a. Increased oxygen consumption and increased mitochondrial effectiveness
   b. Decreased resting HR and increased blood volume
   c. Decreased maximal oxygen consumption and increased muscle atrophy
   d. Increased lung volumes and decreased mitochondrial density
2. How does an elevated hematocrit increase the risk for DVT?
   a. Decreases resistance to blood flow
   b. Increases resistance to blood flow
   c. Triggers release of natural anticoagulants
   d. Triggers release of local catecholamines
3. Which of the following is the predominant response to reduced muscle use from prolonged bed rest?
   a. Muscle atrophy and reduction in contractile force
   b. Slowed break down of actin and myosin
   c. Increased Type II muscle fiber size
   d. Increased Krebs cycle activation and greater aerobic capability
4. Which skeletal sites are most susceptible to bone loss secondary to disuse?
   a. Weightbearing upper limbs
   b. Cervical vertebrae
   c. Weightbearing lower limbs
   d. Shoulder girdle

5. How do PROM exercises primarily benefit a patient confined to bed rest?
   a. By promoting unweighting of bony prominences and preventing osteopenia
   b. By reducing peripheral circulation to LEs
   c. By decreasing osteopenia and improving kinesthetic forces at weightbearing joints
   d. By promoting prevention of pressure ulcers

Answers: 1c, 2b, 3a, 4c, 5d

References

1. Asher RA. The dangers of going to bed. *Br Med J.* 1947;4:967-968.
2. Markey DW, Brown RJ. An interdisciplinary approach to addressing patient activity and mobility in the medical-surgical patient. *J Nurs Care Qual.* 2002;16:1-12.
3. Creditor MC. Hazards of hospitalization of the elderly. *Annals of Intern Med.* 1993;18:219-223.
4. Lamont CT, Sampson S, Matthias R, Kane R. The outcome of hospitalization for acute illness in the elderly. *J Am Geriatr Soc.* 1983;31:282-288.
5. Bloomfield S. Changes in musculoskeletal structure and function with prolonged bed rest. *Med Sci Sports Exerc.* 1997;29:197-206.
6. McArdle WD, Katch FI, Katch VL. *Exercise Physiology: Energy, Nutrition and Human Performance.* Philadelphia, PA: Lippincott Williams & Wilkins; 2001.
7. Hirsch CH, Sommers L, Olsen A, Mullen L, Winograd CH. The natural history of functional morbidity in hospitalized older patients. *J Am Geriatr Soc.* 1990;38:1296-1303.
8. Landefeld CS, Palmer RM, Kresevic DM, Fortinsky RH, Kowal J. A randomized trial of care in a hospital medical unit especially designed to improve the functional outcomes of acutely ill older patients. *N Engl J Med.* 1995;332(20):1338-1344.
9. Bassey E, Bennett T, Birmingham AT, et al. Effects of surgical operation and bed rest on cardiovascular responses to exercise in hospital patients. *Cardiovasc Res.* 1973;7:588-592.
10. Convertino V. Effects of exercise and inactivity on intravascular volume and cardiovascular control mechanisms. *Acta Astronautica.* 1992;27:123-129.
11. Gogia P, Schneider V, LeBlanc AD, et al. Bed rest effect on extremity muscle torque in healthy men. *Arch Phys Med Rehab.* 1988;69: 1030-1032.
12. Crandall C, Johnson V, Convertino VA, et al. Altered thermoregulatory responses after 15-days of head-down tilt. *J Appl Phys.* 1994;77: 1863-1867.
13. Convertino V, Bloomfield S, Greenleaf J. An overview of the issues: physiological effects of bed rest and restricted physical activity. *Med Sci Sports Exerc.* 1997; 29:187-190.
14. Convertino V. Effects of orthostatic stress on exercise performance after bedrest: relation to in hospital rehabilitation. *J Cardiac Rehabil.* 1983;3:660-663.
15. Greenleaf J, Bernauer A, Ertl AC, et al. Work capacity during 30-days of bed rest with isotonic and isokinetic exercise training. *J Appl Phys.* 1989;67:1820-1826.
16. Convertino V. Cardiovascular consequences of bed rest: effect on maximal oxygen uptake. *Med Sci Sports Exerc.* 1997;29:191-196.
17. Saltin B, Bloomqv, Mitchell JH, et al. Response to exercise after bed rest and after training. *Circulation.* 1968;38:1-78.
18. Convertino VA. Value of orthostatic stress in maintaining functional status soon after myocardial infarction or cardiac artery bypass grafting. *J Cardiovasc Nurs.* 2003;18:124-130.
19. Convertino V, Doerr DF, Mathes KL, et al. Changes in size and compliance of the calf following 30 days of exposure to simulated microgravity. *Aviat Space Environ Med.* 1989;60:653-658.
20. Englelke J, Convertino V. Catecholamine response to maximal exercise following 16 days of simulated microgravity. *Aviat Space Environ Med.* 1996;67:243-247.
21. Crandall C, Englelke J, Pawelczyk JA, et al. Power spectral and time based analysis of heart rate variability following 15 days head-down bed rest. *Aviat Space Environ Med.* 1994;65:1105-1109.

22. Convertino VA, Doerr DF, Eckberg DL, et al. Head-down bed rest impairs vagal baroreflex responses and provokes orthostatic hypotension. *J Appl Phys.* 1990;68:1458-1464.
23. Kasper CE, Talbot LA, Gaines JM. Skeletal muscle damage and recovery. *AACN Clin Issues.* 2002;13:237-247.
24. Edgerton VR, Roy RR, Allen DL, Monti RJ. Adaptations in skeletal muscle disuse or decreased-use atrophy. *Am J Phys Med Rehab.* 2002;81:S127-S147.
25. American College of Sports Medicine. *ACSM's Resource Manual for Guidelines for Exercise Testing and Prescription.* 4th ed. Philadelphia, PA: Lippincott Williams & Wilkins; 2001.
26. LeBlanc A, Gogia V, Schneider V, et al. Calf muscle area and strength changes after five weeks of horizontal bed rest. *Am J Sports Med.* 1988;16:624-629.
27. American College of Sports Medicine. *ACSM's Resource Manual for Guidelines for Exercise Testing and Prescription.* Philadelphia, PA: Lea & Febiger; 1993.
28. Kawakami Y, Akima H, Kubo K, et al. Changes in muscle size, architecture, and neural activation after 20 days of bed rest with and without resistance exercise. *Eur J Appl Physiol.* 2001;84:7-12.
29. Hikida RS, Gollnick, Dudley GA, et al. Structural and metabolic characteristics of human skeletal muscle following 30 days of simulated microgravity. *Aviat Space Environ Med.* 1989;60:664-670.
30. Pette D, Staron RS. Transitions of muscle fiber phenotypic profiles. *Histochem Cell Biol.* 2001;115:359-372.
31. Goldspink G. Changes in muscle mass and phenotype and the expression of autocrine and systemic growth factors by muscle in response to stretch and overload. *J Anat.* 1998;194:323-334.
32. Venturoli D, Semino P, Negrini D, et al. Respiratory mechanics after 180 days space mission. *Acta Astronaut.* 1998;42:185-204.
33. Montmerle S, Spaak J, Linnarsson, D. Lung function during and after prolonged head-down bed rest. *J Appl Physiol.* 2002;92:75-83.
34. Vitacca M, Clini E, Spassini W, et al. Does the supine position worsen respiratory function in elderly subjects? *Gerontology.* 1996;42:46-53.
35. Lawrence VA, Hilsenbeck SG, Mulrow DC. Incidence and hospital stay for cardiac and pulmonary complications after abdominal surgery. *J Gen Intern Med.* 1995;10:671-678
36. Daugaard JR, Richter EA. Relationship between muscle fibre composition, glucose transporter protein 4 and exercise training: possible consequences in non-insulin-dependent diabetes mellitus. *Acta Physiol Scand.* 2001;171:267-276.
37. Greenleaf JE. Physiological consequences of reduced physical activity during bed rest. *Exerc Sports Sci Reviews.* 1982;10:84-119.
38. Zorbas YG, Kakurin VJ, Afonin VB, et al. Electrolyte changes in plasma and urine of athletes during acute and rigorous bed rest and ambulatory conditions. *Biol Trace Elem Res.* 2001;79:49-65.
39. Tipton CM, Greenleaf JE, Jackson CG. Neuroendocrine and immune system responses with spaceflights. *Med Sci Sports Exerc.* 1996;28:988-998.
40. Shibasaki M, Wilson TE, Cui J, et al. Exercise throughout 6-degree head-down tilt bed rest preserves thermoregulatory responses. *J Appl Physiol.* 2003;95:1817-1823.
41. Cole MG. Delirium in elderly patients. *Am J Geriatr Psychiatry.* 2004;12:7-21.
42. Siegel MD. Management of agitation in the intensive care unit. *Clin Chest Med.* 2003;24:713-725.
43. Reade MC, Finfer S. Sedation and delirium in the intensive care unit. *N Engl J Med* 2014;370:444-454
44. Peterson JF, Pun BT, Dittus RS, et al. Delirium and its motoric subtypes: a study of 614 critically ill patients. *J Am Geriatr Soc.* 2006;54(3):479-484.
45. Girard TD, Pandharipande PP, Ely EW. Delirium in the intensive care unit. *Critical Care* 2008;12(suppl 3):S3.
46. Covinsky KE, Fortinsky RH, Palmer RM, et al. Relation between symptoms of depression and health status outcomes in acutely ill hospitalized older persons. *Ann Intern Med.* 1997;126:417-425.
47. Szokol JW, Vender JS. Anxiety, delirium, and pain in the intensive care unit. *Crit Care Clin.* 2001;17:821-842.
48. Lanken P. *The Intensive Care Unit Manual.* Philadelphia, PA: WB Saunders; 2014.

49. Kotler DP. Cachexia. *Ann of Intern Med.* 2000;17:622-634.
50. Berek K, Margreiter J, Willeit J, et al. Polyneuropathies in critically patients: a prospective evaluation. *Int Care Med.* 1996;22:849-855.
51. Hund E. Myopathy in critically ill patients. *Crit Care Med.* 1999;27:2544-2547.
52. Lacomis D, Giuliani MJ, Van Cott A, et al. Acute myopathy of intensive care: clinical, electromyographic, and pathologic aspects. *Ann Neurol.* 1996;40:645-654.
53. Partridge BL, Abroms JH, Bazemore C, et al. Prolonged neuromuscular blockade after long-term infusion of vecuronium bromide in the intensive care unit. *Crit Care Med.* 1990;18:1177-1179.
54. Gutmann L. Critical Illness neuropathy and myopathy. *Archiv Neurol.* 1999;56:527-528.
55. Leijten FS, Harinck-de Weerd JE, Poortvliet DC, et al. The role of polyneuropathy in motor convalescence after prolonged mechanical ventilation. *JAMA.* 1995;274:1221-1225.
56. Schweickert WD, Hall J. ICU-acquired weakness. *Chest.* 2007;131 (5):1541-9.
57. Kress JP, Hall JB. ICU-acquired weakness and recovery from critical illness. *N Engl J Med.* 2014;370(17):1626-35.
58. Polkey MI, Lyall RA, Moxham J, et al. Respiratory aspects of neurologic disease. *J Neurol Neurosurg Psychiatry.* 1999;66:5-15.
59. Huether SE, McCance KL. *Understanding Pathophysiology.* St. Louis, MO: Mosby; 1996.
60. Alshekhlee A, Kaminski HJ, Ruff RL. Neuromuscular manifestations of endocrine disorders. *Neurologic Clinics.* 2002;20:35-58.
61. Anagnos A, Ruff RL, Kaminski HJ. Endocrine neuromyopathies. *Neurol Clin.* 1997;15:673-696.
62. Malinoski DJ, Slater MS, Mullins RJ. Crush injury and rhabdomyolysis. *Crit Care Clin.* 2004;20:171-192.
63. Warren JD, Blumbergs PC, Thompson PD. Rhabdomyolysis: a review. *Muscle Nerve.* 2002;25:332-347.
64. Dalakas MC, Hohlfeld R. Polymyositis and dermatomyositis. *Lancet.* 2003;362:971-982.
65. Yazici Y, Kagen LJ. Clinical presentation of the idiopathic inflammatory myopathies. *Rheum Dis Clin North Am.* 2002;28:823-832.
66. Koch S, Spuler S, Deja M, et al. Critical illness myopathy is frequent: accompanying neuropathy protracts ICU discharge. *J Neurol Neurosurg Psychiatry.* 2011;82:287-293.
67. Nordon-Craft A, Moss M, Quan D, Schenkman M. Intensive care unit-acquired weakness: implications for physical therapist management. *Phys Ther.* 2012;92(12):1494-506.
68. Skinner EH, Berney S, Warrillow S, Denehy L. Development of a physical function outcome measure (PFIT) and a pilot exercise training protocol for use in intensive care. *Crit Care Resusc.* 2009;11(2):110-115.
69. Denehy L, de Morton NA, Skinner EH, et al. A physical function test for use in the intensive care unit: validity, responsiveness, and predictive utility of the physical function ICU test (scored). *Phys Ther.* 2013;93(12):1636-1645. doi: 10.2522/ptj.20120310
70. Tipping CJ, Bailey MJ, Bellomo R, et al. The ICU Mobility Scale has construct and predictive validity and is responsive: a multicenter observational study. *Ann Am Thorac Soc.* 2016;13(6):887-893.
71. Zanni JM, Korupolu R, Fan E, et al. Rehabilitation therapy and outcomes in acute respiratory failure: an observational pilot project. *J Crit Care.* 2009;25:254-262.
72. Thrush A, Rozek M, Dekerlegand JL. The clinical utility of the Functional Status Score for the Intensive Care Unit (FSS-ICU) at a long-term acute care hospital: a prospective cohort study. *Phys Ther.* 2012;92:1536-1545.
73. Needham DM, Truong AD, Fan E. Technology to enhance physical rehabilitation of critically ill patients. *Crit Care Med.* 2009;37(10 suppl):S436-S441.
74. Greenleaf JE. Intensive exercise training during bed rest attenuates deconditioning. *Med Sci Sports Exerc.* 1997;29:207-215.
75. Kawakami Y, Muraoka Y, Kubo K, et al. Changes in muscle size and architecture following 20 days of bed rest. *J Gravit Physiol.* 2000;7:53-59.

76. Bamman MM, Clarke MS, Feeback DI, et al. Impact of resistance exercise during bed rest on skeletal muscle sarcopenia and myosin isoform distribution. *J Appl Physiol.* 1998;84:157-163.
77. Akima H, Kubo K, Kanehisa H, et al. Leg-press resistance training during 20 days of 6 degrees head-down-tilt bed rest prevents muscle deconditioning. *Eur J Appl Physiol.* 2000;82:30-38.
78. Bamman MM, Hunter GR, Stevens BR, et al. Resistance exercise prevents plantar flexor deconditioning during bed rest. *Med Sci Sports Exerc.* 1997;29:1462-1468.
79. Haruna Y, Suzuki Y, Kawakubo K, et al. Baroreflex during exercise in different postures before and after 20-days bed rest. *J Gravit Physiol.* 1997;4:S53-S57.
80. Burtin C, Clerckx B, Robbeets C, et al. Early exercise in critically ill patients enhances short-term functional recovery. *Crit Care Med.* 2009;37(9):2499-2505.
81. Fagevik Olsén M, Hahn I, Nordgren S, Lönroth H, Lundholm K. Randomized controlled trial of prophylactic chest physiotherapy in major abdominal surgery. *Br J Surg.* 1997;84:1535-1538.
82. Thomas JA, McIntosh JM. Are incentive spirometry, intermittent positive pressure breathing, and deep breathing exercises effective in the prevention of postoperative pulmonary complications after upper abdominal surgery? A systematic overview and meta-analysis. *Phys Ther.* 1994;74:3-10.

Chapter 5

The Immune System and Infectious Diseases and Disorders

Zoher F. Kapasi, PT, PhD, MBA

The primary function of the immune system is to defend the body against infectious microbes—bacteria, viruses, fungi, protozoa, and multicellular parasites. These microbes can cause disease, and, if they multiply unchecked, they will eventually kill their host. The immune system is effective in curtailing most infections in healthy individuals such that infectious disease is short-lived and leaves little permanent damage. In addition to infectious microbes, even noninfectious foreign substances can elicit immune responses. Finally, the immune system also reacts against many tumors. Note that not all immune system responses are helpful, as in the case of organ or tissue transplant rejection (see Chapter 14). Additionally, excessive or inappropriate activity of the immune system can result in different hypersensitivity states, immune complex disease, or autoimmune disease. This chapter will focus on and briefly review the immune responses useful in combating infections, including general clinical manifestations common to most infectious diseases. While discussion of specific infectious diseases is beyond the scope of this chapter, the physical therapist will be provided with guidelines to follow that apply in treating patients with an infectious disease. These guidelines will include the impact of exercise, a therapeutic intervention, on the immune system and infection.

Immune Response to Infection

The microbes that infect our body come in many different forms, and hence, a wide variety of immune responses are required to deal with each type of infection. However, any immune response involves recognition of the pathogen (ie, disease-causing microbe) or other foreign material, and then a reaction to eliminate it. The different types of immune responses fall into 2 categories: innate and adaptive (Table 5-1). **Innate immunity**, also called **natural** or **native immunity**, is constitutional and does not improve on repeated contact with the same infectious agent. Innate immunity is the body's first line of defense to prevent the entry of pathogens. Through mutation, the microbes can

Malone DJ, Bishop KL, eds. *Acute Care Physical Therapy: A Clinician's Guide, Second Edition* (pp 149-176).

Table 5-1

THE IMMUNE RESPONSE

Innate Immunity	*Adaptive Immunity*	
	Humoral	**Cell-Mediated**
Nonspecific interaction with different antigens, lacks immunologic memory	Specific interaction with different antigens, immunologic memory present	Specific interaction with different antigens, immunologic memory present
Exterior defenses: Skin, mucosa, secretions, nasal hair, ear wax	Mediated by antibodies, present as serum globulins	Mediated by T lymphocytes
Soluble mediators: Complement, acute phase proteins and interferons (IFNs)	Antibodies are produced by plasma cells (differentiated form of B lymphocytes)	Production of helper T cells (CD4+) and cytotoxic T cells (CD8+)
Phagocytes (leukocytes): • Neutrophils (polymorphonuclear [PMN] cells) • Monocytes/macrophages dendritic cells • Eosinophils • Basophils	Globulins having antibody activity are called immunoglobulins	Secretion of lymphokines
Mast cells and platelets (inflammation)	Primary and secondary (memory) antibody response	Primary and secondary (memory) T cell response
Natural killer (NK) cells or large granular lymphocytes		

evolve strategies to evade innate defenses; therefore, our body is equipped with **adaptive immunity**. The 2 features of adaptive immunity, also called **acquired** or **specific immunity**, are specificity and memory. An adaptive immune response is highly specific for a particular pathogen and improves with each successive encounter with the same pathogen. In other words, the adaptive immune system remembers the infectious agent and can prevent it from causing disease later due to an improved immune response. There are 2 types of adaptive immune responses, called **humoral** and **cell-mediated immunity**, which are mediated by different components of the immune system and function to eliminate different types of microbes (Figure 5-1).

INNATE IMMUNITY

The components of innate immunity include exterior defenses, like skin; soluble mediators, like complement, acute-phase proteins, and IFNs; cells that are involved in phagocytosis and inflammation (ie, neutrophils, macrophages, dendritic cells, eosinophils, basophils, mast cells), and NK cells.

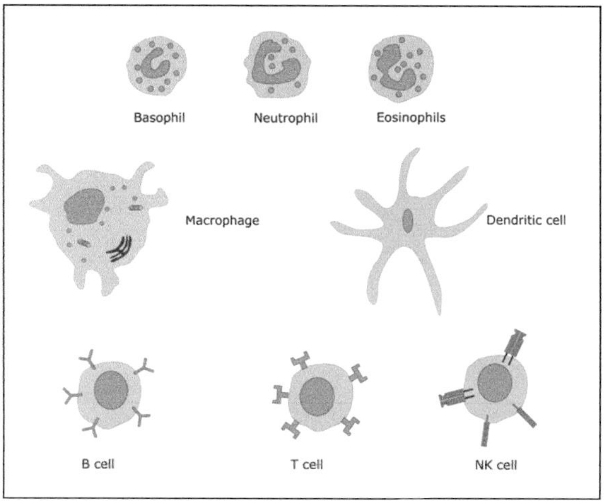

Figure 5-1. Main cells of immune system. (ellepigrafica/Shutterstock.com)

Exterior Defenses

Infection can be avoided by preventing the microbes from gaining access to the body. When intact, the skin is impermeable to most infectious agents. Infection becomes a major problem when there is skin loss, as in burns. In areas where there are openings in the body (eg, mouth, nostrils, ears, eyes), unique protection is provided. For example, saliva and stomach acid destroy organisms ingested through the mouth. Nasal hair and secretions protect against microbes entering the nostrils. A waxy secretion prevents microbes from advancing inside the ear canal. The washing action and presence of lysozyme in tears can kill bacteria in the eye. Finally, protective low pH of vaginal secretions and acidic urine protect the genitourinary (GU) openings. When microbes enter the body by penetrating the skin or the epithelial surface of the respiratory, gastrointestinal (GI), or GU tract, 2 main defensive operations come into play: the destructive effect of soluble mediators and the mechanism of phagocytosis carried out by the phagocytes. Components of the innate immune system are able to distinguish self from non-self by recognizing surface markers such as lipids, polysaccharides, and proteins that do not occur in the host (Figure 5-2).

Soluble Mediators

The complement system is a group of about 20 serum proteins produced by the liver that have an intrinsic ability to recognize microbial components and antibodies (produced by B cells during the humoral immune response) bound to the microbe. The complement system of proteins can lyse the cell membranes of many bacterial species. Complement products released in this reaction attract phagocytes to the site of the reaction (ie, **chemotaxis**). Furthermore, complement components can coat the bacterial surface (ie, **opsonization**) allowing the phagocytes to recognize the bacteria and engulf them. A number of serum proteins increase rapidly during infection and tissue injury and are, therefore, collectively called **acute phase proteins** (C-reactive and mannose binding proteins). The acute phase proteins bind to microbes and promote their uptake by phagocytes (ie, opsonization). IFNs are important in limiting the spread of certain viral infections. IFNα and IFNβ are produced by cells that have become virally infected, and IFNγ is released by certain activated T cells. IFNs induce a state of antiviral resistance in surrounding uninfected tissue cells. The IFNs are produced very early in infection and are the first line of resistance to several viral infections. The ability of the innate immune response to limit microbes early in the

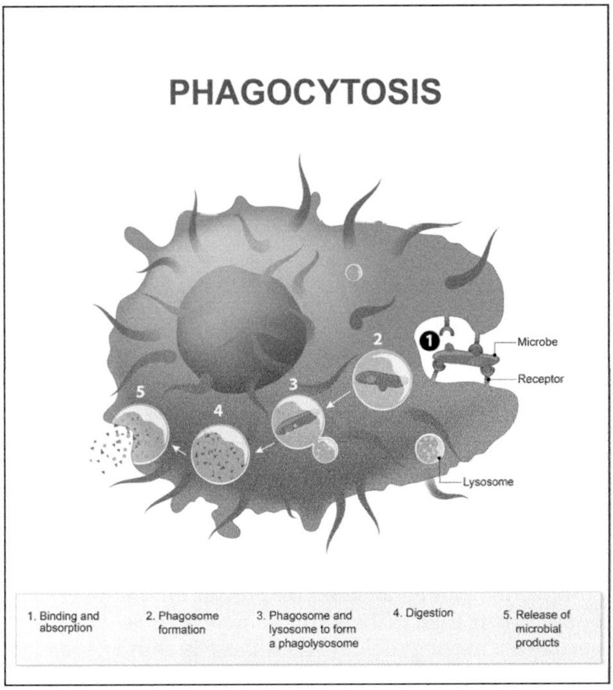

Figure 5-2. Example of innate immunity where a macrophage has recognized an invading microbe as non-self and is destroying the bacteria by phagocytosis. (Designua/Shutterstock.com)

infectious process results from binding of the microbes to the pattern recognition receptors, such as Toll-like receptors on leukocytes, which in turn initiates the signaling events that lead to complement activation and phagocytosis. Invading pathogens contain conserved structures in their cell membranes, termed **pathogen-associated molecular patterns**, which are recognized by the cells of the innate immune system through the pattern recognition receptors.

Neutrophils

The function of ingesting and destroying microbes is mediated by phagocytes, which include **neutrophils**, early in the innate immune response and macrophages later in the response. Because of their multi-lobed nucleus, neutrophils are also called **PMN cells** and are the most abundant leukocytes (white blood cells [WBCs]). Neutrophils are short lived (2 to 3 days) relative to monocytes/macrophages, which may live for months or years. The importance of these cells is evident in individuals with reduced white blood cell numbers, such as following chemotherapy or radiotherapy in cancer or with rare genetic defects that prevent PMN emigration in tissues in response to chemotactic stimuli. Both defects markedly increase susceptibility to infection.

Macrophages

Macrophages are big eaters. Macrophages develop from blood monocytes after monocytes enter into tissues. Macrophages are particularly concentrated in the lung (alveolar macrophages), liver (Kupffer cells), and lining of spleen sinusoids and lymph node medullary sinuses where they are strategically placed to filter foreign material, including microbes. Macrophages persist much longer at sites of inflammation and are the dominant effector cells of the later stages of the innate immune response, 1 or 2 days after infection.

Neutrophils and macrophages both have receptors for complement and antibodies (opsonins), so coating of microbes with opsonins enhances phagocytosis (see Figure 5-2).

Dendritic Cells

Dendritic cells, a heterogeneous family of cells with long dendrite-like cytoplasmic processes, are constitutively present in epithelia and most tissues of the body. Because of their placement and morphology, these cells are poised to detect invading microbes. In addition to phagocytosis, dendritic cells and macrophages process and present antigens in the initiation of immune response acting as a major initiator of the adaptive immune response. Dendritic cells take up microbial protein antigens, transport them to lymph nodes where naive T cells home, and display the protein antigens in a form that the T cells can recognize and thus trigger and direct the adaptive immune response. Thus, dendritic cells act as a bridge between the innate and adaptive immune response.

Eosinophils

Eosinophils are derived from bone marrow like other WBCs and are involved in destroying large parasites that cannot physically be phagocytosed. Eosinophils secrete chemicals that damage the parasite's membrane leading to organism destruction.

Basophils, Mast Cells, and Platelets

These play a role in immunity against microbes by releasing mediators that enhance inflammation. In particular, mediators such as histamine, released by basophils and mast cells, propagate inflammatory reactions controlling parasitic infections.

Natural Killer Cells

NK cells are large, granular lymphocytes that are neither T nor B lymphocytes. The function of NK cells is to kill viruses, other intracellular microbe infected cells, and tumor cells. NK cells account for 15% of blood lymphocytes.

Adaptive Immunity

While innate immunity provides early defense against pathogenic microbes, adaptive immunity is the later reaction. Adaptive immunity enhances the protective mechanisms of innate immunity and directs these mechanisms to sites of infection. Adaptive immune responses to microbes induce effector cells that eliminate the microbes and activate memory cells that protect the individual from subsequent infections, so-called **protective immunity**. There are 2 types of adaptive immune responses: humoral and cell-mediated immunity (Figure 5-3).

Humoral Immunity

Humoral immunity is the mechanism of defense against extracellular microbes (including viruses before they enter a cell) and their toxins. It is mediated by antibodies present in different secretions (humors) such as saliva, blood, or vaginal secretions. Humoral immunity is mediated by B lymphocytes or B cells (called as such because they originate and mature in **bone marrow**, a primary lymphoid organ). Each B cell can recognize a specific antigen and then proliferate and differentiate into

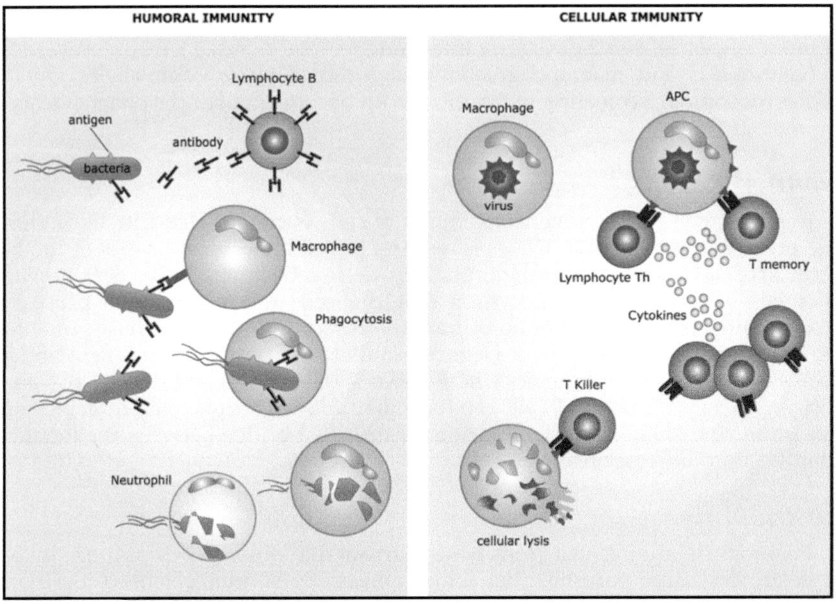

Figure 5-3. The main subdivision of the adaptive immune system: humoral immunity and cellular immunity. (ellepigrafica/Shutterstock.com)

antibody-producing plasma cells or B memory cells. The plasma cells produce antibodies of different isotypes, like IgG, IgA, IgM, IgD, and IgE (serum globulins having antibody activity are called **immunoglobulins** [Ig]). Antibodies combat infections by numerous mechanisms. High-affinity antibodies bind to and neutralize microbes and their toxins. Antibodies of different isotypes perform different effector functions. Some IgG antibodies opsonize microbes and are recognized by phagocytes with subsequent ingestion and degradation of the microbes. IgM and some IgG antibodies bound to microbes activate the complement system and promote phagocytosis and lysis of the microbes. IgA antibodies are secreted through mucosal epithelia and neutralize microbes in the lumens of mucosal organs, such as the GI tract. In pregnant people, some IgG antibodies are transported through the placenta and later IgA antibodies are transported via the breast milk to provide passive immunity to the newborn while the immune system is developing. Memory B cells circulate throughout the body and are responsible for the more rapid and stronger immune response that occurs with repeated exposure to the same antigen.

Cell-Mediated Immunity

Cell-mediated immunity is the mechanism of defense against intracellular microbes that are either ingested by and survive in phagocytes or infect nonphagocytic cells. As antibodies cannot reach inside the cell, cell-mediated immunity is necessary to destroy the microbes inside a cell. T lymphocytes or T cells (called as such because their precursors arise in bone marrow and mature in thymus, primary lymphoid organs) mediate this form of immunity. T cells are classified as CD4 or CD8 T cells (based on distinctive molecules called cluster designation [CD] present on their cell surface). CD4 T cells are generally referred to as **helper T cells** and CD8 T cells are also called **cytotoxic T lymphocytes** (CTLs). CD4 T cells secrete cytokines (protein molecules that encompass molecules such as interleukins, lymphokines, monokines, and IFN) that activate macrophages to destroy microbes and also help B cells augment antibody production. CTLs recognize peptide antigens of microbes, such as viruses, that infect and survive or replicate in the cytoplasm of any nucleated host cell. Once the CTLs recognize the cell in which the microbe is hiding, they secrete granule proteins and express surface molecules that kill the infected cells and, thereby, eliminate a reservoir of infection. Finally, regulatory T lymphocytes are a subset of CD4 T cells whose function is to suppress immune responses and prevent inappropriate responses against self antigens (ie, to maintain self-tolerance). A possibility exists that defects in these cells may result in various autoimmune diseases.

The complexity of the cellular interactions that occur during adaptive immune responses requires specialized microenvironments in which relevant cells can collaborate efficiently. These microenvironments are provided in secondary lymphoid organs. Secondary lymphoid organs include lymph nodes that filter lymph, the spleen that filters blood, and mucosal-associated lymphoid tissues, such as tonsils, adenoids, and Peyer's patches in the small intestine, that handle microbes that enter thorough the nasal and oral cavity. Because only a few lymphocytes are specific for any given antigen, T cells and B cells need to migrate throughout the body in blood and secondary lymphoid organs to increase the probability that they will encounter that particular antigen.

Infectious Disease

Infectious disease occurs when pathogens cause signs and symptoms of illness. The interactions between a host, such as a human, and the microbes that reside on or in the host are not always detrimental and in certain situations may benefit both organisms. Harmless inhabitation of the skin and mucous membranes by these microbes is called **colonization**. Normal flora that reside in the host can become opportunistic pathogens, capable of producing an infectious disease when the immunity of the host is compromised.

Factors Affecting Immunity

Immunity of the host is weakened by several factors. For example, skin and mucous membrane that act as important mechanical and biochemical barriers are compromised in patients with incisions, intravenous or urinary catheters, endotracheal tubes, chest tubes, and other invasive monitoring catheters. Adequate nutrition is necessary to maintain a healthy immune system. Malnutrition (eg, protein-energy malnutrition, vitamin and trace element deficiencies) is a risk factor for development of infections. Chronic illnesses, such as diabetes, cancer, heart disease, and renal failure, are associated with an increased risk of infection. Diabetes alters the host's ability to resist infection. Phagocytosis is impaired with hyperglycemia, and detection of pain from infection may be delayed because of neuropathies. The virulence of some microbes is increased when exposed to hyperglycemic conditions. Circulatory problems associated with cardiac failure or peripheral vascular disease are risk factors for infection because the cellular components of the immune system and antimicrobial agents are dependent on the circulatory system for delivery to the site of infection. Many pathogens thrive in areas with poor tissue perfusion. Age of the host is an important variable in the ability to resist infections. Infants are at an increased risk for infection because of an immature immune system. The elderly are more susceptible to infection because immune function declines with aging, leading to greater morbidity and mortality. The lungs and the urinary tract are the most common sites of infection in the elderly. Infection in the elderly may also be manifested atypically, with absence of fever and sudden onset of confusion. Finally, a host may be immunocompromised due to defects in one or more components of the immune system, as in AIDS wherein the HIV destroys the CD4 T cells. Agents such as antimetabolites, corticosteroids, cyclosporine, and antibiotics can cause immunosuppression. Surgery and anesthesia can also suppress both T and B cell function for up to 1 month postoperatively. Stress has been implicated in predisposing individuals to an infectious process by causing release of stress hormones that are known to depress immune function. Sleep deprivation, similar to stress, depresses cellular immunity.

Transmission of Infection

For infection to be transmitted, the microbe must be transported from an infected source to a susceptible host. The 6 main routes of transmission are as follows:

1. Contact
2. Airborne
3. Droplet
4. Vehicle
5. Vectorborne
6. Nosocomial infection

Contact transmission occurs directly or indirectly. Direct contact is the transfer of microbes that come into physical contact either by skin-to-skin or mucous membrane-to-mucous membrane (eg, sexual contact, biting, touching, kissing). Indirect contact involves transfer of microbes from a source to a host by passive transfer from an inanimate, intermediate object, called a **fomite**. Inanimate objects include assistive devices, goniometer, cuff weights, sphygmomanometer, bedside rail, tray tables, cellphones, or any item that comes in direct contact with the infected person.

Airborne transmission occurs when microbes are so small (<5 µm) that they float on air currents within a room and remain suspended for several hours. They are often propelled from the respiratory tract through coughing or sneezing. A host then inhales the particles directly into the respiratory tract (eg, tuberculosis, chickenpox).

Droplet transmission is different from airborne transmission because droplets are larger particles (>5 µm) and, therefore, do not remain suspended in air but fall within 3 feet of the source. Droplets are produced when a person coughs or sneezes and transmission occurs when droplets containing the microorganisms are propelled a short distance through air and are deposited on another person's conjunctiva, nasal mucosa, or mouth. An example of droplet transmission of a microbe is the influenza virus. People in closest proximity to the infected source have the highest risk for infection through droplet transmission.

Vehicle transmission occurs when infectious organisms (eg, *Salmonella*) are transmitted through a common source (eg, contaminated food, water, intravenous fluid) to susceptible hosts.

Vectorborne transmission of infectious organisms involves insects and/or animals that act as intermediaries between 2 or more hosts. Lyme disease, Rocky Mountain spotted fever, and Creutzfeldt-Jakob disease are examples of vectorborne diseases.

An infection acquired during hospitalization of a patient is referred to as **nosocomial infection**. Nosocomial infections result in prolongation of hospital stays, increases in cost of care, significant morbidity, and can result in death. The most common infections are urinary tract infections (UTIs; usually associated with Foley catheters or urologic procedures) or bloodstream infections. Prevention is of critical importance in controlling nosocomial infections. Please note that to include places other than hospitals and nursing homes where care is provided to patients, such as outpatient surgery centers and dialysis centers, the Centers for Disease Control and Prevention now prefers the term **health care–associated infection** rather than nosocomial.

Clinical Presentation and Management of Infectious Disease

Clinical presentation of infectious disease depends on the type of infecting microbe (eg, bacteria, virus) and the body system affected (eg, GU, GI, nervous system, cardiopulmonary system). The symptoms of an infectious disease may be specific and reflect the site of infection. For example, painful urination (dysuria) can result from a UTIs, a skin rash and red streaks can represent a manifestation of a skin infection, and diarrhea can result from a GI infection. Conversely, systemic symptoms, such as fever, chills, sweating, malaise, and myalgia, are shared by a number of diverse infectious diseases. Elderly persons may experience a change in mentation (eg, confusion, memory loss, difficulty concentrating).

Infections can cause a hypermetabolic state that presents clinically as an increase in heart rate (HR), respiratory rate (RR), and blood pressure (BP). However, BP can decrease secondary to vasodilation from inflammatory responses in the body. Inflammatory response to infection can also lead to an increase in erythrocyte sedimentation rate and leukocyte or WBC count. A differential WBC count (granulocytes—neutrophils, basophils, and eosinophils; lymphocytes and monocytes) can assist in identification of the type of infection. For example, a bacterial infection leads to an increase in neutrophils, whereas a parasitic infection leads to increased eosinophils in blood.

In addition to clinical presentation, diagnosis of infectious disease requires the recovery of a probable pathogen or evidence of its presence from the infected sites of a disease host. In the laboratory, the diagnosis of an infectious agent is accomplished using 3 basic techniques:

1. Culture
2. Serology
3. Direct antigen detection

Culture refers to the propagation of a microbe outside the body using an artificial growth media, such as agar plates or broth. The specimen (eg, urine, feces, sputum, cerebrospinal fluid, pleural fluid, synovial fluid) from the diseased host is inoculated into broth or placed on the surface of an agar plate, and the culture is placed in an incubator until the growth of the microbe becomes detectable. In the case of bacteria, identification is based on microscopic appearance and Gram's stain reaction (positive or negative), shape, texture, and color (ie, morphology) of the colonies. **Serology**, the study of serum, is an indirect means of identifying infectious agents by measuring serum antibodies in the diseased host. **Direct antigen detection** relies on purified antibodies to detect antigens of infectious agents in specimens obtained from a diseased host. Identification of microbes is also done through detection of sequences of DNA or RNA unique to that microbe using techniques like DNA probe hybridization and polymerase chain reaction. Each technique has a different degree of sensitivity regarding the number of microbes that need to be present in a specimen for detection. Most infectious diseases of humans are self-limiting and require little or no medical therapy for a complete cure; however, when therapeutic intervention is essential the choice of treatment may be use of the following:

- Antimicrobial agents (see Pharmacological Information)
- Immunologic therapies with antibody preparations, vaccine, or substances that stimulate and improve the host's immune function, such as cytokines
- Surgery to remove infected tissues

Physical Therapy Implications

Physical therapists and physical therapist assistants need to be aware of 2-tier precautions that have to be followed in an acute-care hospital setting—standard and transmission-based precautions—related to infection control.

Standard precautions are designed for the care of all patients in hospitals regardless of their diagnosis or presumed infection status. Implementation of standard precautions is the primary strategy for successfully controlling nosocomial/hospital-acquired infections. Standard precautions are designed to reduce the risk of transmission of blood-borne pathogens and reduce the risk of transmission of pathogens from moist body substances. Standard precautions apply to:

- Blood
- All body fluids, secretions, and excretions, except sweat, regardless of whether or not they contain visible blood
- Non-intact skin
- Mucous membranes

Standard precautions are designed to reduce the risk of transmission of microbes from both recognized and unrecognized sources of infection in hospitals. Use **personal protective equipment** to implement barrier precautions:

- All health care workers should routinely use appropriate barrier precautions to prevent skin and mucous membrane exposure when contact with blood or body fluids or generation of droplets is anticipated. For whirlpool or pulsatile lavage with suction consider hair coverings, masks, face shields, and protective eyewear to protect mucus membranes of the eyes, nose, and mouth. Shoulder length gloves should be available for those working with whirlpools, but may fill with contaminated water, limiting effectiveness.
- Gloves should be worn for touching blood and body fluids, mucous membranes, and non-intact skin of all persons.
- Gloves should be changed and hands washed after contact with each client.
- Hand cream should be applied after glove removal to prevent skin chapping, which is a potential risk factor for employees. Petroleum-based hand creams or lotions should not be used, which can damage latex gloves.
- Fluid-resistant gowns or aprons should be worn during procedures that are likely to generate splashes of blood or other body fluids.
- Hand hygiene (ie, hand washing or use of alcohol-based hand rubs) should be practiced before and after client contact and after removing personal protective equipment.
- Hands and other skin surfaces should be washed immediately and thoroughly if contaminated with blood or other body fluids. If hands are visibly soiled, they should be washed with soap and water immediately after gloves are removed. However, if hands are not visibly soiled, an alcohol-based hand hygiene product is the preferred method of hand cleansing.
- Sharp instruments, such as scissors or scalpels, should be handled with great care and disposed of in puncture-resistant containers. Needles should never be manipulated, bent, broken, or recapped.
- Pocket masks or mechanical ventilation devices should be available in areas in which cardiopulmonary resuscitation procedures are likely.
- Health care workers who have exudative lesions or weeping dermatitis should refrain from all direct client care and from handling equipment belonging to the client until the condition resolves.
- Eating, drinking, applying lip balm or lipstick, and handling contact lenses is prohibited in any area where clients or their body fluids are present.

Note that hand hygiene has been cited as the easiest and most effective means of preventing nosocomial infection and must be done routinely, even when gloves are used. Before beginning handwashing with soap and water, prepare to have access to a paper towel. This will ensure that once the hands are cleansed, the health care worker does not contaminate his or her hands by touching the paper towel dispenser. Moisten hands before applying soap to ensure that the soap starts lathering as soon as it touches the hands. Avoid using hot water, because repeated exposure to hot water may increase the risk of dermatitis. Effective handwashing technique involves scrubbing for at least 15 seconds (as long as it takes to sing "Happy Birthday" or "Twinkle, Twinkle Little Star" twice). Both sides of both hands must be scrubbed along with wrists, web space between the fingers, and under the nails. Use a paper towel to turn off the faucet and if leaving the room use the paper towel to open the door before discarding the towel. When dealing with antimicrobial-resistant Gram-positive cocci (eg, methicillin-resistant *Staphylococcus aureus* [MRSA], vancomycin-resistant *Enterococci*), an antimicrobial soap is recommended. When using an alcohol-based hand rub, apply product to palm of one hand and rub hands together, covering all surfaces of hands and fingers, until hands are dry. Note that the volume needed to reduce the number of bacteria on hands varies by product. Alcohol-based hand rubs significantly reduce the number of microbes on skin, are fast acting, cause less skin irritation, and take less time to use than traditional hand washing. Health care personnel should avoid wearing artificial nails and keep natural nails less than ¼-inch long if they care for patients at high risk of acquiring infections. Hand hygiene must be practiced after taking gloves off and before touching anything and before and after each and every client (before to protect the client and after to protect yourself and others). Do not touch a chart with gloved hands. Apart from hand hygiene, every health care worker should be adequately immunized against hepatitis B, influenza (every year), measles, mumps, rubella, polio, tetanus, diphtheria, and varicella to control nosocomial infections. As UTIs associated with Foley catheter is a common nosocomial infection, a physical therapist should take certain precautions (over and above the standard precautions) when handling the drainage bag while working with the client. Before turning, moving, or transferring a catheterized person, locate the proximal end of the tubing and either clamp it to the person's gown or hold it to allow necessary slack during movement. This will help prevent the catheter from accidentally and traumatically being pulled out. Avoid raising the drainage bag above the level of the person's bladder to prevent backflow of the urine from the tube toward the bladder. If it becomes necessary to raise the bag during transfers, clamp the tubing to prevent backflow as you move the bag and then release the clamp. Avoid allowing large loops of tubing to dangle from the bedside, wheelchair, or walker. Drain all the urine from tubing into the bag before the person exercises or ambulates.

Transmission-based precautions are designed for patients documented or suspected to be infected or colonized with highly transmissible or epidemiologically important pathogens for which additional precautions beyond standard precautions are needed to interrupt transmission in hospitals. There are 3 types of **transmission-based precautions:**

1. Airborne precautions
2. Droplet precautions
3. Contact precautions

They may be combined for diseases that have multiple routes of transmission. When used either singularly or in combination, they are to be used in addition to standard precautions. Make sure to identify each client's individual transmission precautions and procedures. When in doubt, ask the nursing staff regarding the status of the person in question. Some transmission-based precautions include:

- Private, negative pressure room (airborne transmission isolation room) with doors kept closed (note that airborne transmission isolation room is not required for droplet or contact transmission-based precautions).
- Wear a mask when entering the room (for airborne and droplet transmission-based precautions).

- Limit transport of client from room. Place surgical mask on client when transported.
- Remove gown and gloves before leaving client environment, wash hands immediately with antimicrobial soap, and then do not touch potentially contaminated materials or surfaces as you leave the room (for contact transmission-based precautions).
- Dedicate use of non-critical client care items to only this person (eg, leave the stethoscope, gait belt, cuff weights, goniometer, and assistive devices in the client's room; for contact transmission-based precautions).
- Disinfect equipment with approved disinfectant prior to use with other people (for contact transmission-based precautions).

Optimizing the client's mobility and endurance are frequently the goals of physical therapy in an acute care setting, and, consequently, the physical therapist should be aware of the effects of physical exercise on immune function. A detailed review[1] of these effects is beyond the scope of this chapter; however, the physical therapist should be aware that intense exercise (exercising at >80% of maximum oxygen consumption [VO_{2max}]) is known to suppress immune function, particularly in young individuals. The immune system takes 6 to 24 hours to recover from the acute effects of intense exercise. Each individual client must be evaluated after exercise to determine the perceived intensity of the exercise or intervention session. For example, in the deconditioned older adult with compromised cardiopulmonary function, reduced oxygen transport, and impaired mobility, ambulating from the bed to the bathroom may be perceived by his or her body as intense exercise. However, in a recent study, intense exercise was shown not to have a detrimental effect on immune function and incidence of infections in the elderly.[2] While the suppressive effects of exercise on immune function may differ between young and elderly persons, intense exercise during an infectious episode should be avoided in both young and elderly clients. For anyone (especially competitive athletes) wondering whether or not to exercise in the presence of acute bacterial or viral infection (eg, when manifesting constitutional symptoms), do a **neck check**. If the symptoms are located above the neck, such as stuffy or runny nose, sneezing, or a scratchy throat, exercise should be performed cautiously through the scheduled workout at half the usual intensity and duration. If, after 10 minutes, the symptoms are alleviated, the workout can be completed using the usual exercise prescription (ie, frequency/intensity/duration). If, instead, the symptoms are worse, and the head is pounding or throbbing with every footstep, the exercise program should be stopped, and the person should rest. If there is fever or there are symptoms below the neck, such as aching muscles, a hacking cough, diarrhea, or vomiting, exercise should not be initiated. Finally, because of vasodilation occurring from inflammation associated with infection, patients may experience orthostatic hypotension and hypotension with functional activities. Consequently, frequent BP monitoring and gradual changes in positions, particularly from recumbent to upright positions, are important to promote tolerance to functional activities.

Summary

The immune system protects the body against pathogens by means of innate and adaptive immunity. Infectious disease occurs when the pathogen overwhelms the immune system resulting in signs and symptoms of the disease. Immune function is compromised by several factors, including malnutrition, loss of skin integrity, coexisting chronic illnesses (eg, diabetes, stress), drugs (eg, steroids), and the age of the patient (ie, elderly and children), and may predispose a person to infection. The physical therapist and physical therapist assistants should follow standard and transmission-based precautions to ensure infection control. Moreover, the therapist should understand the impact of exercise on the immune response and tailor mobility and endurance exercise programs to the clinical presentation of the infectious disease the client is manifesting.

Case Study

A 66-year-old male, Mr. O'Baxter, diagnosed with type 2 diabetes, is admitted with fever and a large ulcer on the plantar surface of the right foot. In the past 2 days, the amount of drainage from the ulcer has increased. Physical therapy is consulted for wound management.

Patient/Client History

General Demographics, Social History, and Living Environment

Mr. O'Baxter lives with his wife and children on the third floor of a walk-up apartment building. He is formerly employed as a manager of a construction company. He presently works part time helping in his wife's dry cleaning business.

General Health Status, Social/Health Habits, and Family History

Mr. O'Baxter quit smoking 2 years ago after smoking for 25 years (50 packs/year). He states he enjoys a beer a couple times/week.

Medical/Surgical History

Past medical history includes a positive annual PPD (purified protein derivative) tuberculin skin tests with negative chest x-rays since returning from Vietnam several years ago. Patient completed 6 months of INH (isoniazid) chemotherapy after his positive PPD.

Current Conditions

Mr. O'Baxter is complaining of right foot discomfort, fever, and a noticeable increase in drainage in his right sock and shoe. On physical examination, the patient has a fever of 101.8°F with decreased breath sounds in left apical lung fields and a frequent dry cough. The chest x-ray shows a suspicious 2.5-cm diameter area of consolidation in left apical lobe. The dorsal surface of his right foot is red with induration from mid-foot distally. There is a large callous with an ulcer draining large amounts of malodorous purulent material on the plantar surface of the right foot. The wound is covered with fibrous yellow and black necrotic debris and wound depth is unable to be determined. The patient is on full respiratory precautions until cleared by infection control. Sputum cultures have been sent to the lab.

Activities and Participation

Mr. O'Baxter was functionally independent prior to the foot infection.

Other Clinical Tests

Laboratory findings reveal the following data: hemoglobin (Hb) A1C 9.9% (elevated), WBC 11,560/mm^3 (elevated), creatinine 1.5 mg/dL (elevated), and Ankle Brachial Index of 0.8 (moderate disease).

Systems Review

Cardiovascular and Pulmonary

Resting vital signs (VS) in bed (head of bed raised >45 degrees) are oxygen saturation (SpO_2) 94% on 0.35 F_IO_2 (35%) via face mask, HR 108 beats per minute (bpm), pulse regular, RR 24 breaths/minute with accessory muscle use, BP 108/76 mm Hg, and pain 2/10 with right foot elevated in bed. Breath sounds are decreased in left apical lung fields and a frequent dry cough. Patient is on respiratory precautions. Following transfers and ambulation, his VS were 95% SpO_2, HR 114 bpm, RR 32 breaths/minute, BP 110/76 mm Hg, and pain 4/10.

Integumentary

The dorsal surface of the right foot is red with induration from mid-foot distally. There is a large callous surrounding an ulcer draining large amounts of purulent material on the plantar surface of the right foot. The wound is covered with fibrous yellow and black necrotic debris. The wound measures 5 cm across and 3 cm in width. No depth was measured at this time.

Musculoskeletal

Manual Muscle Test (MMT), range of motion (ROM) of bilateral upper extremities (BUE) and left lower extremity are all within normal limits (WNL). Right lower extremity hip/knee MMT and ROM are also WNL. Ankle motion appears intact, but due to pain on movement did not fully assess.

Neuromuscular

BUE sensation intact, sharp/dull diminished below bilateral knees. Bed mobility (rolling, supine to sit) is independent (Functional Independence Measure [FIM] 7) and non-weightbearing sit-to-stand transfers to a bedside chair requires minimal assistance and verbal cues (FIM 4). He ambulates 10 feet with minimal assistance and a walker (FIM 2).

Communication, Affect, Cognition, Language, and Learning Style

Mr. O'Baxter is awake, alert, and oriented x 4. He does complain of chills and discomfort. His primary language is English.

Tests and Measures

Aerobic Capacity and Endurance

Mr. O'Baxter demonstrated elevated resting HR, RR and apparent respiratory distress with accessory muscle usage. His VS responses during functional examination (transfers, short distance ambulation) were appropriate, although he appears short of breath and uses his accessory muscles during minimal activity, suggesting poor endurance. Laboratory findings support poor diabetes management, probable infection, renal insufficiency, and large vessel disease most likely from complications of diabetes. Await sputum results for tuberculosis/acid fast bacilli screen.

Assistive and Adaptive Devices

Recommend a standard walker for the patient's room to assist with non-weightbearing transfers and eventual ambulation.

Balance, Gait, and Mobility (Including Locomotion)

At this time, transfers and short distance ambulation were attempted. He ambulates 10 feet with minimal assistance and a walker (FIM 2). Patient's static and dynamic balance were fair, but he did require minimal assistance during gait activities.

Pain

Mr. O'Baxter had increased pain with non-weightbearing transfers. This may change with further wound management. Pain control should be optimized prior to and during future therapy sessions.

EVALUATION

Mr. O'Baxter's functional limitations are related to his non-weightbearing status and limited pulmonary reserve. The provision of physical therapy services is challenged by his remaining in a private negative pressure isolation room. Appropriate wound care and medical management should enable this elderly man to return to his home.

DIAGNOSIS

Mr. O'Baxter presents with a respiratory impairment as well as a non-healing wound in his right lower extremity. He needs to remain on full respiratory precautions until his cultures return and rule out tuberculosis. He will have to be treated bedside for wound care.

PROGNOSIS

Diabetes impairs immune function, and chronic illnesses like diabetes are associated with increased infection risk. Furthermore, immune function declines with aging and infection in the elderly is associated with greater morbidity and mortality. Although there is a history of a positive skin test for exposure to tuberculosis, the patient completed preventive drug therapy. However, because the patient's immune system is depressed, there is a possibility for reactivation of the infection. The patient's cough and the small area of consolidation on the chest x-ray made it necessary to put the patient on respiratory precautions. These precautions include housing the patient in a private room with doors closed and continuous negative pressure airflow. Finally, because the patient has a fever, he should be advised to balance rest with activities that are not exhausting. He is restricted to bathroom privileges and ambulation with assistance and within his room only.

INTERVENTION

Recommend aggressive wound care as well as deep breathing and active ROM exercises to prevent possible pneumonia from limited activity. Gait, transfer, and wheelchair training are performed maintaining non-weightbearing until independent with use of walker.

ICF Clinical Reasoning Tool Case Study Summary

Health Condition

HPI: Fever, inflammation of dorsum and large ulcer on plantar surface of right foot, consolidation left apical lobe, type 2 diabetes, leukocytosis, decreased iron, elevated creatinine, hypoxic, neuropathic pain
PMHx: Poorly controlled type 2 diabetes, nonsmoker >2 years, +annual TB skin test

Precautions/Contraindications

Negative CXR (completed 6 months of INH), negative isolation room
Risk management: Active pulmonary TB infection, depression, poor wound healing, CAD, renal insufficiency

Body Structure and Function			*Activity/Task Limitations*			*Participation*		
Impairment/ Problem	*Tests and Measures*	*Intervention*	*Activity*	*Tests and Measures*	*Intervention*	*Participation*	*Tests and Measures*	*Intervention*
• Elevated RR • Decreased breath sounds • Impaired gas exchange • Decreased LE sensation • Impaired ROM and strength • Decreased endurance • Impaired wound healing • Pain • Fever • Edema • Abnormal lab values	• VS including BS and SpO_2 • Pulmonary examination • Sensation testing (monofilament) • Grade pitting edema • ROM/MMT • Wound examination • ABI • Pain • Temperature	• Breathing exercises • Bedside ROM • Progressive resistance exercises • Education on wound care and NWB status • Consult registered dietician and diabetes educator	• ADLs • Bed mobility • Transfers • Gait • Balance	• Functional task analysis • FIM	• Progressive functional mobility training while maintaining NWB status • Supervised OOB activity due to fall risk • Pain and wound management education	• Unable to return to work	• QoL: SF-36 • Disease-specific QoL: DQoL	• Continue physical therapy services • Consult social worker and family regarding discharge plan

(continued)

ICF Clinical Reasoning Tool Case Study Summary (continued)

Personal Factors	*Other Considerations*	*Environmental Factors*
• Age: 66 y/o male • Primary language: English • Married, lives with wife and children • Prior to admission independent with all ADLs and functional level • Formerly employed as manager construction company • Presently works part-time at wife's dry cleaning business • 25-year history of smoking • Self-management of diabetes		Home: • 3rd floor walk-up apartment building Hospital: • Airborne precautions, supplemental oxygen devices, communication, bedside wound care and physical therapy intervention

ABI = Ankle Brachial Index; ADLs = activities of daily living; AM-PAC = Activity Measure for Post Acute Care; CAD = coronary artery disease; CXR = chest roentogram; DQoL = Diabetes Quality of Life Measure; HPI = history of present illness; INH = isoniazid; NWB = non-weightbearing; OOB = out of bed; PMHx = past medical history; QoL = quality of life; SF = Short Form; TB = mycobacterium tuberculosis; y/o = year old.

Adapted from American Physical Therapy Association. *Guide to Physical Therapist Practice*. 3rd ed. http://www.apta.org/Guide/. Updated October 21, 2015. Accessed October 5, 2018 and *Towards a Common Language for Functioning, Disability and Health*. World Health Organization. www.who.int/classifications/icf/icfbeginnersguide.pdf. Published 2002. Accessed April 29, 2019.

Reexamination

Mr. O'Baxter remains on full respiratory precautions, is independent with mobility (FIM 7) within the confines of his room, and bedside wound care continues. He can independently use a wheelchair for locomotion less than 500 feet (FIM 7). Ambulation distance is limited to 150 feet x2 (FIM 7) due to complaints of fatigue and shortness of breath.

Outcomes

Recommend continued outpatient wound care once cleared to leave hospital.

Chapter Review Questions

1. The following is the primary function of the immune system:
    a. Defends against opportunistic infections via phagocytosis
    b. Defends against infectious microbes like bacteria and viruses
    c. Defends against innate immune infections via macrophages
    d. Defends against autoimmune reactions
2. Which of the following best describes the 2 types of immunity?
    a. Neutrophils and soluble mediators
    b. Eosinophils and macrophages
    c. Adaptive and innate
    d. Humeral and lymphokines
3. The clinical presentation of an infectious disease includes:
    a. Malaise, decreased WBCs, and elevated neutrophils
    b. Chills, increased eosinophils in blood, and constipation
    c. Sweating, increased erythrocyte sedimentation rate, and mentation change in the elderly
    d. Myalgia, decreased granulocytes, and hypometabolic state
4. Which of the following are standard and transmission-based precautions for infection control?
    a. Wash hands immediately with alcohol-based hand sanitizer if exposed to blood
    b. Utilize gowns and gloves to avoid airborne pathogens
    c. Gloves and hand washing with alcohol-based sanitizer for all hospital patient contact
    d. Wear gown and gloves when entering a room labeled droplet transmission precautions

5. Which of the following best represents immune system function and infectious diseases?
   a. If patient has a fever, diarrhea, and LE muscle aches, reduce exercise intensity in half
   b. Immune function is enhanced when exercise is performed at greater than 80% maximum oxygen consumption
   c. Immune function requires 6 hours to normalize if exercise is performed at less than 40% maximum oxygen consumption
   d. Use the above the neck check and patient symptoms as a guide to prescribing a reduced exercise intensity

Answers: 1b, 2c, 3c, 4c, 5d

References

1. Goodman CC, Kapasi ZF. The effect of exercise on the immune system. *Rehabilitation Oncology*. 2002;20(1):13-15.
2. Kapasi ZF, Ouslander JG, Schnelle JF, Kutner M, Fahey JL. Effects of an exercise intervention on immunologic parameters in frail elderly nursing home residents. *J Gerontol Series A Biol Sci Med Sci*. 2003;58:636-643.
3. American Physical Therapy Association. *Guide to Physical Therapist Practice*. 2nd ed. Physical Therapy. 2001;81(1):9-746.

Bibliography

Abbas AK, Lichtman AH, Pillai S. *Cellular and Molecular Immunology*. 8th ed. Philadelphia, PA: Elsevier Saunders; 2015.

Common infectious disease worldwide. Infoplease. http://www.infoplease.com/ipa/A0903696.html. Accessed on October 18, 2018.

Copstead LC, Banasik JL. *Pathophysiology*. 3rd ed. St. Louis, MO: Elsevier Saunders; 2005.

Craig CR, Stitzel RE. *Modern Pharmacology with Clinical Applications*. New York, NY: Little, Brown, and Co; 1997.

Deglin JH, Vallerand AH. *Davis's Drug Guide for Nurses*. 8th ed. Philadelphia, PA: FA Davis; 2003.

Goodman CC, Fuller KS. *Pathology: Implications for the Physical Therapist*. 4th ed. St. Louis, MO: Elsevier Saunders; 2015.

Boyce JM, Pittet D; Healthcare Infection Control Practices Advisory Committee; HICPAC/SHEA/APIC/IDSA Hand Hygiene Task Force. Guideline for hand hygiene in health-care settings. Recommendations of the Healthcare Infection Control Practices Advisory Committee and the HICPAC/SHEA/APIC/IDSA Hand Hygiene Task Force. Society for Healthcare Epidemiology of America/Association for Professionals in Infection Control/Infectious Diseases Society of America. *MMWR Recomm Rep*. 2002;51(RR16):1-45.

Karch AM. *Lippincott's Nursing Drug Guide*. Springhouse, PA: Lippincott Williams & Wilkins; 2004.

Grossman SC, Porth CM. *Pathophysiology: Concepts of Altered Health States*. 9th ed. Philadelphia, PA: Lippincott Williams & Wilkins; 2014.

Ritter JM, Lewis LD, Mant TG. *Textbook of Clinical Pharmacology*. London, United Kingdom: Edward Arnold Co; 1995.

Roitt I, Brostoff J, Male D. *Immunology*. 6th ed. London, United Kingdom: Mosby; 2001.

APPENDIX A

DISEASE INFORMATION: COMMON INFECTIOUS DISEASES WORLDWIDE

The following is a list of the most common infectious diseases throughout the world today. Accurate caseload numbers are difficult to determine, especially because so many of these diseases are endemic to developing countries, where many people do not have access to modern medical care. Approximately half of all deaths caused by infectious diseases each year can be attributed to just 3 diseases: tuberculosis, malaria, and AIDS. Together, these diseases cause more than 300 million illnesses and more than 5 million deaths each year.

The list does not include diseases that have received a significant amount of media attention in recent years, such as Ebola hemorrhagic fever or West Nile virus, but which in fact have infected a relatively small number of people.

African Trypanosomiasis (Sleeping Sickness)

African trypanosomiasis is spread by the tsetse fly, which is common to many African countries. The World Health Organization (WHO) estimates that nearly 450,000 cases occur each year. Symptoms of the disease include fever, headaches, joint pains, and itching in the early stage and confusion, sensory disturbances, poor coordination, and disrupted sleep cycles in the second stage. If the disease goes untreated in its first stage, it causes irreparable neurological damage; if it goes untreated in its second stage, it is fatal.

Cholera

Cholera is a disease spread mostly through contaminated drinking water and unsanitary conditions. It is endemic in the Indian subcontinent, Russia, and sub-Saharan Africa. It is an acute infection of the intestines with the bacterium *Vibrio cholerae.* Its main symptom is copious diarrhea. Between 5% and 10% of those infected with the disease will develop severe symptoms, which also include vomiting and leg cramps. In its severe form, cholera can cause death by dehydration. An estimated 200,000 cases are reported to WHO annually.

Cryptosporidiosis

Cryptosporidiosis has become one of the most common causes of water-borne disease in the United States in recent years; it is also found throughout the rest of the world. It is caused by a parasite that spreads when a water source is contaminated, usually with the feces of infected animals or humans. Symptoms include diarrhea, stomach cramps, an upset stomach, and slight fever. Some people do not exhibit any symptoms.

Dengue

WHO estimates that 50 million cases of dengue fever appear each year. The spread of dengue fever is through the bite of the *Aedes aegypti* mosquito. Recent years have seen dengue outbreaks all over Asia and Africa. Dengue fever can be mild to moderate, and occasionally severe, though it is rarely fatal. Mild cases, which usually affect infants and young children, involve a nonspecific febrile illness, while moderate cases, seen in older children and adults, display high fever, severe headaches, muscle and joint pains, and rash. Severe cases develop into dengue hemorrhagic fever, which involves high fever, hemorrhaging, and sometimes circulatory failure.

Hepatitis A

Hepatitis A is a highly contagious liver disease caused by the hepatitis A virus. Spread primarily by the fecal-oral route or by ingestion of contaminated water or food, the number of annual infections worldwide is estimated at 1.4 million. Symptoms include fever, fatigue, jaundice, and dark urine. Although those exposed usually develop life-long immunity, the best protection against hepatitis A is vaccination.

Hepatitis B

Approximately 2 billion people are infected with the hepatitis B virus, making it the most common infectious disease in the world today. More than 350 million of those infected never rid themselves of the infection. Hepatitis is an inflammation of the liver that causes symptoms such as jaundice, extreme fatigue, nausea, vomiting, and stomach pain; hepatitis B is the most serious form of the disease. Chronic infections can cause cirrhosis of the liver or liver cancer in later years.

Hepatitis C

Hepatitis C is a less common, and less severe, form of hepatitis. An estimated 170 million people worldwide are infected with hepatitis C virus; 3 to 4 million more are infected every year. The majority of hepatitis C virus cases are asymptomatic, even in people who develop chronic infection.

HIV/AIDS

AIDS was first reported in mid-1981 in the United States and is believed to have originated in sub-Saharan Africa. The HIV that causes AIDS was identified in 1983, and by 1985 tests to detect the virus were available. The clinical consequences of HIV infection are due to the ability of this retrovirus to target crucial cells of the immune system, the lymphocyte, that expresses the cell surface marker CD4, which serves as a receptor that binds the envelope protein of the virus. Two major types of HIV have been recognized: HIV-l and HIV-2. HIV-l is the dominant type worldwide. HIV-2 is found principally in West Africa, but cases have been reported in East Africa, Europe, Asia, and Latin America. There are at least 10 different genetic subtypes of HIV-l, but their biological and epidemiological significance is unclear at present. Both HIV-l and HIV-2 are transmitted in the same ways. Although the first reported cases involved homosexual men in Los Angeles who were infected through sexual contact, the principal mode of transmission throughout the world is through the exchange of bodily fluids during heterosexual intercourse. HIV is transmitted by sexual contact, intravenous drug users sharing infected hypodermic needles, through transfused blood or its components, and it may also be transmitted from infected mother to infant before, during, or shortly after birth.

HIV infection is characterized by the progressive loss of CD4+ lymphocytes, and immunodeficiency results not only from a lack of effective immunity against HIV itself, but also because the virus damages CD4 cell subsets that are crucial for containing other pathogens. AIDS is the fatal and incurable disease caused by HIV. AIDS attacks and destroys the immune system, gradually leaving the individual defenseless against illnesses that lead to death. These illnesses are referred to as **opportunistic infections** or diseases; in AIDS patients the most common are *Pneumocystis carinii* pneumonia, a parasitic infection of the lungs, and a type of cancer known as **Kaposi's sarcoma**. Other opportunistic infections include unusually severe infections with yeast, cytomegalovirus, herpes virus, and parasites, such as *Toxoplasma gondii* or *Cryptosporidium* . Milder infections with these organisms do not suggest immune deficiencies. Symptoms of full-blown

AIDS include a persistent cough, fever, and difficulty breathing. Multiple purplish blotches and bumps on the skin may indicate Kaposi's sarcoma. The virus can also cause brain damage. People infected with the virus can have a wide range of symptoms—from none, to mild, to severe. At least one-fourth to one-half of those infected with HIV will develop AIDS within 4 to 10 years.

The introduction of highly active antiretroviral (ARV) therapy in 1996 was a turning point for those with access to sophisticated health care systems. Although they cannot cure HIV/AIDS, ARVs and their use in combination (ie, cocktails) have dramatically reduced mortality and morbidity and prolonged and improved the lives of sufferers. With no cure at present, prudence could save thousands of people who have yet to be exposed to the virus. Use of condoms lessens the possibility of transmission, as does the elimination of sharing hypodermic needles. The fate of many will depend less on science than on the ability of large numbers of human beings to change their behavior in the face of growing danger.

Influenza

Several influenza epidemics in the 20th century caused millions of deaths worldwide, including the worst epidemic in American history, the Spanish influenza outbreak that killed more than 500,000 in 1918. Today influenza is less of a public health threat, though it continues to be a serious disease that affects many people. Approximately 20,000 people die of the flu in the United States every year. The influenza virus attacks the human respiratory tract, causing symptoms such as fever, headaches, fatigue, coughing, sore throat, nasal congestion, and body aches.

Japanese Encephalitis

Japanese encephalitis is a mosquito-borne disease endemic in Asia. Around 50,000 cases occur each year; 25% to 30% of all cases are fatal.

Leishmaniasi

Leishmaniasis is a disease spread by the bite of the sandfly. It is found mostly in tropical countries. There are several types of leishmaniasis, and they vary in symptoms and severity. Visceral leishmaniasis (**kala azar**) is the most severe; left untreated, it is always fatal. Symptoms include fever, weight loss, anemia, and a swelling of the spleen and liver. Mucocutaneous leishmaniasis (**espundia**) produces lesions that affect the nose, mouth, and throat and can destroy their mucous membranes. Cutaneous leishmaniasis produces skin ulcers, sometimes as many as 200, that cause disability and extensive scarring. Diffuse cutaneous leishmaniasis is similar to cutaneous leishmaniasis, and infected people are prone to relapses. Approximately 12 million cases of leishmaniasis exist today.

Malaria

Malaria is a mosquito-borne disease that affects 300 to 500 million people annually, causing nearly 3 million deaths. Most common in tropical and subtropical climates, malaria is found in more than 100 countries, including many parts of Central and South America, Africa, Southeast Asia and the Indian subcontinent, and the Middle East. Symptoms include several stages of illness. The first stage consists of shaking and chills, the next stage involves high fever and severe headache, and in the final stage the infected person's temperature drops and he or she sweats profusely. Infected people also often suffer from anemia, weakness, and a swelling of the spleen. Malaria was almost eradicated 30 years ago; now it is on the rise again.

Measles

Measles is a disease that has seen a drastic reduction in countries where a vaccine is readily available, but it is still prevalent in developing countries, where most of the 777,000 deaths (out of 30 million cases) it caused in 2001 occurred. Symptoms include high fever, coughing, and a maculopapular rash; common complications include diarrhea, pneumonia, and ear infections.

Meningitis

Meningitis, often known as **spinal meningitis**, is an infection of the spinal cord and usually the result of a viral or bacterial infection. Bacterial meningitis is more severe than viral meningitis and may cause brain damage, hearing loss, and learning disabilities. An estimated 1.2 million cases of bacterial meningitis occur every year, over 1/10 of which are fatal. Symptoms include severe headache, fever, nausea, vomiting, lethargy, delirium, photophobia, and a stiff neck.

Onchocerciasis (River Blindness)

Onchocerciasis is caused by the larvae of *Onchocerca volvulus*, a parasitic worm that lives in the human body for years. It is endemic in Africa, where nearly all of the 18 million people infected with the disease live. Of those infected, over 6.5 million have developed dermatitis and 270,000 have gone blind. Symptoms include visual impairment, rashes, lesions, intense itching, skin depigmentation, and lymphadenitis.

Pneumonia

Pneumonia has many possible causes, but it is usually an infection of the streptococcus or mycoplasma bacteria. These bacteria can live in the human body without causing infection for years, and only surface when another illness has lowered the person's immunity to disease. *Streptococcus pneumoniae* causes streptococcal pneumonia, the most common kind, which is more severe than mycoplasmal pneumonia. *S pneumoniae* is responsible for more than 100,000 hospitalizations for pneumonia annually, as well as 6 million cases of otitis media and over 60,000 cases of invasive diseases such as meningitis.

Rotavirus

Rotavirus is the most common cause of viral gastroenteritis worldwide. It kills more than 600,000 children each year, mostly in developing countries. Symptoms include vomiting, watery diarrhea, fever, and abdominal pain.

Schistosomiasis

Schistosomiasis is a parasitic disease that is endemic in many developing countries. Roughly 200 million people worldwide are infected with the fluke worm, whose eggs cause the symptoms of the disease. Some 120 million of those infected are symptomatic, and 20 million suffer severely from the infection. Symptoms include rash and itchiness soon after becoming infected, followed by fever, chills, coughing, and muscle aches.

Shigellosis

Shigella infection causes an estimated 600,000 deaths worldwide every year. It is most common in developing countries with poor sanitation. Shigella bacteria cause bacillary dysentery, or shigellosis. Symptoms include diarrhea with bloody stool, vomiting, and abdominal cramps.

Strep Throat

Strep throat is caused by the *streptococcus* bacteria. Several million cases of strep throat occur every year. Symptoms include a sore throat, fever, headache, fatigue, and nausea.

Tuberculosis

Tuberculosis causes nearly 2 million deaths every year, and WHO estimates that nearly 1 billion people will be infected between 2000 and 2020 if more effective preventive procedures are not adopted. The tuberculosis bacteria are most often found in the lungs, where they can cause chest pain and a bad cough that brings up bloody phlegm. Other symptoms include fatigue, weight loss, appetite loss, chills, fever, and night sweats.

Typhoid

Typhoid fever causes an estimated 600,000 deaths annually, out of 12 to 17 million cases. It is usually spread through infected food or water. Symptoms include a sudden and sustained fever, severe headache, nausea, severe appetite loss, constipation, and sometimes diarrhea.

Yellow Fever

Yellow fever causes an estimated 30,000 deaths each year, out of 200,000 cases. The disease has 2 phases. In the acute phase, symptoms include fever, muscle pain, headache, shivers, appetite loss, nausea, and vomiting. This lasts for 3 to 4 days, after which most patients recover. However, 15% will enter the toxic phase, in which fever reappears, along with other symptoms, including jaundice, abdominal pain, vomiting, bleeding from the mouth, nose, eyes, and stomach, and deterioration of kidney function (sometimes complete kidney failure). Half of all patients in the toxic phase die within 2 weeks; the other half recover.

Appendix B

Pharmacological Information: Infectious Diseases and Pharmacology

Antifungals

Action

Antifungal agents can kill susceptible fungi (fungicidal) or stop growth (fungistatic). Antifungals bind and disrupt the cell membrane of the fungi or alter protein or lipid synthesis within the fungi leading to the therapeutic effects.

Side Effects

CNS: Headache, dizziness
CV: Hypotension, dysrhythmias
GI: Vomiting, abdominal pain
Miscellaneous: Arthralgias, myalgias, peripheral neuropathy, skin exfoliation

Common Medications

Systemic: Amphotericin, Diflucan (fluconazole), itraconazole
Local/topical: Ciclopirox; Lotrimin (clotrimazole); Nizoral (keoconazole); Micatin, Desenex (miconazole); nystatin

Anti-Infectives

Aminoglycosides

Action

Aminoglycosides are used for the treatment or prophylaxis of Gram-negative bacterial infections, including *Pseudomonas aeruginosa, Klebsiella pneumonia, Escherichia coli, Serratia, Acinetobacter, Staphylococcus aureus*. Aminoglycosides are bacteriocidal through inhibition of ribosomal protein synthesis.

Side Effects

GU: Nephrotoxicity
Miscellaneous: Ototoxicity, hypersensitivity reactions

Common Medications

Gentamicin, neomycin, streptomycin, tobramycin

Carbapenems

Action

Carbapenems bind to bacterial cell walls resulting in cell death. These are broad spectrum antibiotics that are active against most Gram-positive infectious agents, including *Streptococcus pneumonia, Enterococcus, S aureus*, and Gram-negative infections, including *Pseudomonas aeruginosa, Klebsiella, E coli.* Imipenem may be combined with cilastatin to decrease renal inactivation of drug.

Side Effects

CNS: Seizures, dizziness
CV: Hypotension
GI: Diarrhea, nausea, vomiting, colitis
Miscellaneous: Anaphylaxis

Common Medications

Primaxin (imipenem/cilastatin)

Cephalosporins

Action

Cephalosporins are bacteriocidal to Gram-positive cocci including *S pneumonia, staphylococci,* and *streptococci.* Second- and third-generation cephalosporins have greater Gram-negative bacteriocidal activity.

Side Effects

CNS: Seizures, dizziness
CV: Hypotension
GI: Diarrhea, nausea, vomiting, colitis
Miscellaneous: Anaphylaxis, pain/phlebitis at administration site

Common Medications

First generation: Ancef (cefazolin), Biocef (cephalexin), Keflex (cephalexin)
Second generation: Monocid (cefmetazole), Cefzil (cefprozil), Ceftin (cefuroxime), Kefurox (cefuroxime), Zinacef (cefuroxime)
Third generation: Cefepime, Ceftaz (ceftazidime)

Penicillins

Action

Penicillins are bacteriocidal by preventing bacterial cell wall synthesis. They are commonly prescribed for respiratory and GU infections, sepsis, endocarditis, peptic ulcer disease, sexually transmitted diseases (eg, chlamydia, syphillis, gonorrhea), and Lyme disease. Penicillins are effective against streptococcal, pneumococcal, gonococcal, and meningococcal infections.

Side Effects

CNS: Seizures
GI: Diarrhea, nausea, vomiting, colitis
Miscellaneous: Allergic reactions (eg, rash, bronchospasm), anaphylaxis

Common Medications

Penicillins: Benzylpenicillin (penicillin G), phenoxymethylpenicillin (penicillin V)
Extended-spectrum penicillins: mpicillin, amoxicillin, piperacillin
Penicillinase-resistant penicillins: Methicillin, nafcillin, oxacillin, cloxacillin, dicloxacillin

Fluoroquinolones

Action

Fluoroquinolones are bacteriostatic by inhibiting DNA synthesis. These broad-spectrum agents are prescribed for the prophylaxis and treatment of many Gram-positive pathogens including MRSA and streptococcus pneumonia; Gram-negative activity against *E coli, Pseudomonal aeruginosa,* and *Acinetobacter.* Common in respiratory, GU, and GI tract infections, meningitis, and septicemia.

Side Effects

CNS: Seizures, dizziness, drowsiness, fatigue, headache
CV: Dysrhythmias
GI: Diarrhea, nausea, vomiting, colitis, hepatotoxicity
Miscellaneous: Hyper- and hypoglycemia, tendinitis/tendon rupture, anaphylaxis, skin exfoliation (Stevens-Johnson syndrome)

Common Medications

Cipro (ciprofloxacin), Levaquin (levofloxacin)

Macrolides

Action

Macrolides are bacteriostatic by binding to bacterial ribosomes inhibiting protein synthesis. Macrolides are frequently prescribed for Gram-positive and Gram-negative pathogens. Commonly used in cellulitis, respiratory infections, and chronic bronchitis.

Side Effects

CNS: Dizziness, drowsiness, fatigue, headache
CV: Chest pain, palpitations
GI: Diarrhea, nausea, vomiting, abdominal cramps
Miscellaneous: Angioedema, pain/phlebitis at administration site

Common Medications

Erhythromycin, Biaxin (clarithromycin), Zithromax (azithromycin)

Tetracyclines

Action

Tetracyclines are bacteriostatic by binding to bacterial ribosomes inhibiting protein synthesis of Gram-positive and Gram-negative pathogens. They are frequently prescribed for atypical pneumonias, chronic bronchitis, acne, and periodontitis.

Side Effects

CNS: Dizziness/fatigue
Dermatological: Light sensitivity, rash
GI: Diarrhea, nausea, colitis
Miscellaneous: Ataxia, discoloration of teeth

Common Medications

Tetracycline, Doxy (doxycycline), Minocin (minocycline)

Sulfonamides

Action

Sulfonamides inhibit the bacterial synthesis of folic acid that is essential for growth. These broad-spectrum antibiotics are prescribed for multiple Gram-positive and Gram-negative pathogens. Most notably, these agents are used for UTIs, meningitis, and intestinal and lower respiratory tract infections.

Side Effects

CNS: Fatigue, hallucinations, headache
GI: Diarrhea, vomiting, nausea
Miscellaneous: Hypersensitivity, skin rash, thrombocytopenia, fever

Common Medications

Bactrim (trimethoprim/sulfamethoxazole)

Antiretrovirals

Action

ARVs are used in the management of HIV to improve the CD4 cell counts and decrease viral load. These medications include nucleoside and non-nucleoside reverse transciptase inhibitors and protease inhibitors. Viruses use the infected cell to replicate new viral particles through the process of reverse transcription. Reverse transciptase inhibitors limit viral reproduction. Protease inhibitors limit the cleavage and activation of HIV proteins that are necessary for viral replication, leading to reductions in viral levels in the blood.

Side Effects

CNS: Dizziness, drowsiness, fatigue, headache
CV: Orthostatic hypotension
GI: Abdominal pain, diarrhea, vomiting, nausea
Miscellaneous: Hypersensitivity/anaphylaxis (Stevens-Johnson syndrome), musculoskeletal pain, fat redistribution, peripheral neuropathy, weakness

Common Medications

Nonnucleoside reverse transcriptase inhibitors: Rescriptor (delavirdine), Sustiva (efavirenz), Viramune (nevirapine)
Nucleoside reverse transcriptase inhibitors: Ziagen (abacavir); ddI (didanosine); Videx (didanosine); ddC (zalcitabine); AZT, Retrovir (zidovudine)
Protease inhibitors: Agenerase (amprenavir), Crixivan (indinavir)

Antituberculars

Action

Antituberculars are medications used in the treatment and prevention of tuberculosis. These medications inhibit RNA synthesis by blocking RNA transcription or disrupt formation of the bacterial cell wall.

Side Effects

CNS: Ataxia, confusion, drowsiness, fatigue, headache
GI: Abdominal pain, diarrhea, vomiting, nausea, hepatitis
Miscellaneous: Arthralgias, myalgias, peripheral neuropathy, weakness

Common Medications

Ethambutol, Inh (isoniazid), pyrazinamide, Rifadin (rifampin), Priftin (rifapentine)

Antivirals

Action

Antiviral agents limit replication and spread of viruses through multiple mechanisms. Common viral infections treated by antiviral medications include herpes simplex, herpes zoster (shingles), varicella (chicken pox), influenza, and cytomegalovirus.

Side Effects

CNS: Seizures, dizziness, headache, drowsiness
CV: Dysrhythmias, hypo- and hypertension
GI: GI bleeding, diarrhea, vomiting, nausea
Miscellaneous: Arthralgias, tremor, ataxia, peripheral neuropathy

Common Medications

Avirax, Zovirax (acyclovir); Vitrasert (ganciclovir); Tamiflu (oseltamivir); Valtrex (valacyclovir); Relenza (zanamivir)

CNS=central nervous system; CV=cardiovascular.

Chapter 6

Cardiovascular Diseases and Disorders

Daniel J. Malone, PT, PhD, CCS

Cardiovascular disease (CVD), specifically heart disease and stroke, is the number one cause of death in the United States. Although the rates of death attributable to CVD have declined about 30% over the last decade, the burden of disease remains high and CVD remains the leading cause of morbidity and mortality. CVD includes coronary artery disease (CAD) and heart failure, hypertension (HTN), cerebrovascular disease, congenital heart diseases, and valve dysfunction. Approximately 85.6 million (>1/3) of Americans are living with some form of CVD.[1-3] Physical therapists and physical therapist assistants will absolutely work with patients who have primary and secondary CVD in their practice. This chapter will review basic anatomy and physiology of the cardiovascular system and describe the most common health conditions encountered in the acute care setting. Physical therapist management of CVD will be presented in the context of cardiac rehabilitation. Appendix A will expand on electrophysiology, electrocardiogram (ECG), pacemakers, and defibrillators.

Anatomy and Physiology

The cardiovascular system's primary purpose is to deliver adequate amounts of oxygen and remove waste from the body.[4,5] The heart's pumping action provides the motive force to open the heart's valves and push blood throughout the body. The blood vessels provide the conduit for the distribution and return of blood and waste products to their appropriate destinations. In order to perform its functions, the cardiovascular system works together with the respiratory, neurologic, urinary, digestive, endocrine, and integumentary systems in maintaining homeostasis.[6-8]

Anatomically, the cardiovascular system includes the heart, the pericardium, and all the blood vessels, including the arteries, veins, capillaries, and lymphatics. Physiologically, the therapist must not only consider the anatomy but also the presence of disease, neurological influences, blood fluid volume, medications, and surgery to assess proper function.

Malone DJ, Bishop KL, eds. *Acute Care Physical Therapy: A Clinician's Guide, Second Edition* (pp 177-244).

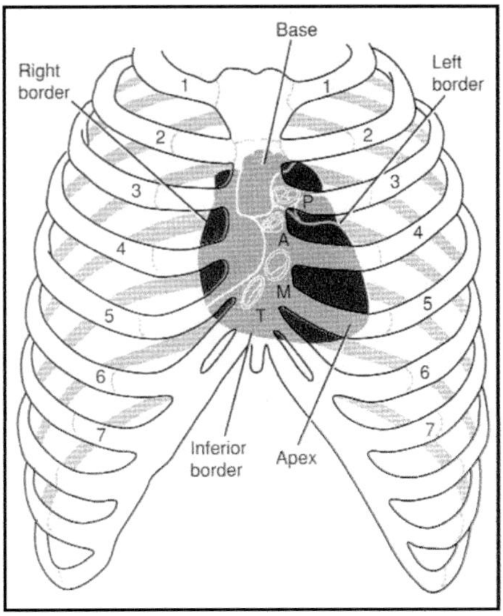

Figure 6-1. Relationship of the heart and the principle valves to the overlying rib cage. (A=aortic valve; M=mitral valve; P=pulmonary valve; T=tricuspid valve.) (Reprinted from Hillegass EA, Sadowsky HS. *Essentials of Cardiopulmonary Physical Therapy.* 2nd ed. Philadelphia, PA: WB Saunders; 2001:30 with permission from Elsevier.)

The heart is located within the **mediastinum** of the thorax, the space superior to the diaphragm and medial to the lungs. It contains the heart encased in its protective layer, the **pericardium**, the great vessels including the aorta, the superior vena cava (SVC) and inferior vena cava (IVC), the pulmonary arteries and veins, as well as the esophagus, the phrenic nerves, and the sympathetic chain ganglia.

Normally, the heart is conical in shape and is roughly the size of the patient's fist. It is located anteriorly in the mediastinum behind the sternum with approximately two-thirds of the heart left of midline. The surface marking of the heart can be identified over the anterior chest wall extending from the second to fifth intercostal spaces from the sternum to the left midclavicular line[1,7,9,10] (Figure 6-1). The **base** of the heart faces posteriorly and consists largely of the left atrium and a portion of the right atrium. The base is the superior portion of the heart and is related to the second intercostal space parasternally. The **apex** is the inferior portion of the heart and is comprised mainly of the left ventricle. The apex projects into the fifth intercostal space in the midclavicular line, the **point of maximal impulse** (PMI). Palpating the PMI determines the relative position of the left ventricle.[9]

Blood Vessels

The blood vessels form a tubular network transporting blood throughout the body. The 3 major types of blood vessels are

1. Arteries, which carry blood away from the heart
2. Veins, which carry blood toward the heart
3. Capillaries, which join the arterial and venous circulations

The arteries continuously branch into progressively smaller diameter arterioles increasing the total surface area of the circulation leading to the capillaries, the site of gas and nutrient exchange. Blood returns to the heart from the capillaries passing through vessels of progressively larger diameters, called **venules** and **veins**.[4] The blood vessels actively control the flow and distribution of blood throughout the body by smooth muscle vasoconstriction or dilatation resulting from the influences of vasoactive substances, hormones, and neurological input (Table 6-1).

Table 6-1

COMMON VASOACTIVE FACTORS

Vasodilation Factors	*Vasoconstriction Factors*
• Vasovagal syncope • Deep pain (eg, joint disruption, crush injury), visceral pain, and distension • Autonomic dysfunction (eg, Parkinson's disease, diabetes) inflammatory mediators, sepsis) • Fever, hyperthermia • Pain medications (narcotic analgesics [eg, opiods]) • Anxiolytics, sedatives • Cardiovascular medications: ¤ Nitrates, calcium channel blockers, beta blockers, vasodilators ¤ Nitric oxide (from vascular endothelium)	• Superficial pain • Endothelin (from vascular endothelium) • Angiotensin II • Beta agonists (eg, norepinephrine, epinephrine, isoproteronol) • Vasopressin (antidiuretic hormone [ADH]) • Cold temperature, hypothermia • Sympathetic nervous system activation (norepinephrine) • Hypoxic vasoconstriction (pulmonary vessels) • Acidosis (peripheral vessels)

All vessels larger than the capillaries consist of 3 distinct layers: the intima tunica, media, and adventitia (Figure 6-2). The innermost layer, the tunica intima, consists of a smooth layer of endothelial cells, supporting connective tissue, and isolated smooth muscle cells. The **endothelium** promotes smooth laminar blood flow and is selectively permeable to different molecules (eg, low-density lipoprotein [LDL] cholesterol). The endothelium secretes and responds to a variety of vasoactive substances that determine the diameter of the vessel lumen (see Table 6-1). The middle layer, the tunica media, consists of multiple layers of smooth muscle cells and elastic tissue. The media is the site of vasoconstriction/vasodilation. The outer layer, the tunica adventitia, consists of collagen and loose connective tissues. The adventitia provides a support structure, binds the vessel loosely to the surrounding connective tissue, and contains nerves and the vaso vasorum, small blood vessels that supply blood and nutrients to the vessel itself.[9,11-13]

The Heart

The heart is a 4-chambered muscular pump divided into right and left halves containing the **atria** and a **ventricle**. The atria receive blood returning to the heart from the veins (ie, IVC, SVC, pulmonary veins), while the ventricles receive blood from the atria and eject into the main arteries (ie, pulmonary artery, aorta, coronary arteries). A muscular wall, the **interventricular septum**, separates the ventricles and contributes to the contractile function of the heart. The right heart pumps to the lungs and is referred to as the **pulmonary circuit,** while the left heart is the **systemic circuit**, pumping to the remainder of the body (Figure 6-3).

The walls of the heart are made up of 3 layers[12]:

1. Endocardium, the inner layer
2. Myocardium, the middle muscular layer
3. Epicardium, the outer protective layer

The innermost layer, the **endocardium**, is a thin layer of endothelial cells supported by underlying connective tissue. This layer repeatedly folds on itself to form

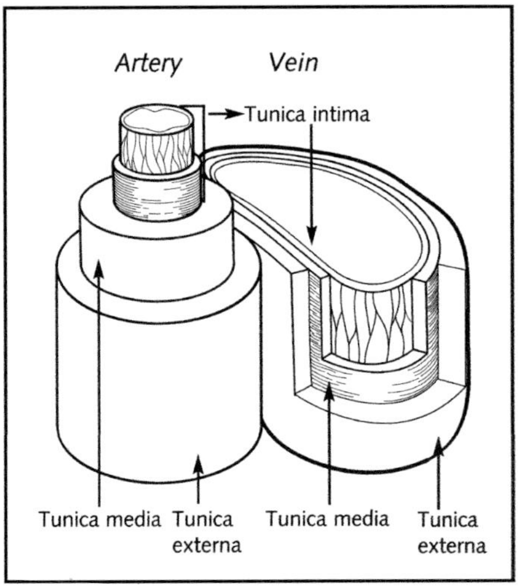

Figure 6-2. Diagram of an artery and vein showing similar structural components but different proportions. (Reprinted with permission from Sheldon LK. *Oxygenation.* Sudbury, MA: Jones and Bartlett; 2001.)

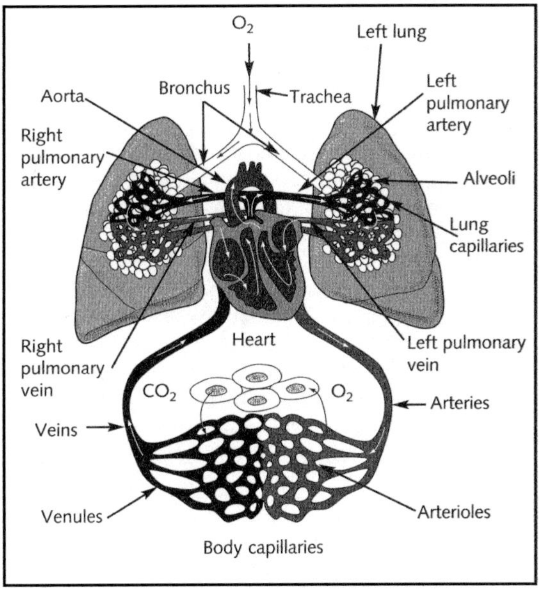

Figure 6-3. Diagram of the vascular circuits: pulmonary circulation and systemic circulation. (Reprinted with permission from Sheldon LK. *Oxygenation.* Sudbury, MA: Jones and Bartlett; 2001.)

the valves of the heart and is continuous with the innermost layer of the blood vessels, the tunica intima. The middle layer, the **myocardium**, is the contractile layer of the heart and is composed primarily of cardiac muscle fibers. The outer layer, the **epicardium**, is a thin membrane that encases the myocardium. The epicardium turns back on itself to form a sac that surrounds the heart, the **pericardium**. Between the layers of the pericardium is a thin layer of pericardial fluid.[11,12]

The **pericardium** is the fibrous sac covering the heart and the root of the great vessels as they enter or leave the heart. This double layered sac consists of the external fibrous pericardium and the inner serous pericardium, which is divided into the inner visceral and outer parietal layers separated by a virtual space containing the pericardial fluid. The pericardium lubricates the moving surfaces of the heart to reduce friction as the heart contracts. The pericardium protects the heart from external trauma and infection and limits distension of the heart with blood volume changes. The pericardium maintains the position of the heart in the thorax preventing excess motion during contraction and distributes contractile forces throughout the heart's chambers supporting the ejection of blood.[14,15]

Pulmonary Circuit

The right atrium receives deoxygenated blood returning from the body by the **SVC** and **IVC**. The SVC drains blood from the head and upper extremities (UEs), and the IVC drains blood from the lower extremities (LEs) and abdomen. Separating the right atrium from the right ventricle is the **tricuspid valve**. The right ventricle receives the blood from the right atrium and pumps blood through the pulmonary valve into the main pulmonary artery, which bifurcates into the right and left pulmonary arteries for transport to the lungs. The pulmonary circuit is a low-pressure, high-capacitance system that receives the entire cardiac output while maintaining pressures that are usually 1/4 to 1/5 of the systemic circulation. The right ventricle has a thicker myocardium than the atria, but is approximately 1/3 the thickness of the left ventricle. This thinner myocardium is due to the lower pulmonary vascular resistance (**PVR**) within the pulmonary circuit compared to the systemic circuit. However, disorders causing high PVR (eg, pulmonary hypertension, pulmonary embolism, left ventricular failure) can lead to right ventricular hypertrophy and failure (cor pulmonale).

Systemic Circuit

The 4 pulmonary veins return blood to the left atrium and the blood passes through the **mitral valve**, traveling to the left ventricle. As noted previously, the left ventricle is roughly 3 times thicker than the right ventricle due to the large systemic/total peripheral vascular resistance (**SVR/TPR**). Blood leaves the left ventricle through the **aortic valve** entering the **aorta** for distribution throughout the body.

Atrioventricular and Semilunar Valves

There are 2 atrioventricular valves, the **tricuspid valve** and **mitral valve**, and 2 semilunar valves, the **pulmonary valve** and **aortic valve**. The valves' primary function is to direct the one-way flow of blood through the pulmonary and systemic circuits. Within the interior of the ventricles are the papillary muscles that attach to the atrioventricular valves via the chordae tendinae. The papillary muscle–chordae tendinae apparatus contracts and provides an inward-directed force during ventricular ejection that prevents the eversion of the atrioventricular valves into the atria.

Conduction System and Electrocardiography

Myocardial cells have the potential for spontaneous electrical activity that can lead to a variety of abnormal heart rhythms. The **sinoatrial node** located in the superior aspect of the right atrium, has the fastest rate of depolarizations and is the usual pacemaker of the heart. Once the sinoatrial node fires, the depolarization wave is transmitted throughout the entire heart over the conduction system as outlined in Figure 6-4. From the sinoatrial node, the impulses travel over Bachman's bundle to the left atrium and down the internodal fasciculi through the right atrium to the ventricles. A connective tissue sheath separates the atria and ventricles. This sheath prevents transmission of the impulse into the ventricles except through the **atrioventricular node**. The **atrioventricular node**, the **atrioventricular bundle** (Bundle of His), and **purkinje fibers** complete the pathway conducting the electrical impulses

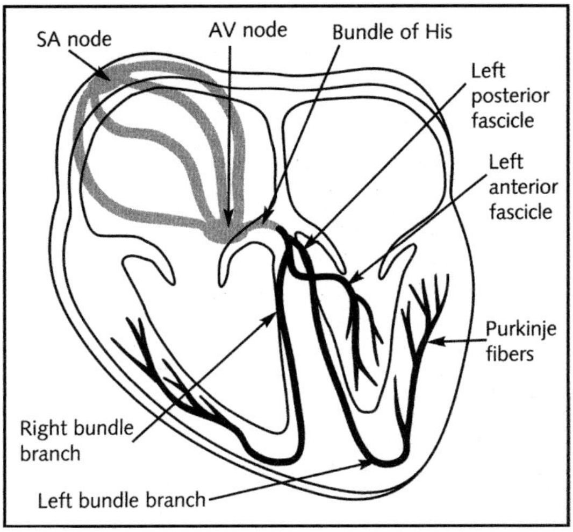

Figure 6-4. Conduction system of the heart. (SA = sinoatrial; AV = atrioventricular.) (Reprinted with permission from Sheldon LK. *Oxygenation*. Sudbury, MA: Jones and Bartlett; 2001.)

throughout the ventricles. The electrical impulse is delayed at the atrioventricular node allowing the atria to fully contract prior to ventricular ejection (systole). This time delay between the atria and ventricles promotes ventricular filling during diastole in order to enhance ventricular systole. Abnormalities in electrical impulse generation or abnormalities in electrical impulse conduction can lead to changes in the heart's rhythm. These dysrhythmias can impair diastolic filling or systolic contraction altering the stroke volume and cardiac output (see Figure 6-16).

The Cardiac Cycle

The cardiac cycle (Figure 6-5) defines the combined electrical and mechanical forces within the heart to complete one heartbeat and consists of one systole (contraction) and one diastole (filling). Systole begins with contraction of the ventricle resulting from electrical stimulation (QRS complex on ECG) traveling through the conduction system. Ventricular contraction generates the pressure required to force open the aortic/pulmonic valves and propel blood into the major arteries. Initially, as the ventricle contracts, all heart valves are closed and there is no movement of blood (**isovolumic contraction**). However, as contraction continues, the intraventricular pressure becomes greater than the pressure within the great arteries, and the aortic/pulmonic valves open and blood is ejected into the aorta and pulmonary arteries. As the ventricles continue to contract and blood flows into the great arteries, ventricular pressure falls below the pressures within the major arteries and the aortic/pulmonic valves close (**S2 heart sound**). With closure of the valves, ejection ends, the ventricles begin to relax, and diastole begins. Diastole begins with all valves closed and as the ventricle continues to relax, the myocardium lengthens, increasing the intraventricular volume and the intraventricular pressures decrease (**isovolumic relaxation**). Ventricular pressure continues to fall and when atrial pressure is greater than ventricular pressure, the mitral/tricuspid valves open and blood flows passively into the ventricles. Passive filling accounts for approximately 80% of the ventricular filling volume. The atria depolarize (P wave on ECG) followed by atrial contraction, providing the active contribution of ventricular filling (approximately 20%). As blood fills the ventricles, intraventricular pressure increases and with the initiation of ventricular contraction (QRS complex on ECG), pressure increases further closing the mitral valve/tricuspid valve (**S1 heart sound**). This signals the end of diastole and the beginning of systole.

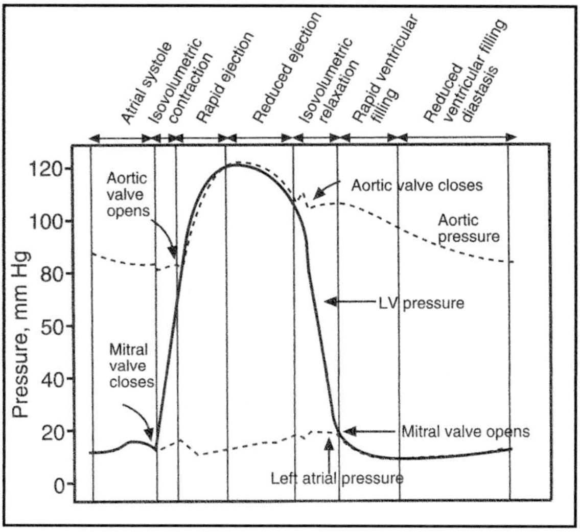

Figure 6-5. The cardiac cycle showing the pressure changes in the left atria, left ventricle, and aorta resulting in the opening/closing of the valves of the heart. (LV = left ventricle.) (Reprinted with permission from Sheldon LK. *Oxygenation*. Sudbury, MA: Jones and Bartlett; 2001.)

The amount of blood ejected from the heart with each ventricular systole, is the **stroke volume**. The stroke volume is highly dependent upon the amount of blood filling the heart prior to ejection. This blood volume is called the **preload** or **end-diastolic volume** (EDV). The amount of blood ejected from the ventricles per minute defines the **cardiac output**. Mathematically, cardiac output (CO) is the product of heart rate (HR) times stroke volume (SV) (CO=HR x SV). One heartbeat typically lasts approximately 0.8 seconds with two-thirds of that time spent in diastole. Increases in HR will shorten the diastolic filling time. This may partially explain the decrease in stroke volume and cardiac output associated with tachyarrhythmias, an abnormal rapid heart rhythm.

Health Conditions

Electrocardiogram/Dysrhythmias

Therapists should be aware of the major dysrhythmias and the impact on cardiovascular physiology and the patient's hemodynamics. The presence of dysrhythmias will influence patient monitoring and the prescription of therapeutic interventions. As outlined in Appendix A in this chapter, most dysrhythmias impact ventricular diastole or systole leading to abnormalities in stroke volume and cardiac output. Dysrhythmias may also impact myocardial oxygen supply and demand. Cardiac dysrhythmia interpretation is not limited to critical care as many patients encountered in the acute care environment require telemetry monitoring.

Coronary Artery Disease/Angina/Myocardial Infarction Revascularization Procedures

Atherosclerosis is a disease affecting the large- and medium-sized arteries. When it occurs in the vessels of the heart, it is known as **coronary artery disease** (CAD). When atherosclerosis occurs in the extremities, aorta, or iliac arteries, it is called **peripheral arterial disease** (PAD) or **peripheral arterial occlusive disease** (PAOD). CAD and cerebrovascular disease are present in a large portion of individuals with

Table 6-2

RISK FACTORS FOR CORONARY ARTERY DISEASE

Modifiable Risk Factors	*Non-Modifiable Risk Factors*
• Smoking • HTN • Hypercholesterolemia • Sedentary lifestyle • Diabetes • Obesity • Diet • Stress	• Age • Sex • Genetics and family history

PAD, and PAD itself sharply increases the risks for cardiac and cerebral events.[16] Atherosclerosis is associated with known risk factors that are amenable to rehabilitation (Table 6-2). Atherosclerosis involves the formation of fibromuscular plaques within the walls of the arteries that limit blood flow. Plaque formation begins with the leaking of blood lipids (LDL cholesterol) and inflammatory cells through the endothelial layer of the vessel forming a fatty streak. Smoking, shear stress related to HTN, age, and diabetes increase the permeability of the tunica intima by damaging endothelial cells of the tunica intima. Smooth muscle cells migrate from the tunica media to this region of damage. This fibromuscular plaque begins to decrease the diameter of the lumen of the blood vessel.[13,17] The result is reduced blood flow, leading to ischemia, and, eventually, cell death. **Angina**, the result of ischemia, is the complaint of pain or pressure commonly behind the sternum, left shoulder, and jaw of patients with CAD. **Myocardial infarction** results in cell damage and death. PAD is a leading cause of **intermittent claudication**, the complaint of LE burning, cramping, or ache associated with walking, is the equivalent to angina but in the LE. PAD also lead to wounds, impaired wound healing, and potential limb loss and amputation.

Angina, myocardial infarction, and intermittent claudication result from an imbalance in oxygen supply and oxygen demand. For example, CAD leads to coronary artery stenosis, a decrease in coronary artery lumen diameter, reducing blood flow and oxygen supply. Other factors that reduce blood flow and oxygen supply include coronary vasospasm and coronary thrombosis. The main determinants of oxygen demand are HR, myocardial contractility, and ventricular wall stress[6,8,14] (Figure 6-6). The ventricular wall stress is related to the ventricular volume and systemic blood pressure (BP). Increases in myocardial oxygen demand are associated with physical work, exercise, and mental stress. Increased oxygen demand combined with limited blood flow will cause myocardial ischemia. The treatments for CAD and PAD are to increase oxygen supply or reduce oxygen demand through various pharmacological and/or surgical procedures as well as risk factors and behavior modifications through cardiac rehabilitation.[1,13,18]

Medical Management/Nonsurgical Intervention

The acute care therapist is an integral member of the health care team involved in the management of cardiovascular disease. Pharmacological intervention involves the use of medications to reduce oxygen demand (eg, beta blockers, calcium channel blockers, angiotensin-converting enzyme [ACE] inhibitors, diuretics) and improve oxygen supply (eg, antiplatelets, anticoagulants, calcium channel blockers; see Appendix B).

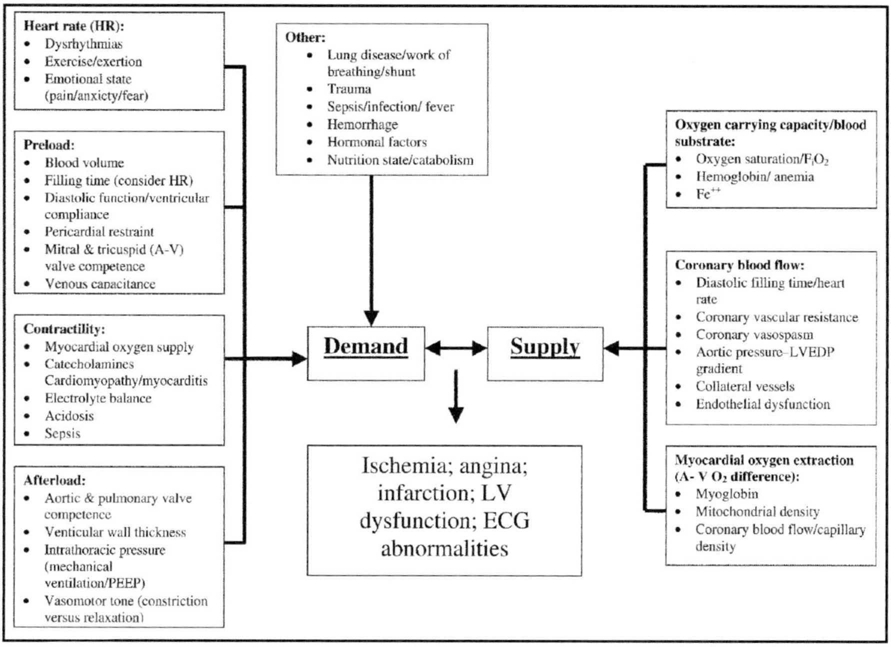

Figure 6-6. Myocardial oxygen supply-demand relationship. (A-V = arteriovenous; Fe^{++} = iron; LVEDP = left ventricular end-diastolic pressure; PEEP = postive end expiratory pressure.) (Adapted from Tibby SM, Murdoch IA. Monitoring cardiac function in intensive care. *Arch Dis Child.* 2003;88:46-52.)

Surgical Intervention/Revascularization Procedures

Percutaneous transluminal coronary angioplasty (PTCA), also called **percutaneous coronary intervention** (PCI), involves the insertion of a balloon-tipped catheter through a peripheral artery (usually femoral or brachial artery), which is guided to the heart and coronary vessels. Once inside the coronary vessel, the catheter is placed so that it straddles the stenotic lesion. The balloon is inflated and the plaque is literally crushed between the vessel wall and the balloon.[13] An **endoluminal stent** may be placed at the site of the atherosclerotic lesion to maintain the patency of the coronary artery (Figure 6-7). The most significant complications associated with PTCA include vascular trauma, perioperative myocardial infarction, and restenosis. Restenosis typically occurs within 6 months after the procedure. Bare metal stents (BMSs) and drug-eluting stents (DES) combined with antiplatelet medications have decreased the incidence of restenosis and thrombus formation. PTCA is usually performed as an outpatient and prolonged hospitalization would occur only if complications have arisen.

Coronary artery bypass grafting (CABG) uses segments of arteries and/or veins to bypass around complete occlusions, multiple plaques not amenable to PTCA, or severe CAD. The vascular segments connect the aorta and a coronary artery distal to the obstruction (Figure 6-8). The vascular segments are often taken from the LEs (saphenous veins), anterior chest wall (internal mammary artery), or forearms (radial artery). The surgical approach is usually a median sternotomy where the sternum is transected from the sternal notch extending below the xiphoid process. The sternum is generally closed with stainless steel sutures either through or around the sternum to provide stability. Postoperative complications include incision pain, dysrhythmias (eg, atrial fibrillation, premature ventricular contractions [PVCs]),

Figure 6-7. Angioplasty and stent placement for CAD. (Adapted with permission from Sheldon LK. Oxygenation. Sudbury, MA: Jones and Bartlett; 2001.)

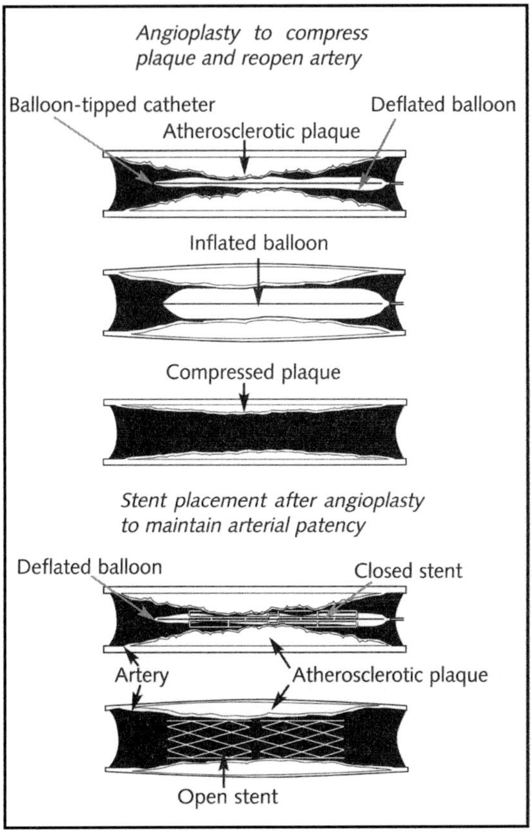

Figure 6-8. Coronary arteries and CABG. (Reprinted with permission from Sheldon LK. Oxygenation. Sudbury, MA: Jones and Bartlett; 2001.)

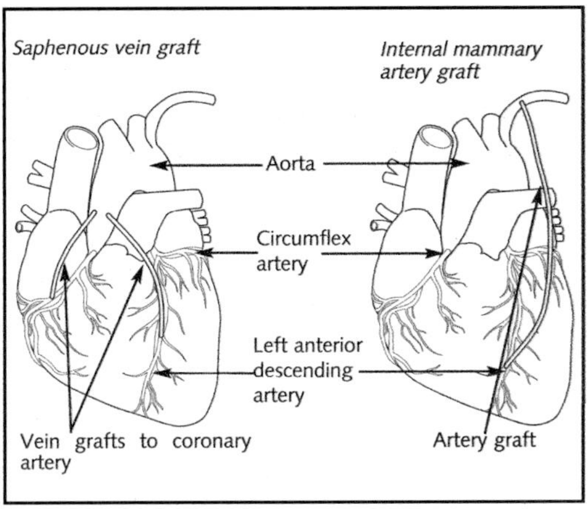

HTN, hyperglycemia, wound infection, cerebral vascular accident (CVA), myocardial infarction, and abnormal lab values.[19,20] The patient will often have a mediastinal chest tube, external pacemaker, and multiple intravascular catheters.

Table 6-3

Classification of Blood Pressure for Adults

Category	*Systolic (mm Hg)*	*Diastolic (mm Hg)*
Normal	< 120	<80
Elevated	120 to 129	<80
Stage 1 HTN	130 to 139	80 to 89
Stage 2 HTN	≥ 140	≥ 90
HTN crisis	≥ 180	≥ 120

Adapted from Whelton PK, Carey RM, Aronow WS, et al. 2017 ACC/AHA/AAPA/ABC/ACPM/AGS/APhA/ASH/ASPC/NMA/PCNA Guideline for the Prevention, Detection, Evaluation, and Management of High Blood Pressure in Adults: Executive Summary: A Report of the American College of Cardiology/American Heart Association Task Force on Clinical Practice Guidelines. *Hypertension*. 2018;71(6):1269-1324.

Transmyocardial revascularization (TMR) uses a laser to create a channel in the ischemic myocardium. This channel facilitates microcirculatory blood flow and possible new vessel formation (neovascularization/angiogenesis) reducing angina symptoms. This procedure is performed for patients with inoperable CAD and chronic angina.[21,22]

Hypertension

HTN has recently been redefined as an elevated BP greater than 130/80 (Table 6-3).[23] The newer guidelines emphasize lifestyle changes in each BP category and leave antihypertensive medications for higher-risk stage 1 and stage 2 HTN. HTN is common, affecting nearly 80 million people, which is 33% of the US population, or approximately 1 in every 3 adults.[2] Early recognition and medical management reduces the risk of CVD and HTN is an important modifiable risk factor for stroke, transient ischemic attack (TIA), CAD, and heart failure.[2,24] BP is the product of cardiac output times the total peripheral resistance (TPR), also called **systemic vascular resistance** (SVR), (BP=CO x TPR) and HTN is an abnormality of TPR regulation. Essential HTN, also known as **primary HTN**, has an unknown cause and accounts for 90% of the cases. Secondary HTN is associated with renal disease (eg, glomerulonephritis, nephritis, diabetic nephropathy), endocrine disorders (eg, acromegaly, hyperthyroidism), adrenal disorders (eg, Cushing's syndrome, aldosteronism, pheochromocytoma), sleep apnea, pregnancy, and acute stress (eg, postoperative, hypoglycemia, alcohol withdrawal).[17] Medical management of HTN includes self-care (eg, diet, sodium restriction, exercise) and medications including diuretics, calcium channel blockers, ACE inhibitors, angiotensin receptor blockers, and vasodilators. The optimal BP target is somewhat uncertain, and a common goal is systolic BP <140 mm Hg. However, recent studies demonstrate that a lower systolic BP goal of <120 mm Hg further reduces cardiovascular morbidity and mortality compared to the standard goal.[25] Although the lower targets do not appear to increase the risk for adverse events, such as orthostatic hypotension and injurious falls, the therapist should consider these potential adverse events.[26]

Cardiomyopathy

The cardiomyopathies are a diverse group of disorders involving the myocardium resulting in mechanical and/or electrical dysfunction and are associated with ventricular hypertrophy or dilatation. These disorders are classified in multiple ways

Table 6-4

CLASSIFICATIONS OF CARDIOMYOPATHIES

Primary Cardiomyopathies		
Genetic	**Mixed**	**Acquired**
• Hypertrophic • Conduction abnormalities • Mitochondrial myopathies • Ion channelopathies	• Dilated • Restrictive	• Inflammatory (myocarditis • Stress provoked (Tako-Tsubo) • Peripartum • Tachycardia-induced
Secondary Cardiomyopathies		
Infiltrative	**Storage**	**Toxicity**
• Amyloidosis • Gaucher's disease	• Hemochromatosis • Fabry's disease	• Alcohol • Chemotherapy/radiotherapy • Lead/mercury
Endocrine	**Autoimmune**	**Neuromuscular**
• Diabetes • Hyper-/hypothyroidism • Pheochromocytoma • Acromegaly	• Systemic lupus erythematosus • Rheumatoid arthritis • Scleroderma	• Duchenne-Becker muscular dystrophy • Neurofibromatosis

Adapted from Maron BJ, Towbin JA, Thiene G, et al; American Heart Association; Council on Clinical Cardiology, Heart Failure and Transplantation Committee; Quality of Care and Outcomes Research and Functional Genomics and Translational Biology Interdisciplinary Working Groups; Council on Epidemiology and Prevention. Contemporary definitions and classification of the cardiomyopathies: an American Heart Association Scientific Statement from the Council on Clinical Cardiology, Heart Failure and Transplantation Committee; Quality of Care and Outcomes Research and Functional Genomics and Translational Biology Interdisciplinary Working Groups; and Council on Epidemiology and Prevention. *Circulation*. 2006 11;113(14):1807-116.

as noted in Table 6-4.[27] Table 6-5 defines cardiomyopathy by morphology (ie, size and function), dilated, hypertrophic, or restrictive.[27,28] Ischemic cardiomyopathy is the most common form of dilated cardiomyopathy and results from CAD and myocardial infarction. The cardiomyopathies each have a distinct pathophysiology but ultimately lead to heart failure as outlined in Table 6-5.[17,27,28]

Valve Disease

Valvular heart disease (VHD) in the adult results from rheumatic fever in childhood, congenital disorders, or degenerative changes. Degenerative changes occur with aging and are most often due to calcification and infections.[28-30]

Valve dysfunction can occur in all valves of the heart but primarily impact the aortic and mitral valves. Valve disorders are generally described as valve stenosis or valve insufficiency resulting in regurgitation (Table 6-6).

Aortic Stenosis

Aortic stenosis is narrowing of the aortic valve opening that obstructs blood flow from the left ventricle into the ascending aorta during ventricular systole

Table 6-5
Signs and Symptoms of Cardiomyopathy

Dilated	*Hypertrophic*	*Restrictive*
• CHF • ECG: Ventricular dysrhythmias, non-specific repolarization abnormalities (ST-T changes) • Left ventricle dilation/ dysfunction • High diastolic pressure/ low cardiac output • Systolic dysfunction (HFrEF)	• Dyspnea, chest pain, syncope • ECG: LVH, exaggerated Q waves • LVH, hypercontractile function • Diastolic dysfunction (HFpEF)	• Dyspnea, fatigue, right-sided CHF • ECG: Non-specific repolarization abnormalities (ST-T segment changes) • Small left ventricle, normal or mildly reduced left ventricle function • Diastolic dysfunction (HFpEF)

CHF = congestive heart failure; HFpEF = heart failure with preserved ejection fraction; HFrEF = heart failure with reduced ejection fraction; LVH = left ventricular hypertrophy.

Adapted from Carabello[31]; Carabello and Crawford [32]; Doherty[78]; Papadakis and McPhee[79]; and Porter and Kaplan.[80]

Table 6-6
Signs and Symptoms of Valve Dysfunction

Aortic Stenosis	*Aortic Insufficiency/Regurgitation*
• Harsh, systolic murmur, often radiating to the neck • ECG: LVH • Dampened peripheral pulses • Angina on exertion, syncope, dyspnea, orthopnea and paroxysmal nocturnal dyspnea (PND)	• Wide pulse pressure • Chest pain • ECG: LVH • Diastolic murmur along left sternal border • PMI in left axilla
Mitral Stenosis	*Mitral Insufficiency/Regurgitation*
• ECG: Atrial fibrillation (common), left atrial enlargement • Prominent S1 heart sound • Right ventricular heave • Dyspnea, orthopnea, PND	• ECG: Left atrial enlargement • Pulmonary congestion (crackles) • Systolic murmur • Palpitations, fatigue, dyspnea, wheezing, orthopnea, PND

(ejection).[29,30] Aortic stenosis is most commonly associated with age and a congenital bicuspid valve (the normal aortic valve has 3 cusps), but may also be associated with rheumatic fever resulting in fibrotic thickening and fusion of the valve leaflets. Factors contributing to aortic stenosis are progressive calcification, hypercholesterolemia, and inflammation. Aortic stenosis occurs more often in men, is generally asymptomatic until middle age or older, and is the most common cardiac valve disorder in the United States.[31] Ventricular strain and increased myocardial oxygen demand result in a pressure overload as the heart attempts to eject against a narrowed opening. Ventricular hypertrophy maintains stroke volume and cardiac output during a prolonged latency period, but chronic obstruction and pressure overload lead to angina, syncope, and, ultimately, systolic heart failure.[28-31] Typical signs and symptoms are listed in Table 6-6.

Aortic Insufficiency/Regurgitation

Aortic regurgitation is retrograde blood flow from the aorta into the left ventricle through an incompetent aortic valve during ventricular diastole. Aortic regurgitation is most often associated with rheumatic heart disease, congenital bicuspid aortic valve, infective endocarditis, HTN, and disorders involving the aortic root (eg, Marfan's syndrome, aortic aneurysm).[13,28] Initially, the left ventricle hypertrophies to maintain stroke volume and cardiac output; however, chronic regurgitation results in progressive diastolic run-off leading to volume overload and left ventricle failure.

Mitral Stenosis

Mitral stenosis is an obstruction of blood flow from the left atrium to the left ventricle because of a narrowed mitral orifice during diastole.[17,28] Mitral stenosis is most commonly associated with rheumatic heart disease. As mitral stenosis reduces left ventricle filling during diastole, cardiac output may be decreased. As mitral stenosis progresses, pressures increase in the left atrium resulting in increased pulmonary vascular pressures, which increases the stress on the right ventricle. Right ventricle function is compromised as it strains to propel blood through the pulmonary circuit due to this increase in afterload. Patients present with symptoms of left ventricle failure due to reduced left ventricle filling and reduced cardiac output, but left ventricle ejection fraction is often normal.[17,32]

Mitral Insufficiency/Mitral Regurgitation

Mitral regurgitation is the retrograde flow of blood from the left ventricle into the left atrium through an incompetent mitral valve during systole. Common causes of mitral regurgitation include rheumatic heart disease, rupture of papillary muscle or chordae tendinae, infective endocarditis, collagen vascular disease, myxomatous degeneration (mitral valve prolapse), and cardiomyopathy-related annular distension.[32,33] The mitral regurgitation induced retrograde flow of blood into the left atrium during systole increases the filling volume of the left ventricle during the next diastole. The increased left ventricle preload allows a forceful systolic contraction and emptying of the left ventricle that maintains stroke volume and cardiac output (see the Starling Law of the Heart). However, left ventricle work and hypertrophy progresses over time and eventual contractile dysfunction leads to symptoms of left ventricle failure.[32,33]

Medical and Surgical Management of Valvular Heart Disease

Repair or Replacement

The decision to manage VHD medically or to proceed with surgical repair or replacement is based on hemodynamics, the ejection fraction, surgical repairability, the presence of comorbid conditions, and patient's age.[34] Goals of maintaining the valve apparatus are to allow sustained ventricular function, reduce operative mortality, promote better late outcomes, lessen need for anticoagulation therapy, reduce endocarditis, and avoid possible failure of prosthetic valves.[32] Valve repair surgeries, when feasible, are viewed as superior to replacement procedures. Minimally invasive techniques, sometimes combined with robotically maneuvered instruments, are becoming more common. Goals of minimally invasive surgeries include reduced blood loss, decreased postoperative pain, and shorter hospital lengths of stay.[35,36] Valve surgery may also involve median sternotomy, partial sternotomy, transverse sternotomy, or limited lateral thoracotomy as the surgical approach.

Stenosis

Valvulotomies enlarge the narrowed opening of a heart valve. A **commissurotomy** involves cutting through the commissures, an abnormal connection between a valve's leaflets, with a knife or by a finger thrust. A **balloon valvotomy** or **valvuloplasty** involves the insertion and inflation of a balloon-tipped catheter across the stenotic valve widening the opening.[36-38] These techniques may be performed in closed fashion through the insertion of a catheter into a large peripheral vessel (vein for mitral valve; artery for aortic valve) or in an open fashion associated with cardiopulmonary bypass.[17,36]

Regurgitation

Annuloplasty involves the placement of a prosthetic ring to recreate the normal annular geometry and decrease the size of the valve opening. Other repair procedures include **chordal transfer** or **shortening**, **artificial chordae tendinae** via sutures, **cusp plication** or **cusp extension**, or **cusp replacement** using autologous pericardium. These procedures attempt to normalize the valvular apparatus by promoting complete closure of the valves, thereby preventing regurgitation.[36,37]

Valve replacement uses either artificial mechanical valves or tissue (also called **bioprosthetic**) valves. Common mechanical valves include the caged-ball type (eg, Starr-Edwards), bileaflet-tilting disc (eg, St. Jude Medical), or the single-tilting disc (eg, Bjork-Shiley). The bioprosthetic valves are usually composed of either porcine or bovine tissue, or homografts, which are preserved human valves.[17,39] Mechanical valves are thrombogenic and, therefore, require that the patient receive long-term anticoagulant therapy.[39] The surgical approach is often a median sternotomy but endovascular techniques are rapidly becoming more common. The percutaneous endovascular valve replacement uses a catheter to deliver an expandable valve to its anatomic location. Catheter-based alternatives, especially mitral valve (transcatheter mitral valve replacement [TMVR]) and aortic valve (transcatheter aortic valve replacement [TAVR)]), were initially reserved for older and higher risk patients but are now being applied to a greater percentage of the population.[40]

Complications after valve surgery include valve thrombosis and embolism, which is often attributable to inadequate anticoagulation, atrial fibrillation, age greater than 70 years, and depressed left ventricle function.[39] Early endocarditis may occur in a minority of patients who acquire perioperative bacteremia arising from skin, wound, or contaminated intravascular devices. Valve failure or regurgitation occurs minimally but may be a complication of prosthetic-valve endocarditis.[39]

Close anatomic relationship between the valves and the conduction tissue may lead to dysrhythmias and are frequently encountered in the early postoperative period.[41] Postoperative bleeding has also been noted at the insertion site with the endovascular techniques.

Aneurysm

An aneurysm is a localized abnormal dilation of a blood vessel, usually an artery. Complications of aneurysms include thrombus, progressive expansion, and rupture. Risk factors for aneurysms include atherosclerosis, HTN, male gender, cigarette smoking, chronic obstructive pulmonary disease (COPD), and older age.[42] Aneurysms may be classified as saccular, a local outpouching, or, more commonly, fusiform, an enlargement of the entire vessel lumen.[30] Clinically, aortic aneurysms are classified according to anatomic features as shown in Figure 6-9. Aneurysms are often asymptomatic, making diagnosis difficult. Dissection involves rupture of

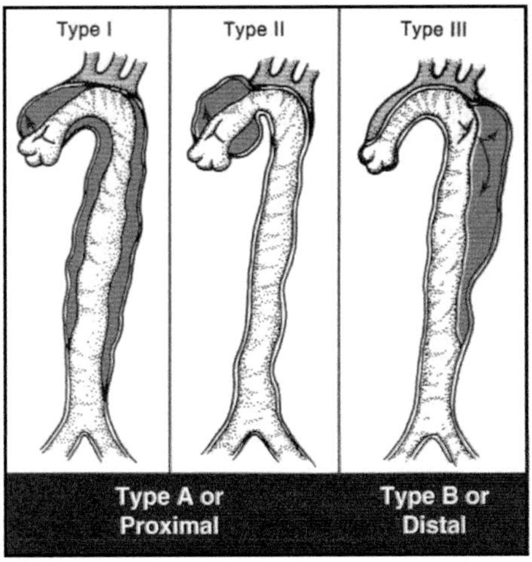

Figure 6-9. The DeBakey classification system for aortic dissection. Type I originates in the ascending aorta and may propagate beyond the aortic arch. Type II is confined to the ascending aorta, and Type III originates in the descending aorta and extends distally. Proximal dissection includes DeBakey Types I and II, while distal dissections are DeBakey III. (Reprinted with permission from Braunwald E. *Heart Disease: A Textbook of Cardiovascular Medicine*. 6th ed. Philadelphia, PA: Elsevier; 2001.)

the tunica intima followed by intraluminal splitting and separation of the medial layers of the vessel by a column of blood.[43] Classic signs and symptoms of aortic aneurysm dissection are related to the size and location of the defect, but typically include severe tearing chest, back, and abdominal pain; differences in measured pulse quality and BP between extremities; signs of decreased cerebral perfusion, including stroke, syncope, and altered mental status; or less, frequently, spinal cord ischemia.[30,43]

Medical Management

Medical therapy is directed to decrease the risk of rupture and slow the progression of dissection by reducing the force of left ventricle contractions and decreasing arterial BP without compromising organ perfusion.[43] Common medications include beta-blockers, nitrates, and vasodilators.

Surgical Management

Surgical repair is performed to prevent rupture at a time that the risk of rupture is greater than the risk of death from the operation.[44] Surgical techniques for aneurysms may be endovascular or a traditional open approach by a thoracotomy for thoracic aortic aneurysm (TAA) or transperitoneal, midline, or left retroperitoneal incision for abdominal aortic aneurysms (AAA). The aim of an open surgery is to excise and replace the dissecting aortic segment. Open repairs use synthetic grafts of woven or knitted Dacron.[43] **Endovascular aneurysm repair** (EVAR) are minimally invasive procedures that use stents and grafts to bridge or buttress the aneurysm. The femoral artery is a common access point for AAA and **TAA endovascular repairs** (TEVAR).

Complications are typically reduced with the endovascular approach; however, AAA and TAA repairs are high-risk surgeries, and complications include death, myocardial infarction, hemorrhage, pulmonary insufficiency, renal failure, impaired bowel function, including paralytic ileus and colonic ischemia, graft infection, and spinal cord injury.[42,45] Spinal cord ischemia is the most significant nonfatal complication and rates of spinal cord injury have decreased with the implementation of cerebrospinal fluid drainage, reimplantation of patent critical intercostal arteries, the use of intraoperative somatosensory evoked-potential monitoring and maintenance of distal aortic perfusion during surgery with the use of atriofemoral (left heart) bypass to the distal aorta.[46]

Endocarditis/Myocarditis

Endocarditis is an infection of the endocardium resulting in fever, valvular vegetations, and valve dysfunction, as well as systemic emboli and CVA. It is most common in patients with underlying heart disease, diabetes, and renal disease requiring hemodialysis, as well as patients with a history of intravenous drug use, hospital-acquired infections and poor dental hygiene.[28,29,46] Common symptoms include fever, fatigue, dyspnea, arthralgias, weight loss, night sweats, heart murmurs, and petechiae on the skin.[28,46] Diagnosis is confirmed by blood cultures and guide antimicrobial therapy. Complications include embolic CVA, abscess formation, valve dysfunction resulting in regurgitation, and conduction disturbances.

Myocarditis is a focal or diffuse inflammation of the myocardium due to viral, bacterial, or fungal infections and secondarily to drugs and immunologic reactions. Myocarditis is most common following a respiratory infection and patient presentation may include chest pain, tachycardia, and symptoms of heart failure including dyspnea, orthopnea, and fatigue.

Pericardial Disease

Pericarditis is an inflammatory process involving the pericardium and the epicardial surface. Pericarditis may occur after an acute myocardial infarction, open heart surgery, uremia due to kidney failure, and viral and bacterial infections. Patients will frequently complain of chest pain and fever, and present with a pericardial friction rub on auscultation. Complications include tamponade physiology and heart failure.

Cardiac tamponade is the accumulation of fluid within the pericardial space, **pericardial effusion**, that compresses the heart and interferes with diastolic filling, reducing stroke volume, cardiac output, and coronary artery blood flow. Patients will present with elevated right atrial pressure (RAP) (ie, jugular venous distention [JVD]), diminished heart sounds, falling BP, and tachycardia. Cardiac tamponade may occur following chest trauma, cancer, renal failure (uremia), and pericarditis. Although uncommon, tamponade may be a complication of epicardial pacemaker wire removal following open heart surgery.

Heart Failure

Heart failure may be defined as the inability of the heart to pump sufficient amounts of blood to meet the physiologic demands of the body.[17,47]

Nearly 6 million Americans are affected with heart failure and the prevalence of heart failure is expected to increase 46% over the next decade.[2] The incidence of heart failure approaches 10/1000 people and is the admitting diagnosis for over 20% of persons older than 65.[2] Heart failure is the final pathway for virtually all forms of heart disease, including CAD/ischemic heart disease, HTN, cardiomyopathies, valve disorders, heart dysrhythmias, and congenital heart disease (Figure 6-10).[17] Clinically, heart failure may be categorized in multiple ways, including high/low output, right/left sided, but the most frequent description is **systolic heart failure**, failure of the ventricular pump, or **diastolic heart failure**, the inability of the heart to fill properly due to altered relaxation increasing ventricular stiffness. Heart failure is also commonly described in relation to the ejection fraction: **heart failure with preserved ejection fraction** (HFpEF) and **heart failure with reduced ejection fraction** (HFrEF). Systolic heart failure decreases the ejection fraction while diastolic heart failure is often associated with a preserved ejection fraction but other mechanism besides ventricular stiffness contribute to the reduced filling of the ventricle in HFpEF.[48,49] The common denominator for all descriptions of heart failure is that the clinical manifestations result from an inadequate cardiac output. The pathogenesis of heart failure is multifactorial resulting from a complex blend of structural, functional, and biological alterations including altered loading conditions, altered energy metabolism, altered

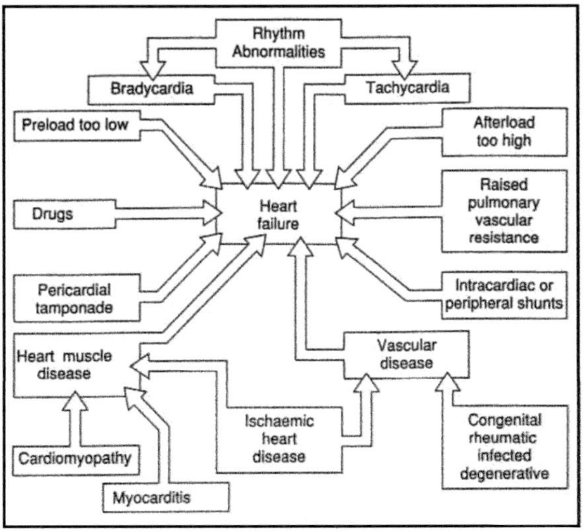

Figure 6-10. Heart failure is the final common pathway of most heart diseases and disorders.

Table 6-7

Pathophysiologic Mechanisms in Heart Failure

Structural	*Functional*	*Biological*
• Hypertrophy • Fibrosis/extracellular matrix changes • Myocyte apoptosis • Left ventricle remodeling • Dilation, increased spherical shape • Wall thinning, aneurysm formation • Coronary artery obstruction/inflammation • Expression of fetal contractile proteins	• Valve dysfunction • Ischemic myocardium • Atrial and ventricular dysrhythmias • Altered right and left ventricle interaction	• Activation of renin-angiotensin-aldosterone system • Activation of sympathetic nervous system • Increased expression of inflammatory cytokines and oxidative stress • Altered calcium handling

Adapted from Jessup M, Brozena S. Medical progress: heart failure. *N Engl J Med*. 2003;348:2007-2018 and Udelson JE. Heart failure with preserved ejection fraction. *Circulation*. 2011;124(21):e540-e543.

neurohumoral activation and signal transduction, abnormal expression and function of contractile proteins, abnormal excitation-contraction coupling, and an altered cytoskeleton (Table 6-7).[3,45] Multiple compensatory mechanisms attempt to increase blood volume and raise cardiac filling pressure to maintain the cardiac output, raise BP, and redistribute blood flow. However, as heart failure proceeds, the heart's ability to contract and relax declines progressively and the failure worsens.[17,47] Common symptoms of heart failure are listed in Table 6-8.

Table 6-8 SIGNS AND SYMPTOMS OF HEART FAILURE
Respiratory Distress
• Dyspnea on exertion (DOE)/shortness of breath (SOB) • Orthopnea • Paroxysmal nocturnal dyspnea • Cough; pink, frothy sputum • ↑ respiratory rate
Physical Exam
• Pulmonary crackles • S3 heart sound • JVD/ ↑ central venous pressure (CVP)/RAP
Reduced Exercise Capacity
• Fatigue/weakness • Limited ability to perform activities of daily living (ADLs) and limited walking ability (6 Minute Walk Test [6MWT])

Medical and Surgical Management

The goals of therapy in patients with heart failure are to improve quality and quantity of life and to prevent progression of the syndrome. These goals are accomplished by correcting the underlying cause (eg, aortic valve replacement secondary to aortic stenosis, antibiotics for endocarditis) and control of the heart failure state. Pharmacologic control of the heart failure state is accomplished through ACE inhibitors, angiotensin receptor blockers (ARBs), diuretics, beta-blockers, inotropic agents, and vasodilators (see Appendix B).[3,17,50,51] These drugs attempt to limit the activation of the renin-angiotensin-aldosterone system and sympathetic nervous system. Medications reduce afterload, correct fluid balance, and improve ventricular contractility to increase the stroke volume and cardiac output.

Surgical interventions for heart failure include heart transplantation (see Chapter 14), CABG, and PTCA, valve repairs/replacement surgeries, and implantation of pacemakers, defibrillators and mechanical circulatory support devices including intra-aortic balloon pump (IABPs), left ventricular assist devices (LVADs), and total artificial hearts (TAHs).[17,22]

IABP is indicated for patients in cardiogenic shock following cardiac surgery or an acute myocardial infarction. The device consists of a balloon-tipped flexible catheter attached to a console. The catheter is usually inserted through the femoral artery and guided to the descending thoracic aorta. The patient's ECG and pressure waveforms are monitored, and the balloon is triggered to inflate during ventricular diastole and deflate during systole. Inflation of the balloon displaces blood and increases diastolic pressure in the arch of the aorta (behind the balloon) increasing blood flow through the coronary arteries. Balloon deflation increases cardiac output by reducing aortic pressures (afterload) prior to ventricular ejection.[17,52] Patients are often critically ill and physical therapy services may not be indicated. Patients may be referred for bed mobility, range of motion (ROM) exercises, airway clearance, and mobilization activities out of the bed. However, if the IABP is inserted into the femoral artery, patient mobility is limited to in-bed activities. Recently, IABP may be inserted into the subclavian or axillary arteries allowing out of bed mobilization

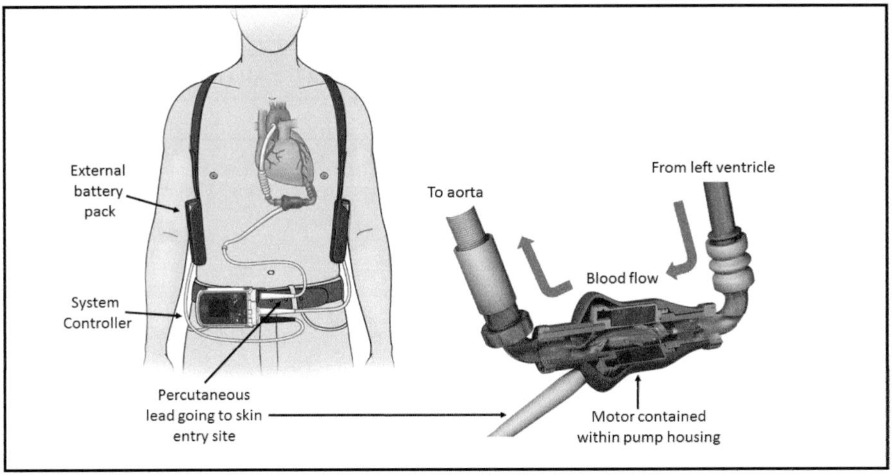

Figure 6-11. HeartMate XVE left ventricular assist system (LVAS). (Reprinted with permission from Thoratec Corp.)

and ambulation.[53,54] Precautions for IABP include maintaining hip flexion less than 70 degrees of the involved limb if inserted into the femoral artery and careful monitoring of all vascular access and patient's hemodynamics.[7] Complications include LE ischemia, line infections, and vascular injuries (eg, aortic dissection/laceration, lymphocele).[17]

Ventricular assist devices (VADs) are designed to unload the right (right ventricular assist device **[RVAD]**) or left (**LVAD**) ventricles and support the pulmonary or systemic circulation by improving cardiac output and end-organ blood flow (Figure 6-11).[17,55] VAD support was previously viewed as rescue therapy as a bridge to transplantation. Now, the VAD can be considered terminal or destination therapy and bridge to heart transplant.[56,57] The implanted LVAD has an outflow line connected to the left ventricular apex where blood is diverted through a pump and returned to the circulation via an aortic inflow line. The RVAD withdraws blood from the right atrium and returns to the main pulmonary artery. Two blood pumps can be used for biventricular support.[17,22,55] VAD support has led to reverse remodeling or improvements in ventricular size, shape, and contractile function leading to device removal in select patients. First generation VADs were pulsatile pumps, while the second generation pumps are continuous axial flow pumps. A pulsatile VAD has a sac and diaphragm that creates a compressible blood chamber. The chamber expands to fill when blood enters and is emptied by the compression of the diaphragm. Nonpulsatile VADs are divided into axial flow pumps (eg, HeartMate II [Thoratec]), in which a propeller pushes blood unidirectionally, and centrifugal pumps (eg, HeartWare [HeartWare Inc]), in which blood comes into the center of the pump, and is spun and accelerated out to the periphery of the plate.[56] Currently, the most common VADs are the second generation axial flow or centrifugal devices. These pumps provide a continuous flow up to 10 liters/minute depending on the revolutions per minute (RPM) of the device. A palpable pulse, BP, or pulse oximetry readings may no longer be recognized because there is no true diastolic or systolic phase of the cardiac cycle with continuous-flow pumps. The therapist or nurse will need to use an ultrasound device to assess the mean arterial blood pressure.[57] Third generation VADs are being studied. These devices are also continuous-flow pumps (axial and centrifugal) but have a noncontact design that is hypothesized to increase durability and reduce thrombosis.[58] VADs are connected to a central console that allows monitoring and recording of device data (eg, device RPMs, output flows [cardiac output]). Physical therapy will be consulted to initiate exercise conditioning with these patients and therapeutic interventions may include progressive mobilization, including treadmill walking and progressive resistive exercises utilizing the principles of phase I to II cardiac rehabilitation programs. Patients will demonstrate improvements in quality of life and exercise capacity.[59-62] VADs can operate on batteries to allow greater mobility, and the therapist must be familiar with emergency procedures in case of battery failure. The therapist must maintain the patency of the drive lines with external pumps to ensure adequate flows and monitor the patient's and device's hemodynamic information (ie, rates, BP, outputs). Complications of VADs include thrombus formation related to blood stasis within the pump or inadequate anticoagulation, CVA, hemorrhage, line infections, gastrointestinal (GI) bleeding, and renal or hepatic insufficiency.[17,63]

Novel mechanical circulatory assist devices (eg, Tandem Heart [Cardiac Assist Inc], Impella 2.5 and 5.0 [Abiomed]) are being used for temporary support of patients who have acute decompensated heart failure or cardiogenic shock similar to IABP. These devices are inserted percutaneously and aim to support the hemodynamic status of the patient. The Tandem Heart is an extracorporeal continuous-flow centrifugal assist device where a cannula is inserted through the femoral vein and advanced across the intra-atrial septum into the left atrium, while the Impella is a catheter-based pump inserted into the femoral artery or through the axillary artery and advanced to the left ventricle. Each of these devices are typically indicated for short-term use (< 14 days).[64] Mobilization out of bed and ambulation have successfully been performed with the axillary approach for insertion of the Impella device.[65]

Left ventricle and **biventricular pacing** have proven effective to improve the electrical and mechanical synchrony for patients with CHF, intraventricular conduction delay, or left bundle branch block. **Synchrony** refers to the normal coordinated, electrically induced contraction of the right and left ventricles. Biventricular pacing synchronizes the right and left ventricles leading to increases in the ejection fraction, stroke volume, and cardiac output.[66] **Automatic implantable cardioverter-defibrillators** (AICDs) are devices used for the prevention of sudden cardiac arrest due to life-threatening ventricular dysrhythmias (eg, ventricular tachycardia, ventricular fibrillation).[67]

Patients who have received a pacemaker or ICD can participate in therapy. The therapist should review the ECG information and standard precautions provided for pacemakers/ICDs (see Appendix A).

Differential Diagnosis of Chest Pain

Chest pain occurs frequently and is usually benign; however, myocardial ischemia is an important consideration because it impacts patient morbidity and is potentially fatal.[68-71] Angina pectoris, or chest pain of cardiac origin, results from myocardial ischemia, which is caused by an imbalance between myocardial oxygen supply and demand (see Figure 6-6).[17] The rapid recognition of chest pain that is cardiac or noncardiac in origin will impact the therapist's clinical decision making. Unstable angina may be a symptom of the onset of acute coronary syndrome leading to eventual myocardial infarction. Physical therapy is contraindicated for patients with unstable angina until the patient has been medically or surgically stabilized. Unstable angina is defined as having 3 possible presentations[13,55]:

1. Symptoms of angina at rest or with minimal exertion
2. New onset of exertional angina
3. Recent acceleration of angina symptoms superimposed on a preexisting pattern of angina

Table 6-9 provides a general schema to determine the origins of chest pain. Patient complaints of chest pain should be forwarded to the nursing and medical team. The evaluation of acute chest pain should begin with a clinical history that focuses on the characteristics of pain, time of onset, and duration of symptoms and an examination of vital signs. Secondary questions should include an assessment of cardiac risk factors and for gastric or pulmonary disease, as well as psychological disorders.[67-70] About 50% of all patients with chest pain and normal coronary anatomy have esophageal reflux or GI motility disorders, approximately 60% have evidence of breathing disorders, and 60% have psychological abnormalities.[68-71]

Physical Therapist Management

Phase I Cardiac Rehabilitation

The principles of cardiac rehabilitation should be used in the treatment of patients with cardiovascular disease. Cardiac rehabilitation is a program of education and exercise established to assist individuals with heart disease in achieving optimal physical, psychosocial, and functional status within the limits of their disease. Cardiac rehabilitation as part of comprehensive risk factor intervention can extend overall survival, improve quality of life, decrease the need for interventional procedures, such as PTCA and CABG, and reduces the incidence of subsequent myocardial infarction.[1] Exercise training improves exercise tolerance, reduces the severity of angina symptoms, and improves both physical and mental functioning.[72,73]

Phase I cardiac rehabilitation is classically described as occurring in the acute care hospital but may be extended to post-acute environments, such as skilled nursing facilities, inpatient rehabilitation facilities, and home health. Rehabilitation begins when the patient is determined to be stable (Table 6-10). Following the history and systems review, a physical examination is performed, which should include a more thorough aerobic capacity (eg, vital sign and symptom responses to activity), circulation (eg, auscultation of heart sounds, ECG analysis, pulse quality), mental function, mobility, ventilation, and respiration (eg, pulse oximetry, auscultation of breath sounds) as noted in Table 1-2, Figure 1-3, and Tables 6-11 and 7-13.[7]

Progression of rehabilitation depends on daily examination findings. Progression may vary from a more rapid increase in activity tolerance in the low-risk patient to a slower progression in higher risk or more debilitated patients.[7] A framework to determine risk stratification is presented in Table 6-12 and contraindications and relative contraindications for exercise training are provided in Table 6-13. These tables combined with the daily examination will guide the therapist to determine an appropriate exercise and activity prescription. The general goal of Phase I cardiac rehabilitation is to enable the patient to tolerate ADLs, including self-care activities, stair climbing, toileting, and walking functional distances (1 to 4 metabolic equivalents [METs] of activity) with minimal to no cardiovascular symptoms and appropriate vital sign responses (Tables 6-14 and 6-15). During Phase I cardiac rehabilitation, education is of paramount importance, and this is a time to initiate risk factor and behavior modification. It is well established that risk factor modification and living a more heart healthy lifestyle can reduce secondary complications and future cardiac events.

Additional Considerations

Physical therapists should review the **ECG**, laboratory values, determine hemodynamic stability through review of vital signs over the past 12 to 24 hours, and examine all wounds and incisions. Common postoperative ECG changes include atrial fibrillation/flutter and premature ventricular beats. Recall that atrial contraction may contribute 20% to the filling of the ventricles during diastole. Abnormal atrial rhythms

Table 6-9

Differential Diagnosis of Chest Pain

Descriptor (Questions to ask)	*Angina Cardiac*	*Other* (eg, pericarditis)	*Musculoskeletal* (eg, subacromial bursitis)	*Gastrointestinal*
Symptoms	Nonfocal, dull, vague	Sharp, cutting, difficulty swallowing	Intense, constant, dull, sometimes throbbing, vague onset	Vague onset, symptoms ↑ related to food consumption
Location	Anything above the waist (classic: substernal, left UE, jaw)	Substernal, may radiate to neck, upper back, upper trapezius, left arm	Anterolateral shoulder region	No effect
Exercise	↑ symptoms	↓ symptoms or no effect	↑ symptoms with motions of involved UE, especially overhead movements	May exacerbate symptoms (eg, peptic ulcers), but often no effect
Rest	↓ symptoms; may awaken from sleep	No effect, sleep delayed	↓ symptoms	No effect; may awaken from sleep
Body position/ROM	No effect	↓ symptoms in quadruped, leaning forward, sitting upright; ↑ symptoms by trunk rotation/side-bending	↑ symptoms with lying on involved side	↑ symptoms with head down positioning (eg, gastroesophageal reflux disease)
Deep breath/cough	No effect	↑ symptoms with any activity that causes chest wall to move	No effect	No effect
Palpation	No effect	Painful over left, anterior/lower chest wall	Painful over bursa; area may be warm/swollen	No effect

(continued)

Table 6-9 (continued)

Differential Diagnosis of Chest Pain

Descriptor (Questions to ask)	*Angina Cardiac*	*Other* (eg, pericarditis)	*Musculoskeletal* (eg, subacromial bursitis)	*Gastrointestinal*
Nitroglycerine	↓ symptoms	No effect	No effect	No effect
Other		History of fever/chills, recent myocardial infarction, complains of weakness	Relief with heat, non-steroidal anti-inflammatory agents	Relief with antacids

Adapted from Heibert J, Coffman S. Presentation: Chest Pain—Now What? Recognition and Management of Angina. Combined Sections Meeting, San Antonio, TX; 2001 and Seidel HM, Ball JW, Benedict GW, et al. *Mosby's Guide to Physical Examination*. 7th ed. St. Louis, MO; Elsevier: WB Saunders Co; 2011.

Table 6-10

Cardiac Rehabilitation and Patient Readiness

Patient is considered stable if:

- No new/recurrent episode of chest pain in 8 hours
- No new signs of decompensated heart failure, including:
  - Dyspnea at rest
  - Bilateral crackles >0.5 of lung
  - Hypotension
- No new significant, abnormal dysrhythmia or ECG changes in past 8 hours
  - If atrial fibrillation: Ventricular rate <110 beats per minute (bpm) at rest
  - Able to speak comfortably with a RR <30 breaths/minute
  - Cardiac index (cardiac output/body mass) >2 L/min/m_2
  - Central venous pressure <12 mm Hg

Adapted from American Association of Cardiovascular and Pulmonary Rehabilitation. *Guidelines for Cardiac Rehabilitation and Secondary Prevention Programs*. 5th edition. Champaign, IL: Human Kinetics; 2013.

(atrial fibrillation/flutter) or a decrease in diastolic filling time (PVC) will decrease ventricular filling, possibly reducing the stroke volume and cardiac output, leading to hypotension/orthostasis and complaints of dizziness. Generally, rehabilitation is held if the patient is experiencing atrial fibrillation/flutter with a rapid ventricular response (HR> 110; sometimes called **uncontrolled atrial fibrillation/flutter**).

Laboratory values are important to monitor because the electrolyte and blood cell counts will impact the intensity and appropriateness of therapy for that day. Special consideration is given to potassium and calcium levels as well as white blood cell (WBC) and hemoglobin concentrations (see Chapter 2). Potassium and calcium are electrolytes that influence myocardial cell electrical activity. When these values are abnormal, dysrhythmias can develop that compromise cardiac output or can be life threatening. The complete blood cell count (CBC) will provide the practitioner with knowledge of oxygen carrying capacity (hemoglobin/hematocrit), presence of

Table 6-11

CARDIOVASCULAR SYSTEM EXAMINATION

Examination Technique	*Description of Technique in Common Health Conditions*	*Examination Findings*
Observation and palpation of chest wall and extremities	• See Table 1-9 regarding grading edema. • See Table 7-13 regarding chest wall and extremity observation and configuration. • See Table 15-1 regarding wound examination and skin inspection.	**↑ accessory muscle hypertrophy**: Chronic respiratory disease, heart failure. **Unilateral edema**: Suspect occlusion of major vein (eg, deep vein thrombosis [DVT]). **Bilateral edema**: Suspect CHF, liver dysfunction, malnutrition, etc
BP	• Warm and clean diaphragm of stethoscope before placement on patient skin. • Review the patient's history to determine if there is a contraindication for BP measurements on a particular extremity (eg, peripherally-inserted central catheter line, recent mastectomy, arterial-venous fistula for hemodialysis, arterial line, recent fracture). • Palpate the brachial pulse (medial to biceps tendon). This is where the diaphragm of the stethoscope will be placed. • Place the appropriate-sized cuff around the upper arm at least 2 fingers (2 to 3 cm) width above the elbow crease. The cuff size will vary depending on the size of the upper arm. The length of the bladder should be twice the width (~80% of the limb circumference). • Raise the UE to heart level and pump the cuff up to >180 mm Hg or until the brachial pulse is absent. • Lower the cuff pressure by 2 to 3 mm Hg per second.	**BP differences**: It is not uncommon for BP to differ by 10 mm Hg between the right and left extremities. The right UE BP is typically higher. Record the higher BP. **False BP reading**: • A cuff too large will underestimate BP. • A cuff too small will overestimate BP. • Auscultatory gap: The period of silence when the Korotkoff sound disappears and reappears 10 to 15 mm Hg lower. Note the first sound as systolic BP. Auscultatory gap may lead to an underestimate of BP. *(continued)*

Table 6-11 (continued) CARDIOVASCULAR SYSTEM EXAMINATION		
Examination Technique	*Description of Technique in Common Health Conditions*	*Examination Findings*
	• Note the first clear Korotkoff sound (systolic BP) and when this sound disappears (diastolic BP). • LE BP measurement: Make sure the cuff fits the LE correctly; in most cases at least a large to extra large adult cuff is needed. LE BP is typically greater than UE BP (note Ankle Brachial Index).	**High BP/HTN**: Typically diagnosed over time; measurement on a single day may not be conclusive **Classification of BP**: See Table 6-3. **Hypotension or blunted BP rise with activity**: Suspect left ventricle pump dysfunction/ heart failure, dehydration, medication side effect
Pulse or heart rate	**Arterial pulses**: A bounding wave of blood that diminishes with increasing distance from the heart. • Palpate a radial pulse using 2 to 3 fingers (not your thumb) on the underside of the forearm. • Follow the patient's thumb from the thenar eminence to just proximal of the wrist crease. • Gently press until a beating sensation is palpated. • Count for a minimum of 15 seconds and then multiply by 4. If there is an irregularity or the pulse feels extremely slow, weak, or fast, count for 30 to 60 seconds and multiply accordingly. • LE pulses (eg, femoral, popliteal, dorsalis pedis) can be palpated if UE pulses are unidentified. • Carotid pulses can be palpated, but only one at a time. Carotid pulses should be avoided during exercise due to risk for vasovagal response (ie, bradycardia and hypotension).	**Pulse rhythm**: • An irregular pulse may accompany or signify a dysrhythmia (eg, atrial fibrillation = irregularly irregular pulse; ventricular bigeminy, sinus arrhythmia = regularly irregular pulse) • The heart rhythm cannot be inferred from the pulse quality; an ECG is required to confirm the presence of a dysrhythmia **Bradycardia**: Pulse rate <60 (eg, cardiac conduction abnormality, hypothyroidism, hypothermia, drug intoxication, athlete) **Tachycardia:** Pulse rate >100 (eg, heart disease, lung disease, fever, hyperthyroidism, anemia, shock, anxiety, exercise) *(continued)*

Table 6-11 (continued) **CARDIOVASCULAR SYSTEM EXAMINATION**		
Examination Technique	*Description of Technique in Common Health Conditions*	*Examination Findings*
	• Apical pulse can be auscultated when peripheral palpation is difficult. • Determine the PMI—left fifth intercostal space, midclavicular region. • Listen and count the number of cardiac cycles and multiply accordingly (each cardiac cycle is one S1 and one S2—see Heart Sounds). Document the: • Calculated pulse rate • Rhythm of the pulse (eg, regular, regularly irregular, irregularly irregular) • Quality of pulse (see Table 1-10) ¤ 4+: Bounding ¤ 3+: Full, strong ¤ 2+: Normal ¤ 1+: Weak, thready ¤ 0: Absent	**Pulses alternans:** • Amplitude of pulse varies between weak and strong beats (eg, heart failure) **Pulses paradoxus:** • Pulse strength falls with inspiration (eg, restrictive pericarditis, pericardial effusion, COPD) **Pulses differens:** • Unequal pulses between left and right extremities (eg, unilateral vascular obstruction) **Bounding pulse (+4):** • Hyperkinetic or strong pulse (eg, aortic rigidity, atherosclerosis, anxiety, fever, hyperthyroidism, exercise)
Auscultation	**Heart sounds**: Listen to determine the S1, the first heart sound ("lub"), and S2, the second heart sound ("dub"). S1 signifies the onset of systole while S2 marks the end of systole/beginning of diastole. Abnormal heart sounds include S3, S4, pericardial friction rub, and heart murmurs (see Table 6-6). • Apical pulse and mitral region: Fifth intercostal space, midclavicular region • Aortic area: Second intercostal space just to the right of sternum • Pulmonic area: Second intercostals costal space just to the left of the sternum	**S1**: Best heard toward the apex of the heart (PMI/mitral region) **S2**: Best heard at the base of the heart (aortic region) **S3** (ventricular gallop): An abnormal heart sound occurring early in diastole (passive filling phase) (eg, CHF). Sounds like "lub-dub-dub." **S4** (atrial gallop): An abnormal heart sound occurring late in ventricular diastole (atrial systole; eg, HTN, myocardial infarction) Sounds like "la-lub-dub." *(continued)*

Table 6-11 (continued) CARDIOVASCULAR SYSTEM EXAMINATION		
Examination Technique	*Description of Technique in Common Health Conditions*	*Examination Findings*
	• Tricuspid area: Fourth or fifth intercostals space border of left sternal area **Arterial bruits**: • A murmur in an artery indicative of turbulent blood flow. • Sites to auscultate include the temporal, carotid, subclavian abdominal aortal, renal, iliac, and femoral arteries	**Pericardial friction rub**: Pericardial inflammation (eg, pericarditis) **Systolic murmurs**: Heard between S1 and S2. Sounds like "lub-swoosh-dub" (eg, aortic and pulmonic stenosis, mitral and tricuspid regurgitation) **Diastolic murmurs**:Heard post S2 preceding S1. Sounds like "lub-dub- swoosh" (eg, mitral and tricuspid stenosis, aortic regurgitation) **Arterial bruits**: May reflect the transmitting of murmurs resulting from aortic or mitral valve disorders (eg, stenosis or regurgitation) may indicate obstructive arterial disease (eg, artherosclerosis, arteritis)
Electrocardiogram review	See Appendix A	
Chest pain	See Table 6-9	**Cardiac**: Angina, myocardial infarction, pericarditis, mitral valve prolapse **Musculoskeletal**: Cervical radiculopathy, shoulder arthritis, rotator cuff injury, costochondritis **Pulmonary**: Pleurisy, pneumothorax **GI**: Hiatal hernia, gastroesophageal reflux disease, esophageal spasm, peptic ulcer, pancreatitis
Adapted from Hillegass[7]; Perloff[9]; Frownfelter and Dean[10]; Irwin and Tecklin[74]; Reid and Chung[75]; Seidel et al[76]; and Watchie.[77]		

infection (WBCs are often elevated post-surgery), and blood coagulation (platelets). The therapist should also be familiar with the coagulation profile of the patient by reviewing the **PT/INR/PTT** (see Chapter 2). If the PT/INR/PTT are elevated, the

Table 6-12

RISK STRATIFICATION IN CARDIAC REHABILITATION

Lowest Risk	*Moderate Risk*	*Highest Risk*
• No significant left ventricle dysfunction (ejection fraction >50%) • No resting/exercise complex dysrhythmias • Uncomplicated myocardial infarction/ CABG/angioplasty • Normal hemodynamics with exercise and recovery • Asymptomatic/absence of angina • Absence of clinical depression	• Moderate left ventricle dysfunction (ejection fraction = 40% to 49%) • Signs/symptoms at moderate levels of exercise (5 to 7 METs) • Moderate risk is assumed for patients who do not meet the low or high risk criteria	• Decreased left ventricle function (ejection fraction <40%) • Survivor of cardiac arrest or sudden death • Complex ventricular dysrhythmia at rest/exercise • Complicated myocardial infarction or CABG • Perioperative ischemia/ myocardial infarction • CHF, shock • Myocardial infarction: Pericarditis • Abnormal hemodynamics with exercise • Flat or decreasing systolic BP • Chronotropic incompetence with ↑ workload • Clinically significant depression

Adapted from *ACSM Guidelines for Exercise Testing and Prescription*. 9th ed. Philadelphia, PA: Lippincott Williams & Wilkins; 2014 and American Association of Cardiovascular and Pulmonary Rehabilitation. *Guidelines for Cardiac Rehabilitation and Secondary Prevention Programs*. 5th edition. Champaign, IL: Human Kinetics; 2013.

patient is at an increased risk of bleeding; however, it should be noted that after valve replacement, myocardial infarction, PTCA or VAD placement, the coagulation profile indices are often maintained in an elevated range to prevent blood clot formation. The therapist should review institutional guidelines or communicate with the physician and nursing staffs to determine optimal ranges for each patient.

Wound and incision examination should include assessing for the presence of infection, inadequate healing, and determining the stability of wound closure. Incisions following open heart surgery heal by primary intention, the tissue surfaces are approximated with stitches, staples, skin glue, or Steri-Strips (3M). Wound infection is suspected if there is excessive, foul-smelling, and/or discolored drainage. It is expected that some serosanguinous drainage may be present. The therapist should determine sternal stability by assessing for presence of a sternal click. The practitioner places 2 fingers on either side of the incision or places a stethoscope over the incision and asks the patient to take a deep breath or cough gently. With a stable sternum, you should feel both sides of the wound rise and fall together and no click/rubbing noise should be auscultated. If there is asymmetry or if a loud click is heard,

Table 6-13

CONTRAINDICATIONS AND RELATIVE CONTRAINDICATIONS TO EXERCISE TRAINING

Contraindications	*Relative Contraindications*
• Unstable angina • Moderate to severe angina • Uncompensated heart failure • Acute aortic dissection • Severe/symptomatic valve dysfunction • Uncontrolled dysrhythmias: ¤ Sustained ventricular tachycardia ¤ Second/third degree heart block ¤ New onset supraventricular tachycardia (SVT) (atrial fibrillation/ flutter, paroxysmal atrial tachycardia) ¤ New onset brady-/tachydysrhythmias with hemodynamic compromise • Drop in systolic BP >10 mm Hg • Resting systolic BP >210; diastolic BP >110 • Inability to monitor pulse or BP • Signs or symptoms of exercise intolerance or poor perfusion, including: ¤ Angina ¤ Marked dyspnea ¤ Pallor ¤ Cyanosis	• Acute myocarditis/pericarditis • Electrolyte abnormalities • Severe HTN (stage 2/3) • New onset brady-/tachyarrhythmias without hemodynamic compromise • Symptomatic valve dysfunction • Inability to monitor ECG • Subjective complaints of fatigue, SOB, wheezing, leg cramps • Systolic BP >210; diastolic BP >110 • Rate of perceived exertion >15 • Peak HR >40 bpm above resting, or 75% of predicted HR maximum

Adapted from American Association of Cardiovascular and Pulmonary Rehabilitation. *Guidelines for Cardiac Rehabilitation and Secondary Prevention Programs*. 5th edition. Champaign, IL: Human Kinetics; 2013

the wound is considered unstable. The surgical team should be notified, and caution should be exercised with UE activities. Finally, patients are often instructed in sternal precautions to limit unnecessary stress on the healing surgical site (Table 6-16).

Postoperative pulmonary complications are a risk following all surgeries due to general anesthesia-induced atelectasis and decreased pulmonary compliance potentially limiting ventilation. Cardiac surgery involving cardiopulmonary bypass may also be associated with increased pulmonary vascular permeability leading to pulmonary edema. Additionally, the incision and patient complaints of chest wall pain will limit chest wall expansion. The sum of these factors leads to impairments in gas exchange and musculoskeletal pump performance. All cardiovascular patients should be involved in an airway clearance and mobility regimen to reduce the incidence of postoperative pulmonary complication.

Table 6-14

Sample Phase I Cardiac Rehabilitation Program/Activity Prescription

Day	*Metabolic Equivalent Level*	*Activity*
Day 1: Intensive care unit	1 to 2	• Bedrest until stable; if stable (eg, acceptable HR/rhythm, BP, symptoms) proceed with: ¤ Supine/sitting UE/LE active range of motion (AROM) exercise (warm up) ¤ Transfer OOB to chair ¤ Consider walking in room ¤ Toileting ¤ Airway clearance techniques (ACTs): Deep breathing, incentive spirometry, cough, or huff ¤ Patient instruction: Supine/sitting exercise, incentive spirometry, sternal precautions
Day 2: Transfer to step down unit	2 to 3	• Sitting UE/LE AROM exercise (warm up) • OOB as tolerated • Walking in room • Continued ACT and patient instruction
Days 3 to 5	2 to 3	• Sitting UE/LE AROM exercises progressing to standing UE/LE AROM warm up exercise • Walking 5 to 10 minutes in the hall, progressing up to 2 to 3 times per day • Continued ACT and patient instruction
	3 to 4	• Shower with seat • Standing warm up exercise • Walking 5 to 10 minutes in the hall, progressing up to 2 to 3 times per day • Initiate stair climbing • Continued ACT and patient instruction

Adapted from American Association of Cardiovascular and Pulmonary Rehabilitation. *Guidelines for Cardiac Rehabilitation and Secondary Prevention Programs*. 5th edition. Champaign, IL: Human Kinetics; 2013.

Table 6-15

Activities of Daily Living and Metabolic Equivalents

Activity	*Method*	*Metabolic Equivalent Level*	*Average Heart Rate Response*
Toileting	• Bed pan • Commode • Urinal (in bed) • Urinal (standing)	• 1 to 2	• 5 to 15 bpm ↑ from resting heart rate (RHR)
Bathing	• Bed bath • Tub bath • Shower	• 2 to 3	• 10 to 20 bpm ↑ from RHR
Walking	Flat surface • 2 mph • 2.5 mph • 3 mph	 • 2 to 2.5 • 2.5 to 2.9 • 3 to 3.3	 • 5 to 15 bpm ↑ from RHR
Stair climbing	1 flight = 12 steps: • Down 1 flight of stairs • Up 1 to 2 flight of stairs	 • 2.5 • 4.0	 • 10 bpm ↑ from RHR • 10 to 25 bpm ↑ from RHR
Upper body exercise	While standing: • UE • Trunk	 • 2.6 to 3.1 • 2 to 2.2	 • 10 to 20 bpm ↑ from RHR
Leg calisthenics		• 2.5 to 4.5	• 15 to 25 bpm ↑ from RHR

Adapted from American Association of Cardiovascular and Pulmonary Rehabilitation. *Guidelines for Cardiac Rehabilitation and Secondary Prevention Programs*. 5th edition. Champaign, IL: Human Kinetics; 2013.

Table 6-16

Sternal Precautions

- Limit bilateral upper extremity (BUE) overhead movements
- Limit UE horizontal adduction across midline and horizontal abduction past the coronal plane
- UE weight lifting is limited to 5 to 10 pounds
- No driving

Restrictions are typically maintained for 6 weeks or until cleared by cardiovascular surgeon or cardiologist. Check with institutional guidelines.

Case Study

Mrs. Hayes is a 74-year-old female with a history of CAD. She had a heart catheterization 8 months ago showing diffuse disease. Her medical management has included beta-blockers, statins, and aspirin. The patient was admitted to the hospital with worsening DOE. She experienced an episode of supraventricular tachycardia (SVT) and atrial fibrillation that was rate controlled with metoprolol and intravenous (IV) procainamide. An echocardiogram revealed an ejection fraction of 40%. She was cardioverted to sinus rhythm. She underwent another cardiac catheterization that revealed a complex left anterior descending/bifurcation stenosis, left circumflex and diagonal stenosis.

On the third hospital day she underwent a CABG using the left internal mammary artery (LIMA) and the saphenous vein from the left lower extremity (LLE). Physical therapy was consulted on postoperative day 1 (hospital day 4).

Patient/Client History

General Demographics, Social History, and Living Environment

Mrs. Hayes has been married for 50 years and lives in a ranch-style home with 4 steps to enter and no handrail. She has 1 son that lives with her with 2 grandchildren (ages 5 and 7). She is a retired postal worker.

General Health Status, Social/Health Habits, and Family History

Mrs. Hayes states she smoked for 40 years and quit 10 years ago when she got short of breath at a work picnic. She enjoys a beer or glass of wine at night when her son gets home from work.

Medical/Surgical History

Mrs. Hayes is a 74-year-old female who has a long history of CAD and is 1 day status post (s/p) CABG. Her medical history includes stable angina for over 2 years, HTN, type 2 diabetes for over 10 years, and she is moderately overweight. She is s/p transmetatarsal amputation of the LLE 4 years ago for complications of a foot ulcer.

Current Condition

Mrs. Hayes is lethargic and complaining of being uncomfortable. She has a nasal cannula, a right radial arterial line with arm board, pneumatic boots on both LE, and a Foley catheter in place. The mediastinal chest tube and central lines have been removed. She remains monitored for oxygen saturation and ECG.

Activities and Participation

Mrs. Hayes used a straight cane to ambulate on all surfaces prior to admission. She could walk a couple blocks but would complain of fatigue. She could complete all ADLs independently but it was becoming "more difficulty." She does not have an orthopedic shoe for the LLE. Her husband drives because she has been having difficulty with her vision lately. They enjoy playing bridge with their church group, but no longer travel outside their hometown. Her prior level of function is classified as New York Heart Association Class III.

Medications

As noted previously, Mrs. Hayes' medications included beta-blockers, statins, aspirin, and procainamide.

Other Clinical Tests

Laboratory results revealed hyperkalemia of 5.6mEq/L (elevated), hyperglycemia with a blood glucose of 200 mg/dL, an elevated HbA1c at 9.0% and elevated WBCs at 14,000.

Systems Review

Cardiovascular and Pulmonary

Resting HR was 90 bpm, BP 100/88, and RR 24 breath/minute. BLE edema was observed.

Integumentary

Mrs. Hayes has a Foley catheter, an arterial line, and a surgical bandage in the center of her thorax with epicardial pacing wires exiting. There appears to be some brownish, dried drainage around the edges of the dressing. The transmetatarsal incision is well-healed. The LLE has a surgical dressing extending from below the knee to just below the groin area.

Musculoskeletal

Gross movements of BUE/BLE were symmetrical but overhead motions were painful and limited. It was also noted that the there was a decrease in ROM of bilateral ankles due to edema.

Neuromuscular

Active and passive movements of BUE/BLE revealed normal tone and no abnormal movement patterns were observed.

Communication, Affect, Cognition, Language, and Learning Style

Mrs. Hayes was awake but lethargic. She was able to recognize where she was and recalled the reasons for her operation. Her primary language is English. She was also able to perform 1- and 2-step directions without cues.

Tests and Measures

Aerobic Capacity and Endurance

Mrs. Hayes demonstrated orthostatic hypotension with transfer into standing. She has tachycardia with an abnormal pulse. She also has tachypnea at rest and has a weak cough. Laboratory results are suspicious for poorly controlled diabetes, which will impact healing, elevated potassium, which could result in dysrhythmias, and elevated WBCs, which may correspond with clinical pulmonary findings, possible infection, or is simply a common postoperative finding. If there is suspicion of perioperative myocardial infarction, cardiac troponins, or other cardiac enzymes should be reviewed (see Chapter 2).

Assistive and Adaptive Technology

Mrs. Hayes currently requires use of bed rails for rolling and it is recommended that she have a rolling walker when she is ready for out of bed (OOB) activities. Sternal precautions are being maintained.

Balance, Gait and Mobility (Including Locomotion)

Bed mobility is moderate assistance of one (Functional Status Score in the ICU [FSS-ICU] 3) with rolling side-to-side using the bed rail. She transferred to dangling with moderate assistance of one. She transferred to standing with moderate assistance of one (FSS-ICU 3). Unable to further examine standing and gait at this time due to orthostasis. Her balance was impaired and she required assistance with her sitting and standing transfers. The Activity Measure for Post Acute Care (AM-PAC) basic mobility score was 10/24.

Circulation (Arterial, Venous, Lymphatic) and Ventilation/Respiration

A more thorough examination of the HR and rhythm revealed atrial fibrillation and a pulse that was irregularly irregular. ROM, Manual Muscle Test (MMT), bed mobility, and transfer to dangling at edge of bed revealed a vital sign response of SpO_2 95%, HR increase from 96 to 110 bpm, and BP remained fairly flat going from BP 100/88 to 94/86 mm Hg. After transferring to standing with assistance, she complained of dizziness and her HR increased to 116 bpm and BP decreased to 86/74 mm Hg. She stood for 30 seconds and was returned to supine. There is pitting edema in her left > right ankle area (+2).

The nursing staff was informed of her vital sign response (ie, orthostatic HTN) and complaints of pain (see following) during the physical therapy examination.

Due to the recent open heart surgery with median sternotomy, resting tachypnea (RR = 24 breaths/minute) and the need for supplemental oxygen, additional tests and measures related to the pulmonary system were included. Her cough is weak and nonproductive with complaints of incision pain. Resting SpO_2 was 92% on 6 liters/minute nasal cannula and the patient exhibited accessory muscle use at rest. Her breath sounds were diminished throughout. The radiologist interpretation of the chest x-ray stated there was a consolidation in the right lower lobe and slight flattening of the diaphragms bilaterally.

Mental Function

Mrs. Hayes was alert, awake and oriented x4. She followed commands easily but appeared fatigued. She has a Richmond Agitation Sedation Score (RASS) of 0.

Muscle Performance

MMT revealed 4/5 for BLE and 4/5 for BUE. The ROM is >90 degrees for bilateral shoulder flexion and abduction but does increase incision pain; the radial board limits wrist movements on the right side, otherwise UEs are within functional limits (WFL). There is a decreased ROM in bilateral ankles due to edema but appears to be functional for standing and gait activities.

Pain

Mrs. Hayes rated her incision pain as 3/10 and this increased with activity and coughing to 6/10.

Sensory Integrity

Due to the history of diabetes, a quick examination of sensation was indicated. Mrs. Hayes had decreased sensation below the knees bilaterally. Proprioception is intact BUE/BLE.

Diagnosis

Laboratory results are suspicious for poorly controlled diabetes, which will negatively impact healing, elevated potassium, which could result in dysrhythmias, and elevated WBC, which may correspond with clinical pulmonary findings, suspicious of infection, or is simply a common postoperative finding. Although there is no evidence at this point, if there is suspicion of perioperative myocardial infarction, cardiac troponins should be reviewed (see Chapter 2).

Mrs. Hayes presents with deconditioning from inactivity prior to surgery and complications related to atrial fibrillation. She may have pneumonia or atelectasis that needs be treated to prevent worsening pulmonary complications and prolonged hospital stay. Mrs. Hayes' mobility status is compromised, and she requires moderate assistance for bed mobility and OOB transfers and demonstrated orthostatic hypotension with standing. Gait needs to be examined when the hemodynamic status is stable. Pain management will need to be coordinated with nursing.

Prognosis

Mrs. Hayes should progress with therapy in conjunction with her medical management (eg, blood glucose control, fluid/electrolyte balance, pain management, titration of medications). Her current activity limitations combined with a presumed short hospital length of stay warrant consultation with social work to start the investigation of a post-acute level of care.

Intervention

Recommend Phase I cardiac rehabilitation as noted in Table 6-14. Mrs. Hayes will perform frequent incentive spirometry and splinted coughing (10x/hour while awake), and progressive mobilization OOB with physical therapy and nursing 3 or 4 times/day once hemodynamically stable. Recommend OOB with nurses a minimum of 45 minutes 3 times/day for all meals. Elevate LE and monitor skin integrity closely. Educate patient and family members on fall precautions due to decreased sensation as well as sternal precautions, importance of airway clearance and OOB activities, including instruction in a home exercise program (AROM at bedside), and cardiac risk factor reduction.

Outcomes

Following 4 days: Foley catheter and arterial line removed. Bulky surgical dressings removed revealing adhesive strips in areas of incisions. MMT grossly 4 to 5/5 BUE/LE, pain 0/10 at rest and 3/10 with activity. Cough when splinted is effective following incentive spirometry. Chest x-ray is clearing. Mrs. Hayes does not require assistance for bed mobility and transfer into standing (FSS-ICU 7) but she does require minimal assistance to transfer to a bedside chair (FSS-ICU 4). Gait with rolling walker requires minimal assistance of one, 50 feet x 2 trials on 3 liters nasal

ICF Clinical Reasoning Tool Case Study Summary

Health Condition

HPI: CAD s/p CABG x 2, bilateral crackles 1/3 bilaterally and 1+ pitting edema, possible pneumonia, leukocytosis, hyperkalemia, elevated blood glucose and HbA1c

PMHx: CAD, stable angina, atrial fibrillation with RVR, SVT requiring cardioversion, heart failure, former smoker, HTN, type 2 diabetes, PAD, and transmetatarsal amputation

Precautions/Contraindications

Precautions: Wound healing (sternum, LLE incision) may be slowed due to diabetes/PAD; fall precautions due to orthostasis combined with decreased sensation, poor balance and vision loss; poor airway clearance due to pain and sternotomy

Body Structure and Function			*Activity/Task Limitations*			*Participation*		
Impairment/ Problem	*Tests and Measures*	*Intervention*	*Activity*	*Tests and Measures*	*Intervention*	*Participation*	*Tests and Measures*	*Intervention*
• Impaired ROM and strength • Decreased endurance • Orthostatic hypotension • Abnormal breath sounds and weak cough • Pain • Abnormal lab values • Decreased vision • Overweight • Impaired wound healing	• ROM/MMT • Grade pitting edema • VS including SpO_2 and ECG • Breath sounds and cough • Pain/numeric scale • Wound examination • Lab values • BMI • Vision assessment	• Bedside ROM • Progressive resistance exercises • Breathing exercises (incentive spirometry)/ splint incision with cough • Education: sternal precautions and falls prevention • Consult registered dietician/ diabetes educator	• ADLs • Bed mobility • Transfers • Gait • Balance	• Functional task analysis • FIM • AM-PAC "6 Clicks" • 2- or 6MWT as able • TUG as able	• Progressive functional retraining following Phase 1 Cardiac Rehab guidelines • Use of assistive technology • Pain control strategies	• Unable to play bridge at church	• HRQoL (SF-36) • PHQ-9 • PSFS	• Continue physical therapy services • Consult social worker and family regarding discharge plan

(continued)

ICF Clinical Reasoning Tool Case Study Summary (continued)

Personal Factors	*Other Considerations*	*Environmental Factors*
• Age: 74 y/o female • Primary language: English • Ambulated with straight cane on all surfaces prior to admission • Orthopedic shoe LLE • Married 50 years, husband drives • 1 live-in son with 2 children (5, 7) • Retired postal worker • 40 year history of smoking, • Transmetatarsal amputation x 4 years ago for foot ulcer		Home: • Ranch-style home • 4 steps to enter, no handrail, uses cane Hospital: • Urinary catheter, arterial line, surgical bandage with epicardial pacing wires

BMI = body mass index; BS = breath sounds; CABG = coronary artery bypass graft; Hb = hemoglobin; HPI = history of present illness; HRQoL = Health-Related Quality of Life; IBW = ideal body weight; MWT = Minute Walk Test; PHQ = Patient Health Questionnaire; PSFS = Patient Specific Functional Scale; PMHx = past medical history; RVR = rapid ventricular rate; SF = Short Form; VS = vital signs; y/o = year old.

Adapted from American Physical Therapy Association. *Guide to Physical Therapist Practice*. 3rd ed. http://www.apta.org/Guide/. Updated October 21, 2015. Accessed October 5, 2018 and *Towards a Common Language for Functioning, Disability and Health*. World Health Organization. www.who.int/classifications/icf/icfbeginnersguide.pdf. Published 2002. Accessed April 29, 2019.

cannula (FSS-ICU 2). Her AM-PAC score increased from 10 to 19/24. She can independently recall her sternal precautions.

Mrs. Hayes is making steady progress but continues to require assistance with ADLs and mobility. She is motivated to return home. The physical therapist recommends transfer to a post-acute facility. Because Mrs. Hayes complains of fatigue following a 30- to 45-minute therapy session, a skilled level of care (ie, sub-acute rehabilitation) is appropriate for continued progression towards functional independence and home discharge. Continuation of the Phase I cardiac rehabilitation principles are recommended.

Chapter Review Questions

1. What are 4 factors that determine myocardial oxygen demand?
   a. Diastolic filling time, mitochondrial density, afterload, and acidosis
   b. Coronary blood flow, LVEDP, venous capacitance, and dysrhythmias
   c. Heart rate, preload, contractility, and afterload
   d. Hormonal factors, aortic pressure gradient, oxygen saturation, and myoglobin
2. Which of the following best represents the clinical presentation of a patient with an exacerbation of heart failure?
   a. S4 heart sound, limited ability to perform ADLs, cough productive of frothy tan secretions
   b. S2 heart sound, DOE, decreased respiratory rate, pleural rub
   c. S1 heart sound, paroxysmal nocturnal dyspnea, orthopnea, cough productive of green secretions
   d. S3 heart sound, JVD, pulmonary crackles, SOB
3. The clinical presentation that is most consistent with cardiac-related chest pain is:
   a. New onset sharp pain, exercise exacerbates pain, patient can elicit pain with palpation
   b. Non-focal, dull, vague, above waist, and body position does not impact intensity of pain
   c. Substernal, related to food consumption, and symptoms worse with head down
   d. Exercise, deep breath, and head down improve
4. Which of the following are modifiable risk factors for coronary artery disease?
   a. Genetics, age, diabetes, stress, and sedentary lifestyle
   b. HTN, diabetes, hyperlipidemia, and smoking
   c. Prior myocardial infarction, aortic aneurysm, and PAD
   d. Gender, family history, high BP, and sleep apnea

5. Which of the following represent signs and symptoms of aortic valve dysfunction:
   a. Angina, PND, orthopnea, and presyncope with exercise
   b. JVD, diastolic murmur, empyema, inspiratory wheeze
   c. Bounding peripheral pulses, soft systolic murmur, right ventricular hypertrophy
   d. Decreased wedge pressure, point of maximal impulse in left axilla, and right atrial enlargement

Answers: 1c, 2d, 3b, 4b, 5a

References

1. Wenger NK, Froelicher ES, Smith LK, et al. *Cardiac Rehabilitation as Secondary Prevention: Clinical Practice Guidelines.* Department of Health and Human Services, Public Heatlth Service, Agency for Health Care Policy and Research and National Heart, Lung and Blood Institute. AHCPR Pub. No. 96-0673. October 1995.
2. Mozaffarian D, Benjamin EJ, Go AS, et al; American Heart Association Statistics Committee; Stroke Statistics Subcommittee. Heart disease and stroke statistics—2016 update: a report from the American Heart Association. *Circulation.* 2016;133(4):e38-e60.
3. Jessup M, Brozena S. Medical progress: heart failure. *N Engl J Med.* 2003;348:2007-2018.
4. Peel G. The cardiopulmonary system and movement dysfunction. *Phys Ther.* 1996;76:448-455.
5. Foss ML, Keteyian SJ. *Fox's Physiologic Basis for Exercise and Sport.* 6th ed. Boston, MA: McGraw-Hill; 1998.
6. Rhoades, RA, Tanner GA. *Medical Physiology.* Baltimore, MD: Lippincott Williams & Wilkins; 1995.
7. Hillegass EA. *Essentials of Cardiopulmonary Physical Therapy.* 3rd ed. St. Louis, MO: Elsevier: WB Saunders; 2011.
8. Guyton AC, Hall JE. *Textbook of Medical Physiology.* Philadelphia, PA: WB Saunders; 2000.
9. Perloff JK. *Physical Examination of the Heart and Circulation.* 3rd ed. Philadelphia, PA: WB Saunders; 2000.
10. Frownfelter D, Dean E. *Principles and Practice of Cardiopulmonary Physical Therapy.* St. Louis, MO: Mosby; 1996.
11. American Association of Cardiovascular and Pulmonary Rehabilitation. *Guidelines for Cardiac Rehabilitation and Secondary Prevention Programs.* Champaign, IL: Human Kinetics; 1999.
12. Powers SK, Howley ET. *Exercise Physiology: Theory and Application to Fitness and Performance.* Dubuque, IA: Brown & Benchmark Publishers; 1997.
13. Cheng JW. Recognition, pathophysiology, and management of acute myocardial infarction. *Am J Health Syst Pharm.* 2001;58:1709-1721.
14. Berne RM, Levy MN. *Cardiovascular Physiology.* 8th ed. St. Louis, MO: Mosby; 2001.
15. Hollinshead WH, Rosse C. *Textbook Anatomy.* 4th ed. New York, NY: Harper & Row; 1985.
16. Criqui MH, Langer RD, Fronek A, et al. Mortality over a period of 10 years in patients with peripheral arterial disease. *N Engl J Med.* 1992;326:381-386.
17. Braunwald E. *Heart Disease: A Textbook of Cardiovascular Medicine.* Philadelphia, PA: WB Saunders; 1997.
18. Ades P. Medical progress: cardiac rehabilitation and secondary prevention of coronary heart disease. *N Engl J Med.* 2001;345:892-902.
19. Matthew JP, Parks R, Savino JS, et al. Atrial fibrillation following coronary artery bypass graft surgery: predictors, outcomes and resource utilization. *JAMA.* 1996;276:300-306.
20. Atlee JL. Perioperative cardiac dysrhythmias: diagnosis and management. *Anesthesiology.* 1997;76:1397-1424.

21. Kantor B, McKenna CJ, Caccitolo JA, et al. Transmyocardial and percutaneous myocardial revascularization: current and future role in the treatment of coronary artery disease. *Mayo Clinic Proc.* 1999;74:585-592.
22. Humphrey R, Arena R. Surgical innovations for chronic heart failure in the context of cardiopulmonary rehabilitation. *Phys Ther.* 2000;80:61-69.
23. Canzanello VJ, Sheps SG. The Sixth Report of the Joint National Committee on Prevention, Detection, Evaluation, and Treatment of High Blood Pressure. *Cardio Rev.* 1998;5(6):272-277.
24. Wolz M, Cutler J, Roccella EJ, et al. Statement from the National High Blood Pressure Education Program: prevalence of hypertension. *Am J Hypertens.* 2000;13:103-104.
25. Wright JT Jr, Williamson JD, Whelton PK, et al; SPRINT Research Group. A randomized trial of intensive versus standard blood-pressure control. *N Engl J Med.* 2015;373(22):2103-2116.
26. Williamson JD, Supiano MA, Applegate WB, et al; SPRINT Research Group. Intensive vs standard blood pressure control and cardiovascular disease outcomes in adults aged ≥75 years: a randomized clinical trial. *JAMA.* 2016;315(24):2673-2682.
27. Davies MJ. The cardiomyopathies: an overview. *Heart.* 2000;83:469-474.
28. Tierney LM, McPhee SJ, Papadakis MA. *Current Medical Diagnosis and Treatment.* Norwalk, CT: Appleton & Lange; 1994.
29. Berkow R. *The Merck Manual of Diagnosis and Therapy.* Rahway, NJ: Merck Sharp & Dome Research Laboratories; 1987.
30. Way LW. *Current Surgical Diagnosis and Treatment.* 9th ed. Norwalk, CT: Appleton & Lange; 1991.
31. Carabello BS. Aortic stenosis. *N Engl J Med.* 2002;346:677-682.
32. Carabello BS, Crawford FA. Medical progress: valvular heart disease. *N Engl J Med.* 1997;337:32-41.
33. Otto CM. Evaluation and management of chronic mitral regurgitation. *N Engl J Med.* 2001;345:740-746.
34. Enriquez-Sarano M. Timing of mitral valve surgery. *Heart.* 2002;87:79-85.
35. Diodato MD, Damiano RJ. Robotic cardiac surgery: overview. *Surg Clin North Am.* 2003;83:1351-1367.
36. Aazami M, Schafers HJ. Advances in heart valve surgery. *J Interventional Cardiol.* 2003;16:535-541.
37. Dreyfus G, Milaiheanu S. Mitral valve repair in cardiomyopathy. *J Heart Lung Transplant.* 2000;19(suppl):S73-S76.
38. Vahanian A. Balloon valvuloplasty. *Heart.* 2001;85:223-228.
39. Vongpatanasin W, Hillis DL, Lange RA. Medical progress: prosthetic heart valves. *N Engl J Med.* 1996;335:407-416.
40. Leon MB, Smith CR, Mack MJ, et al; PARTNER 2 Investigators. Transcatheter or surgical aortic-valve replacement in intermediate-risk patients. *N Engl J Med.* 2016;374(17):1609-1620. doi: 10.1056/NEJMoa1514616
41. Groves P. Surgery of valve disease: late results and late complications. *Heart.* 2001;86:715-721.
42. Shames ML, Thompson RW. Abdominal aortic aneurysms: surgical treatment. *Cardiol Clin.* 2002;20:563-578.
43. Khan I, Nair C. Clinical, diagnostic, and management perspective of aortic dissection. *Chest.* 2002;122:311-328.
44. Dimick JB, Upchurch GR. The quality of care for patients with abdominal aortic aneurysms. *Cardiovascular Surg.* 2003;5:331-336.
45. Bick C. Abdominal aortic aneurysm repair. *Nursing Standard.* 2000;15:47-52,54-56.
46. Isselbacher EM. Thoracic and abdominal aortic aneurysms. *Circulation.* 2005;111:816-828.
47. Mylonakis E, Calderwood SB. Medical progress: infective endocarditis in adults. *N Engl J Med.* 2001;345:1318-1330.
48. Udelson JE. Heart failure with preserved ejection fraction. *Circulation.* 2011;124(21):e540-e543.
49. Kitzman DW, Upadhya B. Heart failure with preserved ejection fraction: a heterogenous disorder with multifactorial pathophysiology. *J Am Coll Cardiol.* 2014;63(5):457-459.
50. Lenfat C. *Report of the Task Force on Research in Heart Failure.* Bethesda, MD: National Heart, Lung and Blood Institute; 1994.

51. Braunwald E, Bristow MR. Congestive heart failure: fifty years of progress. *Circulation.* 2000;102:IV-14-IV-23.
52. Opie LH, Gersh BJ. *Drugs for the Heart.* 5th ed. Philadelphia, PA: WB Saunders; 2001.
53. Bavin TK, Self MA. Weaning from intra-aortic balloon pump support. *Am J Nurs.* 1991;Oct:54-59.
54. Russo MJ, Jeevanandam V, Stepney J, et al. Intra-aortic balloon pump inserted through the subclavian artery: a minimally invasive approach to mechanical support in the ambulatory end-stage heart failure patient. *J Thorac Cardiovasc Surg.* 2012;144(4):951-955.
55. Estep JD, Cordero-Reyes AM, Bhimaraj A, et al. Percutaneous placement of an intra-aortic balloon pump in the left axillary/subclavian position provides safe, ambulatory long-term support as bridge to heart transplantation. *JACC Heart Fail.* 2013;1(5):382-388.
56. Goldstein DJ, Oz MC, Rose EA. Implantable left ventricular assist devices. *N Engl J Med.* 1998;339:1522-1533.
57. Boehmer JP, Popjes E. Cardiac failure: Mechanical support strategies. *Crit Care Med.* 2006;34(9):S268.
58. Wells CL. Physical therapist management of patients with ventricular assist devices: key considerations for the acute care physical therapist. *Phys Ther.* 2013;93(2):266-278.
59. Rodriguez LE, Suarez EE, Loebe M, Bruckner BA. Ventricular assist devices (VAD) therapy: new technology, new hope? *Methodist Debakey Cardiovasc J.* 2013;9(1):32-37
60. Rose EA, Gelijins AC, Moskowitz AJ, et al. Long-term mechanical left ventricular assistance for end-stage heart failure. *N Engl J Med.* 2001;345:2285-2296.
61. Jessup M, Brozena S. Epilogue: support devices for end stage heart failure. *Cardiol Clin.* 2003;21:135-139.
62. Morrone TM, Buck LA, Catanese KA, et al. Early progressive mobilization of patients with left ventricular assist devices is safe and optimizes recovery before heart transplantation. *J Heart Lung Transplant.* 1996;15:423-429.
63. Mancini D, Goldsmith R, Levin H, et al. Comparison of exercise performance in patients with chronic severe heart failure versus left ventricular assist devices. *Circulation.* 1998;98:1178-1183.
64. Slaughter MS, Rogers JG, Milano CA, et al; HeartMate II Investigators. Advanced heart failure treated with continuous-flow left ventricular assist device. *N Engl J Med.* 2009;361(23):2241-2251.
65. Naidu SS. Novel percutaneous cardiac assist devices: the science of and indications for hemodynamic support. *Circulation.* 2011;123(5):533-543.
66. Doersch KM, Tong CW, Gongora E, et al. Temporary left ventricular assist device through axillary access is a promising approach to improve outcomes in refractory cardiogenic shock patients. *ASAIO J.* 2015;61:253-258
67. Gerber TC, Nishimura RA, Holmes DR Jr, et al. Left ventricular and biventricular pacing in congestive heart failure. *Mayo Clinic Proceedings.* 2001;76:803-812.
68. Atlee JL, Bernstein AD. Cardiac rhythm management devices (part 1). *Anesthesiology.* 2001;95:1265-1280.
69. Braunwald E, Jones RH, Mark DB, et al. Diagnosing and managing unstable angina. *Circulation.* 1994;90:613-622.
70. Cooke RA, Smeeton N, Chambers JB. Comparative study of chest pain characteristics in patients with normal and abnormal coronary angiograms. *Heart.* 1997;78:142-146.
71. Lee TH, Goldman L. Primary care: evaluation of the patient with acute chest pain. *Clin Med.* 2000;342:1187-1195.
72. Botoman VA. Noncardiac chest pain. *J Clin Gastroenterol.* 2002;34:6-14.
73. Charlson ME, Isom OW. Care after coronary artery bypass surgery. *N Engl J Med.* 2003;348:456-1463.
74. Irwin S, Tecklin JS. *Cardiopulmonary Physical Therapy: A Guide to Practice.* 4th ed. St. Louis, MO: Mosby; 2004.
75. Reid WD, Chung F. *Clinical Management Notes and Case Histories in Cardiopulmonary Physical Therapy.* Thorofare, NJ: SLACK Incorporated; 2004.

76. Seidel HM, Ball JW, Benedict GW, et al. *Mosby's Guide to Physical Examination*. 7th ed. St. Louis, MO; Elsevier: WB Saunders; 2011.
77. Watchie J. *Cardiopulmonary Physical Therapy: A Clinical Manual*. 2nd ed. St. Louis, MO; Elsevier: WB Saunders; 2010.
78. Doherty GM. *Current Surgical Diagnosis and Treatment*. 13th ed. Norwalk, CT: McGraw-Hill; 2010.
79. Papadakis MA, McPhee SJ. *Current Medical Diagnosis and Treatment*. 53rd ed. McGraw-Hill; 2014.
80. Porter RS, Kaplan JL. *The Merck Manual of Diagnosis and Therapy*. 19th ed. Kenilworth, NJ: Merck Publishing; 2011.

Bibliography

Barold SS, Zipes DP. Cardiac pacemakers and antiarrhythmic devices. In: Braunwald E, ed. *Heart Disease: A Textbook of Cardiovascular Medicine*. Philadelphia, PA: WB Saunders Co; 1997.

Berne RM, Levy MN, eds. Electrical activity of the heart. In: *Cardiovascular Physiology*. 8th ed. St. Louis, MO: Mosby; 2001.

Bubien RS, Ching EA, Kay GN. Cardiac defibrillation and resynchronization therapies. *AACN Clinical Issues*. 2004;15:340-361.

Craig CR, Stitzel RE. *Modern Pharmacology with Clinical Applications*. New York, NY: Little, Brown, and Co; 1997.

Deglin JH, Vallerand AH. *Davis's Drug Guide for Nurses*. 8th ed. Philadelphia, PA: FA Davis Co; 2003.

Gerber TC, Nishimura RA, Holmes DR Jr, et al. Left ventricular and biventricular pacing in congestive heart failure. *Mayo Clinic Proceedings*. 2001;76L:803-812.

Hand H. Common cardiac arrhythmias. *Nurs Stand*. 2002;16:43-58.

Hillegass EA. *Essentials of Cardiopulmonary Physical Therapy*. 3rd ed. St. Louis, MO. Elsevier: WB Saunders; 2011.

Houghton T, Kaye GC. ABC of interventional cardiology: implantable devices for treating tachyarrhythmias. *BMJ*. 2003;327:333-336.

Karch AM. *Lippincott's Nursing Drug Guide*. Springhouse, PA: Lippincott Williams & Wilkins; 2004.

Mammen BA, Irwin S, Tecklin JS. Common cardiac and pulmonary clinical measures. In: Irwin S, Tecklin JS, eds. *Cardiopulmonary Physical Therapy: A Guide to Practice*. 4th ed. St. Louis, MO: Mosby Inc; 2004.

Overbay D, Criddle L. Mastering temporary invasive cardiac pacing. *Crit Care Nurse*. 2004;24:25-32.

Ritter JM, Lewis LD, Mant TG. *Textbook of Clinical Pharmacology*. London, United Kingdom: Edward Arnold; 1995

Timothy PR, Rodeman BJ. Temporary pacemakers in critically ill patients. *AACN Clinical Issues*. 2004;15:305-325.

Zipes DP. Genesis of cardiac arrhythmias: electrophysiological considerations. In: Braunwald E, ed. *Heart Disease: A Textbook of Cardiovascular Medicine*. Philadelphia, PA: WB Saunders; 1997.

Zipes DP. Specific arrhythmias: diagnosis and treatment. In: Braunwald E, ed. *Heart Disease: A Textbook of Cardiovascular Medicine*. Philadelphia, PA: WB Saunders; 1997.

Appendix A

Monitoring Information: The Electrocardiogram, Interpretation, and Antiarrhythmic Devices

Monitoring of the ECG and interacting with patients who require pacemakers or defibrillators is common practice in the acute care setting. This section will provide an overview of electrophysiology and electrocardiography, provide the definitions and examples of common dysrhythmias, and discuss devices used to manage electrophysiological abnormalities.

The Electrocardiogram

The electrical events within the heart initiate the cardiac cycle resulting in myocardial contraction and pressure generation, the opening and closing of the valves, and the ejection of blood. The action potential of the cardiac myocyte is divided into **depolarization**, or the change of the membrane potential from negative to positive, and **repolarization**, or the return to the resting negative steady state. The action potential consists of 5 phases as noted in Figure 6-12. These phases result from changes in the permeability of the cell membrane due to the opening and closing of ion channels. The ion channels allow the diffusion of sodium, potassium, and calcium across the cell membrane changing the membrane potential and resulting in cardiac contraction.

Cardiac myocytes have unique properties: automaticity and conductivity. **Automaticity** is the ability of a cardiac myocyte to discharge an electrical current without stimulation from the nervous system. The pacemaker cells of the sinoatrial node, atrioventricular node, and purkinje system highlight this property (Table 6-17), but other regions of the myocardium can also initiate electrical impulses and take over pacemaker function. **Conductivity** is the ability of myocytes to transmit impulses rapidly to neighboring cells. Cardiac myocytes are connected via intercalated discs that couple the cells both mechanically and electrically, allowing the heart to contract as a unit.

A **dysrhythmia** is an abnormal heart rhythm. Dysrhythmias may result from:

- Disturbance in automaticity: This may involve a speeding up or slowing down of the sinus node (ie, sinus bradycardia/tachycardia), the formation of premature beats (often called **premature complexes** or depolarizations) from the atria, the atrioventricular junction, or the ventricles (PAC/PJC/PVCs).
- Disturbance in conductivity: Conduction may be too rapid (eg, Wolf-Parkinson-White syndrome) or too slow (eg, atrioventricular block).
- Combinations of altered automaticity and conductivity

The **ECG** is a recording of the electrical forces produced by the heart and inscribed on graph paper. The ECG paper is divided into 5 small squares comprising 1 large square. Each small square corresponds to 0.04 seconds and each large square is 0.20 seconds (0.04 seconds x 5 small boxes) as noted in Figure 6-13. Electrodes, placed on the skin of the patient, record the electrical activity that precedes the mechanical contraction and relaxation of the myocardium. Changing the location of the recording electrodes provides different perspectives and different waveforms, enabling the observer to gain a more complete picture of the electrical forces within the heart. The selection of a particular lead configuration is based upon which lead provides the clearest picture or allows the observer to focus on particular regions of the heart. The standard 12-lead ECG consists of tracings from 6 limb leads (I, II, III, aVR, aVL, aVF) and 6 chest leads (V1, V2, V3, V4, V5, V6) (Figure 6-14). The physical therapist should be familiar with a single lead tracing (ie, a rhythm strip) and be able to interpret the HR, rhythm, and presence

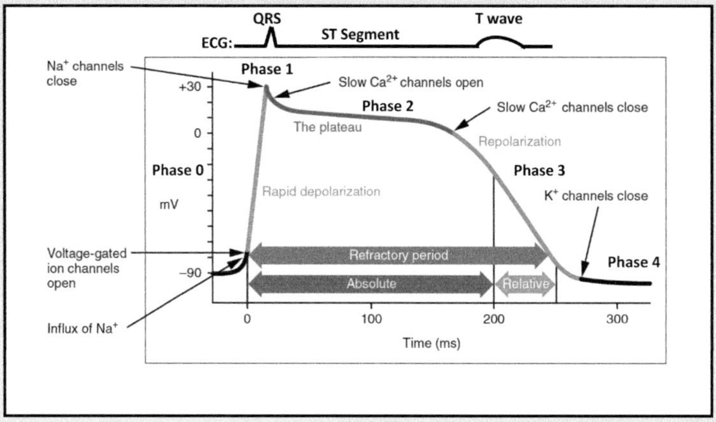

Figure 6-12. Phases of the action potential. Phase 0 (depolarization): Upon stimulation (eg, SA Node), sodium channels open resulting in the rapid movement of sodium into the cell creating a positive intracellular potential; permeability to potassium decreases. Phase 1 (partial repolarization): Sodium channels are closing combined with opening of slow potassium channels leading to the efflux of potassium out of the cell and a slight decrease in the membrane potential. Phase 2 (plateau phase): Calcium channels open leading to calcium movement into the cell, which is balanced by potassium exiting the cell. Phase 3 (rapid repolarization): Sodium and calcium channels are closed as potassium channels continue to open with efflux of potassium out of the cell. Phase 4 (resting membrane potential): The sodium–potassium pump is active moving sodium outward and bringing potassium inward returning the cell to its normal resting negative intracellular potential (-90 mV).

Table 6-17

PACEMAKERS OF THE HEART

Pacemaker	*Intrinsic Rate*
Primary Pacemaker	
SA node	60 to 100
Latent or Secondary Pacemakers	
AV node	40 to 60
Ventricles/purkinje system	20 to 40

(or absence) of dysrhythmias. Once the rhythm strip has been interpreted, it is imperative that the therapist understands the impact of these electrical events on the hemodynamic profile of the patient (Figure 6-15).

Electrocardiogram Interpretation

ECG interpretation begins with identification of the electrical waveforms and intervals, as noted in Figure 6-16, including:

Figure 6-13. The ECG paper displays time on the horizontal axis and voltage on the vertical axis. Note the small and large boxes. (Reprinted from Hillegass EA, Sadowsky HS. *Essentials of Cardiopulmonary Physical Therapy*, page 387, with permission from Elsevier.)

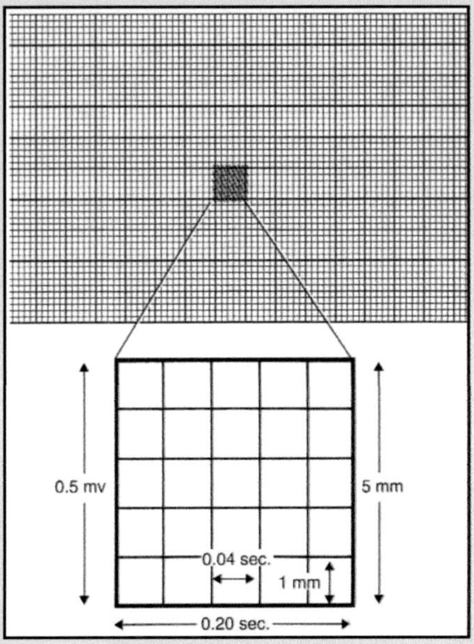

Figure 6-14. The ECG tracing from the chest leads (V1 to V6) showing the changes in the QRS configuration. (Reprinted from Hillegass EA, Sadowsky HS. *Essentials of Cardiopulmonary Physical Therapy*, page 387, with permission from Elsevier.)

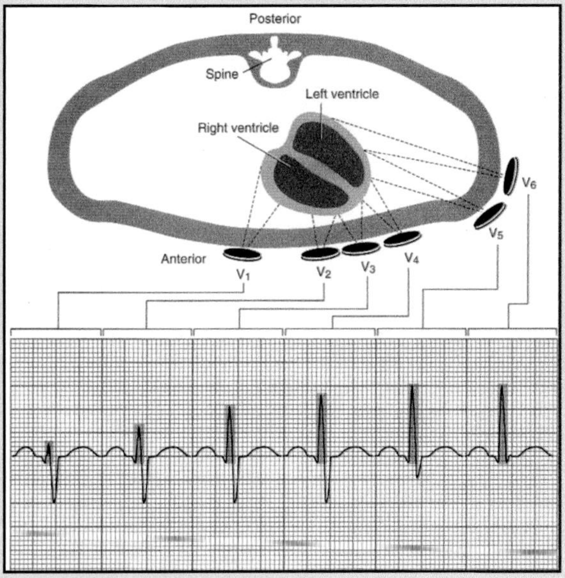

- **P waves**: Atrial depolarization
- **QRS complex**: Ventricular depolarization
- **T wave**: Ventricular repolarization
- **U wave**: Possible repolarization of the Purkinje system (minimal significance)
- **PR interval**: Extends from the beginning of the P wave to the onset of the QRS complex. This interval represents conduction through the atria to the atrioventricular node and the Bundle of His. The PR interval (PRI) is measured from the

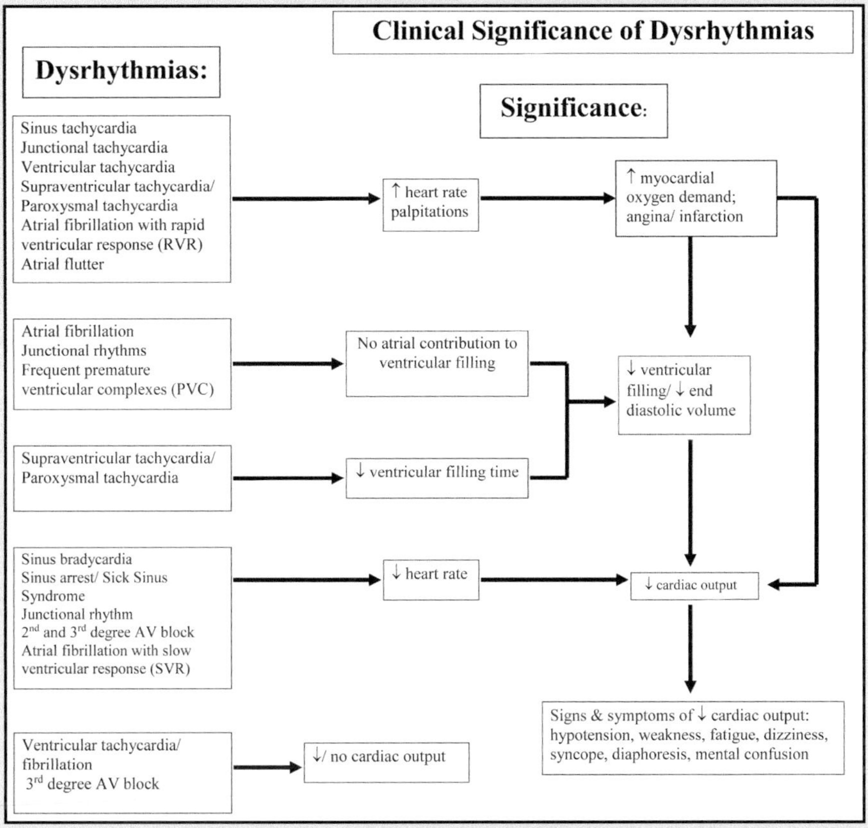

Figure 6-15. Impact of various dysrhythmias on hemodynamic responses and patient complaints. (Adapted from Watchie J. *Cardiopulmonary Physical Therapy: A Clinical Manual.* Philadelphia, PA: WB Saunders; 1995. With permission from Elsevier.)

onset of the P wave to the onset of the QRS complex, and its normal duration is 0.12 to 0.20 seconds.

- **QRS interval**: Extends from the end of the PRI (noted by change in the waveform deflection) and ends with the return to baseline. The QRS interval represents the time it takes for the ventricles to depolarize or conduction from the atrioventricular node, through the Bundle of His, the bundle branches, and the Purkinje system. The normal QRS duration is 0.04 to 0.11 seconds.
- **ST segment**: Interval measured from the end of the QRS complex and the beginning of the T wave. It represents the time during which the ventricles have completed depolarization and repolarization begins. ST segment elevation and depression are observed as an early ECG sign of infarction.
- **Q-T interval**: Extends from the beginning of the QRS complex until the end of the T wave and represents the time interval for ventricular depolarization and repolarization. The normal Q-T interval is 0.32 to 0.40 seconds and prolongation is associated with drug toxicity and increased risk of dysrhythmias.

ECG interpretation should be performed in an organized and systematic fashion. Table 6-18 provides a step-wise approach.

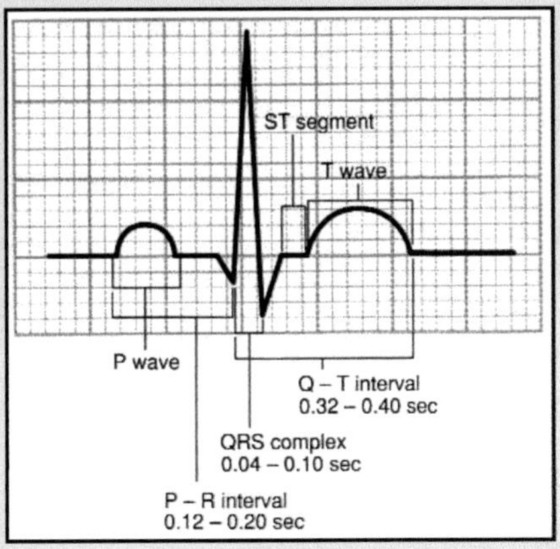

Figure 6-16. Electrical waveforms and intervals of an ECG. (Reprinted from Hillegass EA, Sadowsky HS. *Essentials of Cardiopulmonary Physical Therapy,* page 468, with permission from Elsevier.)

Common Rhythms/Dysrhythmias

Normal Sinus Rhythm

Rate: 60 to 100; sinus bradycardia is a rate less than 60 (Figure 6-17); sinus tachycardia is a rate greater than 100 (Figure 6-18)
Rhythm: Regular

Sinus Arrhythmia

- **Definition**: An irregularity in rhythm in which the impulse is initiated by the sinoatrial node but with phasic quickening and slowing of the impulse formation.
- **Rate**: 40 to 100
- **Rhythm**: Irregular. Impulse is originated in the sinoatrial node but with phasic quickening and slowing of the impulse formation. The irregularity is usually caused by an alternation in vagal stimulation (eg, inspiration—increases rate; expiration—decreases rate).
- **P waves**: Sinus, P followed by QRS.
- **PRI**: 0.12 to 0.20 seconds
- **QRS**: 0.06 to 0.12 seconds
- **Common causes**:
  - Most common type is associated with the respiratory cycle and is usually observed in the young and the elderly. Sinus arrhythmia often disappears with activity.
  - Nonrespiratory sinus arrhythmia may occur in conditions of infection, fever, and medication administration (particularly toxicity with digoxin or morphine).
- **Treatment**:
  - The respiratory type is benign and does not require treatment
  - The nonrespiratory type should be evaluated for the underlying cause and then treated.

Table 6-18

Systematic Approach to Dysrhythmia Interpretation

1. Regularity (also called rhythm):
- Is it regular?
- Is it irregular (check R-R interval)?
- Are there any patterns to the irregularity?
- Are there any ectopic beats; if so, are they early or late?

2. Rate:
- What is the exact rate?
- Is the atrial rate the same as the ventricular rate?

3. P waves:
- Are the P waves regular?
- Is there one P wave for every QRS?
- Is the P wave in front of the QRS or behind it?
- Is the P wave normal or upright in lead II?
- Are there more P waves than QRS complexes?
- Do all the P waves look alike?
- Are the irregular P waves associated with ectopic beats?

4. PRI:
- Are all the PRIs constant?
- Is the PRI measurement within the normal range?
- If the PRI varies, is there a pattern to the changing measurements?

5. QRS complex:
- Are all the QRS complexes of equal duration?
- What is the measurement of the QRS complex?
- Is the QRS measurement within normal limits?
- Do all the QRS complexes look alike?
- Are the unusual QRS complexes associated with ectopic beats?

Adapted from *Dysrhythmia Review Manual*. Nursing Staff Development. University of Pennsylvania Health System. Hospital of the University of Pennsylvania; Hillegass EA. *Essentials of Cardiopulmonary Physical Therapy*. 3rd ed. St. Louis, MO: Elsevier: WB Saunders; 2011; and Mammen BA, Irwin S, Tecklin JS. Common cardiac and pulmonary clinical measures. In: Irwin S, Tecklin JS. *Cardiopulmonary Physical Therapy: A Guide to Practice*. 4th ed. St. Louis, MO: Mosby; 2004.

Sinus Pause or Block

- **Definition**: Occurs when the sinoatrial node fails to initiate an impulse, usually only for one cycle.
- **Rate**: Usually 60 to 100
- **Rhythm**: Underlying rhythm is regular, but occasional pauses are noted
- **P waves**: Sinus, P followed by QRS
- **PRI**: 0.12 to 0.20 seconds
- **QRS**: 0.06 to 0.12 seconds
- **Common causes**:
  - Sudden increases in parasympathetic activity
  - Organic disease of the sinoatrial node (eg, sick sinus syndrome)
  - Other causes may include infection, rheumatic disease, severe ischemia, or infarction to the sinoatrial node, and/or digoxin toxicity.
- **Treatment**:
  - Required only if symptomatic. Remove or correct causative factor.

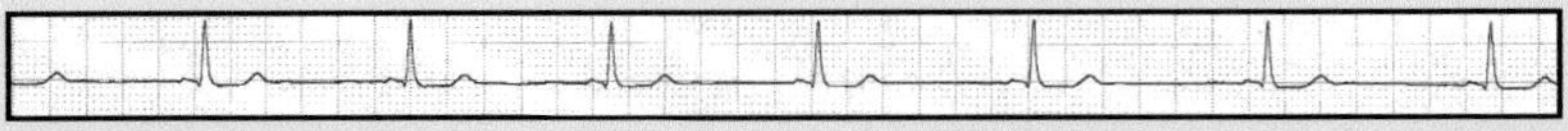

Figure 6-17. Sinus bradycardia.

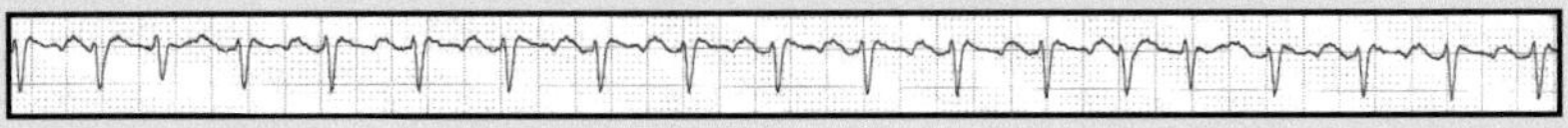

Figure 6-18. Sinus tachycardia.

Atrial Dysrhythmias

Premature Atrial Complexes (PAC)

- **Definition**: An ectopic, or abnormal, focus in either atria that initiates an impulse before the next impulse is initiated by the sinoatrial node. Conduction through the ventricles is normal.
- **Significance**: PACs reflect the irritability of atrial muscle. May reflect a predisposition to other atrial dysrhythmias.
- **Rate**: Underlying rhythm is usually sinus; therefore, rate is 60 to 100.
- **Rhythm**: Irregular. The premature ectopic beat will interrupt the regularity of the underlying rhythm. Note the irregular P-P and R-R intervals if you include the ectopic beat.
- **P waves**: A P wave, differing in morphology from that of the sinus node, occurring before the next expected sinus beat, hence the P-P interval is shorter than the normal P-P interval. PACs originating from the same focus will have similar P waves. A noncompensatory pause is usually present.
- **PRI**: Normal or prolonged. The PRI of the ectopic will probably be different from the PRI of the other complexes.
- **QRS**: Normal or aberrant
- **Assessment**:
  - Pulse: Irregular
  - Identification: By ECG
- **Common causes**:
  - Stimulants, infectious disorders, myocardial infarction
  - Stress, exertion, anxiety drug toxicity
  - Metabolic disorders, cor pulmonale
- **Treatment**:
  - Treat the underlying cause
  - Antiarrhythmic drugs (eg, procainamide, verapamil)

Paroxysmal Atrial Tachycardia (PAT)/Atrial Tachycardia (Figure 6-19)

- **Definition**: A clinical syndrome characterized by repeated episodes (ie, paroxysms) of atrial tachycardia with abrupt onset lasting from a few seconds to many hours.
- **Significance**:
  - May result in a decrease in stroke volume and cardiac output and, eventually, BP.
  - Predisposes to heart failure.
  - Increases myocardial oxygen consumption, which can lead to angina or infarction in ischemic heart disease (ie, CAD).

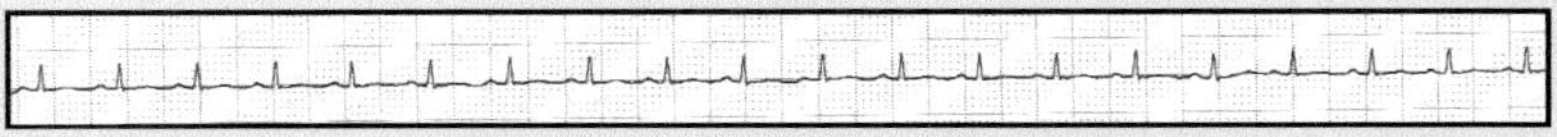

Figure 6-19. Paroxysmal atrial tachycardia/atrial tachycardia.

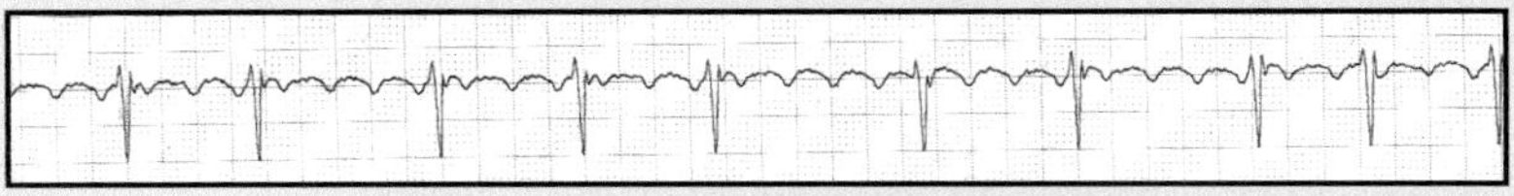

Figure 6-20. Atrial flutter with variable conduction (2:1, 3:1; 4:1).

- **Rate**: Atrial rate is usually 150 to 250
- **Rhythm**: Atrial rhythm is usually regular. The ventricular rhythm is often regular with 1:1 atrioventricular conduction when the atrial rate is <200. With atrial rate >200, 2:1 atrioventricular block (or higher) is common.
- **P waves**: May be difficult to identify because the P wave may be buried within preceding T wave. The P waves will differ morphologically from sinus P waves.
- **PRI**: Normal or prolonged
- **QRS**: Normal
- **Assessment**:
  - Pulse and HR are rapid.
  - Cardiac output and BP may be lower due to reduced ventricular filling time and limited stroke volume.
  - May complain of dizziness, anxiety, generalized weakness, palpitations, chest thumping.
- **Common causes**:
  - Emotional factors (eg, stress)
  - Overexertion, hyperventilation
  - Potassium depletion
  - Caffeine, nicotine, or aspirin sensitivity; digitalis toxicity
  - Rheumatic heart disease, mitral valve dysfunction (ie, mitral valve prolapse)
  - Pulmonary embolism
  - Thyroid disease
- **Treatment**:
  - Identify underlying cause
  - Discontinuation of medications
  - Vagal maneuvers are sometimes performed to increase parasympathetic output (ie, valsalva maneuvers, breath holding, coughing).
  - If episodes are prolonged, medications may be indicated (eg, beta blockers, calcium channel blockers).

Atrial Flutter (Figure 6-20)

- **Definition**: An ectopic atrial focus depolarizes at a rate of 250 to 350 bpm, exciting nearby areas repeatedly forming a reentry pathway. If only one ectopic focus is firing repetitively, the P waves look identical and have a characteristic sawtooth pattern.
- **Significance**:
  - Decrease cardiac output
  - Increased myocardial oxygen demand
  - Predisposition to left ventricle failure

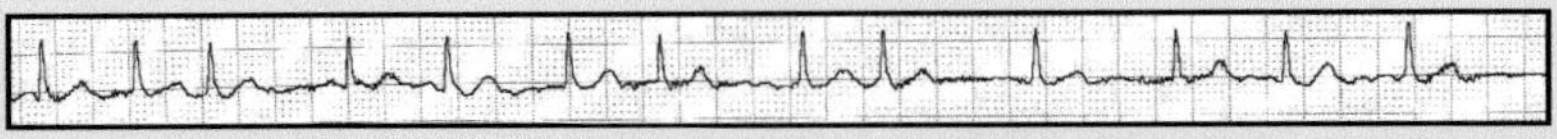

Figure 6-21. Atrial fibrillation. Note the lack of defined P waves, presence of fibrillatory waves, and irregularity.

- **Rate**: Atrial rate is 250 to 350; ventricular rate may vary depending on conduction to the ventricles. Commonly there is a block at the atrioventricular node because of the refractory period resulting in a 2:1 conduction.
- **Rhythm**: Atrial rhythm usually regular. Ventricular rhythm will be regular if a constant degree of atrioventricular block or may be irregular if variable block is present.
- **P waves**: Flutter waves (ie, sawtooth)
- **PRI**: Normal or may vary. Often it is impossible to identify a PRI because of the unusual configuration of the P waves (flutter waves).
- **QRS**: Normal or aberrant
- **Assessment**:
  - Pulse: Regular if conduction is constant. Irregular if conduction ratio varies.
  - If cardiac output is decreased, BP is diminished. Patients frequently complain of angina, palpitations, and/or dizziness.
  - Identification: Via ECG
- **Common causes**:
  - Multiple pathologic conditions including rheumatic heart disease, cardiomyopathy, mitral valve disease, CAD, myocardial infarction, stress, drugs, renal failure, hypoxemia, and pericarditis.
- **Treatment**:
  - With increased ventricular rate, cardiac output may become compromised.
  - Medications:
    - Antiarrhythmic: Verapamil, procainamide
    - Drugs to reduce atrioventricular conduction: Digitalis, beta blockers (propranolol).
  - Cardioversion or pacemaker

Atrial Fibrillation (Figure 6-21)

- **Definition**: An erratic quivering or twitching of the atrial muscle caused by multiple ectopic foci in the atria or multiple reentry pathways. There is a loss of atrial contraction and potential thrombi formation. The atrioventricular node attempts to control the entry of impulses that initiate QRS complexes; therefore, a totally irregular rhythm is present.
- **Rate**: Atrial rate is 400 to 700 (usually cannot be counted). Ventricular rate may be normal, slow, or rapid.
- **Rhythm**: Irregularly irregular ventricular rhythm. Atrial rhythm is unmeasurable because atrial activity is chaotic.
- **P waves**: None of the ectopic foci fully depolarize the atria, so no true P waves are present. There is no organized atrial activity and fibrillatory waves are present.
- **PRI**: Not identified
- **QRS**: Normal or aberrant
- **Assessment**:
  - Pulse: Irregularly irregular
  - Sign/symptoms of decreased cardiac output

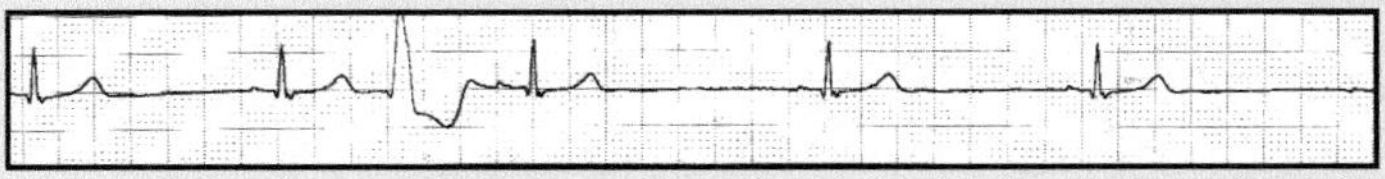

Figure 6-22. A single premature ventricular contraction. Note the underlying rhythm is sinus bradycardia.

- **Common causes**:
  - Multiple factors including age, CHF, ischemia, infarction, cardiomyopathy, digoxin toxicity, drug use, stress or pain, renal failure, or rheumatic heart disease.
- **Treatment**:
  - If loss of atrial activity (ie, atrial kick), cardiac output may be compromised (up to a 20% to 30% decrease). With ventricular response rates <100, the decrease in cardiac output is usually not problematic. With ventricular rates >100, cardiac output may be diminished, and signs and symptoms of hemodynamic compromise may occur (eg, decreased BP/hypotension, complaint of dizziness, palpitations, SOB).
  - Increased potential to develop mural thrombi; therefore, patients are prescribed anticoagulant therapy.
  - Medications: Verapamil, digoxin
  - Cardioversion

Ventricular Dysrhythmias

Premature Ventricular Complexes (Figure 6-22)

- **Definition**: A depolarization that arises in either ventricle prior to the next expected sinus beat. As the impulse originates outside of the normal conduction system, conduction is slowed, resulting in a bizarre and widened QRS complex without a P wave and followed by a complete compensatory pause. PVCs may be identical (**unifocal**—originating from the same foci) or look different (**multifocal**—originating from different foci).
- **Significance**: May indicate a predisposition to developing other lethal dysrhythmias, especially if PVCs existing in the following forms:
  - Frequent: >5/minute
  - Multifocal: Configuration varies (indicates a varying focus)
  - Bigeminy (1:1), trigeminy (2:1), quadrigeminy (3:1)
  - R on T pattern
  - Sequential salvos: Short runs of 2 or 3 beats
- **Rhythm**: Irregular; underlying rhythm usually sinus
- **P waves**: Sinus P waves are usually obscured by the QRS, ST segment, or the T wave of the PVC. The presence of a sinus P wave can be inferred by the presence of a fully compensatory pause.
- **PRI**: Depends upon underlying rhythm. Cannot determine PRI of PVC.
- **QRS**: >0.12 seconds; wide and distorted
- **Assessment**:
  - Conscious sensation: Palpitations, skipping a beat, thumping
  - Pulse: Irregular
  - BP may be lower than usual.
  - Decreased cardiac output: Patient may complain of dizziness, angina, weakness.

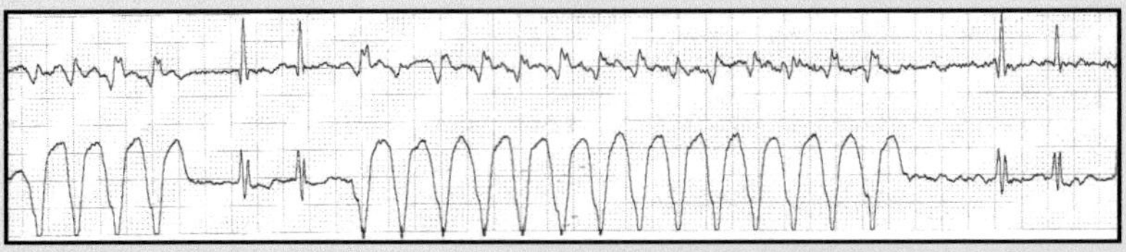

Figure 6-23. Ventricular tachycardia show in 2 different leads. Note that there is a rhythm before/after the ventricular tachycardia. This is an example of non-sustained ventricular tachycardia (NSVT).

- **Common causes**:
  - Caffeine or nicotine sensitivity
  - Electrolyte imbalances (particularly hypo- or hyperkalemia)
  - Cardiac ischemia, cardiomyopathy, myocardial infarction, CHF
  - Chronic lung disease and/or hypoxemia
- **Treatment**:
  - Depends on the underlying cause, frequency, and severity of the PVCs and the associated symptoms. PVCs may indicate increased irritability of the ventricle and may progress to lethal ventricular tachycardia or ventricular fibrillation.

Ventricular Tachycardia (Figure 6-23)

- **Definition**: A series of three or more PVCs in a row. Occurs because of rapid firing by a single ventricular focus with increased automaticity. NSVT is defined as a rate >120 bpm and a duration of <30 seconds.
- **Significance**:
  - Indicates extensive myocardial ischemia and irritability.
  - Decreased cardiac output and BP
  - Unreliable pacemaker.
  - Predisposing to ventricular fibrillation and ventricular standstill
- **Rate**: Ventricular rate 100 to 250
- **Rhythm**: Usually regular
- **P waves**: Absent (buried in QRS complex)
- **PRI**: Absent
- **QRS**: >0.12 sec.; wide and bizarre in appearance.
- **Assessment**:
  - Signs and symptoms of decreased cardiac output:
    - Angina
    - Dizziness
    - Low to no BP
    - Syncope
    - Weak, thready pulse
  - If conscious, may complain of anxiety, confusion, disorientation, thumping, and racing heartbeat.
  - Patient may be unconscious.
- **Common causes**:
  - Ischemia, acute infarction, CAD
  - Respiratory failure (hypoxia), massive pulmonary embolism
  - Electric shock
  - Cardiac pacing
  - Heart block (advanced)

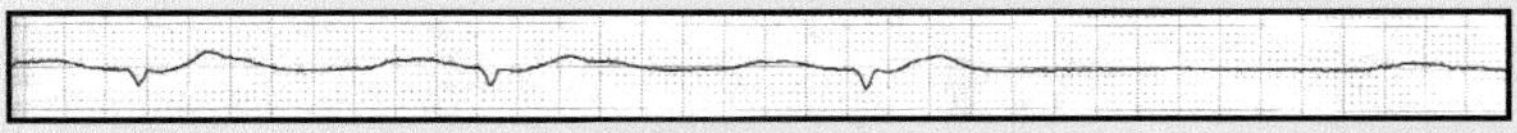

Figure 6-24. Idioventricular rhythm followed by asystole.

- **Treatment**:
  - Emergency situation secondary to compromised cardiac output and BP.
  - Initiate CPR/ACLS (advanced cardiac life support).
  - Immediate cardioversion/defibrillation
  - Immediate pharmacological injection (eg, amiodarone, procainamide, beta blockers, calcium channel blockers)

Ventricular Fibrillation

- **Definition**: Erratic quivering of the ventricular muscle resulting in no cardiac output. As in atrial fibrillation, multiple ectopic foci fire creating asynchrony.
- **Significance**:
  - No cardiac output.
  - Death is inevitable unless the situation is reversed immediately.
- **Rate**: Chaotic
- **Rhythm**: Absent.
- **P waves**: Absent.
- **QRS**: Widened and bizarre, fibrillatory waves present.
- **Assessment:**
  - Pulse: None
  - Heart sounds: None
  - BP: None
  - Unconsciousness
  - Cyanosis
  - Convulsions, pupils dilated
- **Common causes**:
  - Same as ventricular tachycardia.
- **Treatment**:
  - Defibrillation followed by CPR, supplemental oxygen, and medication injection.

Idioventricular Rhythm (Figure 6-24)

- **Definition**: In the absence of a higher pacemaker, the ventricles will function as the dominant pacemaker and initiate a regular impulse at their inherent rate of 20 to 40 bpm.
- **Significance**:
  - Indicates extensive myocardial ischemia and irritability
  - Decreased cardiac output
  - Unreliable pacemaker
  - Predisposing to ventricular fibrillation and ventricular standstill
- **Rate**: Ventricular rate usually 20 to 40; accelerated idioventricular rhythm 40 to 100
- **Rhythm**: Regular
- **P waves**: Absent
- **PRI**: Absent
- **QRS**: >0.12 seconds; wide and distorted

- **Assessment**:
  - Signs and symptoms of decreased cardiac output.
    - Angina
    - Dizziness
    - Low to no BP
    - Syncope
    - Weak, thready pulse
  - If conscious, may complain of anxiety, confusion, disorientation, thumping in chest.
  - Patient may be unconscious.
- **Common causes**:
  - Ischemia, acute infarction, CAD
  - Respiratory failure (hypoxia, massive pulmonary embolism)
  - Electric shock
  - Cardiac pacing malfunction
  - Heart block (advanced)
- **Treatment**:
  - Attempt to increase sinus rate for capture, atropine
  - Antiarrhythmic drugs
  - Treat underlying cause

Asystole (see Figure 6-24)

- **Definition**: There is no electrical pacemaker to initiate measurable electrical flow.
- **Significance**:
  - Cardiovascular collapse/ventricular standstill
  - Death is imminent.
- **Rate**: None
- **Rhythm**: None
- **P waves**: None
- **PRI**: None
- **QRS**: None

Heart Blocks

- **Definition**: Heart blocks are due to delayed, erratic, or absent conduction through the atrioventricular node.

First-Degree Heart Block

- **Rate**: Depends on underlying rhythm
- **Rhythm**: Regular
- **P waves**: Sinus, P followed by QRS
- **PRI**: Lengthened >0.20 seconds. The interval is usually constant, but may vary.
- **QRS**: 0.06 to 0.11 seconds
- **Assessment**:
  - Patients are typically asymptomatic.
- **Common causes**:
  - CAD/myocardial infarction
  - Rheumatic heart disease
  - Digoxin or beta blockers
- **Treatment**: None, unless due to medication reaction

Type I Second-Degree Heart Block (Mobitz Type I; Wenckebach)

- **Definition**: This type of block usually occurs at the atrioventricular node and is highlighted by the prolongation of the PR interval.
- **Rate**: Depends on underlying rhythm; atrial rate will be greater than ventricular rate.
- **Rhythm**: Irregular; the R-R interval will vary
- **P waves**: P followed by QRS until "dropped" beat (QRS).
- **PRI**: Progressively lengthens until one P wave is not followed by a QRS (dropped beat).
- **QRS**: 0.06 to 0.11 seconds
- **Assessment**:
  - Patients are typically asymptomatic.
  - Pulse is irregular. If the block is cyclic, the pulse will be regularly irregular.
- **Common causes**:
  - CAD/myocardial infarction
  - Excessive beta blockade
  - Increased vagal/parasympathetic tone (eg, athlete)
- **Treatment**:
  - None is usually necessary, unless the patient exhibits signs and symptoms of hemodynamic compromise (eg, hypotension, dizziness, SOB).

Type II Second-Degree (Mobitz Type II; Classic Heart Block)

- **Definition**: This type of block occurs typically along the bundle branches or, less commonly, the Bundle of His. This block is associated with a poorer prognosis and may lead to complete heart block.
- **Rate**: Depends on underlying rhythm; atrial rate will be greater than ventricular rate.
- **Rhythm**: Irregular. The R-R interval will vary depending on the constancy of blocked beats.
- **P waves**: All P waves are not followed by QRS. There will be more P waves than QRS complexes.
- **PRI**: The PRI on conducted beats are constant and may be normal (<0.20 seconds) or prolonged (>0.20 seconds).
- **QRS**: May be normal (0.06 to 0.11 seconds), but is often wide (>0.12 seconds).
- **Assessment**:
  - If the block is constant, the pulse will be regular.
  - If the ventricular rate is low, patients may present with hypotension and complain of dizziness.
- **Common causes**:
  - Myocardial infarction
  - Lesion of conducting pathways
- **Treatment**:
  - Pacemaker placement (temporary pacing [eg, transcutaneous or transvenous until a permanent pacemaker can be inserted]).

Third-Degree Heart Block (Complete Heart Block)

- **Definition**: Indicates that all impulses originating from the atria are blocked at the atrioventricular node, the Bundle of His, or the bundle branches. There is an absence of conduction between the atria and ventricles. This is an unstable rhythm.
- **Rate**: The atrial may be equal to or greater than the ventricular rate.
- **Rhythm**: The atria and ventricles are firing independently, and at regular intervals. The P-P interval and the R-R interval are regular.

- **P waves**: The P waves are uniform and usually outnumber the QRS complexes.
- **PRI**: There is no conduction between the atria and ventricles; therefore, there is no PRI.
- **QRS**: If the ventricles are being stimulated from a junctional foci, the QRS will be normal (<0.12 seconds), but if the focus is ventricular, the QRS will be wide (>0.12 seconds).
- **Assessment**:
  - Signs and symptoms of decreased cardiac output (see previously).
- **Common causes**:
  - Myocardial infarction
  - Digoxin toxicity
- **Treatment**:
  - Pacemaker placement (temporary pacing [eg, transcutaneous or transvenous] until a permanent pacemaker can be inserted)

Atrioventricular Junctional Dysrhythmias (Nodal Dysrhythmias)

- **Definition**: Conduction tissue near the atrioventricular node can take over pacemaker function if higher pacemaker sites fail. These rhythms are highlighted by slow HRs and retrograde P waves (eg, upside down [inverted] P waves in lead II, III, and aVF).

Premature Junctional Complexes

- **Rate**: Depends on underlying rhythm
- **Rhythm**: Irregular due to PJC. The R-R interval will vary.
- **P waves**: The P wave of the ectopic beat can come before, during, or after the QRS complex and will be inverted in lead II, III, and aVF.
- **PRI**: If the P wave is before the QRS, the PRI will be less than 0.12 seconds. If the P wave falls with or after the QRS, there is no PRI.
- **QRS**: Normal (<0.12 seconds)

Junctional Escape Rhythm

- **Rate**: Usually between 40 and 60
- **Rhythm**: Regular
- **P waves**: The P waves can come before, during, or after the QRS complex and will be inverted in lead II, III, and aVF.
- **PRI**: If the P wave is before the QRS, the PRI will be less than 0.12 sec. If the P wave falls with or after the QRS, there is no PRI.
- **QRS**: Normal (<0.12 sec)

Accelerated Junctional Rhythm/Junctional Tachycardia

- **Rate**: Usually between 100 to 180
- **Rhythm**: Regular
- **P waves**: The P waves can come before, during, or after the QRS complex and will be inverted in lead II, III, and aVF.
- **PRI**: If the P wave is before the QRS, the PRI will be less than 0.12 seconds. If the P wave falls with or after the QRS, there is no PRI.
- **QRS**: Normal (<0.12 seconds).
- **Assessment**:
  - Cardiac output and BP can be reduced with slow rates or decreased due to limited filling times with tachycardia.
  - Pulses may be weak, thready, and irregular or regular.
  - Patients may complain of dizziness, palpitations, or fatigue.

- **Common causes**:
  - Myocardial infarction, CAD
  - S/p heart surgery
  - Myocarditis
  - Digitalis intoxication
  - Hyperventilation
- **Treatment**:
  - Identify and treat the underlying cause.
  - If rate is slow and patient symptomatic, medications (eg, atropine) or pacemaker are indicated.
  - Often, treatment is not necessary.

Pacemakers, Defibrillators, and Cardioversion

Pacemakers are mechanical devices used prophylactically (eg, post–open heart surgery) to initiate myocardial contractions when intrinsic electrical impulses are insufficient (eg, bradycardia associated with myocardial infarction), the native impulses are not being conducted (eg, second or third heart block), the HR is too slow to maintain an adequate cardiac output (eg, sick sinus syndrome, syncope) or overdriving tachydysrhythmias (eg, atrial flutter). Left **ventricular** and **biventricular** pacing, also known as **cardiac resynchronization therapy** (CRT), is becoming more common in heart failure, left bundle branch block, and intra-ventricular conduction delay. Biventricular pacing attempts to coordinate the electrical and mechanical ventricular activation leading to more efficient ventricular contractions. These devices can be inserted on a temporary or permanent basis. **Temporary pacemaker** implantation is most commonly achieved by transvenous, transcutaneous, or direct placement of electrodes on the epicardial surface of the heart. **Transvenous cardiac pacing** is achieved by threading an electrode through a central vein (eg, subclavian, internal or external jugular or femoral veins) to the endocardial surface of the right ventricle or, less commonly, the right atrium. **Transcutaneous** or **external pacing** is indicated for emergent situations, such as asystole and bradyarrhythmias and involves placement of anterior and posterior electrode pads on the chest. **Epicardial pacing** is common following open-heart procedures, such as CABG, valve repair, or replacement and transplant surgery. The electrodes connecting the pulse generator to the heart are embedded or lightly sutured to the epicardium, the outer surface of the heart, externalized prior to closing the thorax, and secured to the chest wall. **Permanent pacemakers** (PPMs) are usually placed along the left anterior chest wall in an infraclavicular pocket and endocardial leads are affixed to the heart via the cephalic vein as noted in Figure 6-25.

A pacemaker's function is described by a coding system outlined in Table 6-19 that defines the chambers paced and sensed and the pacemaker responses. Sensing is the identification of intrinsic cardiac electrical activity while pacing (or capture) describes the pacemaker's providing electrical stimuli leading to myocardial contraction. For example, a VVI pacemaker will sense and stimulate ventricular activity and is inhibited if sufficient intrinsic ventricular depolarizations are sensed. If native ventricular activity is not sensed, the pacemaker will provide electrical stimulation to the ventricle initiating depolarization. Figure 6-26 provides an example of a ventricle paced rhythm.

Automatic implantable cardioverter-defibrillators (AICD/ICD) are devices that detect life-threatening dysrhythmias, including ventricular fibrillation and ventricular tachycardia, and prevent sudden cardiac arrest (SCA). The ICD provides an electrical shock to temporarily depolarize an irregularly beating heart allowing normal electrical and coordinated contractile activity to resume. ICDs are implanted just as a permanent pacemaker and are generally indicated for those

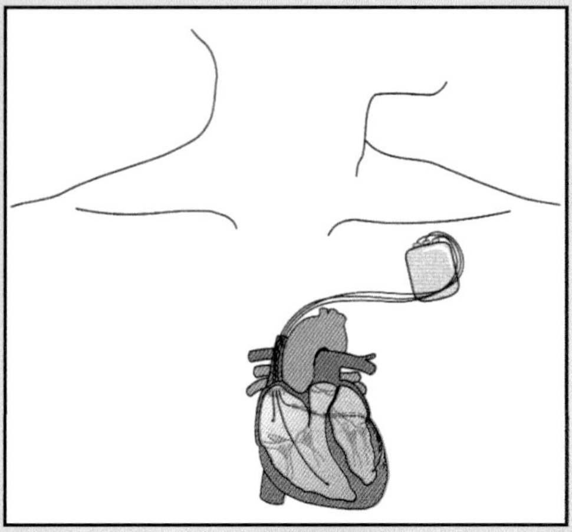

Figure 6-25. PPMs are usually placed along the left anterior chest wall in an infraclavicular pocket and endocardial leads are affixed to the heart via the cephalic vein. Example of permanent pacemaker with 3 leads. (Reprinted from Hillegass EA, Sadowsky HS. Essentials of Cardiopulmonary Physical Therapy, page 468, with permission from Elsevier.)

Table 6-19

NBG Pacemaker Codes

Pacing Location	*Sensing Location*	*Response to Pacing*	*Modulation*	*Antiarrhythmia Function*
A = atrium	A = atrium	O = no response	O = none	O = none
V = ventricle	V = ventricle	I = inhibited	R = rate	P = pacing modulation
D = dual (A & V)	D = dual (A & V)	T = triggered	M = multi-program	S = shock
D = dual (T & I)	C = communicating	D = dual (P & S)		

Adapted from Bernstein AD, Camm AJ, Flecher RD, et al. The NASPE/BPEG generic pacemaker code for antibradyarrhythmias and adaptive-rate pacing and antitachyarrhythmia devices. *Pacing Clin Electrophysiol*. 1987;10:794.

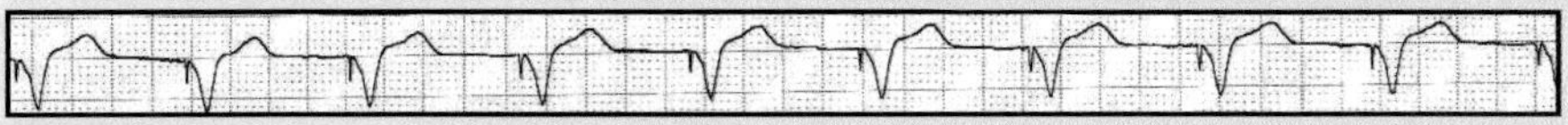

Figure 6-26. Example of ventricular paced rhythm. Note pacemaker spike preceding the wide QRS complexes.

who have survived cardiac arrest due to ventricular tachycardia or ventricular fibrillation, those with recurrent tachydysrhythmias with CAD/myocardial infarction or left ventricle dysfunction, and those with inducible ventricular tachycardia or ventricular fibrillation.[67] As a temporary measure the wearable cardioverter-defibrillator (WCD; LifeVest [Zoll]; Figure 6-27) is worn by patients at risk for SCA, providing protection during their changing condition. Patients should wear the WCD at all times, including while sleeping. The WCD should only be removed when a patient is showering or bathing.

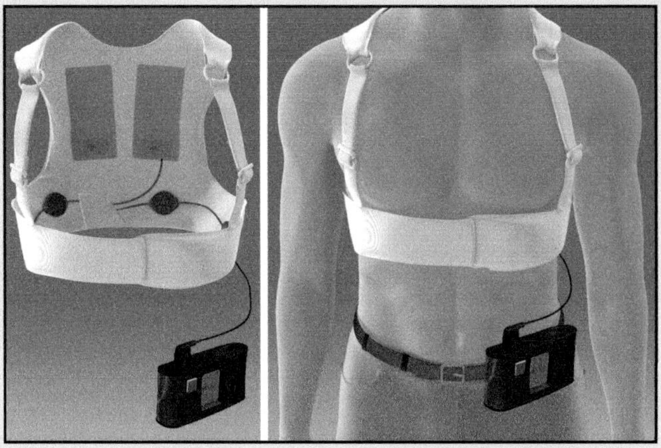

Figure 6-27. Zoll LifeVest.

Table 6-20

PHYSICAL THERAPY CONSIDERATIONS FOR PACEMAKERS AND IMPLANTABLE CARDIOVERTER-DEFIBRILLATORS

Temporary Pacemakers	*Permanent Pacemakers and Implantable Cardioverter-Defibrillators*
• Determine that the epicardial wires are taped securely to the skin to prevent accidental dislodgement. • After epicardial wires are removed, patients should be monitored closely for signs of cardiac tamponade (eg, tachycardia, hypotension). • Patients are frequently maintained on 1 to 2 hours bed rest post-removal.	• Limit weightbearing and heavy lifting (>10 pounds) of the involved UE x 6 to 8 weeks after placement. • Shoulder elevation of the involved UE is limited to <90 degrees x 6 to 8 weeks after placement. • No driving until cleared by physician. • Check incision daily: Redness, swelling, drainage. • Monitor for fever: Temperature >100.5° or develops chills

Cardioversion is similar to defibrillation in concept, but the energy requirements and emergent nature are reduced. Cardioversion can be accomplished through medications (eg, adenosine) or through the application of transcutaneous electrical current. Cardioversion is often performed to terminate dysrhythmias, including atrial fibrillation, atrial flutter, and ventricular tachycardia.

Common physical therapy precautions associated with pacemakers and ICDs are provided in Table 6-20.

Appendix B

Pharmacological Information: Cardiovascular Diseases and Disorders Pharmacology

Nitrates

Action

Produces nitric oxide producing vasodilatation (venous > arterial). The vasodilatation of coronary arteries increases blood supply to ischemic regions. The vasodilatation of peripheral vessels increases venous capacitance resulting in decreased venous return. The net result is improved oxygen supply and reduced oxygen demand. Nitrates are commonly prescribed for patients with ischemic heart disease, angina, heart failure, HTN, and pulmonary edema.

Side Effects

CNS: Dizziness, headache, weakness
CV: Hypotension, syncope, reflex tachycardia
GI: Nausea, vomiting, abdominal pain
Miscellaneous: Flushing

Common Medications

Isordil, Isorbid (isosorbide dinitrate); Imdur (isosorbide mononitrate); Nitrostat, Nitro-Dur, Nitrocot (nitroglycerine)

Calcium Channel Blockers

Action

Calcium channel blockers (CCBs) inhibit the transport of calcium into myocardial (including the sinoatrial and atrioventricular nodes) and vascular smooth muscle cells. The result is slowed pacemaker activity and inhibited excitation-contraction coupling leading to muscular relaxation and vasodilatation. CCB are indicated for patients with ischemic heart disease, coronary vasospasm (Prinzmetal angina), myocardial infarction, HTN, and SVTs.

Side Effects

CNS: Headache, dizziness, fatigue
CV: Bradycardia, tachycardia, palpitations, hypotension, peripheral edema, angina
GI: Nausea, constipation, diarrhea
Miscellaneous: Flushing, sexual dysfunction

Common Medications

Norvasc (amlodipine); Cardizem (diltiazam); Procardia, Adalat (nifedipine); Calan (verapamil); Vascor (bepridil)

Beta Blockers

Action

Beta blockers inhibit the stimulation of the beta 1 (myocardial) and/or beta 2 (pulmonary, vascular) adrenergic receptors. Nonselective agents block both beta 1 and 2; selective agents block only beta 1. Beta blockers decrease HR and BP and are frequently prescribed for those with ischemic heart disease, myocardial infarction, HTN, anxiety, and to decrease progression of heart failure.

Side Effects

CNS: Dizziness, fatigue, anxiety/nervousness
CV: Bradycardia, orthostatic hypotension
GI: Diarrhea, constipation, nausea
Miscellaneous: Arthralgias, back pain, muscle cramp, weakness
Pulmonary: Bronchospasm (nonselective agents)

Common Medications

Non-selective (beta 1 & 2): Coreg (carvedilol); Normodyne, Trandate (labetalol); timolol
Selective (beta 1): Tenormin (atenolol); Lopressor, Toprol (metoprolol)

Angiotensin-Converting Enzyme Inhibitors

Action

ACE inhibitors block the conversion of angiotensin I into the vasoconstrictor Angiotensin II and reduces the production of the sodium and water retaining hormone aldosterone. ACE inhibitors promote vasodilation and fluid loss and are indicated for heart failure, HTN, myocardial infarction and diabetic nephropathy.

Side Effects

CNS: Dizziness, fatigue, headache, insomnia
CV: Hypotension, tachycardia, angina
GI: Diarrhea, nausea
Miscellaneous: Angioedema, fever, weakness
Pulmonary: Cough

Common Medications

Benazapril, Capoten (captopril), Vasotec (enalapril), Monopril (fosinopril), Zestril (lisinopril), Accupril (quiapril), Altace (ramipril)

Angiotensin II Receptor Antagonists/ Angiotensin II Receptor Blockers

Action

Angiotensin II receptor blockers (ARBs) prevent angiotensin II, a vasoconstrictor, from binding to its receptor on the vasculature. ARBs are used in the treatment of HTN. They block the receptor for the vasoconstrictor angiotensin II leading to vasodilation. These medications also reduce the production of aldosterone leading to decreased fluid retention.

Side Effects

CNS: Dizziness, fatigue, headache
CV: Hypotension
GI: Diarrhea, hepatitis
GU: Renal failure
Miscellaneous: Hyperkalemia

Common Medications

Atacand (candesartan), Teveten (eprosartan), Cozaar (losartan), Diovan (valsartan)

Centrally Acting Adrenergic Agonists

Action

Centrally acting adrenergic agonists stimulates the alpha-adrenergic receptors within the CNS, which inhibits peripheral sympathetic outflow. The result is reduced BP, and inhibited HR acceleration. Additionally, these medications provide pain relief.

Side Effects

CNS: Sedation/drowsiness, depression, dizziness
CV: Bradycardia, hypotension, palpitations
GI: Dry mouth, constipation, nausea, vomiting
Miscellaneous: Weight gain, rash, impotence

Common Medications

Catapres (clonidine), methyldopa (Aldomet), reserpine

Diuretics

Action

Diuretics inhibit reabsorption of electrolytes (sodium, potassium, chloride) or increase secretion of electrolytes into loop of Henle or distal tubule of the kidney leading to increased renal excretion of electrolytes and water. Diuretics are prescribed for HTN, pulmonary edema and effusions, and hypervolemia.

Side Effects

CNS: Dizziness, headache
CV: Hypotension (hypovolemia)
GI: Dry mouth, constipation, dyspepsia
Miscellaneous: Electrolyte abnormalities including hyper-/hypokalemia, hyponatremia, hypochloremia, hypomagnesemia, metabolic alkalosis, muscle cramping

Common Medications

Loop diuretics: Bumex (bumetanide), Lasix (furosemide), Demadex (toresemide)
Osmotic diuretics: Mannitol
Potassium-sparing diuretics: Midamor (amiloride), Aldactone (spironolactone)

Thiazide Diuretics: Hydrochlorothiazide

Alpha-Adrenergic Blockers

Action

These medications block the postsynaptic alpha-adrenergic receptors leading to vascular smooth muscle relaxation and vasodilation.

Side Effects

CNS: Dizziness, headache, fatigue
CV: Orthostatic hypotension, tachycardia
GI: Dry mouth, constipation, nausea, vomiting
Miscellaneous: Fluid retention/edema, arthritis/gout, sexual dysfunction, weakness

Common Medications

Minipress (prazosin), Cardura (doxazosin)

Vasodilators

Action

Vasodilators relax the smooth muscle of arteries and veins through varied mechanisms. For example, nitroprusside liberates nitric oxide, a potent vasodilator.

Side Effects

CNS: Dizziness, headache, blurred vision
CV: Hypotension, dyspnea
GI: Nausea, vomiting, pain

Common Medications

Nitropress (nitroprusside), Apresoline (hydralazine), Loniten (minoxidil)

Anticoagulants

Action

Anticoagulants inhibit the clotting mechanism at various points in the clotting cascade (see Figure 2-4). For example, warfarin, an oral anticoagulant, interfere with the hepatic synthesis of Vitamin K-dependent clotting factors (factors II, prothrombin, VII, IX, and X). Heparin, a parenteral (non-oral) anticoagulant, interferes with the conversion of prothrombin to thrombin while dabigatran, a Novel oral anticoagulant (NOAC), directly inhibits thrombin. Rivaroxaban, also a NOAC, inhibits factor Xa. Patients will have the INR/PT (warfarin) or PTT (heparin) monitored to adjust dosage (see Chapter 2).

Side Effects

CNS: Dizziness, headache, bleeding
CV: Edema
GI/GU: Bleeding (GI bleeding, hematuria), nausea, vomiting, anorexia, abdominal cramping, diarrhea
Miscellaneous: Fever

Common Medications

Oral: Coumadin (warfarin)
Parenteral: Heparin; low–molecular weight heparins (dalteparin [Fragmin], danaparoid [Orgaran], enoxaparin [Lovenox])
NOACs: Pradaxa (dabigatran, Xarelto (rivaroxaban), Eliquis (apixaban)

Antiplatelet Agents

Action

Antiplatelet agents disrupt the activation, aggregation or adhesion of platelets through multiple mechanisms. Aspirin inhibits the formation of thromboxane A2, abciximab, a glycoprotein IIb/IIIa inhibitor, blocks fibrinogen receptors on platelets, and clopidogrel blocks adenosine diphosphate receptors on platelets.

Side Effects

CNS: Dizziness, tinnitus, difficulty hearing
CV/Pulmonary: Hypotension, bronchospasm
GI: Bleeding, nausea, dyspepsia, heartburn, abdominal discomfort, hepatotoxicity
GU: Hematuria

Common Medications

Bayer, Ecotrin (aspirin [acetylsalicylic acid]); Aggrastat (tirofiban); Reopro (abcixima); Integrilin (eptifibatide); Plavix (clopidogrel)

Thrombolytics

Action

Thrombolytic agents convert plasminogen to plasmin, which degrades fibrin and dissolve clot. These agents are used in acute coronary syndrome (myocardial infarction), embolic CVA, DVT and clearing of blockage in catheters.

Side Effects

CNS: Bleeding/intracranial hemorrhage
CV: Reperfusion dysrhythmias, hypotension
GI: Bleeding
Pulmonary: Bronchospasm, hemoptysis
Miscellaneous: Allergic reaction, fever

Common Medications

Alteplase (tissue plasminogen activator [t-PA]), streptokinase, urokinase

Antiarrhythmics

Action

Antiarrhythmics interfere with myocardial excitability and automaticity modifying the action potential of the myocytes (see Figure 6-12). These drugs alter the duration of the action potential, slow conduction or prolong the refractory periods and are beneficial for reentry and tachyarrhythmias. These drugs are divided into 4 classifications and most may cause new or worsened dyrhythmias (proarrhythmic effect).

Class IA

Inhibits the fast sodium channels depressing phase 0 of the action potential. Additionally, they prolong the duration of the action potential (similar to Class III).

Common Medications

Quinidine, disopyramide, procainamide

Class IB
Inhibits the fast sodium channels and shortens the action potential selectively in diseased heart tissue.

Common Medications

Lidocaine, Dilantin (phenytoin)

Class IC
Inhibits the fast sodium channels depressing phase 0 and have an affinity to slow conduction and shorten action potential duration of His/pukinje fibers.

Common Medications

Tambocor (flecainide), Rythmol (propafenone), Ethmozine (moricizine)

Class II
Inhibits phase 4 spontaneous depolarization of nodal tissue and indirectly close calcium channels leading to reduced pacemaker automaticity and slower conduction.

Common Medications

Beta blockers: Propranolol, esmolol, acebutolol

Class III
Block outward potassium channels, thereby prolonging the action potential duration and refractory period.

Common Medications

Cordarone (amiodarone), Betapace (sotalol), bretylium

Class IV
CCBs slow conduction and increase the duration of the refractory period of the atrioventricular node by inhibiting the inward calcium channel.

Common Medications

Calan (verapamil), Cardiazem (diltiazem)

Miscellaneous

Atropine: Inhibits the action of postsynaptic acetylcholine diminishing the influence of the parasympathetic nervous system leading to increased HR.
Adenosine: Inhibits both the sinus and atrioventricular nodes by opening potassium channels and indirectly inhibiting the calcium channels.
Digoxin: Augments parasympathetic tone on the atria and atrioventricular node and is prescribed for the treatment of atrial fibrillation.

Lipid-Lowering Agents (HMG CoA Inhibitors—Statins)

Action

Statins inhibit an enzyme (HMG CoA) that is essential for hepatic cholesterol synthesis resulting in reduced LDL and potentially a slight increase in HDL cholesterols.

Side Effects

CNS: Headache, blurred vision, dizziness, insomnia, fatigue
GI: Flatulence, abdominal pain/cramps, constipation, nausea, vomiting, heartburn, elevated liver enzymes
Miscellaneous: Rhabdomyolysis with possible renal failure, arthralgias, rash, muscle cramps

Common Medications

Lipitor (atorvastatin), Lescol (fluvastatin), Mevacor (lovastatin), Pravachol (pravastatin), Zocor (simvastatin)

Inotropes

Action

Inotropic medications increase the intracellular concentrations of calcium in myocytes leading to increased myocardial contractility, prolongation of the refractory period of the atrioventricular node and slower conduction velocities through the sinoatrial and atrioventricular nodes. These agents are indicated for heart failure, atrial fibrillation, SVT

Side Effects

CNS: Fatigue, headache
CV: Dysrhythmias (bradycardia/SVT/Ventricular dysrhythmias), hypotension, chest pain
GI: Nausea, vomiting
Miscellaneous: Thrombocytopenia, weakness

Common Medications

Digitalis, Lanoxin (digoxin), dopamine, dobutamine, Primacor (milrinone)

CNS = central nervous system; CV = cardiovascular; GU = genitourinary.

Chapter 7

Pulmonary Diseases and Disorders

Kathy Lee Bishop, PT, DPT, CCS and Daniel J. Malone, PT, PhD, CCS

Diseases of the respiratory tract are now the third leading cause of death in the United States and are ranked eighth in primary hospital admission diagnoses.[1,2] The most common preventable cause of lung disease remains cigarette smoking; however, environmental and genetic factors can also play a role.[3] The goals of this chapter are to review essential anatomy and physiology of the pulmonary system and to define common pulmonary disorders and the medical and surgical management. Physical therapy examination and interventions, a case study, and chapter review questions are also included.

Anatomy and Physiology

A simple way to consider the pulmonary system is to split the system into the musculoskeletal pump and the gas-exchanging organ.

The Musculoskeletal Pump

The thoracic rib cage, cervical and thoracic spine, and upper pelvic area comprise the bony components of the musculoskeletal pump (Figure 7-1). These bony structures provide the origin and insertion of the respiratory muscles and protect and support the lung tissue.[4-6] Bony or muscular injury, such as a rib or clavicular fracture or a surgical incision, can influence efficiency of the musculoskeletal pump. A tibial fracture can be immobilized internally or covered with a cast, but a rib fracture or a surgical incision in the thorax is not fixated. As the rib cage is in constant motion, patients will complain of difficulty taking deep breaths and soreness with coughing, sneezing, or laughing. The inability to breathe deeply following surgery or trauma increases the risk for atelectasis and pneumonia. A balance of pain medication, early mobilization, and frequent position change can help to optimize ventilation and prevent pulmonary complications.

Malone DJ, Bishop KL, eds. *Acute Care Physical Therapy: A Clinician's Guide, Second Edition* (pp 245-309).

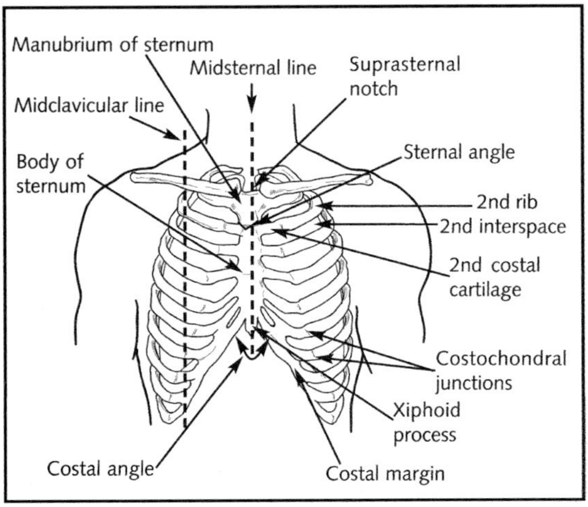

Figure 7-1. Anterior thorax, ribs, and sternum. (Reprinted with permission from Sheldon LK. *Oxygenation*. Sudbury, MA: Jones and Bartlett Publishers; 2001.)

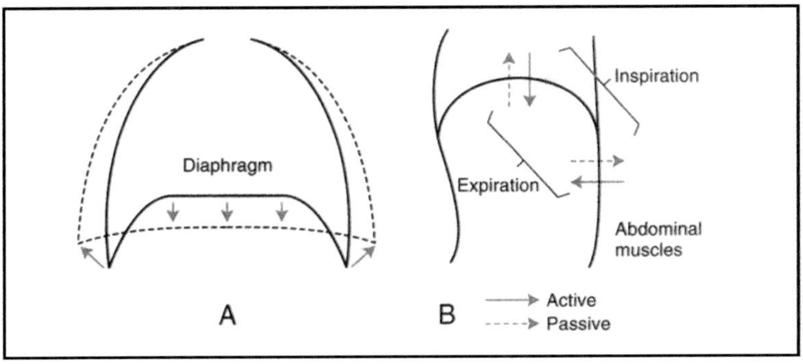

Figure 7-2. (A) On inspiration, the dome-shaped diaphragm contracts, the abdominal contents are forced down and forward, and the rib cage is lifted. The volume of the thorax is, therefore, increased. (B) On forced expiration, the abdominal muscles contract and push the diaphragm up. (Reprinted with permission from West JB, ed. *Pulmonary Physiology and Pathophysiology: An Integrated, Case-Based Approach.* Philadelphia, PA: Lippincott Williams & Wilkins; 2001:3.)

The muscles of respiration alter the configuration of the thoracic cage and produce the pressure fluctuations resulting in inspiration and expiration.[4] These muscles must contract in synchrony on inspiration and relax during a normal expiration. Expiration is normally a passive process resulting from relaxation of the inspiratory muscles and the elastic recoil of the lungs, airways, and chest wall (Figure 7-2). Exceptions to this are forced expiration maneuvers (eg, coughing, sneezing, huffing) and exercise and expiration for patients with increased airway resistance (eg, chronic obstructive pulmonary disease [COPD]). On forced expiration the abdominals, the primary expiratory muscles, and the postural back, cervical, and pelvic muscles contribute to force development (Figure 7-3).[4] Postural muscles stabilize the thorax allowing the abdominals to contract, increasing intra-abdominal pressure, forcing the diaphragm cephalad, increasing thoracic pressure promoting expiration. The expiratory muscles also assist with vomiting leading to complaints of abdominal and postural muscle soreness with severe nausea and prolonged episodes of emesis.

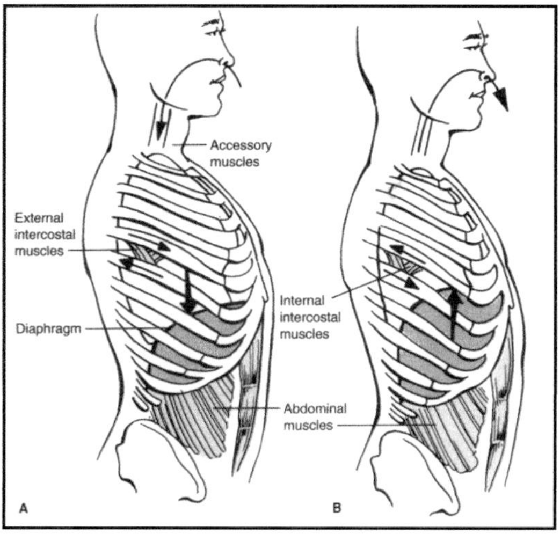

Figure 7-3. Muscles of ventilation. (A) Inspiratory muscles. (B) Expiratory muscles. (Reprinted with permission from Mackin L, Bullock BL. Normal pulmonary function. In: Bullock BA, Henze RL, eds. *Focus on Pathophysiology*. Philadelphia, PA: Lippincott Willams & Wilkins; 2000:533.)

The respiratory muscles must develop force to overcome the resistances of the airways, lung tissue, and chest wall.[4] Airway resistance is impacted by the geometry of the airways (bronchodilation vs constriction) and velocity and type of airflow (laminar vs turbulent, slow vs rapid breathing rate). The majority of airway resistance is due to turbulent airflow in the large bronchi extending from the trachea to the fourth or fifth generation (Figure 7-4). Lung tissue and chest wall resistance refers to the compliance, or ease of expansion, which is influenced by the fluid content of pulmonary tissues and the structural contents of the lung parenchyma and musculoskeletal pump.[4,5] Changes in these factors can increase the work of breathing (WOB), resulting in a greater oxygen consumption for the respiratory muscles. Length tension relationships of the muscles, body positioning, organ size (eg, hepatomegaly, ascites), pregnancy, obesity, scoliotic deformities, chest wall deformities (eg, pectus excavatum), and neurologic disorders (eg, Guillian-Barré, muscular dystrophy, amyotrophic lateral sclerosis) can influence the respiratory muscle function and, therefore, the work of breathing.[6,7]

The primary muscle of inspiration is the diaphragm, and this dome-shaped muscle separates the abdomen from the thorax. [4] The phrenic nerve, originating from cervical nerve roots C3 to C5 (remember "3, 4, 5 stay alive"), innervates the diaphragm.[4,5] The diaphragm is divided into 2 separate domes for the left and the right thoracic cavities. The muscle fans out to attach to the inner surface of the rib cage, the costal diaphragm, and inserts into a central tendon that attaches to the lumbar vertebrae, the crural diaphragm.[6] Contraction of the diaphragm pulls the central tendon downward promoting thoracic expansion. The descent of the diaphragm during inspiration pushes the abdominal organs outward. Interestingly, a patient in respiratory distress may reverse this pattern. This altered pattern where the stomach is drawn inward during inspiration is called **paradoxical breathing**.[8] As noted previously, the shape, position, and function of the diaphragm can be impacted by multiple factors. For example, hyperinflation as seen in COPD can flatten the diaphragm while pregnancy, obesity, and ascites can elevate the diaphragm and restrict diaphragm descent during inspiration.

The accessory muscles of inspiration activate during tasks that challenge the musculoskeletal pump, such as exercise, lung and neuromuscular disease, and chest wall deformities.[4,5,8] This activation reflects an increased WOB and results in greater oxygen consumption of all muscles of inspiration. Table 7-1 lists some of the accessory

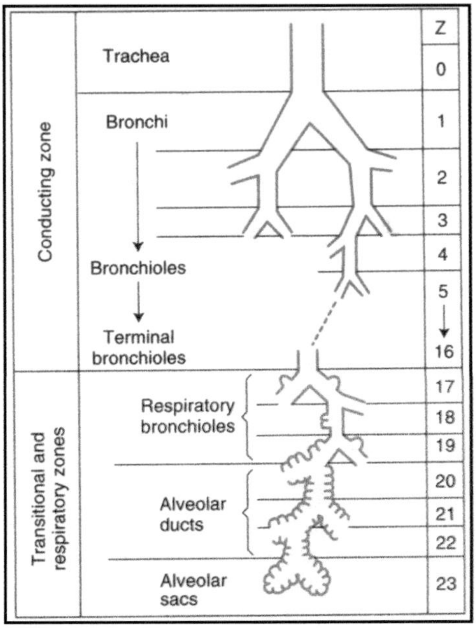

Figure 7-4. Idealization of the human airways to Weibel. (Reprinted with permission from West JB, ed. *Pulmonary Physiology and Pathophysiology: An Integrated, Case-Based Approach.* Philadelphia, PA: Lippincott Williams & Wilkins; 2001:4.)

Table 7-1 ACCESSORY MUSCLES OF INSPIRATION: STERNOCLEIDOMASTOID, ERECTOR SPINAE, TRAPEZIUS, SCALENES
Usage reflects increased work of breathing and oxygen consumption. **Activity that increases ventilation:** Exercise **Disorders with increased airway resistance:** COPD, asthma **Disorders of lung tissue:** Idiopathic pulmonary fibrosis (IPF), pneumonia **Disorders of chest wall:** Scoliosis, ankylosing spondylitis **Disorders altering configuration or force production of diaphragm:** COPD, neuromuscular disease
Adapted from Crystal RG, West JB, Barnes PJ, et al. *The Lung: Scientific Foundations*. New York, NY: Raven Press, Ltd; 1991; Watchie J. *Cardiopulmonary Physical Therapy: A Clinical Manual*. Philadelphia, PA: WB Saunders Co; 1995; and West JB. *Respiratory Physiology—The Essentials*. 3rd ed. Baltimore, MD: Lippincott Williams & Wilkins; 1985.

muscles and conditions that increase demand and the WOB. Many of these conditions can occur simultaneously (eg, a patient with COPD who is exercising) and will have an increase in demand from both the underlying health condition and the exercise.

The Gas-Exchanging Organ

The gas-exchanging organ is composed of the airways that allow air to travel from outside the body to the alveoli and the specialized interface between inspired air and the circulation, the alveolar-capillary membrane. The conducting airways branch repeatedly and extend from the oral-nasal pharynx to the 17th generation of bronchi. The conducting airways do not contribute to gas exchange.

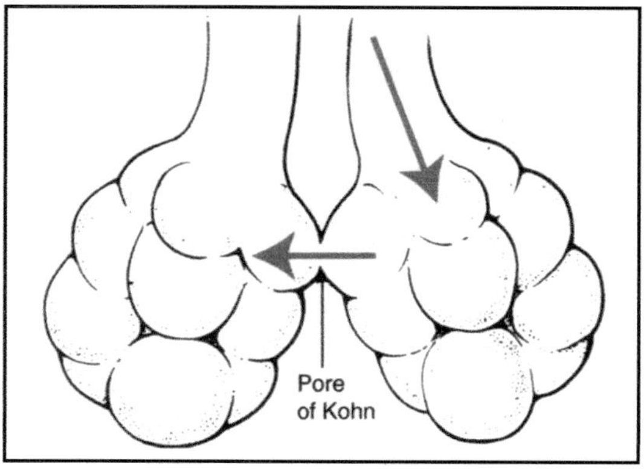

Figure 7-5. Interconnecting alveoli through the pores of Kohn. (Reprinted with permission from Mackin L, Bullock BL. Normal pulmonary function. In: Bullock BA, Henze RL, eds. *Focus on Pathophysiology*. Philadelphia, PA: Lippincott Williams & Wilkins; 2000:531.)

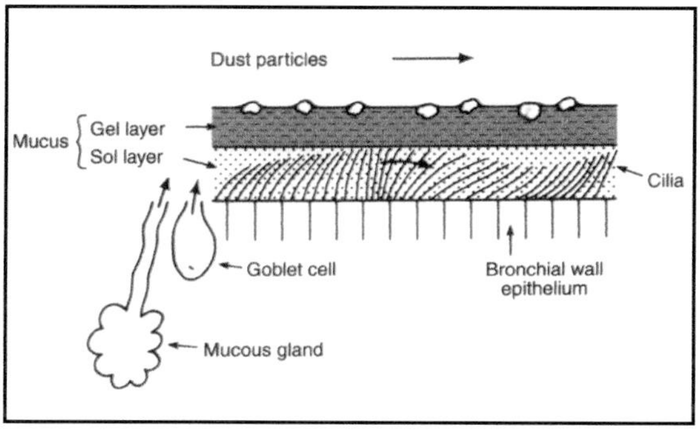

Figure 7-6. Mucociliary escalator. The mucous film consists of a superficial gel layer that traps inhaled particles and a deeper sol layer. It is propelled by cilia. (Reprinted with permission from West JB, ed. *Pulmonary Physiology and Pathophysiology: An Integrated, Case-Based Approach*. Philadelphia, PA: Lippincott Williams & Wilkins; 2001:119.)

The transitional zone consists of respiratory bronchioles, alveolar ducts, and the alveolar sacs and is the site of gas exchange.[4,9] Three specific channels act as a transit area for cells of the pulmonary immune defenses and allow for collateral ventilation, the process of gas passing between adjacent lung units (Figure 7-5). The pores of Kohn connect adjacent alveoli, Lambert's canals connect the alveoli and the respiratory bronchioles, and the channels of Martin go between the respiratory bronchioles.[4]

The **upper respiratory tract** includes the nasopharynx, sinuses, mouth, and larynx above the vocal cords and this portion of the airway acts to warm, humidify, and filter the inspired air. The upper respiratory tract plays an important function as the first line of pulmonary immune defense to prevent infection.[6,9,10] The mucociliary escalator, the second line of immune defense, is a specialized transport system consisting of 2 layers, the gel layer and the sol layer (Figure 7-6). The superficial gel layer is relatively more viscous while the deeper sol layer contains the motile cilia.[11] Inhaled particles imbed within the gel layer and are transported upward by the beating action of the cilia where they are either coughed or swallowed. This protective escalator lines the conducting airways.[6,9] Abnormalities of ciliary function are noted in cystic fibrosis, primary ciliary dyskinesia (Kartagener's syndrome), and some bacterial infections leading to deficient pulmonary defense and increase infection risk.[7,11] Pulmonary defense is completed by immune cells, such as macrophages and neutrophils, that reside in the alveoli (see Chapter 5).[10]

The **lower respiratory tract** consists of the trachea and bronchi, bronchioles, and alveoli. The trachea divides at the carina into the right and left mainstem bronchi as noted in Figure 7-7. This division corresponds anteriorly with the angle of Louis, or sternal angle, the joint between the manubrium and body of the sternum, and

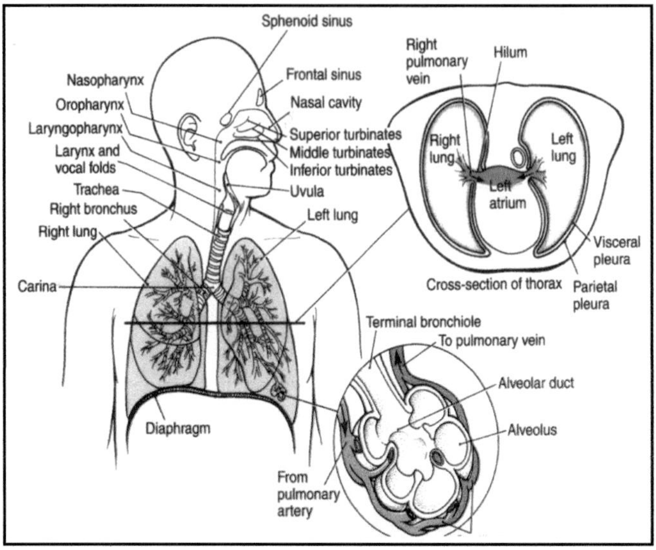

Figure 7-7. The respiratory system. (Reprinted with permission from Mackin L, Bullock BL. Normal pulmonary function. In: Bullock BA, Henze RL, eds. *Focus on Pathophysiology*. Philadelphia, PA: Lippincott Willams & Wilkins; 2000:528.)

posteriorly at the fourth thoracic vertebrae.[12] The sternal angle is an important anatomic landmark for airway clearance when a suction catheter must be inserted into the trachea (see Table 7-17). The right mainstem bronchus is aligned more vertically than the left, increasing the aspiration risk into the right lung.[12] The right lung divides into 3 lobes: middle, upper, and lower. The left lung is divided into 2 lobes: upper and lower. Part of the left upper lobe, the lingula, is considered anatomically similar to the right middle lobe (RML).

The pulmonary circulation serves many purposes, including filtering of blood, participating in gas exchange at the alveolar-capillary junction, providing nutrients to the lungs, and metabolizing blood borne chemicals (eg, conversion of angiotensin I to angiotensin II).[9] The pulmonary circulation is a high-capacity, low-resistance vascular circuit that receives the entire cardiac output. Anatomically, it begins carrying deoxygenated blood from the right ventricle to the main pulmonary artery, branches repeatedly like the airways to the alveolar-capillary junction for gas exchange. Oxygenated blood is carried to the left atrium by the pulmonary veins as noted in Figure 7-8.[9] The bronchial circulation arises from the aorta or from intercostal arteries and supplies oxygenated blood to the conducting airways, pulmonary vessels, nerves, interstitium, and pleura.

The capillary system surrounding the alveoli is well developed to promote optimal exchange of oxygen and carbon dioxide. The alveolar-capillary junction plays a critical role in optimizing gas exchange. The thickness of the alveolar- capillary junction (increased with pulmonary edema or pulmonary fibrosis), the anatomic cross-sectional area (destroyed in emphysema or obstructed by pneumonia), and the oxygen-carrying capacity of hemoglobin may be altered in various health conditions leading to poor gas exchange causing shortness of breath (SOB), fatigue, and decreased physical function. The pulmonary vasculature is sensitive to low oxygen and high carbon dioxide tensions, as seen in poorly ventilated regions of the lung, and will adapt by shunting blood to better ventilated areas. This process is called

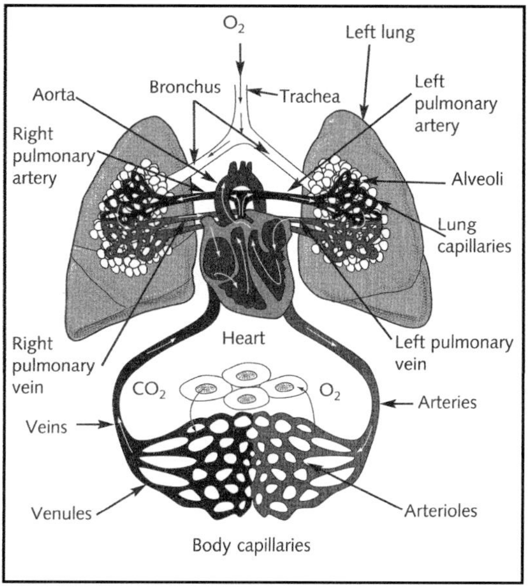

Figure 7-8. The vascular circuits: pulmonic and systemic. (Reprinted with permission from Sheldon LK. *Oxygenation*. Sudbury, MA: Jones and Bartlett Publishers; 2001.)

hypoxic vasoconstriction and tends to improve gas exchange.[9] This adaptive mechanism optimizes the ventilation (V) and perfusion (Q) (V/Q) relationship within the lungs but may become harmful when there is extensive tissue destruction of the lung and/or pulmonary vasculature leading to increased pulmonary vascular resistance (PVR). Increased PVR increases the work of the right ventricle leading to right ventricular hypertrophy, and eventually to right-sided heart failure or **cor pulmonale**. Cor pulmonale may be a complication in many pulmonary disorders, such as end-stage cystic fibrosis, chronic bronchitis, and emphysema.[7]

Physiologically, the V/Q ratio defines the relationship between ventilation and perfusion and is a primary determinate of the gas-exchanging function of the lungs. The mismatch between V and Q is the most common cause of hypoxemia in adults. Hypoxemia is low concentrations of oxygen in the blood and patients with hypoxemia will have low values with pulse oximetry. Regions of low V/Q (Q>V), are known as **shunt** and result in decreased arterial concentration of oxygen (PaO_2) and elevated arterial concentrations of carbon dioxide ($PaCO_2$). Regions of high V/Q (V>Q) are termed **dead space** and result in reduced $PaCO_2$ and an insignificant increase in PaO_2. V/Q matching (V=Q) is optimal for gas exchange. The V/Q ratio can be influenced by posture, exercise and changes in either ventilation or perfusion due to disease, abnormal hemodynamic pressures, and abnormal vasoconstriction or bronchoconstriction.[5,9,12] Table 7-2 shows normal arterial blood gas (ABG) reference values while breathing room air.

Respiratory Control and Innervation

The respiratory control system's primary goal is to maintain adequate oxygen supply and carbon dioxide removal.[5,6,9] Respiratory control is influenced by the autonomic nervous system, chemical and mechanical receptors, and voluntary behaviors. The breathing pattern is usually an automatic function relying on the respiratory centers of the brain stem (ie, medulla, pons) to maintain a normal sequence (ie, breathing pattern, respiratory rate [RR]). However, the cortex (eg, breath holding, volitional

Table 7-2 **ARTERIAL BLOOD GASES**	
Components	*Normal Values on Room Air*
Partial pressure of oxygen (PaO_2)	80 to 100 mm Hg
Partial pressure of carbon dioxide ($PaCO_2$)	35 to 45 mm Hg
Bicarbonate (HCO_3^-)	22 to 28 mEq/L
Acid/base balance (pH)	7.35 to 7.45

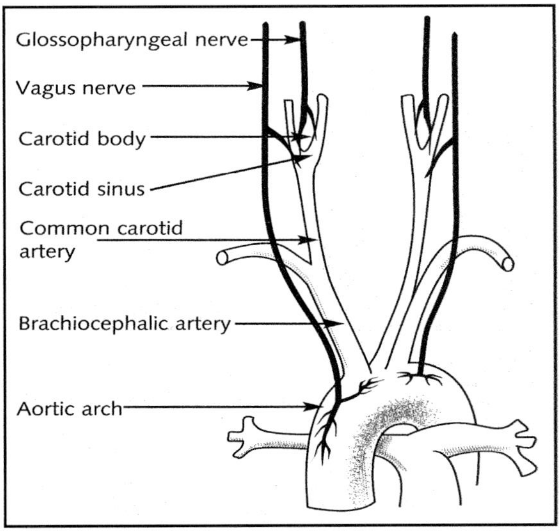

Figure 7-9. Location of peripheral chemoreceptors. (Reprinted with permission from Sheldon LK. *Oxygenation.* Sudbury, MA: Jones and Bartlett Publishers; 2001.)

hyperventilation), hypothalamus, and limbic system (eg, emotional states) can influence the breathing pattern.[9]

The central chemoreceptors, located in the medulla, and peripheral chemoreceptors, within the aortic arch and carotid bodies (Figure 7-9), respond to chemical stimuli and are sensitive to levels of PaO_2 and $PaCO_2$.[5,8,9,12] Elevated $PaCO_2$ increases the hydrogen ion concentration (H^+) of the blood creating an acidosis (ie, decreasing pH) stimulating the central chemoreceptors, while decreased PaO_2 and increased $PaCO_2$ stimulate the peripheral chemoreceptors. The chemoreceptors stimulate the respiratory control center leading to increased rates and depth of breathing. An overview of respiratory control is outlined in Table 7-3. Table 7-4 represents the primary pulmonary reflexes and resulting consequences of stimulation. Similar to control of breathing, the reflexes play a role in breathing patterns that are linked to the stimulated reflex.

HEALTH CONDITIONS

Pulmonary disorders can primarily be divided into obstructive or restrictive disease patterns. The therapist should keep in mind that many pulmonary disorders may be a combination of both patterns, but the pathology was put into one category

Table 7-3

RESPIRATORY CONTROL AND INNERVATION

Primary Goal	*Maintain Adequate Oxygen Supply*	*Carbon Dioxide Removal*		
Influences	Autonomic nervous system	Chemical receptors	Mechanical receptors	Voluntary behaviors
Breathing pattern	Automatic function	Relies on stimulus–respiratory centers	Brain stem Medulla/pons	Normal sequence (RR/breathing pattern)
			Cortex	Breath holding Volitional Hyperventilation Hypoventilation
			Hypothalamus Limbic system	Emotional states
Central chemoreceptors	Increased $PaCO_2$ = increased (H^+) (Acidosis) Stimulating receptors		Medulla	Sensitive to levels of PaO_2 and $PaCO_2$
Peripheral chemoreceptors	Decreased PaO_2 and increased $PaCO_2$ = increased RR and depth More responsive to lower O_2 concentrations		Aortic arch Carotid bodies	
Precautions	Certain disease states V/Q matching Impaired sensitivity of chemoreceptors Increased $PaCO_2$ Reduced PaO_2			Titrate Supplemental Oxygen to target SpO_2 range

Adapted from Watchie[5];Des Jardin[8]; West[9]; and Frownfelter.[12]

for simplification. The patient history, physical examination, and diagnostic testing will confirm the diagnosis. Tables 7-5 and 7-6 and Figure 7-10 provide descriptions of common pulmonary function tests and procedures.

Obstructive Disorders

Chronic Obstructive Pulmonary Disease

COPD, also referred to as **chronic obstructive lung disease** (COLD) or **chronic obstructive airway disease** (COAD), is a slowly progressive disorder characterized by chronic airflow limitation (Figure 7-11).[13] Cigarette smoking is the primary preventable cause of COPD, and 10% to 20% of all smokers are expected to develop

Table 7-4

PULMONARY REFLEXES

Type of Reflex	*Description*
Deflation reflex	Hering-Breuer reflex; stretch receptors in walls of bronchi and bronchioles are stimulated by distention of the lung and influence subsequent respiratory rate and expiration time.
Irritant reflex	Lung compression, deflation, or exposure to noxious gases (mechanical/chemical stimulus) results in cough and bronchoconstriction. Receptors located in subepithelial layer along bronchioles, bronchi, and trachea.
Aortic and carotid sinus baroreceptors	Changes in blood pressure (BP) result in alteration in heart rate (HR) and RR (↑ BP=↓ HR/RR; ↓ BP=↑ HR/RR). Receptors located near aortic arch and carotid sinus.
Juxtapulmonary-capillary receptors (J receptors)	Stimulation causes rapid, shallow breathing. Receptors located in interstitial tissue between alveoli and capillaries.
Stretch reflex	Stimulation (stretch) of skeletal muscle will ↑ strength of contraction. Receptors located in muscle spindles.
Joint/muscle receptors	Stimulation enhances ventilation in preparation for activity. Receptors located in peripheral joints/muscles.

the disease.[14,15] Age, smoking duration, and smoking amount influence COPD development. Clinically, COPD is defined by increased airway resistance, which limits expiration leading to air trapping (ie, **hyperinflation**), increased anterior-to-posterior chest wall diameter (ie, **barrel chest deformity**), and flattened diaphragms. Current classification of severity of airflow limitation for COPD is shown in Table 7-7 and is based on the decline in FEV_1.[16]

Patient presentation depends on disease and symptom severity and common findings include higher RRs, wheezing via auscultation, barrel chest deformity, lower oxygen saturations (SpO_2) on room air, accessory muscle usage, excessive dyspnea on exertion (DOE), and activity limitations, such as limited walk distance and difficulty with activities of daily living (ADLs).

One of the challenges of working with the COPD population is that the levels of dyspnea may not correlate with the disease severity.[16] Recurrent exacerbations result in worsening of symptoms and loss of lung function that may inhibit the individual's return to functional baseline.[17] Exacerbation prevention and disease progression are influenced by many factors including smoking cessation, long-term oxygen usage, prophylactic vaccinations and airway clearance, limiting exposure to communicable diseases, environmental pollutants and allergens, and remaining physically active and participating in pulmonary rehabilitation programs. A simple-to-use, valid tool for tracking changes in patient's self-reported dyspnea is the Modified Medical Research Council (mMRC) Questionnaire for Assessing the Severity of Breathlessness (Table 7-8).[18] This tool is linked to ADLs and can be used to define a patient's prior level of function before an exacerbation. The mMRC can also be used

Table 7-5

Pulmonary Function Tests Definitions

Type of Test	*Definition*
FEV_1	Amount of air expired in the first second of forced exhalation, used to assess obstruction in larger airways
Total lung capacity (TLC)	Amount of gas in lungs at end of maximum inhalation
Residual volume (RV)	Amount of air remaining in lungs following maximum expiration
Inspiratory capacity	Maximal amount of air inspired from resting expiratory levels (V_T + IRV)
Expiratory reserve volume (ERV)	Maximum amount of air expired beyond a normal (quiet) expiration
Inspiratory reserve volume (IRV)	Maximum amount of air inspired above a normal breath
Vital capacity	Maximum amount inspired and expired with a single breath
Tidal volume (V_T)	Normal amount of air ventilated at rest (quiet breathing)
Minute ventilation	Volume of air ventilated in 1 minute (V_T x RR)
Forced expiratory flow % (FEF 25% to 75%)	Maximum mid-expiratory flow rate (average flow rate during the middle 50% of forced vital capacity [FVC]), used to assess obstruction in smaller airways
FEV_1/FVC ratio	Used as general indicator of airway obstruction (normal >75%, obstruction <75%)
Peak expiratory flow rate (PEFR)	Maximum expiratory flow rate
Function residual capacity (FRC)	Volume of air in lungs at the resting expiratory level (RV + ERV)
Diffusing capacity of carbon monoxide (DLCO)	Amount of gas that moves across alveolar-capillary membrane; carbon monoxide single breath technique; provides information regarding the gas exchanging function of the lung
Maximal voluntary ventilation (MVV)	Measures maximal breathing capacity (MBC), used as a marker of respiratory muscle endurance
Maximal inspiratory pressure (MIP), or negative inspiratory force (NIF)	Measures maximal pressure developed during inspiration, measures inspiratory muscle strength
Maximal expiratory pressure (MEP)	Measures maximal pressure developed during expiration, measures expiratory muscle strength

(continued)

Table 7-5 (continued) **PULMONARY FUNCTION TESTS DEFINITIONS**	
Type of Test	*Definition*
Restriction pattern	Reduced lung volumes (V_T, residual volume) and capacities (FRC, vital capacity), preserved flow rates with reduced FEV_1, FVC due to small lung volumes
Obstruction	Increased FRC/residual volume (hyperinflation), limited V_T, reduced flow rates (FEV_1, FVC)

Table 7-6 **TESTS AND PROCEDURES ASSOCIATED WITH THE PULMONARY SYSTEM**	
Test Name	*Clinical Impact for Physical Therapy*
Chest x-ray	Radiographic study to determine the size, shape, and location of the heart; will determine the presence of extravascular fluid (eg, pulmonary edema, pleural effusion), anatomic integrity and alignment of ribs and diaphragm; attempts to localize lung consolidation, hyperdensities (eg, tumor), or translucency (eg, hyperinflation)
Bronchoscopy	Endoscopic procedure allowing direct visualization of the tracheobronchial tree; used to localize airway abnormalities, tumors/lesions, bleeding/hemoptysis, airway stenosis, biopsy, tissue resection, and secretion removal
ABG	Determines adequacy of gas exchange (see Tables 7-2 and 7-4)
Pulmonary function test	Determines restrictive/obstructive patterns and diffusion abnormalities (see Table 7-5 and Figure 7-10)
Thoracentesis	Surgical procedure that drains fluid from pleural space, may be used for biopsy
V/Q scan	Nuclear scan that studies airflow (V) and blood flow (Q) to determine V/Q defects (eg, pulmonary embolism)
Bronchial/alveolar lavage	Fluid is instilled down a patient's airway and removed via gentle suction; allows access to pulmonary fluids and cells of the lower respiratory tract that are unable to be obtained via coughing for COPD; shown in Table 7-7 and is based on the decline in FEV_1[16]

by patients and therapists to identify changes in symptoms, indicating improvement or worsening of ADL performance throughout a hospitalization.

Asthma

Asthma is a reversible or reactive airway disease. The patient has an intrinsic (eg, dust, pollen, pet dander) or extrinsic (eg, medications, infections, exercise, cold air) exposure resulting in airway smooth muscle hyperplasia and hypertrophy,

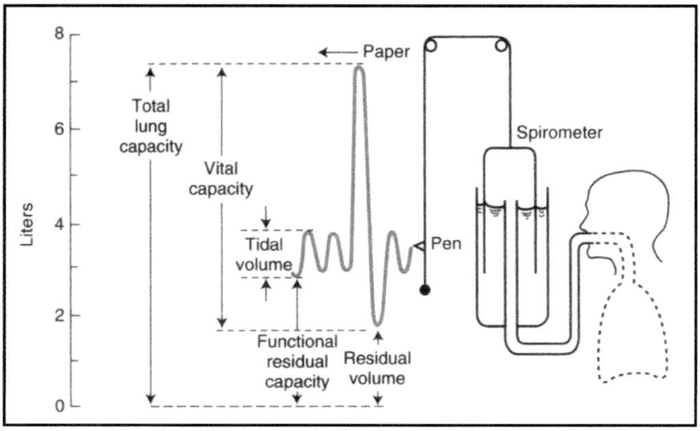

Figure 7-10. Pulmonary function test. Lung volumes. TLC, FRC, and residual volume cannot be measured with the spirometer. (Reprinted with permission from West JB, ed. *Pulmonary Physiology and Pathophysiology: An Integrated, Case-Based Approach.* Philadelphia, PA: Lippincott Williams & Wilkins; 2001:39.)

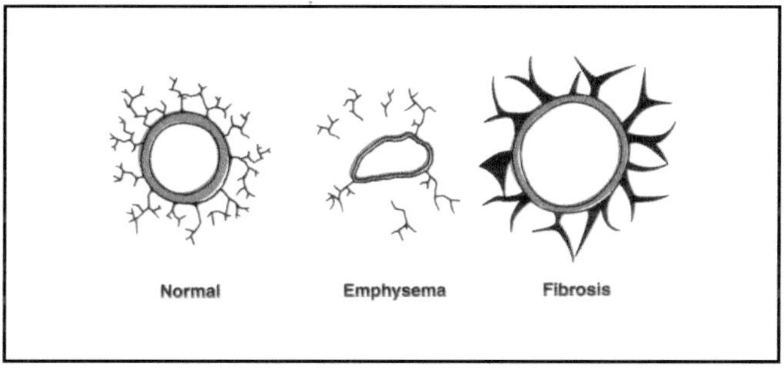

Figure 7-11. Airway caliber in normal lung, emphysema, and interstitial fibrosis. In emphysema, the airways tend to collapse because of the loss of radial traction. By contrast, in fibrosis, radial traction may be excessive, with the result that airway caliber is large when related to lung volume. (Reprinted with permission from West JB, ed. *Pulmonary Physiology and Pathophysiology: An Integrated, Case-Based Approach.* Philadelphia, PA: Lippincott Williams & Wilkins; 2001:78.)

bronchoconstriction, **inflammation** with resultant swelling, and **hypersecretion** of mucus.[8,10,19] The sum of these factors narrows the airways resulting in obstruction as noted in Figure 7-12. Asthma can be life threatening if not managed properly by eliminating trigger exposures and using preventative medications to stabilize inflammation and reduce bronchospasm. Daily medications include bronchodilators and anti-inflammatory agents via meter dose inhalers (MDIs) or intravenous corticosteroids for severe exacerbations. Patients should be instructed in proper technique for MDIs[16] as described in Table 7-9. Asthma-COPD overlap syndrome (ACOS) represents patients who present with clinical features of both asthma and COPD.

Table 7-7

Classification of Severity of Airflow Limitation in Chronic Obstructive Pulmonary Disease (Based on Post-Bronchodilator FEV_1)

In patients with $FEV_1/FVC < 0.70$		
GOLD 1	Mild	$FEV_1 > 80\%$ predicted
GOLD 2	Moderate	$50\% < FEV_1 < 80\%$ predicted
GOLD 3	Severe	$30\% < FEV_1 < 50\%$ predicted
GOLD 4	Very severe	$FEV_1 < 30\%$ predicted

GOLD = Global Initiative for Obstructive Lung Disease.

Table 7-8

Modified Medical Research Council Questionnaire for Assessing the Severity of Breathlessness

Please tick in the box that applies to you (one box only).		
mMRC Grade 0	I only get breathless with strenuous exercise.	
mMRC Grade 1	I get short of breath when hurrying on the level or walking up a slight hill.	
mMRC Grade 2	I walk slower than people of the same age on the level because of breathlessness, or I have to stop for breath when walking on my own pace on the level.	
mMRC Grade 3	I stop for breath after walking about 100 meters or after a few minutes on the level.	
mMRC Grade 4	I am too breathless to leave the house, or I am breathless when dressing or undressing.	

mMRC = Modified Medical Research Council.

Adapted from Modified Medical Research Council Questionnaire for Assessing the Severity of Breathlessness (From the Global Strategy for Diagnosis, Management and Prevention of COPD). Global Initiative for Chronic Obstructive Lung Disease (GOLD). https://www.mdcalc.com/global-initiative-obstructive-lung-disease-gold-criteria-copd. Published 2014. Accessed July 17, 2019.

ACOS prevalence increases with age and may be present in approximately 15% to 45% of patients with COPD.[20]

Emphysema and Alpha-1 Antitrypsin Deficiency

Emphysema is defined anatomically as an irreversible increase in the size of air spaces distal to the terminal bronchioles with destruction of alveolar septa.[7,21] Alveolar destruction reduces surface area for gas exchange. Although emphysema's

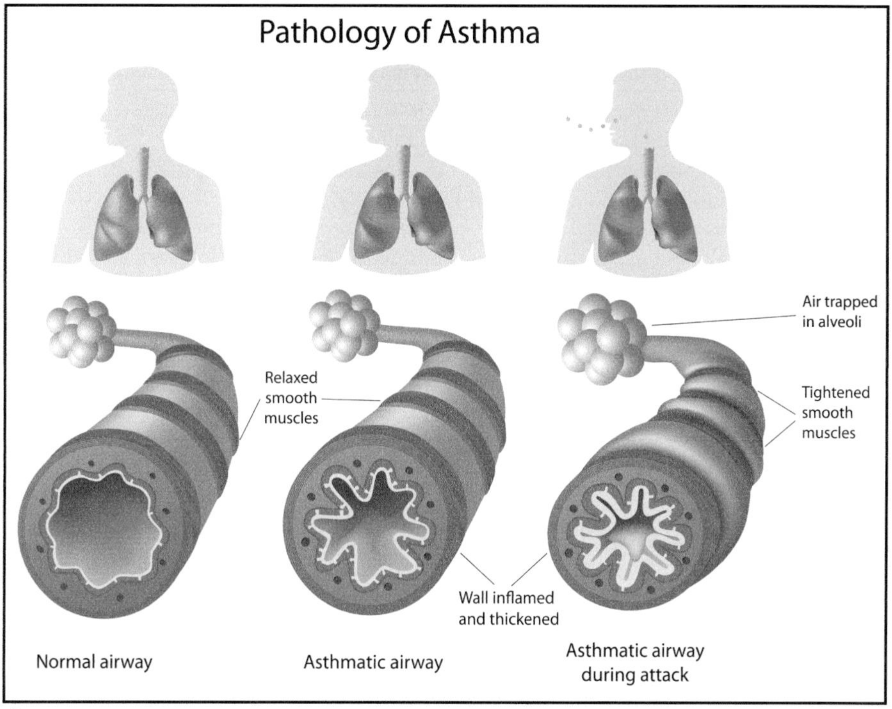

Figure 7-12. Normal bronchiole, bronchiole in asthma, and bronchiole during an asthma exacerbation. (Alila Medical Media/Shutterstock.com)

etiology is unknown, chronic inflammation, oxidative stress, and proteases released from inflammatory cells including macrophages and neutrophils leads to lung destruction.[22] Patients are classically described as "pink puffers" due to malnutrition and cachexia, CO_2 retention with flushing and pursed-lip breathing (PLB). The disease results from loss of the mechanical tethering or distending function of the lung parenchyma. The loss of lung elasticity results in premature **airway collapse** with expiration producing air trapping and wheezing.[22] **Hyperinflation** creates flattening of the diaphragms, use of accessory muscles, development of a barrel chest, and promotes functional decline due to chronic symptoms of SOB and fatigue.

Alpha-1 antitrypsin deficiency (A1AD) is a genetic form of emphysema. Alpha-1 antitrypsin is a glycoprotein that inhibits proteolytic enzymes that damage lung tissue.[12] Patients who are alpha-1 antitrypsin deficient lack this enzyme, the lung architecture will be destroyed over time, and the clinical symptoms of emphysema will develop at an earlier age. Cigarette smoking accelerates the onset of symptoms.

Chronic Bronchitis

Chronic bronchitis is a clinical diagnosis and is defined by complaint of chronic respiratory symptoms for 2 years in a row for 3 consecutive months.[6,8,10]

Patients are classically described as "blue bloaters" due to hypoxemia and cyanosis, and development of peripheral edema. Airway obstruction results from excessive mucus production secondary to hyperplasia and hypertrophy of mucus-secreting cells of the airways.[7] Factors contributing to the development of chronic bronchitis include cigarette smoking and chronic exposures to dust, fumes, and air pollution.[21]

Table 7-9

RECOMMENDED USE OF METER DOSE INHALER

1.	Remove cap from inhaler; shake MDI if prescribed.
2.	Practice controlled breathing (exhale normally).
3.	Place the opening of the MDI 2 finger lengths away from the lips; mouth should be open wide; head should be tilted back slightly
4.	Use a spacer if prescribed by physician or poor technique is demonstrated.
5.	Slowly inhale and at the same time compress the MDI. Press inhaler canister once at beginning of the slow deep breath.
6.	Now hold breath for 8 to 10 seconds.
7.	Reshake MDI if prescribed by instructions.
8.	Wait 3 to 5 minutes or prescribed time by physician.
9.	Repeat steps 3 through 6.
10.	Precautions: Watch for signs of medications being deposited in throat and mouth (eg, thrush, continued complaints of SOB, audible wheezing, continued dyspnea, or thickness in mucus if mucolytic).

Adapted from Lee et al[16]; Casaburi and Petty[136]; Restrepo et al[137]; and Sleuth et al.[138]

In chronic bronchitis, similar to COPD, the decline in functional activity and quality of life is not linear as illustrated in Figure 7-13. Exacerbations and disease progression, poor gas exchange, and anxiety and deconditioning each play a role in symptom development, worsening of activity limitations and poor health-related quality of life.[23] Physical therapists have a tremendous role in slowing down and potentially reversing many of these factors.

Bronchiectasis

Bronchiectasis is the permanent and abnormal widening of bronchi due to chronic infection and inflammation with retained mucus resulting in progressive airflow obstruction.[5,7,12,24] Bronchiectasis can result from ciliary dysfunction (eg, primary ciliary dyskinesia [Kartagener's syndrome], cystic fibrosis), abnormal immune defenses (eg, HIV), genetic defects (eg, cystic fibrosis, killer T cell deficiency) or following prolonged or repeated infectious diseases (eg, tuberculosis, frequent pneumonias).[21] The dilated bronchi become areas for repeated infections and airway destruction. The main clinical manifestation is a productive cough.[24] **Hemoptysis**, or coughing blood, is a complication associated with erosion of the bronchial wall and surrounding pulmonary vessels. Secretions tend to be thick and constant and this population benefits from airway clearance programs.

Cystic Fibrosis

Cystic fibrosis, a defect of chromosome 7, is an inherited autosomal recessive disease affecting the mucus-producing glands in the lungs, sweat glands, digestive tract, and the genitourinary system. To date, over 1800 defects have been identified, and cystic fibrosis is the most common inherited disease in White people.[25] The genetic defect alters the cystic fibrosis transmembrane regulator (CFTR) leading to changes in sodium and chloride transport in the airways resulting in thick, sticky mucus.[25] Patient presentation is variable, but abnormalities may include bronchiectasis, pancreatic insufficiency resulting in impaired dietary fat absorption, malnutrition, diabetes, osteoporosis, and arthropathies. Cystic fibrosis–related diabetes (CFRD) is the most common comorbidity in patients with cystic fibrosis. Complete absence of

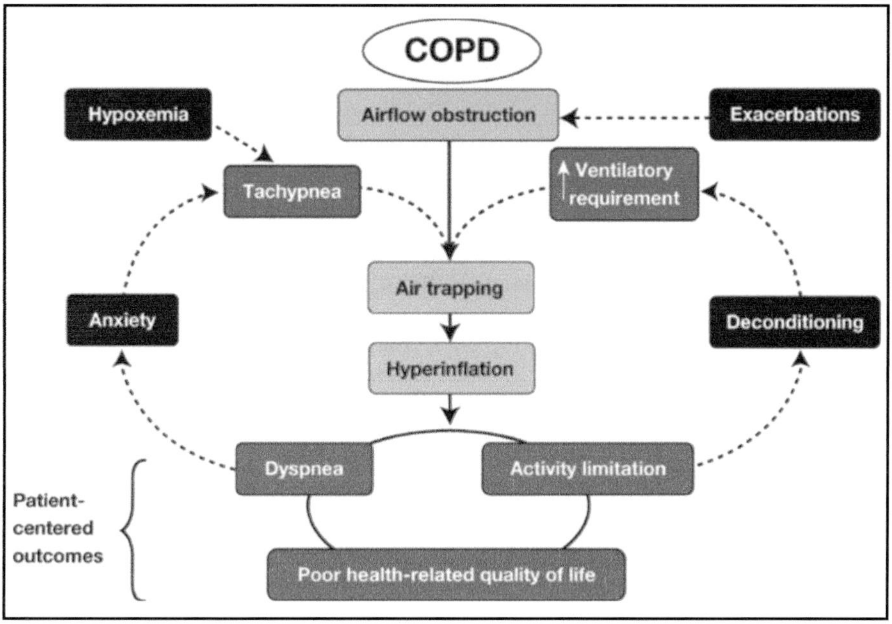

Figure 7-13. The cycle of decline leading to activity limitation in patients with COPD. (Reprinted from The *American Journal of Medicine*, Vol 119, CB Cooper, The connection between chronic obstructive pulmonary disorder and hyperinflation and its impact on exercise and function, 21-31, Copyright 2006, with permission from Elsevier. [3514330981993].)

insulin secretion is uncommon in patients with CFRD.[26] The severity of insulin insufficiency is directly related to the rate of pulmonary function decline. Maintaining normal weight and lean body mass is critical for cystic fibrosis lung function. Patients with cystic fibrosis are susceptible to opportunistic lung infections (eg, *Pseudomonas aeruginosa, Burkholderia cepacia*, non-tuberculous mycobacteria [NTM]), and multi-drug resistant infections are on the rise in cystic fibrosis and contributes to progression of lung inflammation. The median age for survival is 36 years despite advances in cystic fibrosis management. Disease progression ends with respiratory failure, pulmonary hypertension, cor pulmonale, and death.[25,27,28] Worldwide, cystic fibrosis is currently the third most common reason for lung transplantation (see Chapter 14).[29] Therapists must be sensitive to infection control and universal precautions. Equipment should not be shared with other cystic fibrosis patients or those who are immunocompromised. All surfaces must be disinfected. Optimizing airway clearance, nutrition, medication delivery, and exercise are mainstays of care for patients with cystic fibrosis. Awareness of risks for diabetes, osteoporosis, liver dysfunction, and dehydration should be incorporated into the plan of care.[29]

Restrictive Disorders

Interstitial Lung Disease and Pulmonary Fibrosis

Interstitial lung disease (ILD) describes a diverse group of acute and chronic lung disorders involving the interstitium as well as the endothelial and epithelial linings of the vasculature and alveoli.[11,30] The **interstitium** refers to the microscopic anatomic space made up of cellular (ie, fibroblasts, neutrophils) and connective (ie, collagen, elastin, proteoglycans) tissue elements between the alveoli and the pulmonary capillaries.[30-32] ILD development may be:

- Idiopathic (eg, sarcoidosis, collagen vascular diseases, rheumatoid arthritis, systemic lupus erythematosus [SLE], Sjögren's syndrome, bronchiolitis obliterans organizing pneumonia/obliterative bronchiolitis, lymphangioleiomyomatosis [LAM]),
- Related to chronic infections (eg, tuberculosis, Aspergillosis),
- Related to environmental exposures (eg, asbestosis, silicosis, bird fancier's lung)
- Drug induced (eg, chemotherapeutic agents, methotrexate, amiodarone)
- Physical agent induced (eg, radiation exposure, oxygen toxicity)[30]

These disorders typically result in mixed pulmonary restriction and obstructive patterns with pulmonary function testing, impaired gas exchange (decreased DLCO; see Table 7-5), and decreased pulmonary compliance indicating lung stiffness. The most common presenting symptoms are SOB and cough. Resting vital signs may be stable, ambulation and stair climbing can lead to rapid desaturation and disabling dyspnea. The following section will highlight several ILD disorders. The major categories of interstitial lung disorders are listed in Table 7-10.[31]

Idiopathic Pulmonary Fibrosis

Idiopathic pulmonary fibrosis (IPF) is an insidious, progressive restrictive lung disease characterized by interstitial inflammation and fibrosis. IPF has a median survival of 2 to 3 years from initial diagnosis. The pathogenesis of IPF is not clearly understood (see Figure 7-11), but theories have shifted from a state of chronic inflammation to one of abnormal wound healing.[11,31] Patients present with progressive DOE, nonproductive paroxysmal cough (often refractory to antitussives), crackles on auscultation, fatigue, weight loss, hypoxemia, digital clubbing, and, often, severely restricted exercise capacity. Five-year mortality is >40%, primarily due to respiratory insufficiency. Additional causes of death include cardiac ischemia, pulmonary embolism, infections, and neoplasms.[31,32] Diagnosis is confirmed by lung biopsy, radiologic testing, including high-resolution computerized tomography (HRCT), and x-ray.

Medical management has included high-dose corticosteroids, immunosuppressive (eg, azathioprine, cyclosporine) and cytotoxic agents (eg, Cytoxan [cyclophosphamide]), inhibitors of collagen synthesis or fibrosis (eg, colchicine, penicillamine), oxygen therapy, opiates for respiratory distress and dyspnea, and lung transplantation. Recently 2 new drugs (nintedanib and pirfenidone) have been approved for treatment of IPF. These medications both reduce the decline in pulmonary function (FVC), but the impact on overall mortality is still being evaluated.[33,34]

Sarcoidosis

Sarcoidosis is an idiopathic multisystem disease highlighted by the formation of inflammatory granulomas, masses consisting of varied cell types (eg, phagocytes, macrophages, lymphocytes) in the affected organs. Sarcoidosis most commonly affects the lungs and intrathoracic lymph nodes and leads to a progressive restrictive lung disease (reduced lung volumes and flow rates) resulting in SOB, cough, and chest discomfort.[35,36] Therapists need to consider extrapulmonary involvement including cardiac (eg, dysrhythmias, cardiomyopathy, sudden death), neurologic (eg, Bell's palsy, seizures, polyneuropathy, hydrocephalus), and musculoskeletal systems (eg, myopathy, bone cysts, arthritic-type pain).[35] Bronchoscopy, biopsy, and

Table 7-10

Interstitial Lung Disorders: Major Categories

• Idiopathic interstitial pneumonia • IPF • Non-specific interstitial pneumonia (NSIP) • Cryptogenic organizing pneumonia (COP) • Respiratory bronchiolitis interstitial lung disease (RBILD) • Desquamative interstitial pneumonia (DIP) • Acute interstitial pneumonia (AIP) • Lymphoid interstitial pneumonia (LIP)	• Connective tissue disease-associated interstitial lung disease (CTD-ILD) • Sarcoidosis • Hypersensitivity pneumonitis • Iatrogenic pneumonitis/fibrosis (eg, drug-induced ILD, radiation injury) • Eosinophilic ILD (eg, eosinophilic pneumonia) • Occupational lung disease • Inherited disorders (eg, familial pulmonary fibrosis, Hermansky-Pudlak syndrome • Primary disorders (eg, pulmonary langerhans cell histiocytosis)

Adapted from Meyer, KC. Diagnosis and management of interstitial lung disease. *Transl Respir Med.* 2014:2:4.

radiological studies confirm diagnosis. Corticosteroids remain the cornerstone of treatment, and additional medications include cytotoxic and immunosuppressive agents.[36]

Lymphangioleiomyomatosis

LAM is a rare, slowly progressive disease characterized by abnormal smooth muscle cell proliferation affecting women of childbearing age almost exclusively.[37] The smooth-muscle cells are distributed throughout the peribronchial, perivascular, and perilymphatic areas of the lung. Clinically, patients present with a persistent obstructive or mixed pulmonary pattern by pulmonary function test, cough, DOE, recurrent pneumothoraces, and, less commonly, chest pain, and pleural effusions.[37,38] Figure 7-14 shows an example of a pleural effusion. Hormonal manipulation (eg, oophorectomy, progesterone, luteinizing hormone-releasing hormone analogues) and lung transplantation are the basis of treatment.[38]

Tuberculosis

The incidence of **tuberculosis**, an infection with **mycobacterium tuberculosis**, remains a major global health challenge with 8.6 million cases and 1.3 million deaths in 2012.[39] Tuberculosis is typically associated with immunocompromise, poor socioeconomic status, homelessness, alcoholism, and being a health care worker.[40] Tuberculosis is the most common infectious disease in adults worldwide due to the development of multiresistant tuberculosis and HIV.[40] The emergence of multidrug resistant–tuberculosis (MDR-TB) and extensively drug resistant–tuberculosis (XDR-TB) add to the global risk.[40] The **mycobacterium tuberculosis** is contained within an airborne droplet; is spread by coughing, talking, or sneezing; and may be held aloft by air currents.[40] The bacteria bypass the pulmonary defenses of the upper respiratory tract and deposit in the alveolus. Bacilli are ingested by alveolar macrophages, where they multiply, destroying the macrophage. Lysis of the macrophage releases the bacilli triggering a greater immune response from the infected host. Monocytes/macrophages and lymphocytes accumulate at the infection site forming a microscopic lesion or granuloma. The immune response may contain the infection

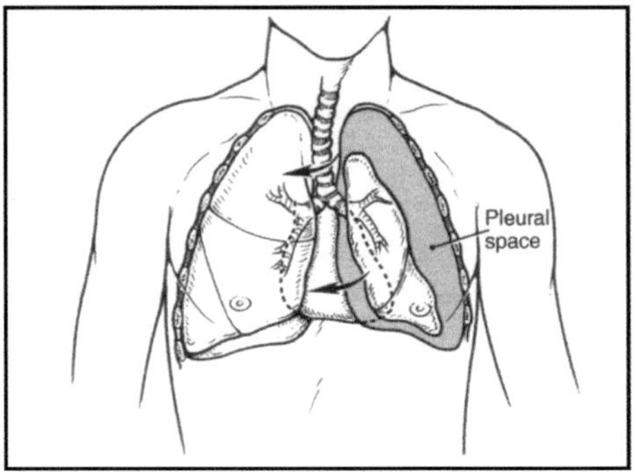

Figure 7-14. Pleural effusion. Shaded area shows fluid collection in the pleural space. Lung tissue is displaced and mediastinal structures are compressed. (Reprinted with permission from Mackin L, Bullock BL. Altered pulmonary function. In: Bullock BA, Henze RL, eds. *Focus on Pathophysiology*. Philadelphia, PA: Lippincott Willams & Wilkins; 2000:574.)

within a fibrotic cavity, tubercle (Ghon complex), or fail, leading to progression and destruction of surrounding lung structures.[11,39] **Reactivation tuberculosis** represents exacerbation of latent infection weeks to years after the primary infection. **Miliary tuberculosis** is widespread infection resulting from bacilli invasion and spread by the circulatory system. Patients with active tuberculosis will present with cough, fever, malaise, and night sweats, and need to be in negative pressure rooms or use designated face masks to prevent infection spread (see Chapter 5).

Extrapulmonary tuberculosis may affect the musculoskeletal system, particularly the spine and weightbearing joints, pericardium, and meninges.[40] The 2 most common forms of NTM infection are mycobacterium avium complex (MAC) and *Mycobacterium abscessus*.[39] Three ways of testing for tuberculosis include the tuberculin skin test, which takes 48 to 72 hours, the acid fast stain, which can be rapidly performed providing data within hours, or the highly sensitive mycobacterial culture, a test that requires 6 to 8 weeks for interpretation.

Cryptogenic Organizing Pneumonia, Bronchiolitis Obliterans Organizing Pneumonia, and Bronchiolitis Obliterans

COP and **bronchiolitis obliterans organizing pneumonia** are rare inflammatory disorders characterized by bronchial fibrosis and intraluminal connective tissue plugs extending into the alveoli.[41,42] Men and women in the fifth and sixth decades are affected similarly. Symptoms include progressive dyspnea, new cough, general malaise, weight loss, and fever. Radiographic examination, lung biopsy, and bronchoalveolar lavage are key to accurate diagnosis. The therapist may see elevated RR and heart rate (HR), decreased pulse oximetry values, and little sputum. Corticosteroids are the mainstay of treatment and prognosis is typically excellent; however, some patients may have permanent fibrotic lung disease.[41-44]

Bronchiolitis obliterans can occur independently or may be a late complication following lung or heart–lung transplant (see Chapter 14). Bronchiolitis obliterans, also termed **obliterative bronchiolitis** or **bronchiolitis obliterans syndrome** (BOS), is the aggressive manifestations of chronic rejection following transplantation.[45] Prevalence post–lung transplant is upwards of 40% by 2 years following transplant.[46] Bronchiolitis obliterans is characterized by irreversible, progressive airway narrowing by granulation tissue.[45] Suspicious clinical findings include progressive DOE, cough, and reduced pulmonary function studies (decreased FEV_1).[47] Specific risk factors for development of bronchiolitis obliterans post-transplant include primary graft failure, cytomegalovirus infection, airway ischemia, human leukocyte antigen (HLA) mismatching, and recurrent, severe acute rejection episodes (see Chapter 14).[46,47]

Respiratory Failure

Respiratory failure can be defined broadly as the impairment of respiratory gas exchange between the ambient air and circulating blood.[19,48] Generally, respiratory failure is categorized as either hypercapnic (ie, increased $PaCO_2$) or hypoxemic (ie, decreased PaO_2) as defined by specific changes in ABGs and may arise either acutely or chronically. Although the causes of respiratory failure are diverse, generally there are 3 pathogenic categories of diseases leading to respiratory failure[49]:

1. Progressive airway obstruction (eg, asthma, emphysema, chronic bronchitis, cystic fibrosis)
2. Altered lung parenchyma (eg, IPF, sarcoidosis)
3. Defects of ventilation caused either by abnormalities of the musculoskeletal pump (eg, spinal cord injury [SCI], flail chest, neuromuscular disease) or dysfunction of the respiratory control center (eg, cerebrovascular accident [CVA], drug overdose)

Each of these disorders can occur individually or may occur in combination (eg, COPD with superimposed pneumonia).

Acute respiratory failure is sudden and the ABG reveals a pH less than 7.35 with the $PaCO_2$ >50 mm Hg (hypercapnea) and PaO_2 <50 mm Hg (hypoxemia).[19] The metabolic system (ie, kidneys) is not able to compensate for the sudden respiratory acidosis. Endotracheal intubation and mechanical ventilation are standard components of treatment.[50] Noninvasive ventilation is being applied as an alternative therapy to minimize invasive procedures. (see Chapters 3 and 4, and discussed later in this chapter)

Chronic respiratory failure can be a late manifestation of pulmonary disorders such as COPD.[19] The regression to failure may develop over days to weeks. Chronic respiratory failure may follow an acute episode of respiratory failure. The roles of therapists on the team weaning a patient from mechanical ventilation following respiratory failure may range from airway clearance and bedside exercise programs to progressive mobilization (see Chapter 3) and discharge planning.

Acute Respiratory Distress Syndrome

Acute respiratory distress syndrome (ARDS) are syndromes consisting of acute, severe alterations in lung structure and function characterized by hypoxemia, low compliance, diffuse radiologic infiltrates, and increased pulmonary vascular endothelial and alveolar epithelial permeability leading to pulmonary edema.[50] Histologically, ARDS is described as a neutrophil-mediated, widespread inflammatory insult to the lung parenchyma and is termed **diffuse alveolar damage** (DAD). The annual incidence of ARDS in the United States may be as high as 190,000 cases with mortality rates ranging between 11% and 68%.[50,51] ARDS is the most severe form of acute lung injury (ALI). The Berlin definition of ARDS is listed in Table 7-11.[50] ARDS may develop after:

- Direct lung injury (eg, pneumonia, aspiration, fat emboli, thoracic trauma, reperfusion pulmonary edema)
- Indirect causes (eg, sepsis, systemic inflammatory response syndrome [SIRS], drug reactions, cardiopulmonary bypass, blood transfusions, pancreatitis)[52]

Regardless of inciting event, intense inflammation is a common pathway leading to pulmonary damage and dysfunction. Neutrophils and alveolar macrophages are not only a line of defense against airborne microbes but are also key in maintaining

Table 7-11 **Berlin Definition of Acute Respiratory Distress Syndrome**	
Timing	<1 week of new or worsening respiratory symptoms or clinical insult
Chest Imaging	Bilateral opacities not related to other causes (eg, effusions, nodules, collapse)
Origin of Edema	Respiratory failure not related to fluid overload or cardiac failure
Oxygenation PaO_2/F_IO_2	Positive end expiratory pressure >5 or continuous positive airway pressure (CPAP) >5 cm H_2O
Mild	200 mm Hg $<PaO_2/F_IO_2<$ 300 mm Hg
Moderate	100 mm Hg $<PaO_2/F_IO_2<$ 200 mm Hg
Severe	$PaO_2/F_IO_2<$ 100 mm Hg

Adapted from O'Sullivan F, Al-Haddad M. Acute respiratory distress syndrome. *Anaesthesia and Intensive Care Medicine*. 2013;14(10):472-474.

the initial acute inflammatory phase and during resolution and recovery phases of ARDS.[52,53] ARDS may be divided into 3 phases of variable duration:

1. Inflammation and exudation (protein rich pulmonary edema)
2. Fibroproliferative
3. Resolution and recovery

The resolution of ARDS is marked by partial or complete return of lung function or long-term fibrosis and gas exchanging abnormalities. Medical management is largely supportive and consists of mechanical ventilation (eg, low stretch/reduced tidal volume protocols, permissive hypercapnea) to alleviate ventilation-induced lung injury (VILI), improve blood gases, and decrease the WOB. Additional treatments include judicious fluid management, anti-inflammatory agents, correction of coagulation disorders, and antibiotics. Physical therapy interventions frequently include positioning and contracture prevention, early mobilization, and patient/family education. Acquired neuromuscular abnormalities are common in this population and often are discovered during physical therapy examination (see Chapter 4).

Pneumonia

Pneumonia is the seventh leading cause of death overall in the United States. The respiratory system is continuously exposed to microorganisms that may lead to disease and pneumonia result from bacterial, viral, fungal, parasitic infection, or even chemical (aspiration) exposures. The human body reacts to this infectious exposure through innate and specific immunity (see Chapter 5) and inflammatory responses by recruitment and activation of alveolar macrophages, neutrophils, lymphocytes, complement, and immunoglobulins (antibodies). This inflammatory process leads to fluid or blood cells filling the alveoli, interstitial tissue, and bronchioles.[8,19,54] Hospitalized patients, the very young or old, and immunocompromised patients are at the greatest risk for developing pneumonia. Impaired functional status has been identified as a risk factor for recurrent pneumonia.[55,56]

Hospital- or health care–acquired pneumonia (HAP/HCAP) and community-acquired pneumonia (CAP) are 2 distinct categories. HCAP is a pneumonia that occurs in an acute care hospital within 2 days or up to 90 days of the admission in absence of symptoms or any signs of pneumonia.[56] Patients can also reside in a long-term care facility or nursing home, attend a hospital-based or hemodialysis clinic, or be receiving wound care, chemotherapy, or IV antibiotic therapy.[56] Risk factors for HCAP are admission to the intensive care unit (ICU), endotracheal intubation, thoracoabdominal surgery, nasogastric tubes, inappropriate use of antibiotics, and altered level of consciousness.[19] **Ventilator-associated pneumonia** (VAP) is a subset of HCAP and develops after endotracheal intubation. The organisms associated with VAP have been isolated to the stomach and oropharynx.[56] VAP is associated with increases in cost of care, morbidity and mortality, and ventilator days.[56] Prevention of VAP includes hand hygiene, mouth care, spontaneous breathing trials, sedation interruption, and elevated head of bed positioning (>45 degrees).[56] The incidence of CAP has remained constant and significantly impacts morbidity, mortality, and overall health care costs. As many as 10% of the patients admitted to the hospital with CAP require intensive care.[54] Annually CAP account for upwards of 4 million physician visits and over 1 million hospital admissions at a cost close to $14 billion dollars a year.[54,55] The dominant mechanism behind CAP remains microaspiration with organisms colonized from the nasopharynx and oropharynx.[57] Some risk factors for CAP include older age, impaired immune function, prior hospital admission with pneumonia and preexisting health conditions, including COPD, chronic liver or renal disease, Parkinson's disease, stroke, dementia, and swallowing problems.[54-57] Nonclinical factors include impaired functional status, current smoking, and chronic alcoholism.[55] Of the nonclinical risk factors for CAP, impaired functional status was associated with a 70% increased risk.

Aspiration pneumonia occurs when a patient cannot protect his or her airway and is a component of both HCAP and CAP. Aspiration is commonly used to denote contents of the upper gastrointestinal (GI) tract that have entered the trachea into the lungs.[57] Risk factors include swallowing dysfunction, altered mental status, esophageal motility disorders, vomiting, enteral feeding, oropharyngeal colonization, drugs, alcohol, anesthesia, CVA, drowning, and trauma. Evidence suggests that being a male smoker and having diabetes in combination with an acute stroke increases the risk for aspiration pneumonia.[57] Aspiration can be further categorized into inert objects (eg, teeth, food, water), chemicals, and bacteria.[19,57] Inert objects may become lodged in the airway causing a local inflammatory response and wheezing. ARDS occurs with a chemical inhalation, such as bile and gastric acid, leading to airway inflammation, fibrosis, and necrosis.[19] Additionally, over 50% of aspirations result in secondary bacterial infections with the most common source of bacteria from the mouth.

Airway clearance, antibiotics, and hydration aid sputum expectoration and improvement in V/Q matching. Therapists may observe elevated RR, HR, accessory muscle use, possible pleuritic chest pain, thick tenacious mucus (bacterial), and decreased pulse oximetry. Radiographic changes may take a few weeks to completely resolve. In the case of inhalation of an inert substance, bronchoscopy may be needed to identify and remove the foreign object.

***Pneumocystis carinii* pneumonia** (PCP) is an opportunistic infection seen in patients with impaired immunity, such as those with AIDS or patients prescribed immunosuppressive therapy.[19] The exact cause is not clearly understood. Exposure may occur in early childhood and an intact immune system controls the infection; however, when immune function is impaired, reactivation of the infection occurs. The clinical course depends on the host and the degree of immune dysfunction. In the non–HIV-infected patient the symptoms can range from a fever and nonproductive cough to diffuse alveolar infiltrates and respiratory failure.[19] The clinical course

Figure 7-15. Clinical features of lung cancer. (Reprinted with permission from Sheldon LK. *Oxygenation*. Sudbury, MA: Jones and Bartlett Publishers; 2001.)

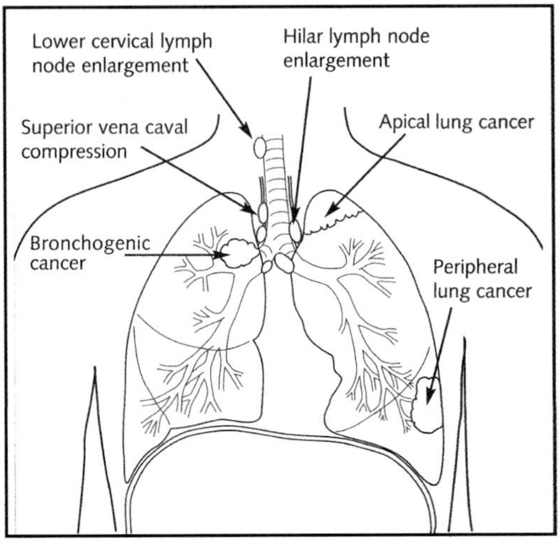

is more sinister in the HIV-infected patient. Radiographic changes may be subtle, combined with a low-grade fever, nonproductive cough, and weight loss.

Lung Cancer

Since 1984 overall lung cancer age-adjusted incidence rates in the United States have stabilized for women with rates for males continuing to decline. Smoking is associated with all lung cancer types (Figure 7-15).[19,58] The 3 cornerstones of treatment are surgery, radiation, and chemotherapy and each can negatively impact lung function resulting in restrictive lung pathology. Patients are at risk for opportunistic infections due to immunocompromise and universal precautions should be observed at all times. Fatigue, cachexia, poor nutrition, altered blood cell counts, frequent bouts of nausea and vomiting, and limited pulmonary reserve can lead to activity limitations and impact the physical therapy care plan (see Chapter 13).

Mesothelioma

Mesothelioma is a rare cancer related to asbestos exposure but is the most common cancer of the pleura.[59] Patients are typically in their 60s and exposure may have occurred 30 to 45 years prior to diagnosis.[52,59,60] Occupational risk is increased in automotive mechanics, ship builders, and asbestos miners and, recently, exposure risk increased following Hurricane Katrina and the 9/11 disaster. The tumor originates mainly on the parietal pleura and progressively spreads to encase the lung surfaces, penetrates the chest wall, infiltrates the diaphragm, and invades mediastinal structures.[59,60] The first manifestation of pleural mesothelioma is a pleural effusion seen as late as 10 to 20 years from exposure. The effusions are typically bilateral and must be sizable enough to cause symptoms (see Figure 7-14).[60] Patients frequently complain of SOB, chest pain, fever, cough, and weakness.

Chest Wall Deformities and Musculoskeletal Disorders

Congenital defects are the primary cause of chest wall abnormalities (eg, pectus excavatum, bifid sternum, scoliosis, Jarcho-Levine syndrome, neuromuscular disorders, lung hypoplasia).[19] Musculoskeletal disorders, abdominal disorders, surgery, and trauma can lead to acquired chest wall abnormalities impacting ventilation and the WOB. Specific examples of chest wall deformities outside of childhood

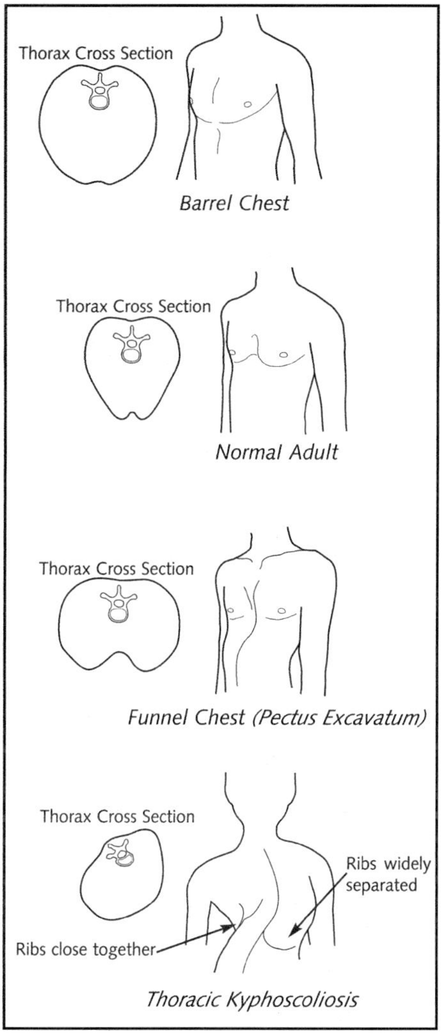

Figure 7-16. Abnormalities of the chest. (Reprinted with permission from Sheldon LK. *Oxygenation*. Sudbury, MA: Jones and Bartlett Publishers; 2001.)

would be rheumatic disorders (eg, ankylosing spondylitis), neuromuscular disorders (eg, Guillain-Barré syndrome, SCI), abdominal conditions (eg, ascites, hepatosplenomegaly), severe upper airway obstruction (eg, laryngeomalacia, subglottic stenosis), surgery (eg, pneumonectomy), or trauma resulting in a flail chest.[61] **Kyphoscoliosis**, **pectus excavatum** (sunken/funnel chest), and **pectus carinatum** (pigeon chest) are chest wall deformities limiting thoracic expansion (Figure 7-16).[62] Lung volumes will be decreased, and some patients may compensate by increasing the respiratory rate. Atelectasis can occur in the areas of lung compression and retained secretions may promote pneumonia.[19] The length tension relationship of the accessory muscles of respiration may be compromised from these chest wall deformities. Flexibility exercise, manual therapy, instruction in stacking breaths, and modifying postures to enhance ventilation can be beneficial.[62]

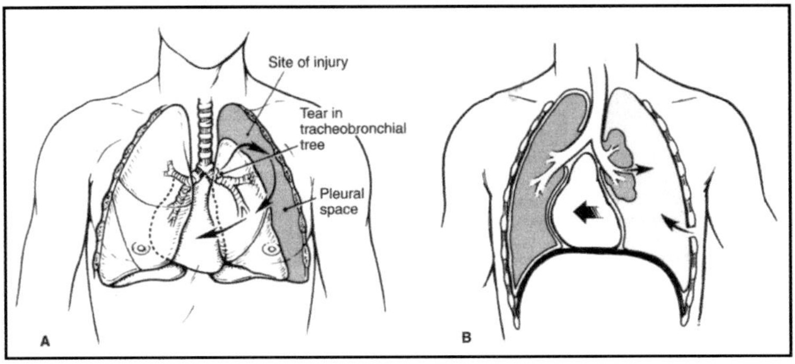

Figure 7-17. Pneumothorax. (A) Atmospheric air entering the pleural space through a tracheobronchial tear. (B) Tension pneumothorax with mediastinal and tracheal shift. (Reprinted with permission from Mackin L, Bullock BL. Altered pulmonary function. In: Bullock BA, Henze RL, eds. *Focus on Pathophysiology*. Philadelphia, PA: Lippincott Willams & Wilkins; 2000:574.)

Neuromuscular disorders, like Guillain-Barré syndrome, SCI, myasthenia gravis, and critical care myopathy/polyneuropathy, as well as degenerative diseases, like amyotrophic lateral sclerosis, muscular dystrophy, and multiple sclerosis can pose a challenge to the therapist in the acute care setting.[63,64] The respiratory muscles may fail to provide adequate force, limiting ventilation, resulting in decreased gas exchange, fatigue, weakness, and dyspnea. Respiratory failure can develop requiring mechanical ventilation. Patients with progressive respiratory failure may benefit from noninvasive ventilation to avoid the complications of intubation.[64] Airway clearance, including assistive cough (see Table 7-16 later in the chapter) and early mobilization, are vital to optimize patient outcomes (see Chapters 3 and 4)

Pneumothorax

A **pneumothorax** literally means "air in the thorax." Air leaks between the visceral and parietal pleural linings of the lungs as noted in Figure 7-17. Pneumothoraces are characterized in multiple ways: **primary spontaneous pneumothorax** typically occurs in 20- to 40-year-old men more than women and is not associated with lung disease; **secondary pneumothorax** is associated with underlying lung disease (eg, COPD); **iatrogenic pneumothorax** can follow a diagnostic or therapeutic procedure (eg, mechanical ventilation, subclavian cannulation, intercostal nerve block); and **traumatic pneumothorax** occurs due to chest trauma (eg, rib fracture, CPR, gunshot wound).[65] **Tension pneumothorax** is a life-threatening condition where air leaks progressively into the thorax resulting in high intrapleural pressures leading to lung collapse, hypoxemia, and cardiac and vascular compression obstructing venous return. The limited venous return results in decreased cardiac output, hypotension, and, potentially, cardiovascular collapse. Patients will frequently complain of acute dyspnea and localized pain. Physical examination may reveal tachycardia, tachypnea, hypoxemia, absent or diminished breath sounds, hyperresonance on chest wall percussion, and tracheal deviation away from the side of lung collapse (see Figure 7-17).[66] A chest x-ray or other radiological studies will confirm diagnosis. Treatments for pneumothorax aim to decrease the intrapleural pressure and expand the lung. This is accomplished by needle aspiration, pleural/chest drainage tubes (see Chapter 3), Heimlich flutter valves for persistent air leaks, pleurodesis, minimally invasive surgery (eg, video-assisted thoracostomy), or open thoracotomy.[65,66] **Pleurodesis** attempts to obliterate the pleural space by producing inflammation and adhesions between the visceral and parietal pleura through mechanical or chemical procedures.

Mechanical pleurodesis involves irritating the pleura with a brush or gauze while chemical pleurodesis uses sclerosing agents, such as talc or tetracycline, to create inflammation. These procedure can be very painful.[66]

Pulmonary Edema

Pulmonary edema is the accumulation of extravascular water in the lungs and typically develops due to increased pulmonary vascular permeability (eg, noncardiogenic pulmonary edema), increased hydrostatic pressures (eg, cardiogenic pulmonary edema), volume overload, or a combination.[67] **Cardiogenic pulmonary edema** (eg, congestive heart failure [CHF]) results from elevated filling pressures in the left ventricle. This elevated pressure is transmitted into the pulmonary veins and promotes the efflux of fluid across the pulmonary capillaries into the lung. **Noncardiogenic pulmonary edema** (eg, ALI/ARDS), results from alterations in the capillary endothelium increasing permeability, allowing increased fluid flux into the lung parenchyma and alveoli. Pulmonary edema leads to fluid-filled alveoli and atelectasis causing hypoxemia. The WOB will also be increased due to surfactant dysfunction, reduced lung compliance, and increased airway resistance.

Pulmonary Emboli

Pulmonary emboli are clots from the systemic venous circulation that obstruct pulmonary arteries and arterioles. Therapists should recognize any sudden complaints of chest pain, dyspnea, and cough. Signs include tachypnea, tachycardia, and crackles via auscultation.[68] Risk factors include genetics and family history (eg, venous thromboembolic disease, antithrombin III deficiency, increased factor VIII), recent surgery or trauma, bed rest and immobilization (eg, plane travel), pregnancy, and oral contraceptives.[68] Lab values such as prothrombin time (PT)/International Normalization Ratio (INR) or partial thromboplastin time (PTT) should be reviewed (see Chapter 2). Diagnosis is accomplished through V/Q scanning, pulmonary angiography, and spiral computed tomography. V/Q scans do not confirm or exclude pulmonary emboli but provide an estimate of likelihood.[68] Lower extremity (LE) ultrasound can detect deep vein thrombosis (DVT) as the cause of the pulmonary emboli. Prevention of DVT and pulmonary emboli are accomplished through prophylactic anticoagulation, pneumatic compression sleeves, and early mobilization.

Rib Fractures and Flail Chest

A **flail chest** is defined as 2 or 3 adjacent ribs fractured in at least 2 places resulting in a free-floating rib segment.[69] Flail chest results from blunt chest wall trauma (eg, motor vehicle accident). The flail segment does not contribute to chest wall expansion during inspiration and complications depend on the size of the flail segment and the associated damage to the lung parenchyma and other organs.[69] Hemothorax, blood in the pleural space, pneumothorax, and pulmonary contusions will contribute to V/Q mismatching, hypoxemia, and increased WOB. Patients complain of pain from rib fractures leading to altered breathing patterns and ineffective coughing with resultant retained secretions, atelectasis, and increased risk for pneumonia and respiratory failure. Physical therapy is consulted for airway clearance (eg, deep breathing/incentive spirometry,[70] effective coughing) and mobilization. Therapists must work closely with the medical team and patient for pain control (eg, intercostal nerve block, epidural analgesia).

Atelectasis

Atelectasis is partial to complete lung collapse due to loss of air volume. Three types of atelectasis are described: absorption, compression, and contraction.[19,22] **Absorption atelectasis** occurs when ventilation is limited to a lung region and the air in the alveoli is absorbed and not replenished as described in Figure 7-18. Absorption

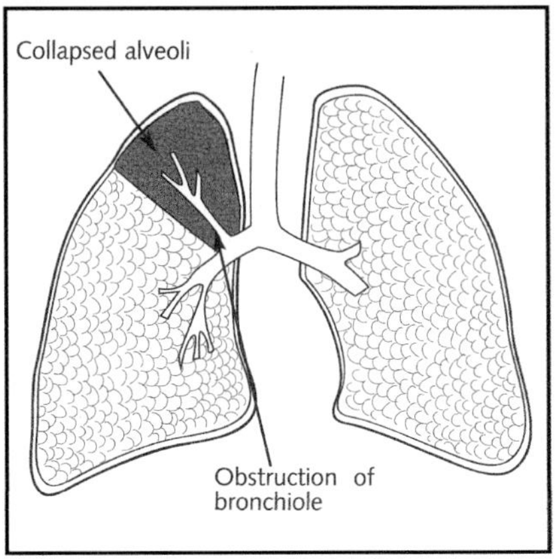

Figure 7-18. Atelectasis due to obstruction. (Reprinted with permission from Sheldon LK. *Oxygenation*. Sudbury, MA: Jones and Bartlett; 2001.)

atelectasis is common post-surgery and in disorders like cystic fibrosis where thick mucus occludes the airway. **Compression atelectasis** occurs when air or fluid occupies the pleural space. Examples include pleural effusion, pneumothorax, hemothorax, or tumor. **Contraction atelectasis** results from decreased pulmonary compliance that limits lung expansion and promotes lung collapse. This is observed in pulmonary fibrosis.[19] Limited evidence is available for routine use of incentive spirometry and deep breathing exercises to prevent primary pulmonary complications, such as pneumonia, atelectasis, bronchospasm, respiratory failure, and prolonged mechanical ventilation.[71] Early mobilization and effective coughing are considered beneficial to reduce atelectasis and development of pneumonia.[72]

Pulmonary Arterial Hypertension

The pulmonary circulation is a high capacitance, low-pressure system and the normal right ventricle is a thin-walled, distensible chamber.[73,74] Pulmonary pressures can increase due to increased pulmonary vascular resistance (PVR) or increased blood flow.[10] Normally, however, pulmonary blood flow can increase 3- to 5-fold with minimal changes in pulmonary artery pressures because of recruitment and distension of the pulmonary vasculature.[75] **Pulmonary arterial hypertension** (PAH) is defined as a mean pulmonary artery pressure >25 mm Hg at rest or >30 mm Hg with exercise. Pulmonary hypertensive diseases can be classified into 5 subgroups[76]:

1. PAH (idiopathic, iatrogenic, heritable, collagen vascular disease, or connective tissue diseases)
2. PAH caused by left heart disease
3. PAH associated with lung diseases or hypoxemia
4. PAH related to chronic embolic/thrombotic disease
5. PAH unclear, multifactorial mechanisms

PAH typically results from increased PVR due to vascular remodeling that includes hypertrophy and migration of smooth muscle, thickening of the intima, and development of occlusive lesions. The vascular remodeling obstructs blood flow and decreases the pulmonary vasculature cross-sectional area.[11,73] The increased PVR creates a chronic pressure overload, which may progress to residual volume dysfunction or cor pulmonale. **Cor pulmonale** denotes residual volume hypertrophy or dilatation due to lung or musculoskeletal pump pathology or impaired respiratory control (eg, sleep apnea/hypoventilation syndrome.[73] Symptoms associated with

PAH are dyspnea, chest pain, dizziness, or syncope. PAH is generally asymptomatic until significant disease is noted.[73]

Risk factors for developing PAH include drug and toxin exposure, female gender, HIV infection, and thyroid disorders. Idiopathic pulmonary arterial hypertension (IPAH) is a rare phenomenon with an estimated 1 to 2 cases per million.[76] The disease has a slight female predominance and usually manifests around a mean age of 36 years. Prognosis and survival are poor if IPAH remains untreated.[73]

Medications are key to treatment for limiting symptoms and end organ damage. Selective vasodilation of the pulmonary vasculature via calcium channel blockers (eg, nifedipine, diltiazem), endothelin receptor blockers (Tracleer [bosentan]), prostanoids (Flolan [epoprostenol]), phosphodiesterase-5 inhibitors (Viagra [sildenafil]), as well as anticoagulation (eg, warfarin, heparin) have been used. Patients are instructed to avoid extreme physical exertion, limit air travel (hypoxia at altitude), and use prescribed supplemental oxygen. Lung transplantation is the primary surgical option long term.[74,76]

Sleep Apnea

Obstructive sleep apnea syndrome (OSAS), or sleep disordered breathing, affects as many as 15% of men and 5% of women in the United States.[77,78] OSAS is associated with the development of systemic hypertension (HTN), PAH, heart failure, dysrhythmias, insulin resistance, and CVAs.[77-79] Prevalence of OSAS in HTN is approximately 50%, 30% in acute coronary syndromes, and as high as 60% in strokes.[77] Upwards of 25% of patients with heart failure have been reported having OSAS.[77,80] OSAS is characterized by episodes of partial or complete occlusion of the upper airway limiting ventilation resulting in repetitive drops in oxygen saturation and fragmented sleep.[81] **Central sleep apnea** differs from OSAS in that there is a periodic cessation of breathing with no respiratory effort followed by hyperventilation.[77] Central sleep apnea is a disorder of the respiratory control of breathing. The apnea-hypopnea index (AHI) refers to the number of obstructive events per hour and is used to quantify OSAS.[77,80] An AHI range of 5 to 15 events per hour defines mild OSAS and ≥30 events per hour defines severe OSAS. A third type of OSAS is called **complex sleep apnea syndrome** (CompSAS). These individuals respond to positive airway pressure for the obstructive issues, but central apnea persists. Central events comprise more than half of the residual sleep disorder and their central apnea index score is >5 events/hour. Prevalence of CompSAS remains variable and is impacted by heart failure, BMI, and narcotics.

Recommended treatments for OSAS include alcohol avoidance, weight loss for obese patients, and CPAP ventilation at night to brace the airways to improve ventilation.[77,80] Oral appliance and postural devices, although beneficial, are not as effective as CPAP. Compliance remains a hurdle with CPAP due to poor fitting masks, skin and eye irritation, and complaints of claustrophobia.[77] Therapists should consider including simple questionnaires to screen for the presence of sleep apnea. The Epworth Sleep Scale is an easily administered standardized measure of tiredness and should be a standard evaluation tools of patients with HTN, obesity, CVA, and heart failure (Table 7-12).[77]

Lung Volume Reduction Surgery

Lung volume reduction surgery (LVRS) was a surgical technique developed in the 1950s for emphysema but abandoned for years because of poor outcomes.[82,83] The surgery reduces the size of the thorax through excision of diseased portions of lung leading to improved elastic recoil and improving the mechanical advantage of the diaphragm and pulmonary function.[82-84] Patients report improved quality of life, reduction in dyspnea, and increased 6 Minute Walk Test (6MWT) distance. Currently, the surgical approach includes video-assisted thoracoscopic surgery, medial sternotomy, or thoracotomy. Because of air leaks resulting in adverse events like pneumonia,

Table 7-12

EPWORTH SLEEPINESS SCALE

Name: ______________________________ Today's date: ______________

Your age (yrs): __________ Your gender (Male = M, Female = F): __________

How likely are you to doze off or fall asleep in the following situations, in contrast to just feeling tired?

This refers to your usual way of life recently.

Even if you haven't done some of these things recently, try to figure out how they would have affected you.

Use the following scale to choose the **most appropriate number** for each situation:

0 = **no chance** of dozing
1 = **slight chance** of dozing
2 = **moderate chance** of dozing
3 = **high chance** of dozing

It is important that you answer each item as best as you can.

Situation	**Chance of Dozing (0-3)**
Sitting and reading	___
Watching TV	___
Sitting inactive in a public place (e.g., a theater or a meeting)	___
As a passenger in a car for an hour without a break	___
Lying down to rest in the afternoon when circumstances permit	___
Sitting and talking to someone	___
Sitting quietly after a lunch without alcohol	___
In a car or bus, while stopped for a few minutes in traffic	___

THANK YOU FOR YOUR COOPERATION

ICU readmission, and prolonged length of stay, further innovations in the surgical procedures have occurred.[83] Additional techniques, like bronchoscopic thermal vapour ablation (BTVA), endobronchial valves, lung volume reduction coils (LVRCs), and biologic lung volume reduction (Bio-LVR), are still under investigation. LVRS has also been used in conjunction or following with lung transplantation.

Noninvasive Positive Pressure Ventilation

Noninvasive positive pressure ventilation (NPPV) is applied to patients with acute exacerbations of COPD and respiratory failure, patients with cystic fibrosis, neuromuscular diseases, chest wall deformities, and OSAS due to high mortality rates with intubation.[85,86] NPPV is used to assist with weaning from invasive ventilation and as bridging therapy for patients awaiting lung transplantation.[87] Increased WOB, inspiratory muscle weakness, and fatigue are the final common denominators for acute respiratory failure. The suggested benefits of NPPV are improvements in gas exchange (decreased PCO_2, increased PaO_2) and decreased WOB. Other benefits include sleep efficiency, quality of life scores, and distance walked.[88,89] NPPV has also been used as an adjunct during exercise and pulmonary rehabilitation.[86,88] Claustrophobia, recent head and neck surgeries, poor appliance fit, poor adherence to medical therapy, inability to protect the airway from aspiration, and cognitive deficits are relative contraindications to NPPV.[88]

Physical Therapist Management

Pulmonary Rehabilitation

Pulmonary rehabilitation is defined as a comprehensive intervention based on a thorough patient assessment followed by patient-tailored therapies that include, but are not limited to, exercise training, education, and behavior change, designed to improve the physical and psychological condition of people with chronic respiratory disease and to promote the long-term adherence to health-enhancing behaviors.[90] Therapists are important members of the multidisciplinary team. Intervention for the patient diagnosed with either primary or secondary respiratory disease covers a broad spectrum of areas. Therapeutic interventions vary from positioning recommendations for the bed bound, medically paralyzed, mechanically ventilated patient to improving exercise capacity via ambulation or even treadmill walking following thoracic surgery. The challenges in the acute care setting are two-fold: first to prevent the complications of immobility (see Chapter 4) and second to examine and intervene in specific aspects of respiratory impairments and the resultant activity limitations and participation restriction. Pulmonary impairments like respiratory muscle weakness, retained sections, poor cough, DOE and desaturation can be treated with early mobility, oxygen supplementation, inspiratory muscle training (IMT), and airway clearance techniques. Postsurgical patients may have specific issues that need to be managed, such as pain or functional mobility restrictions, related to the surgery itself. The examination process (Table 7-13) will guide the physical therapist in determining appropriate intervention to meet these challenges.

Therapeutic Interventions

The examination findings will direct the therapist, but because of the constant changes in physiological, motivational, and emotional conditions, the plan of care must be flexible. Whether the patient is being mechanically ventilated in the ICU or participating in an inpatient pulmonary rehabilitation program, physical therapist services are directed at maximizing functional ability, reducing participation restrictions and, ultimately, enhancing quality of life. There are no established guidelines on precisely where to begin with this patient. Initial interventions are directed at early mobilization while monitoring hemodynamic, pulmonary, and cognitive responses to activity (see Figure 4-3). Interventions are often focused on the activities of bed mobility, transfers, and ambulation while simultaneously monitoring BP, HR, RR, pulse oximetry, and rate of perceived exertion (RPE). Task-specific activities, such as stair climbing or even transfers from sit-to-stand, can be easily fatiguing. How quickly and intensely to progress a patient is dependent on several factors: individual tolerance to activity, patient's goals and motivation, anticipated short-term functional outcomes, caregiver ability, environmental obstacles in the home setting, and resource capability. The profound impact of immobility and bed rest is

Table 7-13

Pulmonary System Examination: Look, Listen, And Feel

Technique	*Description of Technique*	*Examination Findings in Common Diseases/Disorders*
Posture, chest configuration, extremities	• Observe head, shoulder/scapula position (descriptors [ie, rounded, forward, protracted, winged]). • Note ratio of anterior-posterior (A-P) chest wall to lateral costal (A-P should be smaller). • Describe shape of chest wall/thorax (eg, pectus excavatum, pectus carinatum, barrel chest, kyphoscoliosis). • Observe any muscle wasting and/or hypertrophy (accessory muscles). • Observe fingers/toes for cyanosis and clubbing.	• ↑ A-P diameter/barrel chest deformity: Hyperinflation/air trapping (eg, emphysema, asthma, cystic fibrosis, chronic bronchitis) • ↑ accessory muscle hypertrophy: Chronic respiratory disease and respiratory distress • Digital clubbing/cyanosis: May indicate hypoxemia, poor peripheral circulation (eg, emboli, PVD, Raynaud's, vasospasm, cystic fibrosis, chronic bronchitis)
RR	• Measure the RR while the patient is unaware of measurement. • Patients may automatically change the breathing pattern and rate with observation. • Observe the rise and fall of the chest, movement of the shoulders, accessory muscle use, etc. for 15, 30, or 60 seconds and multiply accordingly. • Document rate, depth, accessory muscle use, rhythm, and audible sounds.	• Normal RR: 12 to 20 breaths/minute • ↑ RR ($>$25): Respiratory distress, restrictive lung disease (eg, IPF, pneumonia), exertion/exercise • ↓ RR ($<$12): Respiratory muscle fatigue and pending failure
Respiratory/ breathing pattern	• Observe inhalation and exhalation pattern at rest and with activity. • Determine duration of inspiration to expiration (I:E) ratio. • Note presence or absence of accessory muscle usage, nasal flaring, excessive sighing, etc.	• Normal I:E ratio: 1:2 • ↑ I:E ratio: Obstructive lung disease (eg, emphysema, chronic bronchitis, asthma flare)

(continued)

Table 7-13 (continued)

PULMONARY SYSTEM EXAMINATION: LOOK, LISTEN, AND FEEL

Technique	*Description of Technique*	*Examination Findings in Common Diseases/Disorders*
	• Note specific patterns: ¤ Tachypnea (RR >25): Rapid, shallow breathing ¤ Cheyne-Stokes: Ramping depth changes in V_T with an apneic period ¤ Biot's: Slow, saw-toothed motion of V_T that has apneic periods ¤ Paradoxical: Abdomen is drawn inward during inspiration ¤ Kussmaul: Progressive increase in rate and depth of inhalation ¤ Supraclavicular/intercostals/substernal retractions: Anatomical regions are drawn inward during inspiration	• Tachypnea: ILD (eg, IPF) • Cheyne-Stokes: Critically ill • Biot's: Meningitis • Paradoxical: SCI, diaphragm paralysis, respiratory muscle fatigue, possible pending respiratory failure • Retractions: Respiratory muscle fatigue, possible pending respiratory failure
Auscultation	• Breath sounds: Use diaphragm of stethoscope; warm and clean prior to use; instruct patient to take a large inhalation and relax on exhalation; if unfamiliar with landmarks for lobes/segments, document breath sound finding with external/surface landmarks; use systematic method for comparing lung regions side to side. • Normal breath sounds: ¤ Bronchial: Normal breath sound heard over the mid-sternum and between thoracic vertebrae 4–5 cephalad; abnormal if over other areas of lung fields indicative of consolidation; harsh sounding equal quality on inhalation and exhalation ¤ Normal or vesicular (inhalation >exhalation, should be soft, low pitched); listen away from sternal areas, and spinous processes	• Abnormal breath sounds: ¤ Bronchial: Consolidation, pneumonia, above pleural effusion ¤ Decreased/diminished: COPD (eg, emphysema, chronic bronchitis), asthma flare, pleural effusion, pneumothorax, pulmonary emboli, muscle guarding (eg, thoracic incision pain), stroke, SCI, obesity ¤ Crackles/rales: Atelectasis, pulmonary edema, cystic fibrosis/bronchiectasis, chronic bronchitis, IPF, pulmonary emboli

(continued)

Table 7-13 (continued)

Pulmonary System Examination: Look, Listen, And Feel

Technique	*Description of Technique*	*Examination Findings in Common Diseases/Disorders*
	• Bronchial vesicular: Heard over large airways between scapula and below clavicle, medium sound, inhalation=exhalation; no break in sound between inspiration and expiration • Abnormal breath sounds: ¤ Decreased/diminished: Heard with a low inspiratory volume or minimal air movement and/or hyperinflation ¤ Crackles/rales: Popping sound heard primarily on inhalation; often associated with fluid filled alveoli ¤ Rhonchi/wheezes: Musical sounds heard on exhalation >inspiration ¤ Stridor: Heard on inhalation in larger airways; related to inflammatory process narrowing airway or obstruction narrowing airway ¤ Pleural friction rub: Rough, leathery sound heard on inhalation/exhalation ¤ Egophony: "e" to "a" changes heard over a consolidation ¤ Whispered pectriloquy: Whispered words that are clearer and possibly louder heard over a consolidation ¤ Bronchophony: Spoken word is clear and distinct over a consolidation	¤ Wheezes: Airway obstruction due to inflammation or bronchospasm (eg, COPD, asthma) ¤ Stridor: Upper airway obstruction, epiglottic interference (eg, food particle in airway, acute airway inflammation, bronchoconstriction post-extubation) ¤ Pleural friction rub: Pleural inflammation
Tactile fremitus	• Place hands on each segment of the lung fields to compare right to left and have the patient inspire deeply and exhale easily. • Document areas of fremitus if present/absent. • Vocal fremitus may be felt if hands in place during patient conversation.	• ↑ tactile fremitus: Retained secretions (eg, chronic bronchitis, cystic fibrosis, bronchiectasis, pneumonia) • ↓ tactile fremitus: Pneumothorax, pleural effusion

(continued)

Table 7-13 (continued)

PULMONARY SYSTEM EXAMINATION: LOOK, LISTEN, AND FEEL

Technique	*Description of Technique*	*Examination Findings in Common Diseases/Disorders*
Tracheal position	• Facing patient, move fingertips along clavicle from distal to proximal. • At the proximal point of the clavicle, have the patient relax the neck and look down; trachea should rest midpoint between index fingers/head of clavicles.	• Tracheal deviation toward affected side: Atelectasis • Tracheal deviation away from affected side: Large pleural effusion, tension pneumothorax
Mediate percussion	• Flatten 2 or 3 fingers against the chest wall. • Tap firmly with either your knuckle or 2 fingers of your opposite hand between the distal interphalangeal and proximal interphalangeal joints. • If consolidation or over dense area (eg, bone, pneumonia) should hear a thud/dull-type sound. • If over an area with air, should hear a resonating type sound.	• Dullness: Lung consolidation (eg, pneumonia), pleural effusion, pulmonary fibrosis, atelectasis • Hyperesonance: Pneumothorax, hyperinflation as seen in COPD/asthma exacerbation
Chest wall motion/ expansion	• Anterior/posterior: Place hands in a w-shape position with the thumbs at intercostal spaces 6 or 7 (midaxillary line); keep the hand that borders the posterior rib cage stable and allow the hand closest to the anterior rib cage to move with inhalation; ask the patient to inspire deeply; note change in distance between the 2 thumbs. • Lateral/costal: Place hands in a w-shape position with the thumbs under breast area anteriorly and repeat posteriorly at least 2 intercostal spaces below the angle of the scapulae. • A pliable tape measure or calipers can also be used (note surface landmarks when charting).	• ↓ chest wall expansion: Consolidation/pneumonia, pleural effusion, pneumothorax

(continued)

Table 7-13 (continued)

Pulmonary System Examination: Look, Listen, And Feel

Technique	*Description of Technique*	*Examination Findings in Common Diseases/Disorders*
Diaphragmatic excursion	• Place slightly curled fingertips under each side of the rib cage • Ask the patient to sniff quickly and forcefully • Therapist should palpate hemidiaphragm movement to be equal bilaterally (sometimes difficult to palpate) • To test for posterior diaphragmatic excursion: Use either mediate percussion with deep inhalation and compare side to side	• ↓ diaphragm excursion: Diaphragm weakness/fatigue, ascites, pregnancy • Diaphragm may ascend into thorax with inspiration if paralyzed.
Pitting edema measurement	• 1+: Barely detectable impression when finger is pressed into skin • 2+: Slight indentation; 15 seconds to rebound • 3+: Deeper indentation; 30 seconds to rebound • 4+: >30 seconds to rebound	• +/- edema in extremities with heart failure, renal disorders, pulmonary disorders, prolonged bedrest
Cough	• Have the patient attempt a cough on demand or monitor a spontaneous cough during other parts of evaluation. ¤ Listen for quality and effectiveness of cough; should have a deep inhalation, followed by a forceful exhalation. ¤ Describe sound: Wet, dry, nonproductive, ineffective ¤ Describe secretions: Color, quantity (eg, 1/2 teaspoon, tablespoon, cup), viscosity (stickiness), and odor	• Persistent, productive: Pneumonia, cystic fibrosis/bronchiectasis, bronchitis • Persistent, nonproductive: Pulmonary fibrosis, sarcoid, pneumonitis • Hemoptysis: Pulmonary infarct, cystic fibrosis/bronchiectasis, lung cancer, tuberculosis • Purulent sputum: Bacterial infection • Frothy sputum: CHF, pulmonary edema • Blood-tinged sputum: Tracheal inflammation/suction trauma, infection

(continued)

Table 7-13 (continued)

Pulmonary System Examination: Look, Listen, And Feel

Technique	*Description of Technique*	*Examination Findings in Common Diseases/Disorders*
Pulse oximetry (SpO_2)	• Disinfect probe prior to placing on patient • Place probe on digit (finger or toe) if clothespin-type connection or use disposable probe against the bridge of the nose, ear, or forehead (precaution if allergic to adhesive). • Validate observed pulse with palpated pulse, electrocardiogram, or on monitor (eg, left ventricular assist device, intra-aortic balloon pump). • Determine device limitations/measurement error: Low perfusion states/cold extremities, motion artifact/ambient fluorescent lighting, excessive hand grip, finger nail polish, etc.	• Normal SpO_2: >93% • Abnormal SpO_2: <93%; consider supplemental oxygen if SpO_2 <89%
Outcome Tools for Acute Care		
Activity Measure for Post Acute Care "6 Clicks", 2 Minute Walk Test, 6MWT, Five Time Sit to Stand, Visual Analog Scale (VAS), Dyspnea Index, vital signs, Function in Siting Test, Timed Up and Go, Berg Balance Scale, Functional Independence Measure (FIM), Acute Care Index of Function, Functional Status Score for the Intensive Care Unit		
Questionnaires/Scales		
mMRC, Modified Borg Rate of Perceived Exertion, COPD Assessment Test, St. George Respiratory Questionnaire (SGRQ), UCSD SOB Questionnaire (University of California San Diego Shortness of Breath), Patient Health Questionnaire 9 (PHQ-9), Epworth Sleepiness Scale		

Adapted from Watchie[5]; Frownfelter and Dean[12]; American Thoracic Society[126]; PTNow[127]; Global Strategy for Diagnosis, Management and Prevention of COPD[128]; Hillegass and Sadowsky[129]; Irwin and Tecklin[130]; O'Sullivan and Schmitz[131]; American Thoracic Society[132]; Perloff [133]; Reid and Chung[134]; and Seidel et al.[13]

well documented, and confinement to bed is a common treatment for patients with chronic disease. Bed rest, anesthesia, and surgical incisions of the chest wall diminish pulmonary function resulting in reduced tidal volumes and decreased respiratory muscle strength and expiratory flow rates (FEV_1, FVC), increased pulmonary shunt, and development of atelectasis. Body positioning alone can be an effective means of enhancing oxygen transport by improving V/Q matching in the lung.[91,92] If the patient is medically stable for discharge, yet hospital-based functional goals have not been achieved, the recommendation is made for some level of continued physical therapy services. The patient with respiratory failure may require some level of continued rehabilitation at the time of medical discharge from the hospital.

Body Positioning

Body positioning and mobilization are important therapeutic interventions to prevent and alleviate respiratory complications by increasing oxygen transport and improving arterial oxygenation.[91] Evidence supports side-lying with the affected lung uppermost to improve oxygenation and promote resolution of atelectasis.[93] Prone positioning is supported for patients who present with hypoxemia refractory to other ventilatory strategies. Prone positioning in the ARDS populations has been shown to improve oxygenation and mortality.[94-96] Although the individual response is variable, improvements in PaO_2 may allow reductions in mechanical ventilator settings including the F_IO_2 and inflation pressures to decrease the impact of oxygen toxicity and barotrauma associated with VILI.[94,95]

Positioning may lead to improvements in PaO_2 through improved V/Q matching by redistributing blood flow to previous atelectatic but non-diseased regions, enhanced ventilation uniformity, and reduced pulmonary vascular resistance of previously dependent lung regions.[91,97] Upright positioning can increase peak expiratory flow promoting a more effective cough, and may augment diaphragm excursion promoting inspiration. Complications associated with positioning and mobilization may include accidental removal of endotracheal or tracheostomy tubes, venous or arterial catheters, and feeding tubes. The physical therapist needs to consider hemodynamic instability, transient desaturation, abdominal symptoms, wounds, incision, or skin breakdown, and need for increased sedation or muscle relaxants.[96,97] However, with proper planning, observation, and ongoing monitoring, positioning and mobilization is safe and advantageous for patients with respiratory disease.[96,98]

Breathing Exercises

Breathing exercises are used to alter the patient's breathing pattern by modifying the rate, depth, or distribution of ventilation. Goals include increased alveolar ventilation with resultant increased oxygenation and reductions in carbon dioxide, reduced sensation of dyspnea, and reduced WOB. The breathing strategies commonly administered include diaphragmatic breathing, PLB, segmental breathing, and sustained maximal inspiration breathing exercises, such as incentive spirometry and thoracic expansion exercises. There is insufficient evidence to support one specific type of breathing exercise because studies include small sample sizes, poorly define the breathing exercises used, and include a variety of breathing exercises.[99]

Diaphragmatic Breathing

Diaphragmatic breathing, or **breathing control**, attempts to enhance diaphragmatic motion to reduce accessory muscle usage and normalize the breathing pattern. There is evidence to support chest physiotherapy and deep breathing exercises, such as diaphragmatic breathing, in the early postoperative course following upper abdominal and cardiac surgery.[99,100] Changes in pulmonary function following upper abdominal surgical (UAS) procedures leading to postoperative pulmonary complications include reductions in inspiratory capacity and decreased ventilation at lung bases.[100] Pulmonary complications are also a significant cause of postoperative morbidity following cardiac surgery.[99] Diaphragmatic and sustained maximal inspiration breathing exercises were shown to benefit inspiratory (MIP) and expiratory (MEP) muscle strength. Performing the exercises in seated, leaning forward, or even the standing position are beneficial.[101] Patients with advanced COPD recovering from respiratory failure who were instructed in diaphragmatic breathing demonstrated significant increases in oxygenation along with a decrease in carbon dioxide during the breathing exercise; however, they also showed reduced chest wall coordination, increased dyspnea, and were mechanically less efficient in their breathing.[102,103] The improved gas exchange was demonstrated during the diaphragmatic breathing trial but there was no carryover effect. These studies demonstrate a transient physiologic benefit with diaphragmatic breathing but there was a cost to the patient. Therefore, the physical therapist needs to determine the principle goal to be achieved via the application of the breathing exercise and to determine the effectiveness of their therapeutic intervention.[100]

Pursed-lip Breathing

PLB is believed to increase positive pressure within the airways and buttress the small bronchioles, preventing premature airway collapse. This stenting of the airways should promote effective expiration. This breathing pattern may decrease the RR and increase the tidal volume, improving alveolar ventilation and enhancing the ventilation of previously under-ventilated areas.[104] Mechanical effects of PLB also include slower expiratory flow with an improvement in oxygenation and carbon dioxide removal. PLB is more cost effective from an energy standpoint and may reduce the WOB for select patients, especially those with COPD.

Segmental Breathing

Segmental breathing, also referred to as **localized expansion breathing**, assumes that inspired air can be directed to a specific area of lung by enhancing movement of the thorax overlying that lung region.[105-107] Although limited research demonstrates the efficacy of these techniques, a study demonstrated that regional ventilation can be increased during a unilateral thoracic expansion exercise in trained individuals.[108] Various techniques have been used to increase regional ventilation, including proprioceptive neuromuscular facilitation, joint mobilization, and thoracic flexibility exercises.[106,107]

Deep Breathing and Incentive Spirometry

An **incentive spirometer** is a device that encourages, through visual feedback, the performance of reproducible, sustained maximal inspiration as noted in Figure 7-19. Incentive spirometry continues to be controversial as a primary tool to reduce postoperative pulmonary complications following upper abdominal surgery, thoracic, and post coronary artery bypass grafting.[109-111]

Physical therapy interventions including, PLB, huffing, coughing, and early mobilization, have been demonstrated to improve oxygen saturation and reduce the incidence of postoperative pulmonary complications.[99] Therefore, all patients who are at risk for pulmonary complications should engage in an airway clearance and mobility regimen.

Inspiratory Muscle Training

Respiratory muscle dysfunction often contributes to weaning failure and the need for prolonged mechanical ventilation. When the load placed on the musculoskeletal pump exceeds its capacity, ventilatory failure develops.[112] Conditions that contribute to respiratory muscle dysfunction include sepsis, malnutrition, infection, electrolyte abnormalities (eg, hypokalemia, hypomagnesemia), acid-base disturbances, phrenic

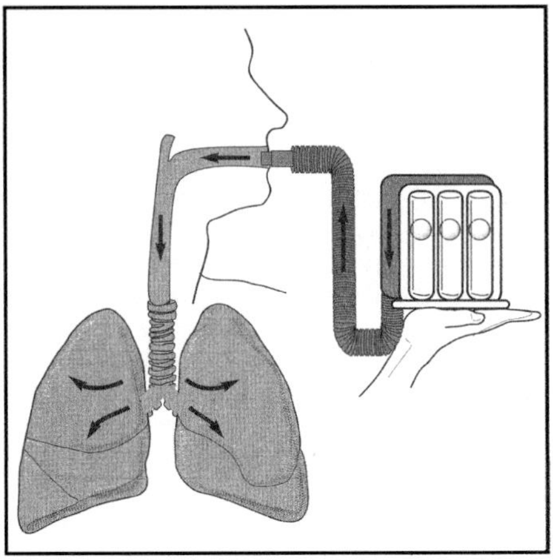

Figure 7-19. How to use an incentive spirometer. (Reprinted with permission from Sheldon LK. *Oxygenation*. Sudbury, MA: Jones and Bartlett Publishers; 2001.)

nerve dysfunction, steroid administration, acquired neuromuscular weakness (eg, steroid myopathy, ICU-acquired weakness), and disuse atrophy. The patient with respiratory failure may present with an increased demand placed on the respiratory system due to airway obstruction (eg, retained secretions, bronchospasm, inflammation), mechanical disadvantage (eg, hyperinflation), reduced lung compliance (eg, pulmonary edema, pulmonary fibrosis), and decreased chest wall compliance (eg, kyphoscoliosis, ankylosing spondylitis).[112-114] Although IMT has been shown to increase the inspiratory muscle strength (MIP), reduce dyspnea, and increase exercise capacity and walking distance in patients with chronic lung disease, the implementation of IMT has not been widely used in the hospitalized or ventilator-dependent population.[115-117] Studies have shown that preoperative IMT improves muscle endurance and reduces risk of postoperative pulmonary complications and length of stay in patients undergoing cardiothoracic surgery.[118,119] Studies have also shown that IMT for patients with respiratory failure may promote successful liberation from mechanical ventilation after failed attempts at standard weaning procedures.[113,120] These studies utilized a threshold training device and emphasized a low repetition, high resistance exercise prescription.[120,121]

Therapeutic Exercise: Range of Motion, Resistance, and Aerobic

Patients diagnosed with advanced lung disease and respiratory failure have often spent some time with enforced bed rest. Deconditioning and the hazards of bedrest (see Chapter 4) are well understood and must not be underestimated by the physical therapist.[122] Gravity alone may be sufficient resistance when initially prescribing an exercise program but progression to isometric, manual resistance, and progressive resistance exercise (PRE) increases strength. Resistive exercise with rubber bands or weights can provide the patient with objective goals for strengthening as number of repetitions increases or band color changes.

Although aerobic training is an important intervention in the long-term management of individuals with chronic lung disease, classic aerobic conditioning has a limited role in the plan of care for the patient with acute respiratory insufficiency. The major aspects of conditioning for this population include functional training activities aimed at improving mobility and ambulation in preparation for discharge. Hospital-based goals are focused on independent mobility while improving activity tolerance. Mobilization sessions must be coordinated with other activities, such as bronchodilator medications and airway clearance, that may reduce the work of breathing. Some patients may benefit from use of exercise equipment, including treadmills and bicycle ergometers, to further challenge endurance. Other rehabilitation interventions, such as neuromuscular electrical stimulation and in bed cycle ergometry, can be used for those patients who cannot tolerate out of bed activities.[123]

Careful monitoring of the patient's vital signs, including pulse oximetry, is imperative before, during, and after each therapy session. The most likely time of critical changes in respiratory and hemodynamic status occurs when the patient progresses from one stage of functional training to another, such as from supine to out-of-bed sitting, then standing, then ambulating. The therapist must control the progression of ambulation to ensure the tolerance of one stage before a patient advances to the next. A Borg dyspnea or fatigue score of 4 to 6 (moderate to very severe) or RPE of 12 to 14 (somewhat hard) is often considered a target training intensity.[90] See Chapter 4 for additional information regarding early rehabilitation programs. Finally, the prescription, instruction, and performance of a home-based exercise program is an important goal for the acute care patient who will be directly discharged to home.

Airway Clearance Techniques

Airway clearance techniques (ACT) have been a mainstay in respiratory care for nearly 50 years.[12] Airway clearance can be as simple as assisting with coughing by splinting an incision to performance of manual techniques, such as percussion, vibration, shaking, or abdominal thrusts. New guidelines do not recommend routine ACT if the patient is able to mobilize secretions with an effective cough or for routine prophylactic postsurgical care.[124] Pulmonary complications after surgery, trauma, or respiratory failure are anticipated due to pain, incisions, chest tubes, fractures, effects of anesthesia, artificial airways, muscular weakness, and immobility. The primary purpose of airway clearance in the acute care setting is to mobilize secretions, improving ventilation and oxygenation, but it should be reserved for patients who are unable to perform these independently or who have restricted mobility. Mobilizing secretions and improving ventilation helps to prevent complications, such as atelectasis and pneumonia, that may prolong hospitalization. Additional benefits may include reduced WOB, improvements in V/Q matching, and decreased dyspnea.[10] The ACT administered will depend on the patient presentation and physical therapy examination findings as noted in Tables 7-13 and 7-14. Obviously, if the patient has an unstable fracture, coagulopathy, osteoporosis, or is hemodynamically compromised, the aggressiveness of the treatment will be moderated. Determining the degree and presumed anatomic locations of pulmonary abnormalities is key to focusing treatment. Proper set up, timing, and administration of ACT and medications, and assistance with coughing or suctioning should be individualized. Mobilizing secretions can be accomplished through deep breathing exercises, bronchial drainage positions, frequent repositioning, manual techniques, and early mobilization as noted in Table 7-15.

Bronchial or **postural drainage** refers to positioning the segment of the lung for gravity to assist secretion drainage. There is a specific position for each segment, but precautions need to be considered. For example, trendelenburg, or head down positioning, should be avoided in patients with gastroesophageal reflux disease (GERD) or elevated intracranial pressures (ICPs). Enteral feeding (tube feeds; see Chapter 11) should be discontinued for at least 1 hour prior to positioning in bronchial drainage positions or before vigorous manual and coughing maneuvers to reduce aspiration risk and abdominal complaints such as nausea.

Percussion is a manual technique where the hand is cupped or small suction cup devices are used to transmit pressure waves through the chest wall to loosen airway secretions. A rhythmic pattern and a hollow-type sound should be generated if the technique is performed correctly. A barrier (eg, towel, gown) should be placed

Table 7-14 **CONCEPTS TO CONSIDER FOR CHOOSING AN AIRWAY CLEARANCE TECHNIQUE**
• Ongoing evaluation of initial treatment choice for effectiveness, efficiency, and adherence • Can the technique meet the goals of treatment without complication? • Can the reatment can be done in any setting or disease state (mild to end-stage)? • Can the technique can be performed with little to no assistance? • Techniques should not overly fatigue the patient. • Age and cognitive level of the individual • Comfort and time efficiency • Cost effective and insurance coverage • Patient motivation
Adapted from Hardy KA. A review of airway clearance: new techniques, indications, and recommendations. *Respiratory Care*. 1994;39(5):440-452; Hardy KA, Anderson BD. Noninvasive clearance of airway secretions. *Respir Care Clin N Am*. 1996;2(2):323-345; and Warnock L, Gates A, van der Schans CP. Chest physiotherapy compared to no chest physiotherapy for cystic fibrosis. *Cochrane Database Syst Rev*. 2013;(9):CD001401. doi: 10.1002/14651858.CD001401.pub2

Table 7-15

AIRWAY CLEARANCE TECHNIQUES

Technique	*Precautions*
Chest physical therapy (CPT): Percussion, vibration, shaking	Osteopenia/osteoporosis, bleeding disorders, elevated ICP, spinal instability or hemodynamic instability; mechanical devices available; patient will need assistance from another person to perform
Bronchial drainage (sometimes called postural drainage)	Gastric reflux, ICP, uncontrolled bleeding, spinal or hemodynamic instability
Forced expiratory technique	Easy to learn; precautions include control flow on exhalation to prevent bronchospasm/airway collapse
Autogenic drainage	Challenging to learn; patients may feel like they need to take deeper breaths
Active cycle of breathing	Gastric reflux, ICP, uncontrolled bleeding, spinal or hemodynamic instability; if quite ill, may need assistance to perform
Assistive/splinted coughing	Pain, osteopenia/osteoporosis, increased ICP, bleeding disorders, chest tubes/incisions/pain (see Table 7-16)
Suctioning	Dysrhythmias, hypoxia, vasovagal response, and bleeding (see Table 7-17)

(continued)

Table 7-15 (continued) **Airway Clearance Techniques**	
Technique	*Precautions*
Aerobic exercise	Modifications to exercise prescription must consider hemodynamics, respiratory status, psychologic factors, and clinical laboratory data
PEP devices: PEP Flutter,[a] TheraPEP,[b] Acapella,[b] Quake,[c] ThresholdPEP[d]	Positioning may alter efficacy of device (eg, flutter must be held upright); patient's inability to generate correct expiratory pressure may impact efficacy of device (eg, TheraPEP requires 10 to 20 cm H_2O); avoid high-pressure PEP if risk of pneumothorax; claustrophobia with facemasks
HFCWO: The Vest,[e] MedPulse System[f]	Must ensure proper fit over lung not stomach/bladder area, claustrophobia, bruising, and complaints of discomfort or SOB, dry mouth, hydration
Intrapulmonary percussive ventilator: Percussionaire[g]	Patient comfort, proper settings for delivery of medications
Cough Assist[h]	Patient comfort, proper fit if artificial airway, may need assistance to set up, pneumothorax risk
PercussiveNeb[i]	Patient comfort, proper fit if artificial airway, may need assistance to set up, pneumothorax risk
[a]AxcanScandipharm Pharmaceutical Co; [b]DHD Health Care; [c]Thayer Medical; [d]HealthScan Products Inc; [e]Hill-ROM; [f]Electromed, Inc; [g]Percussionaire Corp; [h]JH Emerson Co; [i]Vortran Medical Technology 1, Inc	
Adapted from Strickland et al[72]; Hardy[139]; Hardy and Anderson[140]; and Pruitt and Jacobs.[141]	

between the patient's skin and the therapist's hand. Precautions include osteopenia, osteoporosis, pain, coagulopathies, bronchospasm, and hemoptysis. Additionally, therapists should avoid percussing over bony prominences and the floating ribs.

Vibration and **shaking** are performed during the expiratory phase only. These maneuvers aid the forward movement of secretions loosened by percussion and drainage positions. Vibration is a fine movement, whereas shaking is more vigorous. Precautions are similar to those for percussion.

Chest physical therapy (CPT) is the combination of postural drainage, percussion, and vibration/shaking.

Rib springing is an effective method to enhance ventilation, specifically inspiration where a controlled thrust at the end of expiration enhances the volume of the next breath. This technique utilizes the muscle spindles of the intercostals to enhance muscular contraction and is beneficial when the patient is unable to follow cues for taking a deep breath.

Incentive spirometers are devices to practice deep breathing exercises while providing feedback on inspiratory volumes. Typically, the patient is encouraged to use the incentive spirometry devices hourly followed by coughing or huffing. As noted previously, there is little evidence to show the benefit of incentive spirometry in the acute care setting.[111]

Alternative ACTs are valuable in the acute care setting. These techniques include high-frequency chest wall oscillation (HFCWO), positive expiratory pressure (PEP) devices, active cycle of breathing, and autogenic drainage (see Table 7-15). Autogenic drainage requires a high level of concentration and breathing control and may be too challenging to instruct and master in the acute care setting. HFCWO has been administered in the ICU and hospital ward as an alternative to standard CPT. HFCWO applies airway vibration to break up mucus and alters airflow to create "mini-coughs" that move the secretions toward the trachea. Vests should be individually sized and checked for proper fit, and the skin should be inspected for redness after treatment. Frequency is set to mobilize mucus peripherally to the more central airways. In theory, lower frequency settings (5 to 10 Hz) loosen secretions in the periphery with higher frequency ranges mobilizing secretions cephalad (10 to 15 Hz and 15 to 20 Hz). Pressure in the vest should be set by type of vest used (chest vs full vest) and patient comfort. Less than 5 is recommended for the chest vest and greater than 4 is recommended for the full-size vest. Patients may complain of chest wall soreness, claustrophobia, dry mouth, and fatigue. A shirt or other barrier should be placed between the patient's skin and the vest.

PEP devices depend on the patient's ability to control the breathing pattern, maintain a good seal with the mouthpiece or face mask, and generate sufficient positive pressure. There are several devices available including TheraPEP, Threshold PEP, Acapella, Flutter, and Quake. The patient typically generates 10 to 15 mm Hg of pressure for 5 to 10 seconds to recruit collateral ventilation and mobilize secretions. Some of the devices require the patient to generate a set flow rate, volume, and pressure, and are dependent on position to be beneficial. Advantages of the PEP devices are that they are simple to learn, portable, give feedback, and in some cases are even fun. If the patient is unable to follow directions, or requires physical assistance, PEP devices are not as beneficial as the more traditional forms of chest physical therapy (eg, percussion, vibration) or HFCWO.

Secretion Removal

Once the secretions are mobilized, they must be removed by coughing or suctioning. A cough follows a logical sequence: the patient must inhale a large volume of air, the glottis must close, a pressure gradient is created between the abdominal and thoracic cavities, and then the glottis must open with sequential contraction of the abdominal muscles causing the forceful expulsion of air.[10] The phases and effectiveness of the cough can be impacted by pain, muscle weakness, poor coordination, chest tubes, positioning, patient cognition, sedation, and artificial airways. Therefore, proper pain medication and splinting will improve cough. Common assisted cough techniques are described in Table 7-16.

Suctioning can stimulate a cough or directly remove retained secretions. Suctioning is an invasive procedure and may cause airway trauma, hypoxemia, dysrhythmias, or a vasovagal response (eg, bradycardia, hypotension). Suctioning should be the last intervention chosen, instead of the first, to assist with mucus clearance unless the airway and oxygenation are severely compromised (Table 7-17).

Table 7-16

ASSISTED COUGH TECHNIQUES

Technique	*Description*
Splinted cough	Used to support incision area. Patient or therapist braces the incision using a pillow, blanket, or extended hand while the patient attempts a cough. Gentle pressure is applied for bracing only.
Quad cough (abdominal thrust)	Similar to Heimlich maneuver used in CPR. As the patient attempts a cough,the heel of the therapist's hand is thrust inward and upward above the umbilicus but below the xiphoid process. The upward thrust must be coordinated with the patient's expiration/cough. If the patient is intubated, suctioning should occur with the abdominal thrust. If the patient has a recent incision, a blanket or a towel can be used to apply pressure instead of a heel thrust. The blanket or towel is held taut across the abdominal area on the cough, acting as a brace for the abdominal cavity during the cough cycle.
Combined quad cough and thoracic bracing	Use the hand/heel thrust as described in quad cough combined with a downward pressure across the upper anterior rib cage with the other forearm (mid to upper sternal area). There is a downward motion toward the upward thrusting hand/heel on exhalation. This should be done only when timed with an attempted cough by the patient. Precautions include fractured ribs, central lines (eg, pulmonary artery catheter, central venous pressure, dialysis ports), osteopenia/osteoporosis, innervated abdominals, and bleeding disorders.
Thoracic splinting combined with cough	Used with patients with intact spinal cord. As the patient coughs, the therapist applies firm pressure to the chest wall and can even vibrate during the cough. Thoracic splinting is coordinated with the patient's exhalation/cough.
Bilateral rib compression	Can be used with intact spinal cord. The therapist places hands on each side of the thoracic rib cage, but avoids floating ribs. As the patient inspires/expires, the therapist gets in sequence with the patient's rib cage movements. The therapist asks the patient to cough, and during exhalation, the therapist brings his or her hands downward and inward augmenting the movement of the rib cage. Timing is key.
Cough combined with ACTs	An assistive cough can be facilitated using any of the following ACTs: vibration, shaking, PEP devices (eg, PEP, Flutter, TheraPEP, Acapella, Quake, ThresholdPEP), HFCWO (eg, The Vest). The therapist can either apply the pressure (vibration/shaking) on exhalation/cough or the patient can be instructed to "forcefully huff or cough" into the device (eg, PEP, Flutter, TheraPEP, Acapella Choice, Quake, ThresholdPEP). HFCWO is also beneficial to perform an assistive cough maneuver to help brace the rib cage.
Positioning	Optimize the patient's position to enhance the cough phases. For example, to facilitate inspiration, have the patient extend the trunk and neck, add rib springing/proprioceptive neuromuscular techniques; for expiration, promote patient trunk and neck flexion; expiratory flow rates and cough effectiveness are increased with upright positioning. *(continued)*

Table 7-16 (continued) ASSISTED COUGH TECHNIQUES
Precautions
All assisted coughs require caution. The physical therapy examination should identify comorbidities that would modify patient positioning and the technique chosen (eg, osteopenia/osteoporosis, recent thoracic and/or abdominal surgeries, agitation, thoracic and abdominal innervation, feeding tubes/timing of supplemental feeds, corticosteroids, bleeding disorders, pain, ICP).
Adapted from Frownfelter D, Dean E. *Principles and Practice of Cardiopulmonary Physical Therapy.* St. Louis, MO: Mosby-Year Book, Inc; 1996; Hillegass EA, Sadowsky HS. *Essentials of Cardiopulmonary Physical Therapy.* 2nd ed. Philadelphia, PA: WB Saunders; 2001; and Pruitt B, Jacobs M. Clearing away pulmonary secretions. *Nursing*. 2005;July:37-41.

Table 7-17

ENDOTRACHEAL SUCTIONING (VIA ARTIFICIAL AIRWAY)

Evaluate Patient for Ineffective Cough/Inability to Clear Secretions (Auscultate Lung Fields)	*Considerations and Precautions*
1. Explain rationale and procedure to patient. 2. Prepare sterile work area for suctioning; gloves, catheter, and saline (if used); size and length of catheter should be determined by the size of ETT, size of patient, and amount and thickness of secretions. 3. Pre-oxygenate using 100% F_IO_2 prior to, during, and following airway suctioning. 4. Visually measure length of catheter for depth of insertion not to exceed carina (use Angle of Louis/sternal angle as visual landmark or second rib). 5. Insert sterile catheter until resistance and withdraw 1 cm. Apply suction no longer then 8 to 10 seconds at a pressure of 80 to 100 mm Hg as catheter is withdrawn from airway. (Recommend therapist hold breath to simulate patient's breath hold during suctioning.) 6. Repeat depending on volume of secretions, patient's hemodynamic and respiratory responses, and note time to recovery to baseline status. 7. Document procedure, secretion color/viscosity/amount, patient hemodynamic response, any adverse reactions, and recommendations for follow-up sessions.	• Sterile instilled (2 to 3 ccs) saline may be beneficial for cough stimulation. Some evidence relates that instilled saline may lead to increased pulmonary infections. Use instilled saline cautiously or not at all. • Universal precautions (goggles/gloves/gown if indicated) • Observe for: ¤ Red blood with cough (hemoptysis) ¤ Prolonged bronchospasm or wheeze ¤ Dysrhythmias ¤ Vasovagal response with insertion of catheter (eg, bradycardia, hypotension) ¤ Elevated BP due to irritation ¤ Transient or prolonged decline in oxygenation

Case Study

Mrs. Andrews is a 75-year-old (y/o), woman admitted with complaints of (c/o) SOB and pain in her right hip and arm following a fall earlier today at her home. She was evaluated in the emergency department and admitted to the orthopedic service with a right hip fracture (fx) requiring open reduction internal fixation (ORIF), right upper extremity (RUE) radius fx that was treated by casting. Physical therapy was consulted for evaluation and treatment postoperative day 1.

Patient/Client History

General Demographics, Social History, and Living Environment

Mrs. Andrews is a retired paralegal and has been married for 51 years. She lives in a 2-story home with 5 steps to enter and a handrail. The bedroom and full bathroom are on the second floor and a half bath is on the first floor. She does not drive, but her husband, who is 79, continues to drive.

General Health Status, Social/Health Habits, and Family History

Mrs. Andrews is overweight with a body mass index (BMI) of 38. She quit smoking 3 years ago when she was diagnosed with COPD but admits to smoking 2 packs/day for more than 35 years. She states she enjoys 2 cocktails with dinner each night, and she does not participate in any type of exercise routine. Her hobbies include playing bridge on Thursdays and canasta on Saturdays. She and her husband have 2 grown children with 5 grandchildren who all live locally. Her family history is unremarkable.

Medical/Surgical History

Mrs. Andrews is diagnosed with oxygen dependent (2 L/minute via nasal cannula) COPD, HTN, osteoporosis, and is obese.

Current Condition

Mrs. Andrews c/o SOB and pain on any movement in bed. Her chest x-ray is suspicious for RML pneumonia. Mrs. Andrews has a urinary catheter in place to monitor output volume. She is receiving 2 L of O_2 via nasal cannula and has received some pain medication for 7/10 pain with any movement. Her activity status is OOB as tolerated, non-weightbearing (NWB) on her right lower extremity (RLE) and partial weightbearing on RUE.

Activities and Participation

Prior to admission, Mrs. Andrews was independent with ambulation with a cane on all surfaces and ADLs. She reports she can walk around the house, but more than 1 block is "pushing it." She reports needing minimal assistance with instrumental activities of daily living (IADLs), such as housecleaning and food shopping. Her husband also assists with some household tasks, and they both are retired. Her mMRC score at time of admission was rated a 2.

Medications

Mrs. Andrews' medications include metoprolol for HTN, prednisone (corticosteroid), and albuterol (bronchodilator) inhaler 2 puffs twice/day. She is given an oral non-steroidal anti-inflammatory drug for pain prior to therapy.

Other Clinical Tests

ABGs on 3 liters were pH 7.34, PCO_2 52, PO_2 62, HCO_3^- 32 the morning of her evaluation.

Systems Review

Cardiovascular and Pulmonary

Resting vital signs in supine are HR 110 bpm, BP 108/60 mm Hg, RR 20 breaths/minute, SpO_2 93% on 2 L via nasal cannula, RPE 2 using the modified Borg Scale, and breathing pattern demonstrates obvious accessory muscle use.

Integumentary

Mrs. Andrews was placed on a pressure-relieving, low air-loss mattress. She has been wearing pneumatic compression stockings on bilateral lower extremities (BLEs) since her surgery. Her surgical wound site is not visualized secondary to the dressing. Her right forearm has some bruising areas and her skin appears dry.

Musculoskeletal

Gross movements of her left upper extremity (LUE) and left lower extremity (LLE) appeared normal but Mrs. Andrews was unable to move her RUE/RLE due to pain and the cast.

Neuromuscular

Sensation to light touch and gross proprioception were intact LUE/LLE and RLE. The patient reports 8/10 on a 0 to 10 VAS for pain in any movement of the RLE. Rest and elevation relieve the pain.

Communication, Affect, Cognition, Language, and Learning Style

Mrs. Andrews is awake, alert, and oriented to person, place, and time. She reports feeling anxious about moving because of the fear of pain. Her primary language is English.

Tests and Measures

Aerobic Capacity and Endurance

Compared to her resting vital signs (VS), Mrs. Andrews demonstrated tachycardia, and exaggerated BP response, oxygen desaturation, and complained of severe SOB with mobilization out of bed (see Circulation [Arterial, Venous, Lymphatic] and Ventilation and Respiration for specifics). These changes reveal a limited cardiopulmonary reserve and poor endurance.

Assistive and Adaptive Devices

Patient performed a stand-pivot with maximal assistance of 2 therapists. A bedside commode has been ordered with an elevated seat, as well as a long- handled reacher.

Balance, Gait, and Mobility (Including Locomotion)

Mrs. Andrews was able to transfer from bed to a chair. She performed a stand-pivot with maximal assistance of 2 (FIM 1). Mrs. Andrews practiced the incentive spirometer and performed ankle pumps and ADLs (ie, washed her face and hands) in the elevated chair prior to transfer back to bed. She was able to sit out in the chair for 35 minutes total. Gait assessment (FIM 0) was held due to HTN, tachycardia, and oxygen desaturation accompanied by c/o pain and severe SOB.

Circulation (Arterial, Venous, Lymphatic) and Ventilation/Respiration

Mrs. Andrews' pulse was strong and regular. She did not have any pitting edema noted in her extremities. As mentioned previously, her HR and BP changed dramatically transitioning from supine to sit out of bed: HR 110-132, BP 108/60-156/88.

Following the transfer OOB, the SpO_2 was 86% on 3 liters, RR increased to 30 breaths/minute and continued accessory muscle use was noted. Her modified Borg RPE rating was 6-8 with activity. After 2 minutes in sitting, Mrs. Andrews' VS were SpO_2 89% on 2 liters, RR 24 breaths/minute, and continued accessory muscle use. Her VS returned to baseline after 5 minutes. Her breath sounds were distant bilaterally and absent in the area under her right axilla. While sitting, incentive spirometery was practiced and she achieved 400 mL as the best of 3 trials.

Mental Function

Mrs. Andrews was alert, awake and oriented x4. She followed commands easily but appeared anxious.

Muscle Performance

Manual muscle testing of the LUE and LLE revealed strength of 4/5 in all major muscle groups. Mrs. Andrews is unable to lift her RUE cast without assistance and unable to flex or abduct her RLE without assistance. Active range of motion (AROM) appears grossly within normal limits (WNL) for LUE and LLE. Her RLE was not formally assessed secondary to pain with motion and RUE limited to angle of cast and length of cast.

Pain

As noted previously, the patient reports 8/10 on a 0 to 10 numeric pain rating scale for pain any movement of the RLE.

Evaluation

The patient is an older, frail female currently hospitalized secondary to a fall resulting in a femoral neck fracture, ORIF, a humeral fracture status-post (s/p) cast, and a possible RML pneumonia. Past medical history (PMHx) is remarkable for HTN, COPD, osteoporosis, and obesity.

Diagnosis

As noted previously, the patient demonstrated HTN, tachycardia, tachypnea with moderate drop in SpO_2, and increase in accessory muscle use. Her ABG suggests respiratory acidosis. The patient presents with activity limitations due to pain, impaired muscle function, impaired pulmonary function, including gas exchange, and increased WOB related to her COPD and possible RML pneumonia.

Prognosis

Complete healing of femur and radius fracture should allow return to prior level of function, but she will most likely need a different assistive device from admission. The patient will require acute inpatient rehabilitation, most likely a lower intensity subacute rehabilitation facility upon discharge from the hospital due to the limited pulmonary reserve. This prognosis is also based on current mobility deficits, pain, her challenging home environment, and the limited assistance her husband can provide. Her SOB, pain, tachycardia, anxiety, risks for falls, and possible pneumonia will slow her progress.

Intervention

Daily physical therapy intervention with short-term goals of increasing OOB tolerance and decreasing level of assistance required for bedside mobilization are appropriate. In addition to these functional goals, optimizing cough effectiveness and mobilizing secretions are important. Early mobilization to decrease effects of bed rest will also enhance airway clearance. Manual techniques should be utilized with caution due to the risk for rib fracture from potential steroid-induced osteoporosis. Airway clearance will focus on deep breathing exercises (incentive spirometry) and effective coughing. PLB and pacing during functional activities will decrease the WOB as well as normalize the breathing pattern. Pain control and frequent position changes may increase her inspiration volume to augment effective coughing. Additional interventions included ADL and functional training, assistive and adaptive device training, and therapeutic exercise. Interventions will be performed with the target intensity of 4 to 6 on the modified Borg RPE scale while closely monitoring the VS responses. An interval-like training approach is used where short periods of activity/exercise are combined with short rest periods to control DOE. Patient education will continue, including the use of pain medication prior to therapy sessions, skin integrity, weightbearing restrictions, and a bedside ROM exercise program. This session Mrs. Andrews practiced incentive spirometry and transfers and performed ankle pumps. ADLs (ie, washed her face and hands) were attempted while in the elevated chair prior to transfer back to bed. She was able to sit in the chair for 35 minutes total.

Outcomes

Reexamination after 3 treatment sessions revealed the same level of assistance for transfers OOB and continued tachycardia and HTN, but she maintained her SpO_2 >91% on 2 lpm. Complaints of SOB decreased (Borg scale = 4 with activity) and pain was reported to be 5 on the numeric pain scale after receiving pain medication 45 minutes prior to the therapy session. The physical therapist recommended 2 short therapy sessions (typically 20 to 30 minutes) in addition to getting OOB with the nurses at least 1 other time during the day. OOB time will be >2 hours.

Mrs. Andrews was seen by the acute care physical therapy service for 7 days after the initial physical therapy exam, at which point she was transferred to a skilled nursing facility. She continued using her oxygen, but the urinary catheter was discontinued, and she was transferring onto the elevated bedside commode with moderate assistance of 2. Pain and antianxiety medication continued to be required prior to OOB activities. The patient required moderate assistance of 2 (FIM 1) for all transfers due to her difficulty with using the RUE. Once standing and her RUE was placed in the cuff of the rolling platform walker, she could ambulate 10 feet x 2 with moderate assistance of 1 (FIM 2). SOB, anxiety, and pain continued to limit her functional progression, but was improving. Her RML pneumonia responded to antibiotics and airway clearance.

ICF Clinical Reasoning Tool Case Study Summary

Health Condition								
HPI: Right hip fracture s/p ORIF, RUE radius fx casted, pain, possible RML pneumonia PMHx: COPD—oxygen dependent 2 L NP, moderately obese, sedentary lifestyle, hypoxemia, HTN, osteoporosis, +ETOH.								
Precautions/Contraindications								
Pain, fall risk, chronic steroid use may impact wound/bone healing, beta blocker may impact HR response to functional activity/transfers, NWB RLE, partial weightbearing RUE, universal precautions								
Body Structure and Function			*Activity/Task Limitations*			*Participation*		
Impairment/ Problem	*Tests and Measures*	*Intervention*	*Activity*	*Tests and Measures*	*Intervention*	*Participation*	*Tests and Measures*	*Intervention*
• Poor pulmonary reserve abnormal breath sounds • Need for ACTs • Impaired oxygenation • Decreased ROM and strength • Decreased endurance • Pain • Weight exceeds IBW	• Chest assessment • Cough • ROM/MMT • VS including SpO_2, RPE • NPRS • BMI	• Breathing exercises, incentive spirometry • Bedside ROM Progressive resistance exercises • Education on effective coughing, PLB and pacing with functional tasks, falls/safety • Consult physician regarding oxygen titration • Consult registered dietician	• ADLs • Bed mobility • Transfers • Gait	• Functional task analysis • FIM • RPE and mMRC score	• Progressive/ interval functional retraining following pulmonary rehabilitation guidelines • Oxygen titration	• Unable to do house cleaning or grocery shopping • Unable to play bridge or canasta	• mMRC • PHQ-9	• Continue physical therapy services • Consult social worker, occupational therapist, and registered dietician

(continued)

ICF Clinical Reasoning Tool Case Study Summary (continued)

Personal Factors	*Other Considerations*	*Environmental Factors*
• Age: 75 y/o RH, female • Primary language: English • Retired paralegal • Married x 51 years; 79 y/o husband • Husband drives, patient does not drive • I with gait and ADLs all surfaces with cane prior to admission • 2 grown children live locally with 5 grandchildren • Former smoker x 70 pk/yrs, quit x 3 years • Anxious and fearful of pain with movement		Home: • 2 story house, 5 steps to enter with handrail • Bedroom/full bath on 2nd floor; 1/2 bath on first • Oxygen delivery device Hospital: • Urinary catheter, 3 L via NP, surgical bandage, elevated chair, bedside commode

ETOH = ethanol; HPI = history of present illness; I = independent; IBW = ideal body weight; MMT = Manual Muscle Test; NP = nasal prongs; NPRS = Numeric Pain Rating Scale; pk/yrs = packs per years; PMHx = past medical history; RH = right handed; ROM = range of motion.

Adapted from American Physical Therapy Association. *Guide to Physical Therapist Practice*. 3rd ed. http://www.apta.org/Guide/. Updated October 21, 2015. Accessed October 5, 2018 and *Towards a Common Language for Functioning, Disability and Health*. World Health Organization. www.who.int/classifications/icf/icfbeginnersguide.pdf. Published 2002. Accessed April 29, 2019.

Chapter Review Questions

1. Which of the following best represent the 2 most common pulmonary complications following thoracic or abdominal surgery?
   a. Atelectasis and pneumonia
   b. Impaired cough and pleuritis
   c. Bronchiolitis and empyema
   d. Pulmonary edema and aspiration
2. The following is the best definition for pulmonary edema:
   a. Air in thorax
   b. Right sided heart failure
   c. Accumulation of extravascular water in lungs
   d. High intrapleural pressure leading to hypoxemia
3. The following best represents the type of assistive cough used following abdominal surgery:
   a. Quad cough
   b. Bilateral rib compression
   c. Combined quad cough and thoracic splinting
   d. Splinted cough
4. How does upright positioning improve oxygenation?
   a. Decreases ventilation perfusion matching
   b. Resolves atelectasis in nondependent lung fields
   c. Increases peak expiratory flow rate by promoting more effective coughing
   d. Increases ventilation uniformity and reduces pulmonary vascular resistance
5. Which of the following pulmonary disorders would lead to a pulmonary restriction pattern on pulmonary function testing?
   a. Atelectasis and chronic bronchitis
   b. Pulmonary edema and emphysema
   c. Pleural effusion and alpha1 antitrypsin deficiency
   d. Pneumonia and pulmonary contusion

Answers: 1a, 2c, 3d, 4c, 5d

References

1. Hoyert DL, Xu J. Deaths: preliminary data for 2011. *Natl Vital Stat Rep.* 2012;61(6):1-51.
2. Pfunter A, Wier LM, Stocks C. Most frequent conditions in U.S. hospitals, 2011. HCUP Statistical Brief #162. *Agency for Healthcare Research and Quality.* https://hcup-us.ahrq.gov/reports/statbriefs/sb162.pdf. Published September 2013. Accessed January 31, 2019.
3. Chronic obstructive pulmonary disease (COPD). Patient information series. *Am J Respir Crit Care Med.* 2005;171:3-4.
4. Crystal RG, West JB, Barnes PJ, et al. *The Lung: Scientific Foundations.* New York, NY: Raven Press, Ltd; 1991.
5. Watchie J. *Cardiopulmonary Physical Therapy: A Clinical Manual.* Philadelphia, PA: WB Saunders Co; 1995.

6. Cohen M, Michel TH. *Cardiopulmonary Symptoms in Physical Therapy Practice*. New York, NY: Churchill Livingstone; 1988.
7. Rubin E, Farber JL. The respiratory system. In: Rubin E, Farber JL, eds. *Essential Pathology*. 2nd ed. Philadelphia, PA: JB Lippincott Co; 1995.
8. Des Jardins T. *Clinical Manifestations of Respiratory Disease*. 2nd ed. Chicago, IL: Year Book Medical Publishers, Inc; 1990.
9. West JB. *Respiratory Physiology—The Essentials*. 3rd ed. Baltimore, MD: Lippincott Williams & Wilkins; 1985.
10. West JB. *Pulmonary Pathophysiology—The Essentials*. 3rd ed. Baltimore, MD: Lippincott Williams & Wilkins; 1987.
11. Toews GB. Host defense. In: Albert RK, Spiro SG, Jett JR, eds. *Comprehensive Respiratory Medicine*. San Diego, CA: Harcourt Brace; 1999.
12. Frownfelter D, Dean E. *Principles and Practice of Cardiopulmonary Physical Therapy*. 3rd ed. Philadelphia, PA: Mosby; 1996.
13. Qaseem A, Wilt TJ, Weinberger SE, et al. Diagnosis and management of stable chronic obstructive pulmonary disease: a clinical practice guideline update from the American College of Physicians, American College of Chest Physicians, American Thoracic Society, and European Respiratory Society. *Ann Intern Med*. 2011;155:179-191.
14. Dewar M, Whit Curry R. Chronic obstructive pulmonary disease: diagnostic considerations. *Am Fam Physician*. 2006;73:669-676,677-678.
15. Mulhall P, Criner G. Non-pharmacological treatments for COPD. *Respirology*. 2016;21:791-809.
16. Lee H, Kim J, Tagmazyan K. Treatment of stable chronic obstructive pulmonary disease: the GOLD guidelines. *Am Fam Physician*. 2013;88(10):655-663
17. Garcia-Aymerich J, Farrero E, Felez MA, Izquierdo J, Marrades RM, Anto JM. Risk factors of readmission to hospital for a COPD exacerbation: a prospective study. *Thorax*. 2003;58:100-105.
18. Modified Medical Research Council Questionnaire for Assessing the Severity of Breathlessness (From the Global Strategy for Diagnosis, Management and Prevention of COPD). Global Initiative for Chronic Obstructive Lung Disease (GOLD). https://www.mdcalc.com/global-initiative-obstructive-lung-disease-gold-criteria-copd. Published 2014. Accessed July 17, 2019.
19. Bullock BA, Henze RL. *Focus on Pathophysiology*. Philadelphia, PA: Lippincott Williams & Wilkins; 2000.
20. Global Initiative for Asthma. 2015 asthma, COPD, and asthma-COPD overlap syndrome. https://ginasthma.org/asthma-copd-and-asthma-copd-overlap-syndrome-acos. Accessed July 17, 2019.
21. Pannettieri RA. Chronic obstructive pulmonary disease. In: Grippi MA, ed. *Pulmonary Pathophysiology*. Philadelphia, PA: Lippincott Williams & Wilkins; 1995.
22. Corwin EJ. *Handbook of Pathophysiology*. 2nd ed. Philadelphia, PA: Lippincott Williams & Wilkins; 2000.
23. O'Donnell DE, Gebke KB. Examining the role of activity, exercise, and pharmacology in mild COPD. *Postgrad Med*. 2014;126(5):135-145.
24. King PT. The pathophysiology of bronchiectasis. *Int J Chron Obstruct Pulmon Dis*. 2009:4:411-419.
25. Dodge JA. A millennial view of cystic fibrosis. *Dev Period Med*. 2015;XIX(1):9-13.
26. Moran A, Becker D, Casella SJ, et al. CFRD Consensus Conference Committee. *Diabetes Care*. 2010;33(12):2677-2783.
27. Floto RA, Olivier KN, Saiman L, et al. US Cystic Fibrosis Foundation and European Cystic Fibrosis Society consensus recommendations for the management of non-tuberculous mycobacteria in individuals with cystic fibrosis: executive summary. *Thorax*. 2016;71:88-90.
28. Sood N, Paradowski LJ, Yankaskas JR. Outcomes of intensive care unit care in adults with cystic fibrosis. *Am J Respir Crit Care Med*. 2001;163:335-338.
29. Braun AT, Merlo CA. Cystic fibrosis lung transplantation. *Curr Opin Pulm Med*. 2011;17:467-472.
30. Raghu G. Interstitial lung disease—a clinical overview and general approach. In: Fishman AP, Elias JA, Fishman JA, Grippi MA, Kaiser LR, Senior RM, eds. *Fishman's Pulmonary Diseases and Disorders*. 3rd ed. New York, NY: McGraw-Hill;1998.
31. Rafii R, Juarez MM, Albertson TE, Chan AL. A review of current and novel therapies for idiopathic pulmonary fibrosis. *Thorac Dis*. 2013;5(1):48-73. doi:10.3978/j.issn.2072-1439.2012.12.07
32. Britton J. Idiopathic pulmonary fibrosis. In: Albert RK, Spiro SG, Jett JR. eds. *Comprehensive Respiratory Medicine*. San Diego, CA: Harcourt Brace; 1999.
33. Canestro WJ, Forrester Sh, Raghu G, Ho L, Devine BE. Drug treatment of idiopathic pulmonary fibrosis. *Chest*. 2016;149(3):756-766.

34. Loveman E, Copley VR, Scott DA, Colquitt JL, Clegg AJ, O'Reilly KMA. Comparing new treatments for idiopathic pulmonary fibrosis—a network meta-analysis. *BMC Pulm Med.* 2015;15:37.
35. Moller DR. Sarcoidosis. In: Albert RK, Spiro SG, Jett JR, eds. *Comprehensive Respiratory Medicine*. San Diego, CA: Harcourt Brace; 1999.
36. Judson MA. Advances in the diagnosis and treatment of sarcoidosis. *F1000Prime Rep.* 2014;6:89. doi: 10.12703/P6-89
37. Ryu JH, Doerr CH, Fisher SD, Olsen EJ, Sahn SA. Chylothorax in lymphangioleiomyomatosis. *Chest.* 2003;123:623-627.
38. King TE, Crausman RS. Pulmonary lymphangioleiomyomatosis. In: Fishman AP, Elias JA, Fishman JA, Grippi MA, Kaiser LR, Senior RM, eds. *Fishman's Pulmonary Diseases and Disorders*. 3rd ed. New York, NY: McGraw-Hill; 1998.
39. Park CK, Kwon YS. Respiratory review of 2014: tuberculosis and nontuberculous mycobacterial pulmonary disease. *Tuberc Respir Dis.* 2014;77:161-166
40. Boughton WA, Bass JB. Tuberculosis and disease caused by atypical myocbacteria. In: Albert RK, Spiro SG, Jett JR, eds. *Comprehensive Respiratory Medicine*. San Diego, CA: Harcourt Brace; 1999.
41. Cordier JF. Update on cryptogenic organizing pneumonia (idiopathic bronchiolitis obliterans organizing pneumonia). *Swiss Med Wkly.* 2002;132:588-591.
42. Husain SJ, Irfan M, Zubairi AS, Salahuddin N. Rapidly-progressive bronchiolitis obliterans organizing pneumonia. *Singapore Med J.* 2004;45(6):283-285.
43. Nagai S, Izumi T. Bronchiolitis obliterans with organizing pneumonia. *Curr Opin Pulm Med.* 1996;2(5):419-423.
44. Chapman HA. Disorders of lung matrix remodeling. *J Clin Invest.* 2004;113(2):148-157.
45. Keller CA, Cagle PT, Brown RW, Noon G, Frost AE. Bronchiolitis obliterans in recipients of single, double, and heart-lung transplantation. *Chest.* 1995;107:973-980.
46. Husain AN, Siddiqui MT, Holmes EW, et al. Analysis of risk factors for the development of bronchiolilitis obliterans syndrome. *Am J Respir Crit Care Med.* 1999;159:829-833.
47. Bando K, Paradis IL, Similo S, et al. Obliterative bronchiolitis after lung and heart-lung transplantation: an analysis of risk factors and management. *J Thoracic Cardiovasc Surg.* 1995;110:4-14.
48. Lanken PN. Pathophysiology of respiratory failure. In: Grippi MA, ed. *Pulmonary Pathophysiology.* Philadelphia, PA: Lippincott Williams & Wilkins; 1995.
49. MacIntyer NR. Respiratory mechanics in the patient who is weaning from the ventilator. *Respir Care.* 2005;50(2):275-284.
50. O'Sullivan F, Al-Haddad M. Acute respiratory distress syndrome. *Anaesthesia and Intensive Care Medicine.* 2013;14(10):423-476.
51. Blank R, Napolitano LM. Epidemiology of ARDS and ALI. *Crit Care Clin.* 2011;27:439-458.
52. Monahan L. Acute respiratory distress syndrome. *Curr Probl Pediatr Adolesc Health Care.* 2013;43:278-284.
53. Aggarwal NR, King LS, D'Alessio FR. Diverse macrophage populations mediate acute lung inflammation and resolution. *Am J Physiol Lun Cell Mol Physiol.* 2014;306:L709-L725.
54. Restrepo MI, Faverio P, Anzueto A. Long-term prognosis in community-acquired pneumonia. *Curr Opin Infect Dis.* 2013;26(2):151-158.
55. Dang TT, Eurich DT, Weir DL, Marrie TJ, Majunder SR. Rates and risk factors for recurrent pneumonia in patients hospitalized with community-acquired pneumonia: population-based prospective cohort study with 5 years of follow up. *Clin Infect Dis.* 2014;59(1):74-80
56. Ottosen J, Evans H. Pneumonia challenges in definition, diagnosis, and management of disease. *Surg Clin N Am.* 2014;94:1305-1317.
57. DiBardino DM, Wunderink RG. Aspiration pneumonia: a review of modern trends. *J Crit Care.* 2015;30:40-48.
58. Lewis DR, Check DP, Caporaso NE, Travis WD, Devesa SS. US lung cancer trends by histologic type. *Cancer.* 2014;120:2883-2892.
59. Roach HD, Davies GF, Attanoos R, Crane M, Adams H, Phillips S. Asbestos: when the dust settles-an imaging review of asbestos-related disease. *RadioGraphics.* 2002;22:S167-S184.
60. Norbet C, Joseph A, Rossi SS, Bhalla S, Gutierrez FR. Asbestos-related lung disease: a pictorial review. *Curr Probl Diagn Radiolol.* 2015;44(4):371-382.
61. Koumbourlis AC. Chest wall abnormalities and their clinical significance in childhood. *Paediatr Respir Rev.* 2014;15:246-255.
62. Hodgkin JE, Celli BR, Connors GL, eds. *Pulmonary Rehabilitation: Guidelines to Success.* 3rd ed. Philadelphia, PA: Lippincott Williams & Wilkins; 2000.

63. Hermans G, Van den Berghe G. Clinical review: intensive care unit acquired weakness. *Crit Care*. 2015;19:274.
64. Bach JR. *Pulmonary Rehabilitation: The Obstructive and Paralytic Conditions*. Philadelphia, PA: Hanley & Belfus, Inc; 1996.
65. Vanderschueren R. Pneumothorax. In: Albert RK, Spiro SG, Jett JR, eds. *Comprehensive Respiratory Medicine*. San Diego, CA: Harcourt Brace and Co; 1999.
66. Peters JI, Sako EY. Pneumothorax. In: Fishman AP, Elias JA, Fishman JA, Grippi MA, Kaiser LR, Senior RM, eds. *Fishman's Pulmonary Diseases and Disorders*. 3rd ed. New York, NY: McGraw-Hill; 1998.
67. Schuster DP. Pulmonary edema. In: Fishman AP, Elias JA, Fishman JA, Grippi MA, Kaiser LR, Senior RM, eds. *Fishman's Pulmonary Diseases and Disorders*. 3rd ed. New York, NY: McGraw-Hill; 1998.
68. Herold CJ, Bankier AA, Burghuber OC, Minar E, Watzke HH. Pulmonary embolism. In: Albert RK, Spiro SG, Jett JR, eds. *Comprehensive Respiratory Medicine*. San Diego, CA: Harcourt Brace; 1999.
69. Davignon K, Kwo J, Bigatello LM. Pathophysiology and management of the flail chest. *Minerva Anestesiol*. 2004;70(4):193-199.
70. Pieracci FM, Lin Y, Rodil M, et al. A prospective, controlled clinical evaluation of surgical stabilization of severe rib fractures. *J Trauma Acute Care Surg*. 2016;80:187-194.
71. Lunardi AC, Paisani DM, Marques da Silva CCB, Cano DP, Tanaka C, Carvalho CRF. Comparison of lung expansion techniques on thoracoabdominal mechanics and incidence of pulmonary complications after upper abdominal surgery. A randomized controlled trial. *Chest*. 2015;148(4):1003-1010.
72. Strickland SL, Rubin BK, Dresher GS, et al. AARC clinical practice guidelines: effectiveness of nonpharmacologic airway clearance therapies in hospitalized patients. *Respir Care*. 2013;58(12):2187-2193.
73. Fishman AP. Pulmonary hypertension and cor pulmonale. In: Fishman AP, Elias JA, Fishman JA, Grippi MA, Kaiser LR, Senior RM, eds. *Fishman's Pulmonary Diseases and Disorders*. 3rd ed. New York, NY: McGraw-Hill; 1998.
74. Via G, Braschi A. Pathophysiology of severe pulmonary hypertension in the critically ill patient. *Minerva Anestesiol*. 2004;70(4):233-237.
75. Jones A, Evans T. Pulmonary hypertension. In: Albert RK, Spiro SG, Jett JR, eds. *Comprehensive Respiratory Medicine*. San Diego, CA: Harcourt Brace; 1999.
76. Taichman DB, Mandel J. Epidemiology of pulmonary arterial hypertension. *Clin. Chest Med*. 2013;34:619-637.
77. Lattimore JDL, Celermajer DS, Wilcox I. Obstructive sleep apnea and cardiovascular disease. *J Am Coll Cardiol*. 2003;41:1429-1437.
78. Khan MT, Franco RA. Complex sleep apnea syndrome. *Sleep Disord*. 2014;2014:798487.
79. Maeder MT, Schoch OD, Rickli H. A clinical approach to obstructive sleep apnea as a risk factor for cardiovascular disease. *Vasc Health Risk Manag*. 2016;12:85-103.
80. Medical Advisory Secretariat. Polysomnography in patents with obstructive sleep apnea. An evidence-based analysis. *Ont Health Technol Assess Ser*. 2006;6(13):1-38.
81. Mayer P, Dematteis M, Pepin JL, et al. Peripheral neuropathy in sleep apnea: a tissue marker of the severity of nocturnal desaturation. *Am J Respir Crit Care Med*. 1999;159:213-219.
82. Benditt JO. Surgical therapies for chronic obstructive pulmonary disease. *Respir Care*. 2004;49(1):53-61.
83. Trotter MA, Hopkins PM. Advanced therapies for COPD—what's on the horizon? Progress in lung volume reduction and lung transplantation. *J Thorac Dis*. 2014;6(11):1640-1653
84. Gelb AF, McKenna RJ, Brenner M, Epstein JD, Zamel N. Lung function 5 yr after lung volume reduction surgery for emphysema. *Am J Respir Crit Care Med*. 2001;163:1562-1566.
85. Plant PK, Owen JL, Elliott MW. Non-invasive ventilation in acute exacerbations of chronic obstructive pulmonary disease: long term survival and predictors of in-hospital outcome. *Thorax*. 2001;56:708-712.
86. Burns KEA, Meade MO, Premji A, Adhikari NKJ. Noninvasive ventilation as a weaning strategy for intubated adults with respiratory failure: a Cochrane systematic review. *CMAJ*. 2014;186(3):E112-E122.
87. Kotsimbos T, Williams TJ, Anderson GP. Update on lung transplantation: programmes, patients, and prospects. *Eur Respir Rev*. 2012;21:126,271-305.
88. Hill NS. Noninvasive ventilation for chronic obstructive pulmonary disease. *Respir Care*. 2004;49(1):72-87.

89. Wijkstra PJ, Lacasse Y, Guyatt GH, et al. A meta-analysis of nocturnal non-invasive positive pressure ventilation in patients with stable COPD. *Chest.* 2003;124:337-343.
90. Spruit MA, Singh SJ, Garvey C, et. al. An official American Thoracic Society/European Respiratory Society statement: key concepts and advances in pulmonary rehabilitation. *Am J Respir Crit Care Med.* 2013;188(8):e13-e64
91. Ross J, Dean E. Integrating physiologic principles into the comprehensive management of cardiopulmonary dysfunction. *Phys Ther.* 1989;69(4):255-259.
92. Stiller K. Physiotherapy in intensive care: towards an evidence-based practice. *Chest.* 2000;118:1801-1813.
93. Ibanez J, Raurich JM, Abizanda R, et al. The effect of lateral positions on gas exchange in patients with unilateral lung disease during mechanical ventilation. *Intensive Care Med.* 1981;7:231-234.
94. Abroug F, Ouanes-Besbes L, Dachraoui F, Ouanes I, Brochard L. An updated study-level meta-analysis of randomised controlled trials on proning in ARDS and acute lung injury. *Crit Care.* 2011;15:R6.
95. Nakos G, Tsanagaris I, Kostanti E, et al. Effect of the prone position on patients with hydrostatic pulmonary edema compared with patients with acute respiratory distress syndrome and pulmonary fibrosis. *Am J Respir Crit Care Med.* 2000;161:360-368.
96. Guerin C, Reignier J, Richard JC, et al. Prone positioning in severe acute respiratory distress syndrome. *New Engl J Med.* 2013;368:2159-2168.
97. Mure M, Lindhal S. Prone position improves gas exchange, but how? *Acta Anaesthesil Scand.* 2001;45:150-159.
98. Offner PJ, Haenal JB, Moore EE, et al. Complications of prone ventilation in patient with multisystem trauma with fulminant acute respiratory distress syndrome. *J Trauma.* 2000;48:224-228.
99. Westerdahl E. Optimal technique for deep breathing exercises after cardiac surgery. *Minerva Anestesiol.* 2015;81:678-683.
100. Grams ST, Ono LM, Noronha MA, Schivinski CIS, Paulin E. Breathing exercises in upper abdominal surgery: a systematic review and meta-analysis. *Rev Bras Fisioter.* 2012;16(5):345-353.
101. Urell C, Emtner M, Hedenstrom H, Tenling A, Breidenskog M, Westerdahl E. Deep breathing exercises with positive expiratory pressure at high rate improve oxygenation in the early period after cardiac surgery—a randomised controlled trial. *Eur J Cardiothorac Surg.* 2011;40:162-167.
102. Gosselink RA, Wagenaar RC, Rijswijk H, et al. Diaphragmatic breathing reduces efficiency of breathing in patients with chronic obstructive pulmonary disease. *Am J Respir Crit Care Med.* 1995;151:1136-1142.
103. Vitacca M, Clini E, Bianchi L, Ambrosino N. Acute effects of deep diaphragmatic breathing in COPD patients with chronic respiratory insufficiency. *Eur Respir J.* 1998;11:408-415.
104. Thoman RL, Stoker GL, Ross JC. The efficacy of pursed lips breathing in patients with chronic obstructive pulmonary disease. *Am Rev Respir Dis.* 1966;93:100.
105. Castro AA, Calil SR, Freitas SA, Oliveira AB, Porto EF. Chest physiotherapy effectiveness to reduce hospitalization and mechanical ventilation length of stay, pulmonary infection rate and mortality in ICU patients. *Respir Med.* 2013;107:68-74.
106. Polastri M, Venturini E, Pastore S, Dell'Amore A. Do chest expansion exercises aid re-shaping the diaphragm within the first 72 hours following lung transplantation in a usual interstitial pneumonia patient? *Physiother Res Int.* 2015;20(3):191-196.
107. Hanekom S, Louw QA, Coetzee AR. Implementation of a protocol facilitates evidence-based physiotherapy practice in intensive care units. *Physiotherapy.* 2013;99:139-145
108. Tucker B, Jenkins, Cheong D, et al. Effect of unilateral breathing exercises on regional lung ventilation. *Nucl Med Commun.* 1999;20:815-821.
109. Freitas ERFS, Soares BGO, Atallah JR. Incentive spirometry for preventing pulmonary complications after coronary artery bypass graft (review). *Cochrane Database Syst Rev.* 2012;(9):CD004466.
110. do Nascimento P Jr, Modolo NSP, Guimaraes MMF, Braz LG, El Dib R. Incentive spirometry for prevention of postoperative pulmonary complications in upper abdominal surgery. *Cochrane Database Syst Rev.* 2014;(2):CD006058. doi: 10.1002/14651858.CD006058.pu3
111. Carvalho Cr, Paisani DM, Lunardi AC. Incentive spirometry in major surgeries: a systematic review. *Rev Bras Fisioter.* 2011;15(5)343-350.
112. Polkey MI, Moxham J. Clinical aspects of respiratory muscles dysfunction in the critically ill. *Chest.* 2001;119:926-929.

113. Sprague SS, Hopkins PD. Use of inspiratory strength training to wean six patients who were ventilator dependent. *Phys Ther.* 2003;83:171-181.
114. Reid WD, Dechman G. Considerations when testing and training the respiratory muscles. *Phys Ther.* 1995;75:971-982.
115. Sturdy G, Hillman D, Green D, et al. Feasibility of high-intensity, interval based respiratory muscle training in COPD. *Chest.* 2003;123:142-150.
116. Koessler W, Wanke T, Winkler G, et al. 2 years' experience with inspiratory muscle training in patients with neuromuscular disorders. *Chest.* 2001;120:765-769.
117. Sanchez RH, Montemayor RT, Ortega RF, et al. Inspiratory muscle training in patients with COPD: effect on dyspnea, exercise performance, and quality of life. *Chest.* 2001;120:748-756.
118. Neto MG, Martinez BP, Reis HFC, Carvalho VO. Pre- and postoperative inspiratory muscle training in patients undergoing cardiac surgery: systematic review and meta—analysis. *Clin Rehabil.* 2017;31(4):454-464.
119. Mans CM, Reeve JC, Elkins MR. Postoperative outcomes following preoperative inspiratory muscle training in patients undergoing cardiothoracic or upper abdominal surgery: a systematic review and meta-analysis. *Clin Rehabil.* 2015;29(5):426-438.
120. Martin DA, Davenport PD, Franceschi AC, et al. Use of inspiratory muscle strength training to facilitate ventilatory weaning: a series of 10 consecutive patients. *Chest.* 2002;122:192-196.
121. Johnson JL, Cowley AJ, Kinnear WJ. Evaluation of the THRESHOLD trainer for inspiratory muscle endurance training: comparison with the weighted plunger method. *Eur Resp J.* 1996;9:2681-2684.
122. Convertino VA, Bloomfield SA, Greenleaf JE. An overview of the issues: physiological effects of bedrest and restricted physical activity. *Med Sci Sports Exerc.* 1997;29(2):187-190.
123. Connolly B, O'Neill B, Salisbury L, Blackwood B. Physical rehabilitation interventions for adult patients during critical illness: an overview of systematic reviews. *Thorax.* 2016;0:1-10.
124. Strickland SL, Rubin BK, Drescher GS, et al. AARC clinical practice guideline: effectiveness of nonpharmacologic airway clearance therapies in hospitalized patients. *Respir Care.* 2015;60(7):1071-1077.
125. American Physical Therapy Association. *Guide to Physical Therapist Practice.* 3rd ed. http://www.apta.org/Guide/. Updated October 21, 2015. Accessed October 5, 2018.
126. Epworth Sleepiness Scale. American Thoracic Society. http://www.thoracic.org/members/assemblies/assemblies/srn/questionaires/ess.php. Reviewed June 2016. Accessed May 6, 2019.
127. Functional limitation reporting (FLR) under Medicare: tests and measures for high-volume conditions. PTNow. http://www.ptnow.org/FunctionalLimitationReporting/TestsMeasures. Accessed May 6, 2019.
128. Global Strategy for Diagnosis, Management and Prevention of COPD 2014. http://www.goldcopd.org.Accessed August 1, 2019.
129. Hillegass EA, Sadowsky HS. *Essentials of Cardiopulmonary Physical Therapy.* 2nd ed. Philadelphia, PA: WB Saunders; 2001.
130. Irwin S, Tecklin JS. *Cardiopulmonary Physical Therapy: A Guide to Practice.* 4th ed. St. Louis, MO: Mosby; 2004.
131. O'Sullivan SB, Schmitz TJ, eds. *Physical Rehabilitation: Assessment and Treatment.* 5th ed. Philadelphia, PA: FA Davis; 2004.
132. Patient Health Questionnaire. American Thoracic Society. http://www.thoracic.org/members/assemblies/assemblies/srn/questionaires/phq-9.php. Reviewed June 2016. Accessed May 6, 2019.
133. Perloff JK. *Physical Examination of the Heart and Circulation.* 3rd ed. Philadelphia, PA: WB Saunders; 2000.
134. Reid WD, Chung F. *Clinical Management Notes and Case Histories in Cardiopulmonary Physical Therapy.* Thorofare, NJ: SLACK Incorporated; 2004.
135. Seidel HM, Ball JW, Benedict GW, et al. *Mosby's Guide to Physical Examination.* St. Louis, MO: Mosby; 2003.
136. Casaburi R, Petty TL, eds. *Principles and Practice of Pulmonary Rehabilitation.* Philadelphia, PA: WB Saunders; 1993.
137. Restrepo RD, Alvarez MT, Wittnebel LD, et al. Medication adherence issues in patients treated for COPD. *International Journal of COPD.* 2008:3(3)371-384.

138. Sleuth B, Ayala GX, Gillette C, et al. Provider demonstration and assessment of child device technique during pediatric asthma visits. *Pediatrics*. 2011;127(4):642-648.
139. Hardy KA. A review of airway clearance: new techniques, indications, and recommendations. *Respir Care*. 1994;39(5):440-452.
140. Hardy KA, Anderson BD. Noninvasive clearance of airway secretions. *Respir Care Clin N Am*. 1996;2(2):323-345.
141. Pruitt B, Jacobs M. Clearing away pulmonary secretions. *Nursing*. 2005;July:37-41.

Bibliography

Dahlen B. Treatment of aspirin-intolerant asthma with antileukotrienes. *Am J Respir Crit Care Med*. 2000;161:S137-S141.

Drugs.com. www.drugs.com. Accessed July 17, 2019.

Global Initiative for Asthma. Global strategy for asthma management and prevention. www.ginasthma.org. Published 2016. Accessed January 31, 2019.

Grimes GC, Manning JL, Patel P, Via RM. Medications for COPD: a review of effectiveness. *Am Fam Physician*. 2007;76:1141-1148,1151.

Hurt K, Bilton D. Inhaled interventions in cystic fibrosis: mucoactive and antibiotic therapies. *Respiration*. 2014:88:441-448.

Kallsrom TJ. Evidence-based asthma management. *Respir Care*. 2004;49(7):783-792.

Lipworth BJ. Phosphodiesterase-4 inhibitors for asthma and chronic obstructive pulmonary disease. *Lancet*. 2005;365:167-175.

Nursing2011 Drug Handbook. 31st ed. Philadelphia, PA: Lippincott Williams & Wilkins; 2011.

Respitory medications. Global RxPh. http://www.globalrph.com/respiratory.htm. Published 2017. Accessed January 31, 2019.

Appendix

Pharmacological Information: Pulmonary Diseases and Disorders Pharmacology

Medications that Promote Bronchodilation

Adrenergic Agents/Beta Agonists/Sympathomimetics/Combination

Action

Adrenergic agents stimulate the beta adrenergic receptors in the bronchial smooth muscle (beta 2 receptors) resulting in increased levels of cyclic adenosine monophosphate (cAMP). cAMP causes smooth muscle relaxation as well as inhibition of inflammatory mediator release (eg, mast cells); steroid combination incorporates alternate anti-inflammatory mechanisms; beta agonists are used chiefly as aerosol inhalants with oral and IV applications available. Recommend short acting anticholinergic or beta 2 agonist first line bronchodilator for group A COPD. Whereas patients from group D recommend inhaled corticosteroid and long-acting beta 2 agonist and/or long-acting anticholinergic.

Side Effects

CNS: Muscle tremor, headaches, anxiety, dizziness, hyperactivity, nervousness, restlessness

CV: Tachycardia, HTN, dysrhythmias, palpitations, angioedema, angina, hypokalemia

GI: Nausea, heartburn, bad taste

Miscellaneous: Muscle cramps, increased mortality related to overuse of short-acting beta agonists in asthma, spacers, and reservoir devices helpful

Pulmonary: Increased bronchial hyperresponsive on methacholine challenge with regular use of beta 2 agonists

Common Medications

Short-acting beta 2 agonists: Proventil, Ventolin (albuterol); Tornalate (bitolterol); Xopenex (levalbuterol); Maxair (pirbuterol); Alupent (metaproterenol)

Long-acting beta 2 agonists: Brovana (arformoterol tartrate), Foradil (formoterol), Arcapta Neohaler (indacaterol maleate), Serevent (salmeterol), Brethaire (terbutaline), ephedrine, epinephrine, adrenalin, Micronefrin (racemic epinephrine), Isuprel (isoproterenol)

Combination: Advair Diskus (fluticasone propionate and salmeterol)

Anticholinergic Agents/Combination

Action

Anticholinergic agents facilitate bronchodilation by decreasing acetylcholine activity. Normally, parasympathetic activation and acetylcholine release promote bronchial smooth muscle contraction. Additionally, these agents may reduce bronchial secretions. Anticholinergic agents reduce intracellular concentration of cyclic guanosine monophosphate (cyclic GMP) leading to decreased calcium release from the sarcoplasmic reticulum and smooth muscle relaxation.

Side Effects
CNS: Blurred vision, confusion, dizziness, nervousness, headache
CV: Tachycardia, palpitations, cough, HTN, angina, angioedema
GI: Dry mouth, constipation, GI upset
Miscellaneous: Reduce sputum volume without changing viscosity, paradoxical bronchospasm, glaucoma, hypersensitivity reaction

Common Medications
Atrovent (ipratropium bromide), Tudorza Pressair (aclidinium bromide), Spiriva (tiotropium)
Combination (inhaled-beta 2 agonist and anticholinergic): Combivent (albuterol and ipratropium), Anoro Ellipta (umeclidinium and vilanterol inhalation powder)

Methylxanthines

Action
Xanthine derivatives (similar to caffeine) promote bronchodilation through smooth muscle relaxation. Proposed mechanisms include elevations of cAMP by inhibition of phosphodiesterase (an enzyme that breaks down cAMP), antagonisms of adenosine, enhanced release of catecholamines, and inhibition of prostaglandins. Methylxanthines also may have anti-inflammatory effects in airways and may augment respiratory muscle function and respiratory drive.

Side Effects
CNS: Tremors, headaches, insomnia, neuromuscular irritability, seizures, nervousness, fever
CV: Tachycardia, dysrhythmias, hypotension, palpitations
GI: Vomiting, nausea, hyperglycemia, hypokalemia
Miscellaneous: Narrow therapeutic range (5 to 15 µg/mL) leading to risk of toxicity

Common Medications
Theobid, Theolair, Theo-Dur, Anhydrous Slo-Phyllin (theophylline); Phyllcontin, Truphylline (aminophylline); Choledyl (oxtriphylline)

Medications for Treatment of Airway Inflammation

Cromolyn Sodium

Action
Cromolyn sodium prevents inflammation of airway by inhibiting release of inflammatory mediators in respiratory mucosa and stabilize mast cells.

Side Effects
CNS: Dizziness, headache
GI: Nausea, abdominal pain, esophagitis, bad taste
Miscellaneous: Anaphylaxis, can be used alone or in combination with bronchodilators and anti-inflammatory steroids
Pulmonmary: Transient cough

Common Medications
Intal, Nasalcrom (cromolyn sodium); nedocromil (Tilade)

Leukotriene Modifiers

Action

Leukotriene modifiers have 2 main actions: inhibition of leukotriene formation or antagonism of leukotriene receptors. Leukotrienes are phospholipid inflammatory mediators synthesized from arachidonic acid that promote bronchoconstriction and mucus production.

Side Effects

CNS: Headaches
CV: Cough
GI: Nausea, abdominal pain
Miscellaneous: Hepatotoxicity, useful in treatment of aspirin-intolerance in asthma

Common Medications

Zyflo (zileuton), Accolate (zafirlukast), Singulair (montelukast), Onon (pranlukast)

Corticosteroids

Action

Corticosteroids are medications that inhibit inflammatory and immunologic processes. These agents are postulated to decrease the synthesis and release of a variety of mediators (eg, prostaglandins, leukotrienes, histamine) within lymphocytes, eosinophils, neutrophils, and mast cells.

Side Effects

CNS: Depression, euphoria, headache, restlessness
CV: HTN, angioedema, vasculitis
Endocrine: Hyperglycemia
GI: Peptic ulcers, nausea, vomiting
Miscellaneous: Osteoporosis, myopathy, weight gain, skin fragility/tears, immunosuppression, paradoxical bronchospasm, glaucoma, candidiasis, fluid retention/edema, Cushingoid appearance (eg, moon face/buffalo hump)

Common Medications

Beclovent, Vanceril, Qvar (beclomethasone-inhaled); Flovent (fluticasone); Alvesco (ciclesonide); Asmanex (mometasone furoate inhaled); Medrol (methylprednisolone); Deltasone (prednisone); Prelone (prednisolone); Pulmicort (budesonide inhaled); Azmacort (triamcinolone); AeroBid (flunisolide inhaled)
Combination (inhaled-beta 2 agonist and corticosteroid): Advair (fluticasone and salmeterol), Breo Ellipta (fluticasone furoate and vilanterol inhalation powder), Dulera (mometasone furoate and formoterol fumarate), Symbicort (budesonide and formoterol), Combivent Respimat (ipratropium and albuterol)

Phosphodiesterase-4 Inhibitors

Action

Act by increasing intracellular concentrations of cAMP resulting in a broad range of anti-inflammatory effects.

Side Effects

CNS: Suicidal (rare), insomnia, headache
GI: Decreased weight, decreased appetite, diarrhea, nausea, abdominal pain
Miscellaneous: Not recommended with severely weakened immune system.

Common Medications

Daxas, Daliresp (roflumilast)

Smoking Cessation Drugs

Action

These agents replace nicotine by providing an influx of nicotine to help diminish cravings: nicotine receptor agonists, nicotine receptor blockers, and non-nicotine receptor agents. (Bupropion may potentiate effects of dopamine and norepinephrine in brain). Delivered via patch, gum, lozenge, nasal spray, and inhalers.

Side Effects

CNS: Mild headache, insomnia, dream abnormalities, dizziness, seizure
CV: Angina, dysrhythmias (avoid if recent myocardial infarction or CVA)
GI: Nausea, vomiting, anorexia, dry mouth, constipation, abdominal pain
Miscellaneous: Recommend counseling and social support to improve success rate, skin irritation with patch, loss of strength, excess gas in stomach, loss of taste, avoid if skin sensitivities to adhesive, combination therapy now available

Common Medications

Zyban (bupropion), Nicorette (nicotine polacrilex), Inversine (mecamylamine), Prozac (fluoxetine), Rexulti (brexpiprazole), Chantix (varenicline)

Medications Specific for Respiratory Secretions

Mucolytics

Action

Mucolytics decrease viscosity of mucus and promote expectoration by various mechanisms. For example, pulmonary infections and secretions attract leukocytes that degenerate, releasing large volumes of DNA. N-acetylcystein lyses mucus proteins, and rhDNAse assists in the clearance of airway DNA, decreasing airway obstruction.

Side Effects

CNS: Dizziness, headache
CV: Tachycardia, hypotension or HTN, chest pain
GI: Irritation of mouth and throat, nausea, vomiting
Miscellaneous: rhDNAse not proven efficacious with COPD and chronic bronchitis
Pulmonary: Bronchospasm, mucosal irritation, cough

Common Medications

rhDNAse/Pulmozyme (recombinant human deoxyribonuclease I/dornase alfa); Mucomyst, Mucomyst-10 (N-acetylcysteine)

Expectorants

Action

Expectorants facilitate mucous clearance and increase secretion of airway water, thin sputum in upper respiratory tract.

Side Effects

CNS: Dizziness, headache
GI: Diarrhea, nausea, vomiting, stomach pain
Miscellaneous: Rash

Common Medications

DuroTuss, Anti-Tuss,Humibid (guaifenesin)

Antitussives

Action

Antitussives bind at opiate receptor site in the CNS suppressing the cough reflex. Additionally, these agents may provide pain relief.

Side Effects

CNS: Suppression of cough reflex, sedation, drowsiness, lethargy, anxiety, dysphoria, mood changes, blurred vision

CV: Hypotension, bradycardia orthostatic hypotension risk with injection, chest tightness

GI: Constipation, nausea and vomiting

Pulmonary: Respiratory depression

Common Medications

Dilaudid (hydromorphone hydrochloride); TussiCaps (hydrocodone and chlorpheniramine polistirex); Solotuss (carbetapentane); Zonatuss, Tessalon Perles (benzonatate)

Inhaled Antibiotic Therapy

Action

Inhaled antibiotic therapy ensures high concentrations of chosen effective antibiotic to site of infection to facilitate maximum efficacy and long-term treatment with minimal systemic absorption and reduction in risks of toxicity

Side Effect

CNS: Headache, tinnitus, ototoxicity, dysgeusia

Miscellaneous: Bronchospasm, cough, hoarseness, dyspnea, pulmonary exacerbations, hemoptysis, productive cough, musculoskeletal chest pain, myalgia

Common Medications

Tobi (tobramyacin), Colobreathe (colistin)

Neuromuscular Blocking Agents

Action

Neuromuscular blocking agents impede or prevent transmission at the neuromuscular junction resulting in paralysis. Two classes are depolarizing agents or nondepolarizing agents.

Depolarizing agents react with receptors at muscle end-plate and results in overstimulation, so that the end-plate is unable to respond to further excitation. Prolonged exposure reduces receptor sensitivity manifested as flaccid paralysis. Often used for intubation.

Nondepolarizing/competitive agents bind at the muscle endplate's acetylcholine receptors resulting in a competitive, reversible blockade. These agents inhibit excitation potentials at endplate preventing the motor unit from reaching threshold.

Side Effects

CNS: Agents do not affect sensorium (agents are not anesthetics/analgesics), individuals are conscious and can feel pain

CV: Bradycardia, hypotension

GI: Increased gastric pressure with abdominal fasciculations

Miscellaneous: Prolonged paralysis/myopathy (associated with coadministration of corticosteroids/antibiotics/sedatives), hyperkalemia with depolarizing agents, antibiotics (eg, aminoglycosides, macrolides)

Pulmonary: Apnea, increased airway secretions, bronchoconstriction

Common Medications
Non-depolarizing: Norcuron (vecuronium), Pavulon (pancuronium), Tacrium (atracurium)
Depolarizing: Anectine, Quelicin, Sucostrin (succinylcholine)

Specific for Antifibrotic Agents

Action
Inhibits vascular endothelial growth factor, fibroblast growth factor receptor, and platelet-derived growth factor. Binds competitively to adenosine triphosphate and blocks signaling at the intracellular level for transformation, migration, and proliferation of fibroblasts.

Side Effects
CNS: Headaches
CV: HTN, arterial thrombosis, myocardial infarction
GI: Diarrhea, nausea, abdominal pain, vomiting, decreased appetite, GERD
Miscellaneous: Increased liver enzymes, bronchitis, weight loss, hypothyroidism, photosensitivity

Common Medications
Esbriet (pirfenidone), OFEV (nintedanib)

CNS = central nervous system; CV = cardiovascular.

Chapter 8

Musculoskeletal/Orthopedic Diseases and Disorders

Joseph Adler, PT, DPT, CCS

The acute care physical therapist will work with patients diagnosed with a variety of musculoskeletal-related health conditions but most therapists will provide care for patients with degenerative joint disease, spine pathology, and acute fracture related to trauma, and all of these health conditions may require surgical interventions. The physical therapist responsible for the examination, intervention, and physical therapy plan of care of the patient with orthopedic pathology must be familiar with several important and common issues, such as weightbearing and range of motion (ROM) restrictions, surgeon-specific activity protocols, and how to gait train a patient with multiple fractures, as well as appropriate indications for orthotic devices. Because patients frequently require assistive technologies, as well as specialized education in mobility, including ambulation, the physical therapist plays a vital role in the multidisciplinary team management of the patient with acute musculoskeletal dysfunction.

Elective Surgery

Protocols for postoperative orthopedic management often vary with different surgeons. When to initiate ROM activities, how much weightbearing is allowed and when, or if braces may be removed are all examples of surgeon-specific preferences. Prior to mobilizing the postoperative patient, the physical therapist should be confident that activity status and restrictions are documented and orders clarified.

Primary, or first time, total joint replacements are often progressed along institutional guidelines or clinical pathways.[1-3] Guideline or pathway outcomes center on improving functional outcomes, decreasing length of stay, and decreasing cost while mandating clinical activity, such as number of times per day physical therapy intervention should occur and what milestones are expected on a given postoperative day. Although the average length of stay has decreased over the past decade for elective joint replacements,[4] the evidence-based literature provides inconsistent data

Malone DJ, Bishop KL, eds. *Acute Care Physical Therapy: A Clinician's Guide, Second Edition* (pp 311-350).

on the impact of these guidelines on total cost and function at the time of discharge from the hospital.[2,5-7]

The most common joint replacements performed are **total knee arthroplasties** (TKAs) and **total hip arthroplasties** (THAs). According to the American Academy of Orthopedic Surgeons (AAOS) over 260,000 TKAs and 168,000 THAs are performed annually in the United States.[8] Progressive increase in arthritic pain, decline in physical function, and lack of response to conservative management are the primary reasons degenerative joints are replaced.[9] The degenerative process can be inflammatory, as in rheumatoid arthritis, non-inflammatory, as in osteoarthritis or related to post-traumatic arthritis, as noted in Table 8-1.

Rheumatoid arthritis is an autoimmune, polyarticular disease process of unknown etiology that targets the synovial membrane. The synovium hypertrophies, causing joint effusions, ligamentous damage, and eventual joint destruction. Episodes of relapse and remission are common. It is estimated between 1 and 3 million persons are affected with rheumatoid arthritis worldwide.[10] **Osteoarthritis** tends to be more prevalent in individuals over 50 years of age, directly affects articular cartilage, and may be caused by either mechanical or biochemical factors. Traumatic injuries that affect joint integrity or ligamentous structures (often with accompanying vascular damage) are also a cause of joint replacements. Although the predisposing conditions are different, physical therapy approach to acute TKA remains essentially the same, but therapists should anticipate greater challenges in the early mobilization of patients with multiple joint involvement (rheumatoid arthritis) or multiple system involvement (trauma).

Total Knee Arthroplasty (Figure 8-1)

Postoperative, hospital-based physical therapy intervention focuses on early mobilization, functional training, ROM, and discharge planning. Early, full weightbearing with an assistive device should be expected, although postoperative pain can be a limiting factor. The physical therapist will collaborate with the surgical and nursing staff in the prevention of deep vein thrombosis (DVT) and pulmonary emboli, as well as reduction of postoperative swelling and pain management.[11] The use of a continuous passive motion (CPM) machine during the immediate postoperative acute care phase is common, and the physical therapist may play an important role in the set-up and management of the device. However, there is mounting evidence suggesting that the use of a CPM for patients immediately following uncomplicated TKA provides no benefit across a spectrum of outcome measures.[12] The degrees of motion and when to increase those values are generally physician prescribed or protocol driven. CPM usage may provide an early benefit of increased ROM, particularly in the absence of time availability of a therapist. As greater knee ROM presumably provides greater functional ability, CPM may also impact hospital length of stay. When long-term follow-up has been performed, however, there appears to be no significant difference in ROM, pain, or function when comparing CPM as an adjunctive ROM therapy to physical therapy intervention without CPM.[13-15]

In addition to the physical therapist's focus on motor function and functional training, therapeutic exercise and patient/family education begin immediately. Surgeon preference is often based on a combination of literature-based outcomes and clinical experience, which is why one surgeon may want a regimen of quad sets, active assisted ROM, and a knee immobilizer worn until the patient can perform an independent straight leg raise, while another wants no brace, no quad sets, and active motion only in sitting. Once again, the therapist must be familiar with the surgeon's preferences.

Functional goals during the hospital phase will diverge depending on the immediate discharge disposition of the patient.[16,17] There may be specific institutional mechanisms where patients are transferred to a skilled orthopedic rehabilitation

Table 8-1

LOWER EXTREMITY JOINT ARTHROPLASTY

	Knee Arthroplasty	*Hip Arthroplasty*
Primary Diagnostic Indications	• Osteoarthritis • Rheumatoid arthritis • Post-traumatic arthritis	• Osteoarthritis • Rheumatoid arthritis • Post-traumatic arthritis • Proximal hip fracture ¤ Hemiarthroplasty indicated
Surgical Approach	• Anterior	• Posterolateral • Anterolateral • Two incisions ¤ Minimally invasive
Hardware	• Cobalt chrome femoral component • Metal-backed polyethylene tibial component	• Metallic femoral stem/head • Polyethylene acetabular liner
Acute Care Physical Therapy	• Early mobilization • ROM • Education ¤ Weightbearing ¤ Gait • CPM ¤ Monitor ¤ Progress • Discharge planning	• Early mobilization • Gentle strengthening • Education ¤ Hip precautions ¤ Weightbearing ¤ Gait • Discharge planning

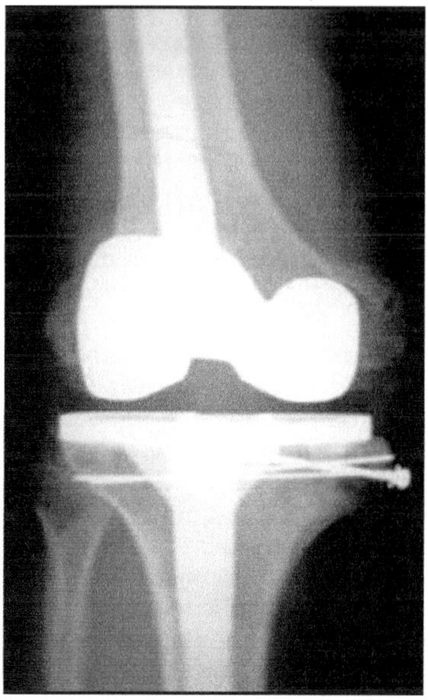

Figure 8-1. Total knee arthroplasty performed for hemophiliac arthropathy with medial tibial structural autograft and press-fit stems. (Reprinted with permission from Canale ST. *Campbell's Operative Orthopaedics*. 10th ed. St. Louis, MO: Mosby Inc; 2003.)

unit. If this process does not exist, then an early determination must be made with the patient whether functional goals can be achieved (eg, stair management, bathroom self-care) to allow for discharge to home. In an increasingly cost-conscious health care environment, therapists are asked to make this discharge recommendation after only 1 or 2 sessions and must take into consideration factors such as falls risk, patient goals, insurance restrictions, and patient tolerance for ongoing therapy.

Examination of the patient after knee replacement focuses on functional mobility, muscle performance, and knee ROM. Goniometric measurements of knee flexion and extension are common data collected throughout the hospital stay and become part of objective documented progress. Other baseline data to collect are integumentary and joint integrity and patient reports of pain. Ninety degrees of passive knee flexion is generally expected prior to discharge from the hospital. If, after several weeks or months, stiffness, pain, and lack of functional ROM persist, manipulation under anesthesia may be indicated (Table 8-2).[18,19]

Total Hip Arthroplasty (Figure 8-2)

The components of total hip replacements are made from metal alloys, high-grade plastics, and polymeric materials. Implants are either cemented in place, not cemented, or a hybrid of the 2. The needs and individual circumstances of each patient determine the surgeon's choice of procedure.[8] A non-cemented prosthesis has a specialized, porous surface texture that stimulates bone growth. These non-cemented femoral stems have small openings allowing for bone to attach and grow through. Because the soft-tissue capsule and musculature surrounding the hip joint are cut and entered to replace the degenerative joint, patients are placed on what are commonly referred to as **hip precautions** postoperatively. These precautions attempt to limit excessive motion of the hip and prevent dislocation of a joint that does not have normal restraints to motion due to surgery. Patients are educated on these precautions that may last weeks to months, throughout the hospital stay.[20,21] Specific precautions are dependent on the surgical approach. The hip joint is approached either posterolaterally, anterolaterally, or by 2 smaller incisions, front and back. Posterolateral approach precautions are no hip flexion past 90 degrees, no adduction past neutral (or midline), and no internal rotation. The anterolateral and 2-incision approaches primarily restrict hip extension especially with external rotation.[22,23] Rotation at the hip joint is a relative motion created by either motion of the leg in relation to the trunk (femoral head on acetabulum) or the trunk in relation to the leg (acetabulum on the femoral head). Patients must be cautioned about common activities that involve twisting motions of the trunk, such as reaching across the body to answer the phone while lying in bed. As surgical techniques and technology advance therapists are encountering the 2-incision, or minimally invasive, approach. Although the prosthetic components are the same as traditional approaches, 2 smaller incisions are made, 1 anterior and 1 posterior. The soft tissue capsule is still violated, but less muscle is incised to enter the hip joint. Proponents of this relatively newer technique report less blood loss, reduced hospitals stays, and quicker return to function.[8]

Several studies have examined the forces applied to the hip joint during functional activity, and these data often influence postoperative strengthening protocols.[24,25] Ankle pumps and quad and glute sets are usually initiated with first patient contact postoperatively as these are gentle yet active. Depending on the institution, the patient will have between 1 and 3 physical therapy sessions daily, according to patient tolerance. As out of bed endurance increases, supported standing exercises (in the parallel bars or at a walker) for the operated hip begin. Gentle, active, antigravity hip flexion, abduction, and extension, while maintaining precautions, have been a standard and effective hospital-based regimen at our institution. The goal of these exercises is to prevent postoperative stiffness and pain while improving functional strength for bed mobility, transfers, stair climbing, and ambulation. Unless

Table 8-2

SUMMARY OF PHYSICAL THERAPY AND KNEE ARTHROPLASTY

- Generally, physical therapy begins postoperative day 1.
- Patients are usually weightbearing as tolerated with an assistive device.
- Active range of motion (AROM) and strengthening begin immediately and are generally accompanied by surgeon-specific protocols.
- Although not achieved by all patients, a knee flexion ROM goal for the acute phase is 0 to 90 degrees.
- Discharge planning begins with the initial examination (see Chapter 1).
- Assist surgical and nursing team with postoperative complication prevention:
  - Breathing exercises to promote lung function (see Chapter 7)
  - Active exercise, weightbearing as indicated, and out of bed activity to prevent thromboembolic disease
- Physical therapy intervention:
  - Education
  - Mobility
  - ROM
  - Discharge recommendations

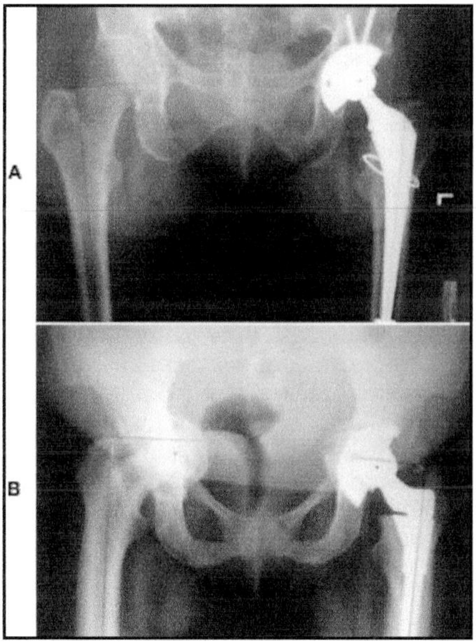

Figure 8-2. Total hip arthroplasty. Note relation of femoral neck orientation to vertical height. (A) Valgus femoral neck with large vertical height. (B) Varus femoral neck with large femoral offset. (Reprinted with permission from Canale ST. *Campbell's Operative Orthopaedics*. 10th ed. St. Louis, MO: Mosby Inc; 2003.)

discharged to an inpatient rehabilitation unit, the expectation is that the patient will be independent with a home exercise program, safe with all aspects of household level mobility and knowledgeable about precautions prior to discharge home.

The weightbearing status of the patient depends on several factors: implant type, surgeon preference, and any intraoperative events or findings. Traditionally, a primary difference between cemented and non-cemented prostheses was that cemented allowed for earlier, full weightbearing, whereas greater time is required for bone to attach to porous implants requiring restricted weightbearing. Long-term studies, however, have demonstrated the durability of both types of hip replacements, and therapists will treat patients who are full weightbearing, regardless of implant type. The physical therapist should expect to use a bilateral assistive device initially, regardless of implant type, to safely mobilize the patient at the bedside. Cemented implants are allowed weightbearing to tolerance, yet do not generally progress to a cane until outpatient follow-up with the surgeon. Non-cemented implants require more restrictive initial weightbearing, as a longer time is required for bone to attach to the implant. These patients may be partially weightbearing (approximately 50% of full), toe-touch, or minimally weightbearing (approximately 10%), or non-weightbearing (NWB), depending on surgeon protocol.

A physical therapist will collaborate with other health care team members (eg, nurses, occupational therapists) on patient education regarding the restricted motions of the hip during functional activities, and are a fundamental component of post-surgical rehabilitation. Patients usually wake up after surgery with some type of pillow or wedge between their legs preventing adduction past mid line. Often, this is accompanied by a knee-immobilizer on the operated leg to further prevent unwanted knee and hip flexion. Use of assistive technologies, such as long-handled reachers, shoehorns, leg lifters, elevated toilet seats, and walkers are all part of early postoperative instructions. This equipment should promote successful performance while maintaining designated precautions with dressing, bathing, hygiene, and feeding.

Problems encountered with hip replacements are pain that results from loosening of the cement/prosthesis interface as well as dislocation. Remediation of these problems includes relocation under anesthesia, application of preventative dislocation braces, and surgical revision or reimplantation. Long-term follow-up, however, demonstrates excellent clinical results for most patients regardless of the type of implant used (Table 8-3).[26,27]

Total Shoulder Arthroplasty

Total shoulder arthroplasty (TSA) is the most common upper extremity (UE) arthroplasty and the third most commonly encountered joint replacement by physical therapists after TKA and THA.[28,29] Surgical intervention is indicated when conservative treatments are no longer effective and pain limits functional activity to an unacceptable degree. The primary diseases affecting the glenohumeral joint are degenerative arthritis, traumatic arthritis, osteonecrosis, rheumatoid arthritis, and rotator cuff arthropathy. Shoulder replacement can include total or hemiarthroplasty when there is no glenoid involvement, as in proximal humeral fractures.[30] Typical hospital length of stay after shoulder replacement is 2 to 3 days with instruction on early shoulder mobilization beginning postoperative day 1. Patients are instructed in passive forward flexion and external rotation and encouraged to perform these exercises independently several times per day. Active hand and elbow motion will maintain strength and minimize edema. Use of ice for pain and edema control is encouraged. Hip level activity of the involved arm is allowed but without lifting, pushing, carrying, or pulling. Patients can expect several months of rehabilitation for TSA as they progress through phases of strengthening and ROM exercises. Intensity of outpatient rehabilitation will, of course, be dependent on the individual goals of the patient.[29]

Spinal Surgery

The acute care therapist typically encounters 3 types of spinal surgery: discectomy combined with laminectomy, decompression, and fusion. These procedures are all encountered in both the cervical and lumbar spines (see Tables 9-20 through 9-22).[31]

Table 8-3

SUMMARY OF PHYSICAL THERAPY AND HIP ARTHROPLASTY

- Physical therapy usually begins postoperative day 1.
- Multiple factors dictate weightbearing status; therefore, determine proper weightbearing status prior to initial examination.
- Education regarding hip precautions accompanies every session.
- AROM and strengthening begins immediately but may have surgeon restrictions.
- Discharge planning begins with the initial examination (see Chapter 1).
- Assist surgical and nursing team with postoperative complication prevention:
  - Breathing exercises to promote lung function (see Chapter 7)
  - Active exercise, weightbearing as indicated, and out of bed activity to prevent thromboembolic disease
- Physical therapy intervention:
  - Education
  - Mobility
  - Strengthening
  - Discharge recommendations

Lumbar disc disease (primarily the lower segments of L4–L5 and L5–S1) is the most prevalent cause of surgical intervention and increased morbidity in the United States, with thoracic disease accounting for <1% of herniated disc disease.[32] Approximately 285,000 fusions are performed in the United States annually, with slightly more than half in the lumbar region.[8] As with other chronic orthopedic health conditions, patients seek surgical treatment when conservative measures (eg, non-steroidal anti-inflammatory drugs, outpatient physical therapy, steroid injections) no longer are effective in controlling pain as physical function becomes impaired to an unsatisfactory degree.[33]

Sources of low back pain can be intervertebral disc herniation, stenosis of either the central vertebral canal or foramina, and degenerative disc disease with accompanying spondylolisthesis. Decompression of neural structures via excision of protruding or herniated interdiscal material (**discectomy**), removal of bone (**decompression**), and stabilization of hypermobile vertebrae (**fusion**) are primary indications for spinal surgery.[31]

Discectomy

This is the least invasive of the 3 types of procedures, often referred to as **microdiscectomy** because microscopic lenses are used to visualize the operating field. Discectomies are typically accompanied by laminectomies. In the absence of complications, patients usually require 1 overnight stay in the hospital. Orthotic bracing is not indicated in the acute phase.[34]

Laminectomy

This is a more involved surgical procedure than discectomy, particularly when more than 1 vertebral level is involved. The term **hemilaminectomy** refers to 1 side of a vertebral level (left or right) that is excised. Orthotic bracing is not indicated in the acute phase.

Decompression

Decompression is a procedure whereby the posterior elements of the vertebral column are removed, including lamina and spinous process. Foramens are widened to relieve pressure on neural elements.

Fusion

When vertebrae are fused, the spine can be approached either anteriorly or posteriorly. When both approaches are performed, they either occur during the same surgery or can be separated by days during the same hospitalization. Fusion material is a combination of hardware (eg, pedicle screws, cages) and bone. Bone may come from a bone bank (allograft) or from the patient (autogenous). Autogenous grafts are usually harvested from the iliac crest. This donor site is frequently painful during the postoperative hospital phase and may require the use of an ambulatory assistive device to mitigate an antalgic gait pattern.[35]

Orthotic bracing is often ordered by the surgeon after fusion to provide external support. The type of brace and wearing schedule will vary with the surgeon and evidence-based literature is equivocal about long-term outcomes.[36] Instruction about the brace is given initially by the orthotist who fabricates and issues the brace, but subsequent education and training during functional activities is done by the therapist. The therapist needs to have a good working knowledge of proper application and fit of prescribed braces. The orthotist may fit the brace in supine but not sit or stand the patient. Improperly fitting braces may either be too high under the axilla/throat/neck area or too long across the hips, limiting hip flexion and upright sitting. Postoperative edema may also cause a brace that was measured preoperatively to appear improperly sized. When these situations are encountered, the therapist should contact the fabricating orthotist for modifications. When the L5–S1 junction is fused, a brace with a thigh piece extension may be prescribed and requires more intensive education and training prior to discharge due to an inability to sit with hips flexed at 90 degrees.

Spinal Precautions

Regardless of the type of surgery, therapists will instruct patients in **spinal precautions** postoperatively. Spinal precautions typically involve some limitations for bending, lifting, and twisting (BLT). There is scant evidence that has examined the application of spinal precautions and yet patients are frequently educated on them.[37] A log rolling technique is used to get out of bed. The hips and shoulders roll as 1 unit, protecting against painful spinal rotation. Excessive trunk flexion is cautioned against when sitting. Extended periods of sitting generally cause pain and stiffness and should be limited, and lifting is restricted. Patients do not usually have weightbearing restrictions after spinal surgeries, but ambulatory assistive devices can provide stability during walking activities and give confidence to the patient. Physical therapy intervention focuses on functional mobility, patient education, pain management, and assistance with appropriate discharge planning. Therapeutic exercise that addresses strength or flexibility deficits, other than gentle active ROM of the extremities, are generally not initiated in the acute care setting and should only be applied judiciously (Table 8-4).

TRAUMA

Physical therapy intervention for the acutely injured orthopedic patient varies widely. In smaller facilities the therapist may primarily encounter isolated extremity fractures or dislocations, whereas the therapist working in a larger trauma center will encounter patients with multiple injuries who have sustained fractures to multiple extremities, spine,

Table 8-4

Summary of Physical Therapy and Spinal Surgery

• Therapists educate patients in: ¤ Log rolling ¤ Avoiding heavy lifting ¤ Avoiding prolonged sitting ¤ Brace application and wearing schedule (if appropriate) • Patients are usually full weightbearing. • Expect pain from autogenous bone graft (use assistive device as needed). • Stair climbing is not contraindicated. • Assist surgical and nursing team with postoperative complication prevention: ¤ Breathing exercises to promote lung function (see Chapter 7) ¤ Active exercise, weightbearing as indicated, and out of bed activity to prevent thromboembolic event • Physical therapy intervention: ¤ Education ¤ Mobility ¤ Discharge recommendations
See also Table 9-22.

and pelvis. Injuries from gunshot wounds, unfortunately, are consuming large resources of orthopedic surgery departments that work in urban trauma centers.[38,] Therapists work under difficult conditions of multi-system trauma as well as related criminal activity. Working with orthopedic injury as a result of trauma becomes more challenging in the presence of other body-system injuries, particularly traumatic brain injury, and often necessitates recommendations for continuing levels of in-patient rehabilitation care. This section examines frequently seen orthopedic injuries associated with trauma.

Spine Trauma

When the spine is involved in acute trauma, the surgical team asked to evaluate the patient must determine whether bony and/or neurological injury has occurred, if the spine is stable, and if not, how to appropriately manage the instability. To evaluate the spine a combination of diagnostic imaging (ie, x-ray, computed tomography [CT] scan, and magnetic resonance imaging [MRI]) and clinical exam is used to assess the extent of the injury. Anatomically, the spine can be divided into 3 columns: anterior, middle, and posterior (Figure 8-3). When 2 or more columns are injured, ligamentous damage generally occurs and the spine is considered unstable. To stabilize the spine, surgical internal fixation, external rigid bracing, or both are required (Figure 8-4). The physical therapist must understand what structures are involved in the injury, what procedures have been performed, whether and what type of bracing is indicated, and whether a definitive plan has been clearly documented.

Transverse or Spinous Process Fractures

These are often seen in high-energy impact injuries, such as motor vehicle crashes (MVC) and falls from heights. These injuries typically do not require surgical fixation or weightbearing restrictions. Pain with motion is common, especially during the rotational movements that occur during bed mobility. These fractures do not require bracing from a stability standpoint but may be indicated to reduce pain and promote greater functional mobility.

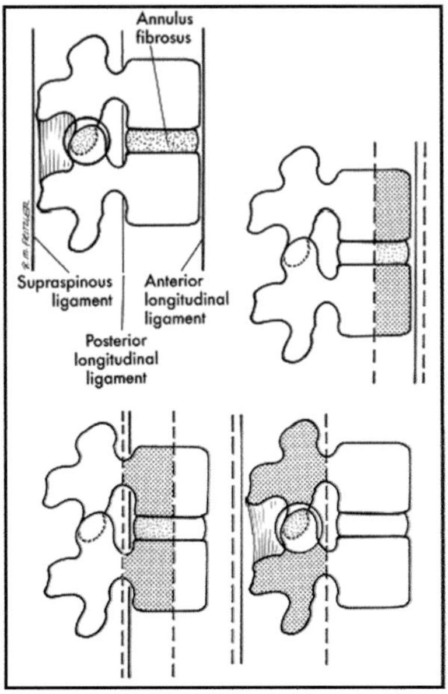

Figure 8-3. The 3-column concept of spinal injury. (A) Anterior column contains the anterior longitudinal ligament, the anterior half of the vertebral body, and the anterior portion of the annulus fibrosis. (B) The middle column consists of the posterior long ligament, the posterior half of the vertebral body, and the posterior aspect of the annulus fibrosus. (C) The posterior column includes the neural arch, the ligamentum flavum, the facet capsules, and the interspinous ligaments. (Reprinted with permission from Canale ST. *Campbell's Operative Orthopaedics*. 10th ed. St. Louis, MO: Mosby Inc; 2003.)

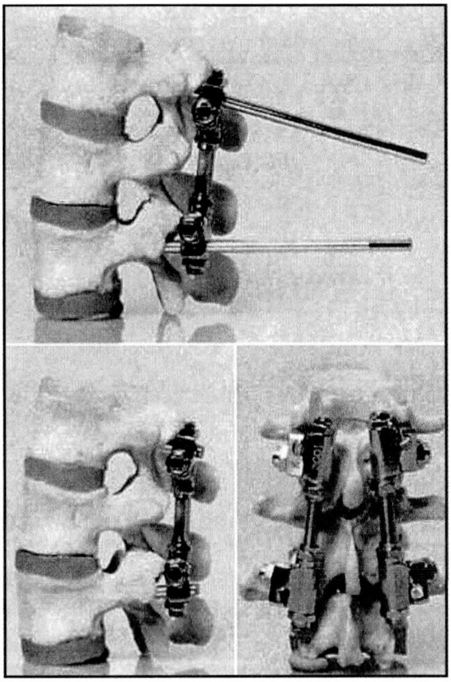

Figure 8-4. Example of Cotrel-Dubousset instrumentation for spinal fracture-dislocations and unstable burst fractures. (Reprinted with permission from Canale ST. *Campbell's Operative Orthopaedics*. 10th ed. St. Louis, MO: Mosby Inc; 2003.)

Table 8-5 SUMMARY OF PHYSICAL THERAPY AND SPINAL TRAUMA
• When the spine is injured, the therapist must be assured that the spine is cleared for mobility. • When braces/orthotics are ordered, the therapist must understand the wearing schedule (ie, hours on/off, activity limitations, time in sitting). • The therapist should be attentive to signs and symptoms of possible neurological impairment resulting from spine injury
See also Tables 9-21 and 9-22.

Ligamentous Injury

Ligamentous injury of the spine is more commonly seen in the cervical spine than in either the thoracic or lumbar regions. Flexion/extension x-rays, sometimes in combination with CT scans, can confirm excessive spinal motion and is typically managed by rigid bracing for 6 to 12 weeks (see Table 8-10 later in this chapter). Weightbearing restrictions during ambulation are generally not required. Patient education must include proper application and wearing schedule.

Compression or Burst Vertebral Body Fractures

A burst fracture is a comminuted compression fracture of the vertebral body that can include retropulsion of fragments into the spinal canal.[40] These injuries occur from pure flexion moments with little or no rotation and are commonly seen in high energy injuries, such as falls from great heights or gunshot wounds. They often require rigid bracing and surgical intervention to maintain spinal extension (see Figure 8-4). Weightbearing during ambulation is not restricted but can obviously be impaired by pain.

Multiple-Level Injury

When multiple levels of the spine are involved (eg, L2–L4, T10–T12) clinical experience has shown that pain is significantly increased with functional mobility. The physical therapist must collaborate with the medical/surgical team to optimize pain management and scheduling of therapy. When multi-level injures combine with spinal instability (2-column involvement) surgical intervention is required. Bracing may or may not be indicated after surgery depending on surgeon preference (Table 8-5). Physical therapy intervention and education must address prevention of the known postoperative complications of pneumonia, DVT, infection, and pressure-related skin breakdown.

Pelvis (Figure 8-5)

Injuries to the pelvis can involve several anatomical areas including the acetabulum, ilium, and pubic rami. For the sake of convenience, the sacrum will be included, although anatomically it is not part of the pelvis proper.

As the acetabular cup is composed of several bones fused together, fracture nomenclature often refers to either the anterior or posterior column. Small chip or non-displaced fractures generally do not require surgical intervention but may require weightbearing restrictions on the side of the injury and necessitate use of an assistive device during ambulation to safely unload pressure. Larger, displaced, or comminuted fractures, as seen in fracture/dislocations in MVCs when the head of the femur is posteriorly displaced, require internal fixation. When dislocation occurs,

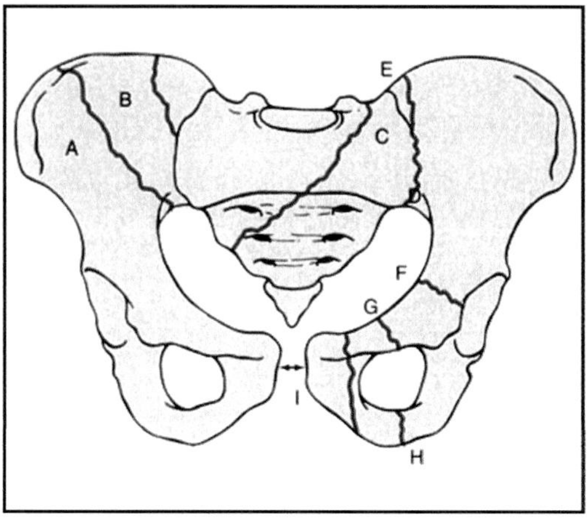

Figure 8-5. The Letournel and Judet classification of pelvic fractures. (A) Iliac wing fractures. (B) Ilium fractures with extension to the sacroiliac joint. (C) Transsacral fractures. (D) Unilateral sacral fractures. (E) Sacroiliac joint fracture-dislocation. (F) Acetabular fracture. (G) Pubic ramus fractures. (H) Ischial fractures. (I) Pubic symphysis separation. (Reprinted from Browner BD, Jupiter JB, Levine AM, Trafton P. *Skeletal Trauma: Basic Science, Management, and Reconstruction.* 5th ed. 2015, with permission from Elsevier.)

whether or not a fracture is present, patients are often NWB acutely and placed on the same postoperative hip precautions as seen after hip replacement surgery because the capsular ligaments have been stretched.

The superior and inferior pubic rami may be fractured individually or together. These injuries typically do not require surgical fixation or weightbearing restrictions but are very painful. The therapist should anticipate pain with bed mobility and standing. Collaboration with the medical and nursing team in aggressive pain management is fundamental to enable the patient maximum mobility, thus preventing possible secondary bed rest–associated complications. Because of the anatomical position of the rami, the pain associated with movement tends not to respond to orthotic management (ie, bracing that could provide compressive support).

When the sacrum is involved in bony injury, surgeons will often refer to either left- or right-sided involvement. If the fracture extends into the sacroiliac joint, a weightbearing restriction usually applies. In severe injury, bars or a plate will be used for fracture fixation. This patient may be allowed out of bed and allowed to ambulate with an assistive device as tolerated. The immediate complication the therapist confronts is usually pain as the patient attempts to flex the trunk to attain a functional sitting position. This inability to achieve a sitting position may necessitate dependent transfers initially and often has an impact on discharge recommendations. These types of injuries often require 2-person assist during the acute phase (for rolling, sitting, and all out of bed transfers) as well as aggressive pain management, especially prior to therapy intervention.

When major trauma has occurred to the pelvis, disrupting the anatomical structure known as the **pelvic ring**, the use of external or internal fixation is generally required.[33,34] These patients are functionally limited by pain, as well as mechanically blocked by the fixation bars from achieving a functional sitting position. Dependent or assisted transfers to a reclining wheelchair that has an adjustable back angle should be employed to facilitate out of bed benefits (cardiovascular and pulmonary) and UE activity (wheelchair propulsion). When major trauma has occurred to the pelvis, the therapist should anticipate associated injuries to the perineal area that may involve painful mobility-limiting edema.[41]

Extremities

Nearly all components of the appendicular skeleton can be fractured during trauma. This section is not meant to be an exhaustive list but rather to emphasize commonly seen fractures and how therapists can appropriately intervene in the acute care setting for both UE and lower extremity (LE) injuries. Common fracture terminology and hardware are provided in Tables 8-6 and 8-7 and Figure 8-6.

Upper Extremity

UE fractures include digits, carpal bones, radius, ulna, humerus, clavicle, and scapula. The physical therapist should anticipate the use of a shoulder sling, particularly with more proximal fractures, that will provide support and comfort during out of bed activities. The patient should be educated in removing the sling while in bed or seated and positioning the extremity to minimize the effects of gravity-induced swelling. Active or active assisted shoulder motion, when allowed, should be taught to minimize the stiffness that will accompany long-standing shoulder immobility and internal rotation. Figure-of-8 slings may be indicated for clavicle fractures or sternoclavicular dislocations. These braces are fit over both shoulders maintaining the scapulae in an adducted, retracted position.

When examining a patient with any UE fracture, there are several concerns the physical therapist must address: is there active motion and intact sensation distal and proximal to the injured segment, and does a weightbearing restriction exist? If a restriction does exist, what impact will it have on mobility, especially in the context of other extremity fractures? An example to illustrate this point is presented in Table 8-8.

Humeral fractures may be splinted and placed in a shoulder sling post-injury without surgical intervention. Humeral fractures are generally NWB as any axial load through the hand/wrist or forearm will be transmitted proximally. Consider this patient fully NWB through the entire UE but remember to encourage hand/wrist and elbow motion where applicable. Anticipate and seek collaboration with occupational therapy for most UE injuries, especially when the dominant hand is involved.

Fractures of the forearm can be isolated to the radius, ulna, or both. These may be internally or externally fixated. As discussed in the case example (see Table 8-8), when the fracture is in the distal third of the forearm, regardless of type of fixation, the patient may be allowed to bear weight through the proximal third of the forearm/elbow on a platform attachment to a crutch or walker.

Lower Extremity

The physical therapist intervenes with a wide range of LE fractures and must be scrupulous in several different areas: reliably verifying the weightbearing status, assessing wound status during functional activities, applying appropriate bracing (if indicated), and selecting the most appropriate assistive device based on weightbearing, activity restrictions, and current functional ability.

Femur

Physical therapists will treat patients who have fractured all parts of the femur: proximally at the neck or intertrochanteric line, mid-shaft, or distally, with or without involvement of the knee joint.[35] Proximal fractures are most often internally fixed (ORIF) while femoral neck fractures often receive a hemiarthroplasty (**hemi** as opposed to **total**; if the acetabulum is unaffected by injury or degenerative joint disease there is no need to replace it). Mid-shaft and distal femoral fractures are either internally fixed, often with an intramedullary rod, or externally fixed when significant soft tissue damage is present (Figure 8-7). The femur is usually casted, whether or not surgical fixation has occurred, for distal fractures. The cast is often flexed at the knee to keep the foot off the floor and assist with NWB transfers and ambulation.

Hip Fracture

The therapist working in acute care orthopedics should anticipate treating the elderly patient who has fallen and broken his or her hip. Much research focuses on

Table 8-6 FRACTURE TERMINOLOGY	
Type	*Description*
Open	• Violation of the skin • Often associated with high-energy injury • Increased risk of infection • Stabilized with external or internal fixation • Requires immediate sterile irrigation, debridement, and antibiotics
Closed	• No violation of the skin
Nondisplaced	• Fracture segments not displaced relative to each other
Displaced	• Fracture segments displaced relative to each other
Simple	• Two fractured parts
Comminuted	• Three or more fractured parts
See Figure 8-3.	

Table 8-7 FRACTURE HARDWARE	
Type	*Description*
Dynamic hip screw	• Commonly used to stabilize intertrochanteric hip fractures • One large screw with a side plate and several small screws
Intramedullary hip screw	• Generic term for a longitudinal rod placed within the medullary canal • Stabilizes diaphyseal long bone fractures • Combination of intramedullary rod and dynamic hip screw • Stabilizes intertrochanteric hip fractures
Percutaneous pin	• Pin placed through the skin • Stabilizes bone, fracture, or joint
Open reduction internal fixation (ORIF)	• Term used when skin must be opened and hardware placed to reduce and stabilize a fracture
External fixation	• Structure of connected pins and bars inserted externally through the skin • Generally used to stabilize high-energy, comminuted fracture with significant soft tissue damage • Allows access for wound care

hip fracture in the elderly, as it is a tremendous financial and societal burden.[42-47] The common orthopedic surgical interventions for hip fractures are ORIFs and hemiarthroplasties with determination of procedure based on several factors: prior activity level of the patient (independent community dweller vs wheelchair bound or minimally ambulatory) and quality of bone (soft osteoporotic bone does not hold

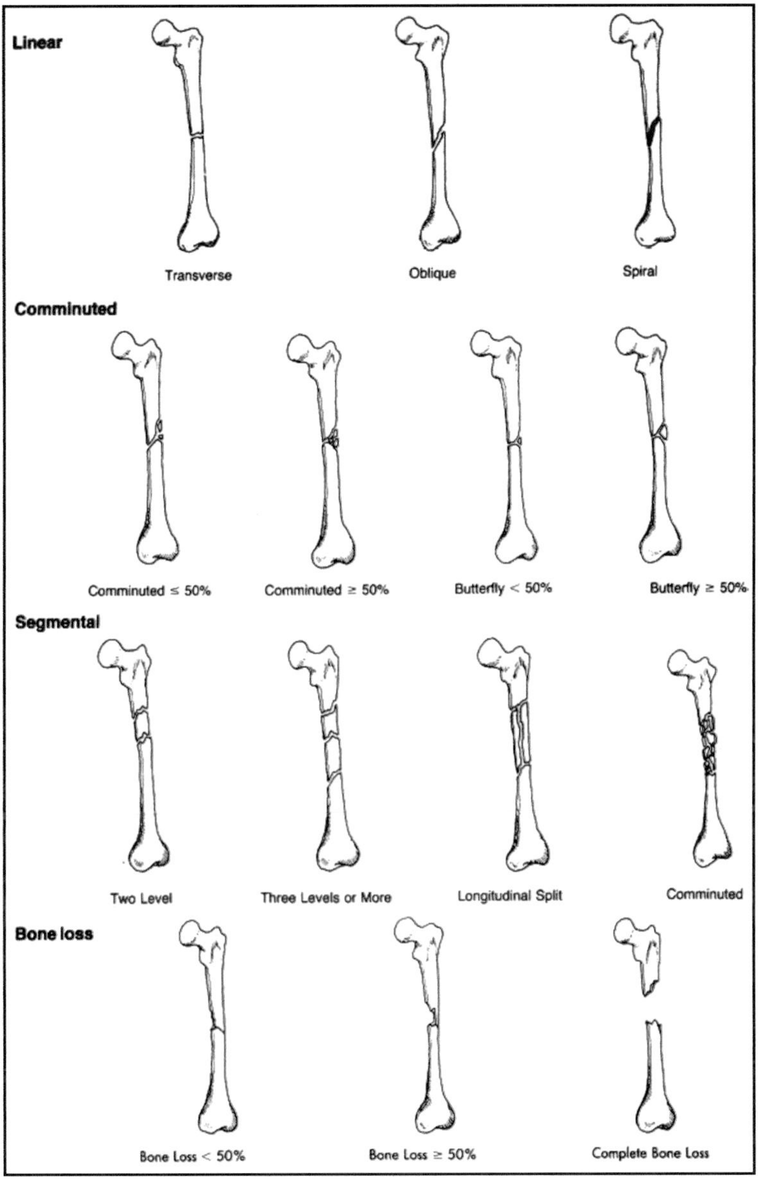

Figure 8-6. Classification of long bone fractures. (Reprinted with permission from Canale ST. *Campbell's Operative Orthopaedics.* 10th ed. St. Louis, MO: Mosby Inc; 2003.)

screws well). When treating the elderly patient who has fractured a hip, the physical therapist encounters several challenging issues: presence of comorbid conditions, weightbearing restrictions complicating mobility, fear and depression regarding loss of independence, and poor tolerance to narcotic pain medication, often resulting in acute delirium. Therapists working with this population are challenged to mobilize

Table 8-8

Case Example

A 24-year-old female is in an MVC and sustains fractures of the left femur and the right distal radius. Both require ORIF. A physical therapy consult is placed. The postoperative activity order states "NWB LLE [left lower extremity] and NWB RUE [right upper extremity]." Based on the orders as written, this patient should not be allowed to ambulate because, for most patients, it is neither safe nor feasible to maintain NWB on one LE without using both UEs. Functional goals will focus on transfers and wheelchair mobility.

Further discussion by the physical therapist with the orthopedic surgeons regarding weightbearing restrictions, however, changes the activity status of her RUE to include weightbearing through the proximal forearm/elbow. Now that she can use both UEs she has the opportunity to ambulate with a platform attachment on either a walker or crutch. This patient now has ambulation goals. The difference between having ambulation goals and having only transfer goals often influences discharge disposition.

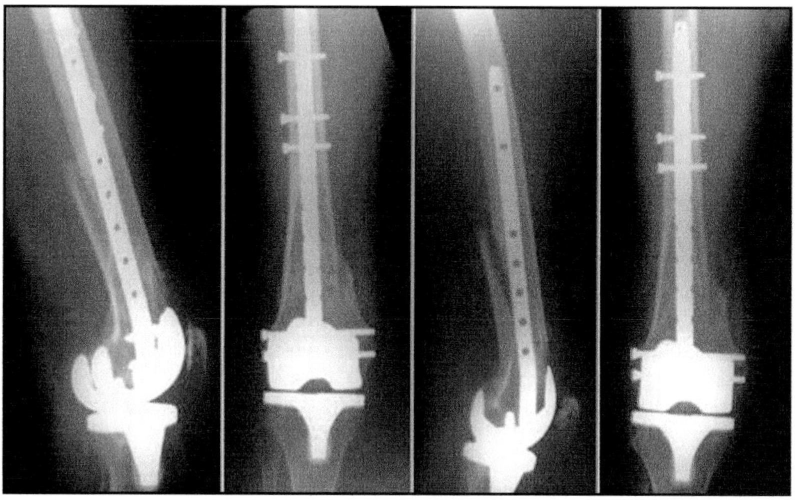

Figure 8-7. Supracondylar intramedullary nail used for fixation of femur fracture. (Reprinted with permission from Canale ST. *Campbell's Operative Orthopaedics*. 10th ed. St. Louis, MO: Mosby Inc; 2003.)

these patients quickly because much literature supports early return to ambulation as an important indicator of return to pre-hospital function.[48,49]

Knee

Injuries involving the knee, including patellar or quadriceps tendon ruptures or patellar fractures, are usually managed surgically and then braced or casted, postoperatively.[50] Postoperative immobilization frequently requires knee immobilizers, dial-lock knee braces, or cylinder-type casts made of either plaster or fiberglass with the foot and ankle left free to move. The therapist should anticipate pain if knee flexion occurs with weightbearing. The use of knee immobilizers and other foam and metal braces may not completely prevent unwanted knee flexion with axial loading. Clinical experience has shown that cylinder casting provides the greatest functional stabilization of full knee extension. This type of injury, once surgically fixed and externally immobilized, allows full weightbearing. The therapist should prepare for difficult sit-to-stand transfers, especially in the complicated instance of bilateral involvement, because the patient is at a considerable biomechanical disadvantage while attempting to rise to, or lower from, a standing position. Use of hospital bed height elevation is generally required secondary to lack of knee flexion. In fact, when considering recommendations for post-hospital discharge a hospital bed that elevates can make the difference between dependent and independent bed mobility and transfers.

Foot/Ankle Complex

Closed fractures of the foot/ankle complex (ie, metatarsals, malleoli, calcanei) that require surgical fixation often have too much traumatic edema to either internally fix or cast immobilize acutely. This patient remains splinted (posterior half cast) and is strictly NWB. If the injury is isolated and unilateral in the absence of significant comorbidities, this patient generally has good potential for gait training. If there is bilateral involvement, the patient must be instructed in NWB transfers to a wheelchair and commode. This type of transfer requires adequate UE strength to achieve independence or minimal dependence. Expect this individual to be non-ambulatory for several months and require ongoing episodes of physical therapy for ROM, strengthening, and gait training as bone healing progresses.

External Fixation

When high-energy fractures occur in combination with extensive soft tissue damage, external fixation devices are applied.[51] External fixators are made of titanium pins and rods inserted externally through the skin and connected to each other to provide fracture stabilization. External fixators of the LE can span either the length of the femur or tibia or cross the knee joint (Figure 8-8). Distal tibia fractures may require fixation extending from the lower third of the leg across the ankle joint.

Mobilizing patients with external fixators can be intimidating. The physical therapist should keep in mind that most individuals have never seen an external fixation device, and the sight of pins and rods protruding from the skin can be anxiety producing. When assisting a patient out of bed, clinical experience has demonstrated that patient comfort is increased if the injured limb is moved by the rods of the external fixation device rather than by supporting the skin and soft tissue underneath.

The therapist should examine the limb for excessive or purulent drainage from the pin sites, as well as pistoning (up and down motion) of the pins. Skin movement around pin sites is normal and may mimic a pistoning pin, but a loose pin no longer provides fracture stabilization and should be attended to immediately. The therapist must stop activity and contact the surgical team, as readjustment may be required.

Many LE external fixators are constructed to prevent heel breakdown because patients spend so much time in bed. Elongated pins connected to the fixators project posteriorly at the foot/ankle so the heel rests without contact when the patient is supine. Although this provides excellent prophylactic pressure relief, these pins add depth and width to the fixation device and can complicate ambulation. When lower leg external fixation devices are applied around the foot and ankle, standard practice at our institution is to custom mold a footplate (held in place by rubber exercise band attached to the pins) with the intent of maintaining neutral dorsiflexion and preventing ankle or forefoot contractures.

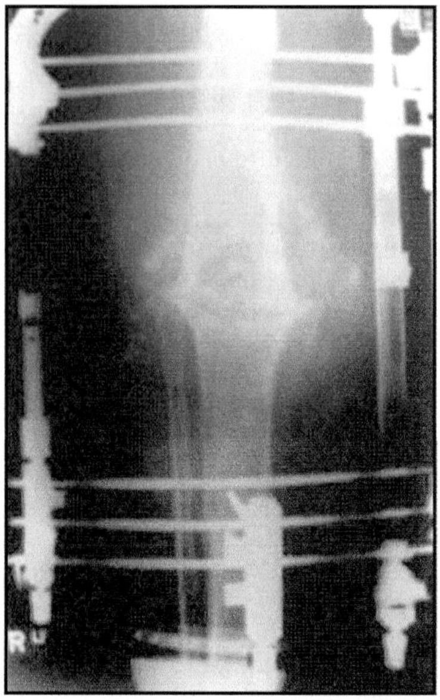

Figure 8-8. Knee arthrodesis with biplanar external fixation secondary to persistent infection. (Reprinted with permission from Canale ST. *Campbell's Operative Orthopaedics*. 10th ed. St. Louis, MO: Mosby Inc; 2003.)

Infection/Non-Healing Fractures

With any surgical procedure, and particularly in the presence of open traumatic wounds, there is a risk of infection.[52] A worrisome complication after joint replacement or fracture repair is persistent infection, poor healing, or nonunion with bone loss or separation (see Figures 8-6 and 8-8). It is common in large trauma centers for the orthopedic surgery service to treat patients for non-healing, malaligned, or nonunion fractures. For open fractures, risk of infection increases linearly based on size of soft tissue damage and length of time from fracture to initial debridement.[53] Acute **osteomyelitis** is an infection of bone that requires hospitalization for a variety of treatments, including sterile debridements, intravenous antibiotics, hyperbaric oxygen therapy, skin grafting, and removal of infected implanted hardware or bone.[54]

Physical therapists will treat previously injured patients who have had some training in ambulation with an assistive device and who now return to the hospital because of infection. A new episode of hospital-based gait and mobility training may be required. Physical therapy is generally indicated prior to discharge because of a NWB status, pain, and possible acute deconditioning secondary to inactivity.

Ridding the patient of infection is the primary medical goal, and several medical/surgical approaches are taken, including serial sterile debridements in the operating room, the use of implanted antibiotic beads or cement restricted weightbearing on the affected extremity, superficial wound management, direct current electrical stimulation,[55] and intravenous antibiotics. New hardware may have to replace infected rods, nails, or prosthetic implants.[56] In cases of chronic infection, where long-term antibiotic use, multiple operative procedures, and even use of bone stimulators, have failed, segments of bone may need to be completely removed. These osteotomies may include fusions and are often seen at the knee and ankle. The Girdlestone procedure at the hip removes a segment of infected, or non-healed, proximal femur and purposefully allows scar tissue to form in order to stabilize the joint.[57] Despite the lack of a true hip joint, independent ambulation can be a realistic long-term goal. The patient may present, ultimately, with a limp and require heel lifts secondary to a leg-length

Table 8-9

SUMMARY OF PHYSICAL THERAPY AND JOINT INFECTIONS

- Chronic and acutely infected joints or hardware often require hospitalization.
- Patients usually have had physical therapy in the past for gait training.
- A new episode of physical therapy intervention is frequently required prior to discharge.
- Procedures frequently encountered:
  - Hardware removal or exchange
  - Osteotomies
  - Joint fusions/arthrodesis
  - Multiple operative debridements
  - Antibiotics; may have central intravenous line placement (eg, peripherally inserted central catheter [PICC])
- Physical therapy intervention:
  - Assess mobility/gait
  - If orthotic is management required, instruct patient in use
  - Bedside exercise program if a long-term hospital stay anticipated

discrepancy. When osteotomies are performed, surgeons may apply skeletal traction to maintain alignment. A removable pin is placed either through the proximal tibia or the distal femur with weights and pulleys hung over the foot of the patient's bed. The therapist must be aware of the activity status because this patient may be allowed to come out of traction to participate in therapy (Table 8-9).

ORTHOTICS

Orthopedic management of acute fracture includes support, comfort, and immobilization; therefore, the use of orthotic devices is commonplace. The physical therapist must understand indications for use in the acute care setting, application, and implications for function.[58] The tables of this section are arranged by anatomical area and, although not an exhaustive listing, give the reader an idea of commonly used devices, frequently encountered brand names, and indications.

For any orthotic device, proper fit is essential. A brace can appear well-fitting in a static position but shift during functional activities. Therapists will assist patients by educating them as to the reason for the brace, how it should be applied, when it should be worn, and how to monitor the skin underneath the brace. A frustrating complication of orthotic use is the occurrence of preventable problems, such as skin breakdown under a brace secondary to lack of vigilant observation.

When outside vendors provide service to patients in the hospital, collaboration can be more difficult. The therapist should attempt to coordinate fittings or adjustments with the outside vendor to enable more efficient patient care.

Beside the use of orthoses, the acute care physical therapist will encounter the use of cast immobilization. Gait and mobility training are impacted by the weight of the cast and the degree to which the immobilization provides comfort. The physical therapist must be alert to complaints of a tight-fitting cast, such as acute pain or paresthesias within or distal to the cast. Contact the surgical team immediately because pressure relief may be indicated and can be performed by either bivalving the cast or cutting a window in the area in question.

Spine

As a general rule, no matter what segment of the spine requires bracing, the primary question to ask is "Does the orthosis attempt to stabilize an unstable area or is it meant for comfort?" When stabilization is required, rigid bracing is indicated. If pain is present but no underlying anatomical structures are at risk, soft material can be appropriate. The important difference is that soft braces can be removed without risk of injury, but rigid braces should have specific wearing schedules that the patient or caregiver must understand, including whether or not the brace can be removed in bed. Common cervical and thoracolumbar orthoses are provided in Tables 8-10 and 8-11 (see also Table 9-20).

Extremities

A wide variety of extremity orthoses exist, most that immobilize, but some that allow degrees of motion. Depending on the institution, either physical or occupational therapists may be responsible for custom molding certain extremity braces. The physical therapist will be challenged to assist the patient and the surgical team with recommending the most appropriate, cost-effective device. Common UE orthoses are provided in Table 8-12 and LE orthoses are provided in Table 8-13.

Foot/Ankle Complex

Orthotic shoes and braces are used to support, relieve pressure, or facilitate weightbearing at the foot and ankle.[59] Custom molded orthotic shoes that accommodate deformity are generally not fabricated during the acute care phase of injury and require outpatient follow-up. Despite the various, and often confusing, array of brand names, the physical therapist must focus on the goal of foot/ankle bracing. For example, is the orthosis for short or long term? Is support or pressure relief required? How much and where is weightbearing allowed? By answering these questions, the therapist should be able to recommend the appropriate orthotic device as noted in Table 8-14.

Clinical experience has found the use of ankle air splints or casts to be effective in assisting with weightbearing and mobility in the appropriate patient. When the foot and ankle are injured during trauma to other limbs, ankle sprains or ligamentous injury often go unnoticed until the patient first gets out of bed and attempts to bear weight. If physical examination (eg, tenderness to palpation, painful resisted movement, ecchymosis) supports the clinical diagnosis of ligamentous injury, a recommendation for an ankle splint should be made. These splints are either air or foam filled, 2-piece plastic, and have Velcro strap closures. They are designed to fit into a regular shoe or sneaker but may be limited secondary to acute edema.

Assistive Devices

All therapists who work in the hospital setting are familiar with the prescription of assistive devices to address mobility impairment and dysfunction. With an orthopedic population, therapists are frequently asked to train patients with various types of devices as outlined in Table 8-15. Choosing which device to use is often determined by several factors. The therapist must know what, if any, weightbearing restrictions exist as any condition requiring less than full, LE weightbearing necessitates a bilateral device, such as a walker or crutches. As many types of walkers and crutches exist, the clinical decision to use one device instead of another is influenced by the demonstrated ability to safely use the device based on the demands of the discharge environment.

Table 8-10

CERVICAL ORTHOSES

Indications	Type
Rigid	
Indications	**Type**
• Unstable cervical spine at C1–C2	• Halo: ¤ Pins inserted externally into skull ¤ Pins attached to plastic and padded-lined vest
Semi-Rigid	
Indications	**Type**
• Stable fractures • Nonoperative ligamentous injury • Postoperative • Prescribed wearing schedule	• Miami-J: ¤ Two-piece ¤ Hard plastic ¤ Gortex liner ¤ Velcro strap closure ¤ Opening for tracheostomy • Philadelphia: ¤ Two-piece ¤ Hard plastic ¤ Foam ¤ Velcro strap closure • Cervical thoracic orthosis (CTO) or cervical thoracic lumbar orthosis (CTLO): ¤ Any brace that has both cervical and thoracic components or extensions ¤ Stabilize cervical and high thoracic injury • Sternal occipital mandibular immobilizer (SOMI): ¤ Three-piece: Sternal pad or yoke, anterior mandibular support, occipital support ¤ No rolling of patient required to apply brace
Soft	
Indications	**Type**
• Symptom management and pain control • Flexible wearing schedule • Indicated after trauma to control pain in the absence of bony or ligamentous injury	• Foam and fabric with Velcro strap closure

Table 8-11

THORACOLUMBAR ORTHOSES

Indications	Type
Rigid	
Indications	**Type**
• Stable fractures • Nonoperative ligamentous injury • Postoperative • Prescribed wearing schedule	• Thoracic lumbosacral orthosis (TLSO): ¤ Indicated for mid-thoracic and lumbar injuries ¤ Usually 2-piece ¤ Hard plastic ¤ Velcro straps ¤ Custom molded or prefabricated • SOMI: ¤ Stabilize cervical and high-level thoracic injury ¤ No rolling of patient required to apply brace ¤ Mandibular and occipital attachments • Jewitt hyperextension brace: ¤ Maintains extension, prevents flexion ¤ Used frequently for compression fractures ¤ Sternal and pubic anterior pads ¤ Posterior lumbar pad ¤ No lateral bars allows for lateral bending • Boston overlap: ¤ One piece, flexible plastic ¤ Velcro straps ¤ Opens anteriorly at midline
Semi-Rigid	
Indications	**Type**
• Combination of soft fabrics and metal or plastic • Symptom management • Pain control in the absence of instability	• Corset: ¤ Fabric with side and posterior metal stays, lace-up sides or front ¤ Often tolerated better than rigid braces, particularly in the geriatric population ¤ More support than soft binders
Soft	
Indications	**Type**
• Symptom management • Pain control in the absence of instability • Flexible wearing schedule	• Abdominal binder • Fabric with Velcro closure anteriorly

Table 8-12
UPPER EXTREMITY ORTHOSES

Rigid	
Indications	**Type**
• Nonoperative fractures requiring external immobilization • Postoperative stabilization • Prescribed wearing schedule	• Sarmiento fracture brace: ¤ Stabilize proximal or mid-shaft humeral fractures ¤ Two-piece ¤ Hard plastic ¤ Velcro strap closure ¤ Prefabricated • Custom-molded immobilizers: ¤ Gutter splint ° Static splint ° Maintains functional position ° Protects postoperative procedures (eg, skin grafts) ¤ Wrist cock-up splint ° Static splint ° Maintains functional wrist position ° Radial nerve palsy/paresis ° Prevents wrist contracture in presence of external fixation
Semi-Rigid	
Indications	**Type**
• Components allow for static (or resting) immobilization, as well as dynamic ROM	• Hinged or dial-lock elbow brace: ¤ Lock in full extension or any degree of elbow flexion ¤ Foam with metal stays ¤ Velcro strap closures
Soft	
Indications	**Type**
• Most often indicated for symptom management and pain control in the absence of instability • Flexible or prescribed wearing schedule • Shoulder slings may cause shoulder stiffness and decreased ROM while maintaining shoulder in adduction and internal rotation	• Shoulder slings: ¤ For clavicle, scapular, or humeral fractures ¤ Used to unweight heavy splints or casts of radius/ulna and wrist fractures • Figure-of-8: ¤ For clavicle fractures ¤ Attempts to align fracture segments ¤ Maintains scapulae retracted and adducted • Shoulder abduction: ¤ Large foam wedge at hip with over-the-shoulder strap ¤ Used often for postoperative shoulder and humeral fractures ¤ Maintains shoulder/extremity in abducted, "gunslinger" position

Table 8-13
Lower Extremity Orthoses

Rigid	
Indications	**Type**
• Postoperative stabilization • Prescribed wearing schedule	• Hip abduction brace: ¤ Usually prefabricated ¤ Hip spica appearance ¤ Indicated for acute and/or multiple hip dislocations after hip replacement ¤ Degree of hip flexion and abduction controlled by external hip joint locking mechanism ¤ Hard plastic, shoulder and waist straps, thigh cuff • Fracture brace: ¤ Custom molded ¤ Usually 2-piece hard plastic with Velcro strap closure ¤ Often seen for the nonunion, non-healing fracture
Semi-Rigid	
Indications	**Type**
• Stabilization of fractures, either nonoperative or surgically repaired • Ligamentous injuries of the knee • Support for weightbearing activities • Prescribed or flexible wearing schedule	• Dial-lock hinged: ¤ Bledsoe, Exo-Tec, Don Joy ¤ Stabilize postoperative fracture stabilization or nonoperative ligamentous injury ¤ Foam padding, medial and lateral metal stays ¤ Velcro strap closure, adjustable dial locks at knee joint ¤ Allows for any degree of knee flexion ROM, often locked in full extension acutely ¤ Indicated for more long-term use than knee immobilizer • Knee immobilizer: ¤ Foam, posterior metal stay, adjustable medial and lateral metal stays, Velcro strap closure ¤ Attempts to lock knee in full extension with no motion ¤ Used frequently in acute care for multiple scenarios: ° Stabilize distal femoral or proximal tibial fractures ° Protect postoperative procedures (eg, skin grafts) ° Provides knee stability for weightbearing in the presence of quadriceps weakness
Soft	
Indications	**Type**
• Used very infrequently in acute care	• ACE bandages: ¤ Compressive, elastic wrap ¤ Holds dressings in place, provides comfort but no stability

Table 8-14

FOOT AND ANKLE ORTHOSES

Rigid	
Indications	**Type**
• In the presence of ankle dorsiflexion weakness, facilitates normal swing-through during swing phase of gait	• Ankle foot orthosis (AFO): ¤ Usually prefabricated in acute care setting ¤ Flexible plastic ¤ Velcro strap closure below fibular head ¤ Fits inside shoe • The term MAFO refers to a molded ankle foot orthosis, which is custom made. A MAFO is a definitive, long-term brace, fabricated either in the outpatient or inpatient rehabilitation setting. Not indicated during acute care phase secondary to wound issues, edema fluctuations and, often, evolving injury status.
Semi-Rigid	
Indications	**Type**
• For minimally or non-ambulatory patients while in bed: ¤ Provides heel pressure relief ¤ Prevents heel cord contracture ¤ Maintains neutral hip rotation • For ambulatory patients: ¤ Facilitates swing-through ¤ Not a long-term device	• AFO: ¤ PRAFO [Pressure Relief Ankle Foot Orthosis], multipodus splint, oscar boot ¤ Foam/fabric lining, flexible plastic shell, thick rubber sole
Shoes	
Indications	**Type**
• For weightbearing activities • To relieve pressure on fore- or hind foot • Provide comfort and/or support • Used to protect wounds	• Heel weightbearing (forefoot relief): ¤ Barouk shoe: Thick heel wedge ¤ DARCO wedge: Thick heel with forefoot protective plate • Postoperative shoe: ¤ Usually open-toed, hard-soled, fabric, and Velcro • Cast shoe or boot: ¤ Open- or closed-toed ¤ Thick sole for weightbearing

Table 8-15

Common Assistive Devices

Bilateral	
Indications	**Type**
• For use with restricted LE weightbearing • Provide stability during ambulation • Must be used in conditions of: ¤ NWB (0%) ¤ Minimal or toe-touch weightbearing (~10%) ¤ Partial weightbearing (~50%) • Percentages (eg, 10%, 50%) refer to percent of total body weight. Sometimes restrictions are given in absolute pounds, regardless of body weight.	• Crutches: ¤ Axillary ° Most commonly issued ° Wooden or aluminium ¤ Forearm or Canadian ° Lofstrand is a brand name of forearm crutches • Walkers: ¤ Standard, no wheels ¤ Wheeled or rollator ¤ Usually front wheeled, no brakes • Forearm platforms can attach to either crutches or walkers to allow proximal weightbearing in the presence of a distal UE fracture.
Unilateral	
Indications	**Type**
• Increase stability during ambulation • Relieve pressure on contralateral side	• Straight point cane • Wide or large base quad cane • Narrow or small base quad cane
Wheelchairs	
Indications	**Type**
• When ambulation is not safe or functional • When wheelchair propulsion is performed with one leg, or both, consider a shorter ground-to-seat height, referred to as hemi-height to get the foot closer to floor.	• Standard: ¤ 16-inch seat depth, 18-inch width ¤ Removable or swing-away arm rests ¤ Leg rests, with calf pads, usually elevating ¤ Rear anti-tippers ¤ Consider wheel-lock (brake) extensions, when one extremity has activity restrictions • Custom: ¤ Generally not indicated during acute phase of injury or rehabilitation

Coordination, fear, prior use of device, pain, ability to learn new skills, and family/caregiver assistance are all considerations in the final recommendation. The physical therapist must determine the ability of the patient to maintain a given weightbearing restriction during functional activities and then direct intervention accordingly. Practically, this often means restricting an activity until further appropriate training can take place, possibly in settings after hospital discharge. Often an activity must wait until the weightbearing restriction is lifted. Ambulation for an older individual with a long-leg cast may not be realistic but transferring independently to a wheelchair or bedside commode might be. The reader is referred to the table on assistive ambulatory devices for types and indications (see Table 8-15).

Summary

The acute care therapist who works with patients with musculoskeletal-related health conditions will intervene for patients with a variety of diagnoses and age ranges. In the examination, evaluation, and formulation of the physical therapy plan of care, the therapist will use many skills, including patient/caregiver education, mobility training, and discharge planning.[53] Attention to surgeon-specific protocols, as well as knowledge of orthotic devices, is critical for safe and effective collaborative patient care. This chapter is meant as a guide to common, hospital-based orthopedic conditions and is not an exhaustive compendium. For areas not addressed, such as spinal cord injury, the reader is encouraged to review Chapter 9 and other texts detailing acute orthopedic and traumatic conditions.

Case Study

Mrs. Jackson, a 58-year-old female, restrained driver, was involved in a head-on-collision against a pole after skidding on ice during a winter storm. This patient was transported from the scene by a helicopter to a Level I Trauma center. After evaluation in the emergency department, she was admitted to the hospital. Three days after admission, a physical therapy consult was ordered.

Patient/Client History

General Demographics, Social History, and Living Environment

Mrs. Jackson was working full time as an accountant, is married, and lives in a split-level 2-story home with 3 steps to enter and a handrail. The bedroom and bathroom are 6 steps up from the family room, and the powder room is 6 steps down. One grown daughter lives out of state. Her husband was a passenger in the car. He was treated for multiple facial lacerations and a fractured left wrist and required a 1-night hospital stay. He was discharged to home.

General Health Status, Social/Health Habits, and Family History

Mrs. Jackson is overweight with a body mass index (BMI) of 30. She admits to smoking half to 1 pack per day and "social" drinking. She denies drug use. She does not consider herself active and has no regular exercise routine. Hobbies include movies, knitting, and travel. Her family history is unremarkable and unrelated to the current condition.

Medical/Surgical History

Mrs. Jackson has hypertension (HTN), hypercholesterolemia, and is obese. Surgical history includes a caesarean section, gallbladder removal (cholecystectomy), and left arthroscopic knee surgery 3 years ago.

Current Conditions

Mrs. Jackson is status post (s/p) MVC. There was loss of consciousness (LOC) requiring intubation for airway protection by the emergency medical technician (EMT) at the scene. Injuries diagnosed upon arrival to the hospital include a left-side hemopneumothorax, a distal right lower extremity (RLE) tibial fracture, and several (L1–L3) lumbar spinous process fractures.

A chest tube was place in the trauma bay to evacuate blood and air from the left pleural space. Orthopedic surgery performed an ORIF to stabilize the tibia fracture. The patient spent 1 day in the intensive care unit (ICU) after surgery where she was extubated without complication and received a blood transfusion for a hemoglobin (Hb) level of 6.8 g/dL. She was transferred to the general care ward on 2 liters of oxygen via nasal cannula, with a Foley catheter, a morphine patient-controlled analgesia (PCA) pump for pain control, and a posterior, ACE wrapped splint immobilizing her distal RLE. She has a chest tube in her left flank draining to a pleurovac collection system connected to 15 cm H_2O suction. Her activity status is out of bed as tolerated, NWB on her RLE.

Activities and Participation

Prior to admission, the patient was independent with all aspects of mobility and activities of daily living (ADLs)/instrumental activities of daily living (IADLs) without the use of an assistive device. Currently, the patient is NWB on the RLE, allowed out of bed ad lib, and is requires assistance for all mobility secondary to pain and NWB status.

Medications

She takes metoprolol (a beta blocker) for HTN, atorvastatin (a statin) for high cholesterol, and a non-steroidal anti-inflammatory for "aches and pains" as needed.

Systems Review

Cardiovascular and Pulmonary

Resting heart rate (HR) 90 beats per minute (bpm), blood pressure (BP) is 150/78 mm Hg, respiratory rate (RR) 20 breaths/minute.

Integumentary

Her surgical wound site is not visualized secondary to the dressing; the chest tube site is sutured and appears clean, dry, and intact (C/D/I). Her right toes are visible, mildly edematous, and show brisk capillary refill. Based on body habitus and lack of mobility, the patient has been placed on a pressure relieving, low air-loss mattress. She has been wearing a pneumatic compression stocking on her left calf.

Musculoskeletal

Gross myotome assessment and AROM of bilateral upper extremities (BUEs) and LLE appears normal except left upper extremity (LUE) shoulder strength limited by pain at chest tube site and the RLE was not formally assessed secondary to pain with motion.

Neuromuscular

Sensation to light touch and gross proprioception are intact throughout. Patient reports "tingling" sensation at the right foot/ankle.

Communication, Affect, Cognition, Language, and Learning Style

Mrs. Jackson is awake, alert, and oriented to person, place, time, and situation. She reports feeling anxious about moving because of the pain. Her primary language is English. She reports that she likes to be told what is going to happen prior to moving.

Tests and Measures

Aerobic Capacity and Endurance

As noted in the Mobility Assessment section that follows, the patient demonstrated orthostatic hypotension (drop in BP of 20 mm Hg with symptoms) with standing at the bedside. Compensatory tachycardia was noted, with mild drop in oxygen saturation (SpO_2).

Assistive Technology

Mrs. Jackson was assisted into a standing position with use of a standard walker. The patient was able to assist with bed mobility by grabbing an overhead trapeze bar. A bedside commode has been ordered as well as a long-handled reacher.

Balance, Gait and Mobility (Including Locomotion)

Mrs. Jackson required moderate assistance to transition from supine↔sitting at the edge of the bed (Functional Independence Measure [FIM] 3) and maximal assistance to complete the sit↔stand transfer (FIM 2) and maintain abbreviated standing with a standard walker.

Mrs. Jackson required maximal assistance (FIM 2) to maintain standing for 30 seconds with a standard walker. A gait assessment was not performed at this time due to symptomatic orthostatic hypotension (FIM 0). Her Activity Measure for Post Acute Care (AM-PAC) "6 Click" Basic Mobility score is 8/24. The highest ICU Mobility Scale (IMS) was 4 (standing).

Circulation (Arterial, Venous, Lymphatic) and Ventilation/Respiration

After sitting at the edge of the bed and standing to a walker, her vital signs (VS) are: BP 150/78-116/68 mm Hg, HR 90-126 bpm, SpO_2 94%-90%. Patient reports feeling lightheaded after standing and is returned to bed. VS return to baseline.

The SpO_2 is 97% on 2 liters per minute (l/m) at rest. Auscultation of breath sounds reveals decreased breath sounds at bilateral lung bases (left decreased more than right) with no adventitious sounds. Incentive spirometry averages 500 mL. Chest tube on left is draining serosanguinous fluid.

Mental Function

The patient was alert, cooperative, and could follow commands easily.

Muscle Performance

Muscle strength was 5/5 in all major muscle groups of bilateral UE/LE with the exception of the RLE which was not formally assessed secondary to pain with motion.

Pain

Using a visual analogue scale, the patient reports RLE 5/10 pain at rest (aching) and 8/10 (sharp) while moving. Rest and RLE elevation relieve the pain.

Evaluation

Mrs. Jackson is a middle-aged female currently hospitalized secondary to an MVC sustaining orthopedic and chest wall trauma. Patient medical history (PMH) is remarkable for HTN and obesity. Orthostatic hypotension is potentially associated with opioid analgesics and blood loss secondary to hemopneumothorax and traumatic fractures. Pulmonary function is impaired by pneumothorax and subsequent chest tube insertion leading to chest wall pain with limited ventilation and decreased breath sounds.

Diagnosis

Mrs. Jackson presents with impairments in AROM/strength and activity limitations, including deficits with transfers and gait related primarily to pain with movement. She will require ongoing physical therapy services to facilitate safe discharge.

Prognosis

Complete tibia fracture healing should allow return to independent mobility and full-time employment without the need of an assistive device. However, it is anticipated that the patient will require acute inpatient rehabilitation upon discharge from the hospital based on current mobility deficits, pain, and her challenging home environment. Additionally, the patient may require ongoing episodes of physical therapy, including outpatient services, once allowed to bear weight on her RLE.

Intervention

Daily physical therapy intervention with short-term goals of increasing out of bed tolerance and decreasing level of assistance required for bedside mobilization. Interventions include functional training (eg, bed mobility, transfers, toilet and gait training, wheelchair management), assistive technology training, including use of walker and reacher, and orthotic device training (eg, posterior splint). Therapeutic exercises (eg, UE/LE AROM, resistive exercises) and patient instruction (eg, use of PCA, skin integrity, incentive spirometry, weightbearing restriction, bedside ROM exercise program, smoking cessation) were initiated and progressed throughout the episode of care.

ICF Clinical Reasoning Tool Case Study Summary

Health Condition

HPI: Restrained driver s/p head-on MVC, left-sided hemopneumothorax, distal RLE tibial fracture s/p ORIF, L1–L3 lumbar spinous process fractures, blood transfusion for low Hb

PMHx: Overweight, HTN, hypercholesterolemia, and sedentary lifestyle; prior surgeries: caesarean section, cholecystectomy, and left knee arthroscopy

Precautions/Contraindications

Orthostatic hypotension, safety/fall risk due to LOC and pain, husband may not be able to help due to her LUE fracture, medication for cholesterol may cause additional musculoskeletal pain, may have weakness from previous LLE surgery, universal precautions

Body Structure and Function			Activity/Task Limitations			Participation		
Impairment/ Problem	*Tests and Measures*	*Intervention*	*Activity*	*Tests and Measures*	*Intervention*	*Participation*	*Tests and Measures*	*Intervention*
• Impaired endurance • Impaired sensation • Pain • Decreased ventilation and chest wall movement due to pain and CT • Weight exceeds IBW • Abnormal lab values	• Chest assessment • ROM/MMT • Sensation • VS including SpO_2 and ECG • Pain/numeric scale • BMI • Lab values	• Breathing exercises (incentive spirometry, deep breathing, PLB) • Assisted/ braced cough • Pain management • Education for risk for falls/ safety • Consult registered dietician	• ADLs • IADLs • Bed mobility • Transfers • Gait	• Functional task analysis • FIM • AM-PAC "6 Clicks" • RPE • Pain scale • PSFS	• Progressive/ interval functional retraining • Careful monitoring of VS due to orthostatic hypotension and cardiovascular risk factors	• Unable to go out to movies and travel • Unable to knit due to impaired concentration	• MMSE/ MoCA • FAQ • PSFS	• Continue physical therapy services • Consultsocial worker • Family meeting to discuss discharge plans

(continued)

ICF Clinical Reasoning Tool Case Study Summary (continued)

Personal Factors	*Other Considerations*	*Environmental Factors*
• Age: 58 y/o female • AAO x 3 • Primary language: English • Full time accountant • Married; husband passenger in car with multiple facial lacerations and fractured left wrist but released after a 1-night hospital stay • 1 grown daughter lives out of state • Independent prior to MVC • Anxious and fearful of pain with movement • Smoker x 1/2 pack/day, social drinker		Home: • Split-level 2 story house, 3 steps to enter with handrail, bedroom/bathroom 6 steps up with a family room, powder room 6 steps down Hospital: • 2 L NP, urinary catheter, chest tube, PCA pump, ACE wrap splint immobilizer, bedside commode, OOB/NWB RLE

AAO = awake, alert, oriented; ADL = activity of daily living; CT = chest tube; ECG = electrocardiogram; FAQ = Functional Activities Questionnaire; HPI = history of present illness; HTN = hypertension; IADL = instrumental activity of daily living; IBW = ideal body weight; MMSE = Mini-Mental State Examination; MoCA = Montreal Cognitive Assessment; MMT = manual muscle test; NP = nasal prongs; OOB = out of bed; PMHx = past medical history; PSFS = Patient Specific Functional Scale; RPE = rate of perceived exertion; s/p = status post; y/o year old.

Adapted from American Physical Therapy Association. *Guide to Physical Therapist Practice*. 3rd ed. http://www.apta.org/Guide/. Updated October 21, 2015. Accessed October 5, 2018 and *Towards a Common Language for Functioning, Disability and Health*. World Health Organization. www.who.int/classifications/icf/icfbeginnersguide.pdf. Published 2002. Accessed April 29, 2019.

Outcomes

Patient received a fluid bolus after the first physical therapy session secondary to orthostasis. Reexamination the following day revealed the same level of assistance required for bed mobility and standing but an appropriate VS response, including an elevation in HR, BP, and stable SpO_2 without complaint of cardiopulmonary symptoms. Mrs. Jackson was able to transfer to the bedside chair and walk approximately 20 feet with maximal assistance of 2 (FIM 1). The IMS improved from 4 to 7 (walking with assistance of 2).

The patient was treated for 5 additional sessions at which point she was transferred to inpatient rehabilitation. Her chest tube, Foley catheter, and oxygen were all discontinued, and she has been converted from the PCA to oral analgesics. The patient required minimal assistance to transfers from supine to sit (FIM 4), moderate assistance for sit to stand (FIM 3), and was ambulating 30 feet x 2 with a rolling walker and moderate assistance (FIM 2). Her AM-PAC "6 Click Basic Mobility score increased from 8 to 14/24. The IMS improved from 7 to 8 (walking with assistance of 1). Pain continued to limit her function, particularly at her lumbar spine and tibia, but was successfully medically managed with a pain scale rating of 1 at rest and 4 with mobility.

Chapter Review Questions

1. What are 2 indications for TKAs/THAs?
   a. Lack of response to conservative joint management and decline in physical function
   b. Traumatic injury and avascular necrosis of the fibular head
   c. Long-term increase in muscle pain and loss of sensation around the joint
   d. Degenerative joint disease and stable pain level
2. Which of the following best represents the pathology of rheumatoid arthritis?
   a. Autorecessive polyarticular disease process
   b. Synovial atrophy and episodes of relapse and remissions
   c. Joint effusions, ligamentous damage, and joint destruction
   d. Traumatic, mechanical, and redundant joint injury
3. What is the benefit of using the log rolling technique following spinal surgery?
   a. Avoids using pelvic area as pivot point for transfer
   b. Avoids using thoracolumbar extension
   c. Avoids using spinal rotation
   d. Avoids using valsalva maneuver
4. Which of the following best represent care team goals after arthroplasty?
   a. Prevent DVT, pulmonary embolism, infection, and reduce pain
   b. Prevent pneumonia, wound dehiscence, atelectasis, and enhance swelling
   c. Prevent decubiti, pulmonary infarction, fever, and reduce pain
   d. Prevent keloid formation, impact of bed rest, orthostasis, and promote function

5. What are 2 physical therapy examination findings that would lead to the prescription of a walker as part of a discharge plan?
   a. NWB on LLE and poor static balance in standing
   b. Full weightbearing BLE and fair dynamic balance in sitting
   c. Partial weightbearing LUE and poor dynamic balance in standing
   d. NWB RUE and good dynamic balance on stairs

Answers: 1a, 2c, 3c, 4a, 5a

References

1. Kim S, Losina E, Solomon DH, Wright J, Katz JN. Effectiveness of clinical pathways for total knee and total hip arthroplasty: literature review. *J Arthroplasty*. 2003;18(1):69-74.
2. Pearson SD, Kleefield SF, Soukop JR, Cook EF, Lee TH. Critical pathways intervention to reduce length of hospital stay. *Am J Med*. 2001;110(3):175-180.
3. Tayrose G, Newman D, Slover J, Jaffe F, Hunter T, Bosco J III. Rapid mobilization decreases length-of-stay in joint replacement patients. *Bull Hosp Jt Dis*. 2013;71(3):222-226.
4. Rana AJ, Iorio R, Healy WL. Hospital economics of primary total knee arthroplasty at a teaching hospital. *Clin Orthop Relat Res*. 2011;469(1):87-94.
5. Hip and knee reconstruction. In: Pellici PM, Tria AJ, Garvin KL eds. *Orthopaedic Knowledge Update*. Rosemont, IL: American Academy of Orthopaedic Surgeons; 2000.
6. Pennington JM, Jones DPG, McIntyre S. Clinical pathways in total knee arthroplasty: a New Zealand experience. *J Orthop Surg*. 2003;11(2):166-173.
7. Orest MR. Total joint replacement literature review. *Acute Care Perspectives (American Physical Therapy Association)*. 2004;13(1):10-12.
8. AAOS Department of Research and Scientific Affairs. *Summary and resources for osteoarthritis of the hip & knee*. American Academy of Orthopaedic Surgeons. http://www.aaos.org/wordhtml/research/oainfo/oainfo.htm. Accessed on April 2, 2006.
9. Vaupel G, Cacanindin N, Wong J. Total knee replacement. In: Maxey L, Magnusson J, eds. *Rehabilitation for the Post Surgical Orthopedic Patient*. St. Louis, MO: Mosby; 2001:268-287.
10. Gartland JJ. Disorders of joints. In: Brinker MR, Miller MD, eds. *Fundamentals of Orthopaedics*. Philadelphia, PA: WB Saunders Co; 1987:122-148.
11. Bullock DP, Sporer SM, Shirreffs TG. Comparison of simultaneous bilateral with unilateral total knee arthroplasty in terms of perioperative complications. *J Bone Joint Surg*. 2003;85(10):1981-1986.
12. Boese CK, Weis M, Phillips T, Lawton-Peters S, Gallo T, Centeno L. The efficacy of continuous passive motion after total knee arthroplasty: a comparison of three protocols. *J Arthroplasty*. 2014;29(6):1158-1162. doi: 10.1016/j.arth.2013.12.005
13. Milne S, Brosseau L, Robinson V, et al. Continuous passive motion following total knee arthroplasty. *Cochrane Database Syst Rev*. 2003;(2):CD004260. doi: 10.1002/14651858.CD004260
14. Beaupre LA, Davies DM, Jones CA, Cinats JG. Exercise combined with continuous passive motion or slider board therapy compared with exercise only: a randomized controlled trial of patients following total knee arthroplasty. *Phys Ther*. 2001;81(4):1029-1037.
15. Harvey LA, Brosseau L, Herbert RD. Continuous passive motion following total knee arthroplasty in people with arthritis. *Cochrane Database Syst Rev*. 2014 6;(2):CD004260. doi: 10.1002/14651858.CD004260.pub3
16. Munin MC, Rudy TE, Glynn NW, Crossett LS, Rubash HE. Early inpatient rehabilitation after elective hip and knee arthroplasty. *J Am Med Assoc*. 1998; 279(11):847-852.
17. Forrest GP, Roque JM, Dawodu ST. Decreasing length of stay after total joint arthroplasty: effect on referrals to rehabilitation units. *Arch Phys Med Rehabil*. 1999;80(2):192-194.
18. Maloney WJ. The stiff total knee arthroplasty: evaluation and management. *J Arthroplasty*. 2002;17(4):71-73.
19. Chiu KY, Ng TP, Tang WM, Tau WP. Review article: knee flexion after total knee arthroplasty. *J Orthop Surg* (Hong Kong). 2002;10(2):194-202.

20. McDonald S, Page MJ, Beringer K, Wasiak J, Sprowson A. Preoperative education for hip or knee replacement. *Cochrane Database Syst Rev.* 2014;(5):CD003526. doi: 10.1002/14651858.CD003526.pub3
21. Jordan RW, Smith NA, Chahal GS, Casson C, Reed MR, Sprowson AP. Enhanced education and physiotherapy before knee replacement; is it worth it? A systematic review. *Physiotherapy.* 2014;100(4):305-312. doi: 10.1016/j.physio.2014.03.003
22. Mirza AJ, Lombardi AV Jr, Morris MJ, Berend KR. A mini-anterior approach to the hip for total joint replacement: optimising results: improving hip joint replacement outcomes. *Bone Joint J.* 2014;96-B(11 suppl A):32-35. doi: 10.1302/0301-620X.96B11.34348
23. Onyemaechi N, Anyanwu E, Obikili E, Ekezie J. Anatomical basis for surgical approaches to the hip. *Ann Med Health Sci Res.* 2014;4(4):487-494. doi: 10.4103/2141-9248.139278
24. Given-Heiss DL, Krebs DE, Riley PO, et al. In vivo acetabular contact pressures during rehabilitation. Part II post-acute phase. *Phys Ther.* 1992;72(10):700-705.
25. Stricland EM, Fares M, Krebs DE, et al. In vivo acetabular contact pressures during rehabilitation. Part I acute phase. *Phys Ther.* 1992;72(10):691-699.
26. Berger RA, Kull LR, Rosenberg AG, Galante JO. Hybrid total hip arthroplasty: 7-10-year results. *Clin Orthop.* 1996; Dec (333):134-146.
27. Kavanagh BF, Wallrichs S, Dewitz M, et al. Charnley low-friction arthroplasty of the hip. Twenty-year results with cement. *J Arthroplasty.* 1994;9(3):229-234.
28. Singh JA, Ramachandran R. Hospital volume predicts outcomes and complications after total shoulder arthroplasty in the United States. *Arthritis Care Res (Hoboken).* 2015;67(6):885-890. doi:10.1002/acr.22507
29. Jain NB, Higgins LD, Guller U, Pietrobon R, Katz JN. Trends in the epidemiology of total shoulder arthroplasty in the United States from 1990-2000. *Arthritis Rheum.* 2006;55(4):591-597.
30. Kelly MJ, Leggin BG. Shoulder rehabilitation. In: Iannotti JP, Williams GR, eds. *Disorders of the Shoulder: Diagnosis and Management.* Philadelphia, PA: Lippincott Williams & Wilkins; 1999:1012-1014.
31. Parker SL, Godil SS, Mendenhall SK, Zuckerman SL, Shau DN, McGirt MJ. Two-year comprehensive medical management of degenerative lumbar spine disease (lumbar spondylolisthesis, stenosis, or disc herniation): a value analysis of cost, pain, disability, and quality of life: clinical article. *J Neurosurg Spine.* 2014;21(2):143-149. doi: 10.3171/2014.3.SPINE1320
32. Lauremann WC, Goldsmith ME. Spine. In: Miller MD, Brinker MR, eds. *Review of Orthopaedics.* 3rd ed. Philadelphia, PA: WB Saunders; 2000:353-378.
33. Nygaard OP, Kloster R, Solberg T. Duration of leg pain as a predictor of outcome after surgery for lumbar disc herniation: a prospective cohort stud with 1-year follow up. *J Neurosurg.* 2001;95 (2 suppl):281-282.
34. Gruskay JA, Fu M, Basques BA, et al. Factors affecting length of stay and complications after elective anterior cervical discectomy and fusion: a study of 2164 patients from the American College of Surgeons National Surgical Quality Improvement Project Database (ACS NSQIP). *Clin Spine Surg.* 2016;29(1):E34-E42. doi: 10.1097/BSD.0000000000000080
35. Canale ST. *Campbell's Operative Orthopaedics: Part XII Spine.* 10th ed. St. Louis, MO: Mosby Inc.; 2003.
36. Elliott RE, Tanweer O, Boah A, et al. Is external cervical orthotic bracing necessary after posterior atlantoaxial fusion with modern instrumentation: meta-analysis and review of literature. *World Neurosurg.* 2013;79(2):369-374. doi: 10.1016/j.wneu.2012.03.022
37. Carragee EJ, Helms E, O'Sullivan GS. Are postoperative activity restrictions necessary after posterior lumbar discectomy? A prospective study of outcomes in 50 consecutive cases. *Spine (Phila Pa 1976).* 1996;21(16):1893-1897.
38. Brown TD, Michas P, Williams RE, et al. The impact of gunshot wounds on an orthopedic surgical service in an urban trauma center. *J Orthop Trauma.* 1997;11(3):149-153.
39. Wright DG, Levin JS, Esterhai JL, Heppenstall RB. Immediate internal fixation of low-velocity gunshot-related femoral fractures. *J Trauma.* 1993;35(5):678-681.
40. Patel AI, Lonner BS, Hoppenfield S. Cervical spine compression and burst fractures. In: Hoppenfield S, Vasantha LM, eds. *Treatment & Rehabilitation of Fractures.* Philadelphia, PA: Lippincott Williams & Wilkins; 2000:535-544.
41. Hasankhani EG, Omidi-Kashani F. Treatment outcomes of open pelvic fractures associated with extensive perineal injuries. *Clin Orthop Surg.* 2013;5(4):263-268. doi: 10.4055/cios.2013.5.4.263
42. Craik RL. Disability following hip fracture. *Phys Ther.* 1994;74(5):387-398.

43. Khasragi FA, Lee EJ, Christmas C, Wenz JF. The economic impact of medical complications in geriatric patients with hip fracture. *Orthopedics.* 2003;26(1):49-53.
44. Melton LJ III. Adverse outcomes of osteoporotic fractures in the general population. *J Bone Mineral Res.* 2003;18(16):1139-1141.
45. Nurmi I, Narinen A, Luthje P, Tanninen S. Cost analysis of hip fracture treatment among the elderly for the public health services: a 1-year prospective study in 106 consecutive patients. *Arch Orthop Trauma Surg.* 2003;123(10):551-554.
46. Mangione KK, Craik RL, Palombaro KM, Tomlinson SS, Hofmann MT. Home-based leg strengthening exercise improves function 1 year after hip fracture: a randomized controlled study. *J Am Geriatr Soc.* 2010;58(10):1911-1917.
47. Coburn M, Sanders RD, Maze M, Rossaint R; HIPELD Investigators. The Hip Fracture Surgery in Elderly Patients (HIPELD) study: protocol for a randomized, multicenter controlled trial evaluating the effect of xenon on postoperative delirium in older patients undergoing hip fracture surgery. *Trials.* 2012;13:180. doi: 10.1186/1745-6215-13-180
48. Mossey JM, Mutran E, Knott K, Craik R. Determinants of recovery 12 months after hip fracture: the importance of psychosocial factors. *Am J Public Health.* 1989;79(3):279-286.
49. Magaziner J, Fredman L, Hawkes W, et al. Changes in functional status attributable to hip fracture: a comparison study of hip fracture patients to community-dwelling aged. *Am J Epidemiol.* 2003;157(11):1023-1031.
50. Browner BD. *Skeletal Trauma: Basic Science, Management, and Reconstruction.* 3rd ed. Philadelphia, PA: WB Saunders; 2003.
51. Freudigman PT, Ziran BH. Orthopedic injuries. In: Peitzman AB, Rhodes M, Schwab CW, Yealy DM, eds. *The Trauma Manual.* Philadelphia, PA: Lippincott-Raven; 1998.
52. Lamagni T, Elgohari S, Harrington P. Trends in surgical site infections following orthopaedic surgery. *Curr Opin Infect Dis.* 2015;28(2):125-132.
53. Heier KA, Infante AF, Walling AK, Sanders RW. Open fractures of the calcaneus: soft-tissue injury determines outcome. *J Bone Joint Surg Am.* 2003;85-A(12):2276-2282.
54. Conway J, Mansour J, Kotze K, Specht S, Shabtai L. Antibiotic cement-coated rods: an effective treatment for infected long bones and prosthetic joint nonunions. *Bone Joint J.* 2014;96-B(10):1349-1354. doi: 10.1302/0301-620X.96B10.33799
55. Brighton CT, Shaman P, Heppenstall RB, et al. Tibial nonunion treated with direct current, capacitive coupling and bone graft. *Clin Orthop.* 1995;321:223-234.
56. Lew DP, Waldvogel FA. Osteomyelitis. *Lancet.* 2004;364(9431):369-379.
57. Lane JM, Glasser DB, Cammisa FP. Tumors. In: Steinberg, M, ed. *The Hip and Its Disorders.* Philadelphia, PA: WB Saunders; 1991:493.
58. Shurr DG, Cook TM. *Prosthetics and Orthotics.* East Norwalk, CT: Appleton & Lange; 1990.
59. Buonomo LJ, Klein JS, Keiper TL. Orthotic devices. Custom-made, prefabricated, and material selection. *Foot Ankle Clin.* 2001;6(2):249-252.

Appendix

Pharmacological Information: Musculoskeletal/Orthopedic Diseases and Disorders Pharmacology

Biphosphonates

Action

Biphosphonates are used in the treatment and prevention of osteoporosis. They may also be used to reduce bone pain and decrease risk of fracture in patients with bone metastases and Paget's disease. These medications stabilize and increase bone mineral density by inhibiting the activity of osteoclasts and stimulating the activity of osteoblasts.

Side Effects

CNS: Headache
CV: Dysrhythmias/tachycardia, HTN
GI: Abdominal discomfort, dyspepsia, acid reflux, nausea, vomiting
Miscellaneous: Hypokalemia, muscle weakness, musculoskeletal pain, osteonecrosis of jaw, atypical femur fracture (long term-use)

Common Medications

Fosamax (alendronate), Didronel (etidronate), Aredia (pamidronate)

Corticosteroids

Action

Systemic corticosteroids are often prescribed as an anti-inflammatory agent but are also used in the management of adrenocortical insufficiency, allergic, hematologic, neoplastic, and autoimmune diseases. These medications decrease inflammation and immune function through a variety of mechanisms including the reduced synthesis and release of mediators (eg, prostaglandins, leukotrienes, histamine) from lymphocytes, eosinophils, neutrophils, and mast cells.

Side Effects

CNS: Depression, euphoria, headache, restlessness
CV: HTN
Endocrine: Hyperglycemia
GI: Peptic ulcers
Miscellaneous: Osteoporosis, myopathy, weight gain, skin tears, immunocompromise

Common Medications

Betamethasone, cortisone, dexamethasone, hydrocortisone, methylprenisolone, prednisone

Disease Modifying Anti-Rheumatic Drugs

Action

Disease modifying anti-rheumatic drugs (DMARDs) are a varied group of medications used in rheumatology to slow disease progression. The drugs decrease bone and cartilage destruction by influencing mediators, metabolites, and immune responses involved in inflammation and autoimmune reactions.

Side Effects

CNS: Fatigue, headache, dizziness
CV: Chest pain, hypotension, HTN, tachycardia
GI: Abdominal pain, nausea, vomiting, constipation, diarrhea, dyspepsia
Miscellaneous: Arthralgia, myalgias, alopecia, rash
Pulmonary: Upper respiratory tract infections, cough

Common Medications

Anti-tumor necrosis factor (TNF): Enbrel (etanercept), Remicade (infliximab)
Immune modulation: Arava (leflunomide)
Cytostatic-cytotoxic drugs: Imuran (azathioprine), Cytoxan (cyclophosphamide), Rheumatrex (methotrexate)
Miscellaneous: Gold preparations

Gout Agents

Action

Gout agents decrease the hyperuricemia (ie, elevated blood uric acid concentration), local inflammation, and pain associated with the acute bouts of gout. Medications may inhibit uric acid synthesis (eg, allopurinol), alter immune responses (eg, cholcicine), and inflammation (eg, non-steroidal anti inflammatory drugs [NSAIDs], corticosteroids).

Side Effects

CNS: Drowsiness
GI: Diarrhea, nausea, vomiting
GU: Renal insufficiency, hematuria
Miscellaneous: Allergic reactions, bone marrow depression (leukopenia, thrombocytopenia), aplastic anemia

Common Medications

Allopurinol, colchicine, corticosteroids (see previously)

Non-Steroidal Anti-inflammatory Agents

Action

NSAIDs are used as anti-inflammatory medications (eg, osteoarthritis/rheumatoid arthritis), analgesics (mild to moderate pain), antipyretics (fever reduction) and anti-platelets agents (eg, myocardial infarction). These medications inhibit the enzyme cyclooxygenases (COX-1, COX-2) that decreases the synthesis of prostaglandins leading to their anti-inflammatory function and to a lesser extent the thrombaxanes leading to inhibition of platelets.

Side Effects
CNS: Headache, dizziness, drowsiness
CV: Prolonged bleeding times, edema
GI: Erosive gastritis, peptic ulcer disease, bleeding, dyspepsia/heart burn, nausea, vomiting
GU: Diminished sodium excretion and fluid retention, renal insufficiency (azotemia, oliguria)
Miscellaneous: Allergic reactions (bronchospasm), hyperkalemia, tinnitus

Common Medications
Salicylates: Ecotrin, Zorprin, Bufferin (aspirin); Advil, Motrin, Nuprin (ibuprofen); Indocin (indomethacin); Aleve, Anaprox, Naprosyn (naproxen)
COX-2 inhibitors: Celebrex (celecoxib), Vioxx (rofecoxib)

Opioids

Action
Opioids are a class of medications that alter the perception and responses to pain. Opioids potentiate the activity of endogenous opioid peptides (eg, eukephalins, endorphins) by binding to receptors with the CNS, reducing the release of the neurotransmitters dopamine and serotonin and inhibiting nociceptive peptides such as substance P, resulting in blockage of pain transmission.

Side Effects
CNS: CNS depression/sedation, confusion, dizziness, hallucinations, seizures
CV: Hypotension, bradycardia
GI: Constipation, nausea, vomiting
Miscellaneous: Flushing, sweating, physical dependence, tolerance
Pulmonary: Respiratory depression, bronchospasm

Common Medications
Stadol (butorphanol), codeine, fentanyl, hydrocodone, Demerol (meperidine), methadone, morphine, Oxycontin (oxycodone), Percocet (oxycodone and acetaminophen), Percodan (oxycodone and aspirin)

Skeletal Muscle Relaxants and Anti-Spasticity Agents

Action
Skeletal muscle relaxants and anti-spasticity agents are a diverse group of medications that impact neuromuscular activity. Agents may act within the CNS by inhibiting release of excitatory neurotransmitters (eg, baclofen) or presynaptic inhibition (eg, benzodiazepines). Agents may also act peripherally by inhibiting neuromuscular transmission through inhibition of acetylcholine release by nerve terminals (eg, botulinum toxin) or by blocking calcium release from the sarcoplasmic reticulum thereby uncoupling muscle excitation-contraction coupling (eg, dantrolene sodium).

Side Effects
CNS: Dizziness, drowsiness, fatigue, headache
CV: Hypotension, edema, dysrhythmias
GI: Constipation, dyspepsia, nausea
Miscellaneous: Dry mouth

Common Medications
Centrally acting: Lioresal (baclofen), Valium (diazepam), Flexeril (cyclobenzaprine)
Direct acting: Dantrium (dantrolene sodium), neuromuscular blocking agents (see Chapter 9, Pharmacological Information)

CNS = central nervous system; CV = cardiovascular; GI = gastrointestinal; GU = genitourinary.

Chapter 9

Neurologic and Neurosurgical Diseases and Disorders

Colleen Chancler, PT, MHS and Heather Dillon Anderson, PT, DPT, NCS

PART I: NEUROLOGY

Neurologic dysfunction encompasses many different disorders, including diagnoses based on a cluster of symptoms. The physical therapist and physical therapist assistant are commonly involved in the care of the patient from the intensive care unit (ICU) to the time of discharge to the next level of care. While examination and treatment strategies are numerous, the physiological response of the patient needs to be considered in each interaction because many neurological conditions and comorbidities arise in patient care. Progress can often be seen with direct therapy intervention and is an exciting part of the overall care of the patient.

Anatomy and Physiology

Anatomically, the **cerebral cortex** is described by dividing the surface area into the following lobes: frontal, parietal, temporal, occipital, limbic, and insular. The frontal lobe is generally described as the executor of human function. It is responsible for organizing behavior, shaping self-awareness, and controlling the actions of the body.[1] The parietal lobe serves as the sensory integrator for pain, temperature, detection of taste, and touch; it also coordinates the process of reading.[1] The temporal lobe contains the primary auditory center along with regions that are responsible for emotion, memory, and speech.[2,3] The occipital lobe contains the primary visual cortex and the visual association area (Figure 9-1).

The **brainstem** is a stalk-like structure, located in the posterior cranial fossa, that forms the rostral continuation of the spinal cord; this junction is marked by the foramen magnum.[4,5] The brainstem is covered posteriorly by the cerebellum and houses the fourth ventricle.[6] It consists of the medulla oblongata, pons, and midbrain. Each region has specialized responsibilities while sharing common fiber tracts.[2,7] These tracts carry somatosensory impulses as well as voluntary motor signals.[8] In addition,

Malone DJ, Bishop KL, eds. *Acute Care Physical Therapy: A Clinician's Guide, Second Edition* (pp 351-420).

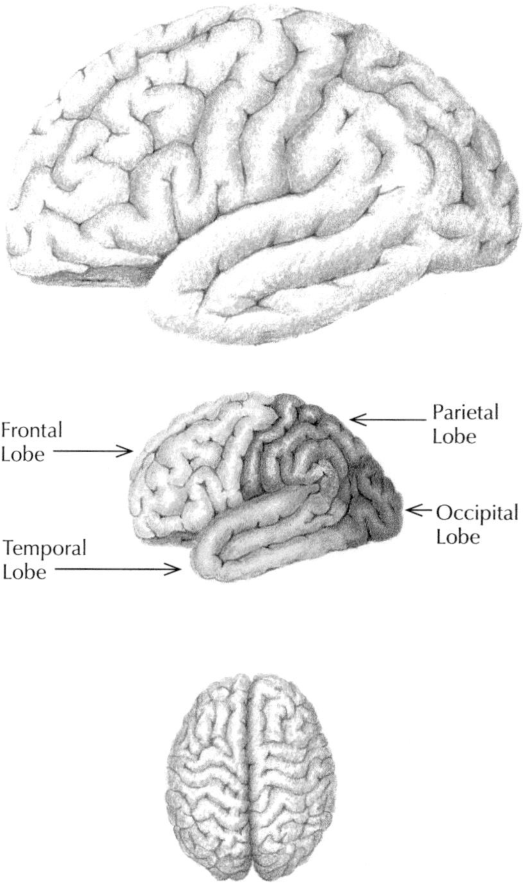

Figure 9-1. Cerebral lobes. (Reprinted with permission from Gutman SA. *Quick Reference Neuroscience for Rehabilitation Professionals. The Essential Neurologic Principles Underlying Rehabilitation Practice*. Thorofare, NJ: SLACK Incorporated; 2001:7.)

all but one of the 12 cranial nerves are located within the brainstem.[3] The brainstem connects to the cerebellum by 3 pairs of cerebellar peduncles that enable the transmission of information.[6]

The **cerebellum** lies posterior to the medulla and pons and is separated from them by the fourth ventricle. It connects to the brainstem via the paired inferior, middle, and superior cerebellar peduncles.[3,5] The cerebellum also contains 4 pairs of cerebellar nuclei deep to its surface.[2] The cerebellum is responsible for coordinating movements and balance by influencing the timing and force of voluntary muscular contractions (Figure 9-2).[2,4]

Four main arteries furnish the blood supply to the brain (Figure 9-3). These arteries include the paired vertebral arteries, which supply the brainstem, cerebellum, and posteroinferior cerebrum and the paired internal carotid arteries (ICAs), which supply the anterior, superior, and lateral cerebral hemispheres.[2,8,9]

The blood supplied by the paired **vertebral arteries**, the first branches off the subclavian arteries, is considered the **posterior circulation** and carries approximately 1/3 of the blood supply to the brain. Each vertebral artery has 3 main branches: the anterior and posterior spinal arteries and the posterior inferior cerebellar artery

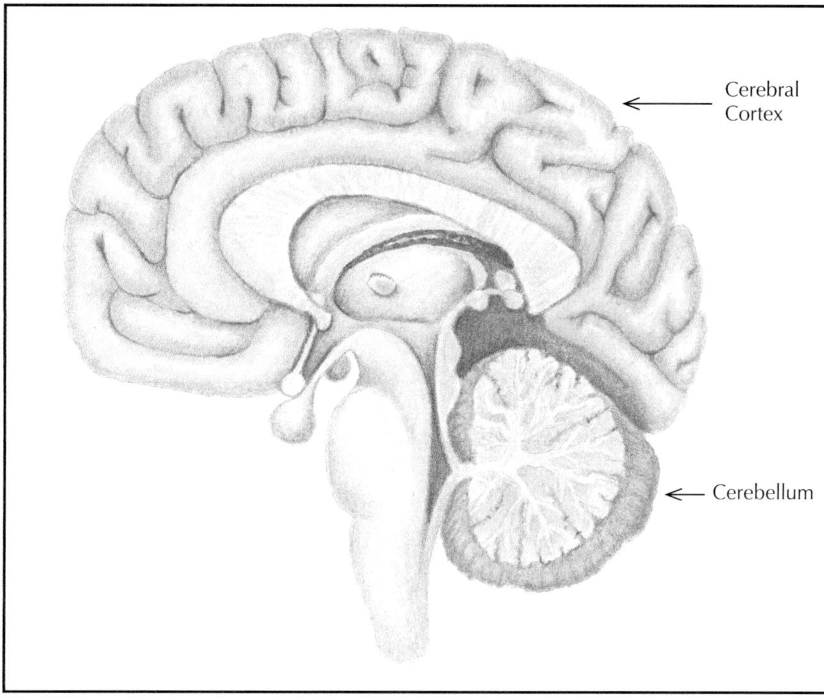

Figure 9-2. Midsagittal cross section of the brain. (Reprinted with permission from Gutman SA. *Quick Reference Neuroscience for Rehabilitation Professionals. The Essential Neurologic Principles Underlying Rehabilitation Practice*. Thorofare, NJ: SLACK Incorporated; 2001:13.)

(PICA). All 3 branches supply blood to the medulla. In addition, the PICA also supplies the inferior cerebellum.[2,10]

A stroke within the distribution of the vertebral artery may cause the following signs and symptoms[2,9-11]:

- **Wallenberg's syndrome**, also known as **lateral meduallary syndrome**, which involves pain, numbness, impaired sensation over half of the face, ataxia, vertigo, nystagmus, diplopia, dysphagia, muscular weakness or paralysis, numbness on the lateral side, and impaired pain and temperature on the contralateral side. This syndrome may also include ipsilateral **Horner's syndrome** (eg, miosis, ptosis of the upper lid, elevation of the lower lid and anhidrosis on the affected side of face).[11]
- **Medial medullary syndrome**, which involves ipsilateral paralysis of the tongue, contralateral paralysis of the upper extremity (UE) and lower extremity (LE) (facial muscles typically spared) and contralateral impairment of touch and position sense.
- Pain in the face, nose or eye; ipsilateral numbness and weakness of the face, nystagmus.
- Decreased coordination, dizziness, staggering gait
- Dysphagia and/or dysarthria

The **basilar artery** and its branches, which include the anterior inferior cerebellar artery (AICA) and superior cerebellar artery, supply the pons and the cerebellum.[6] At the junction of the midbrain and pons, the basilar artery divides into the

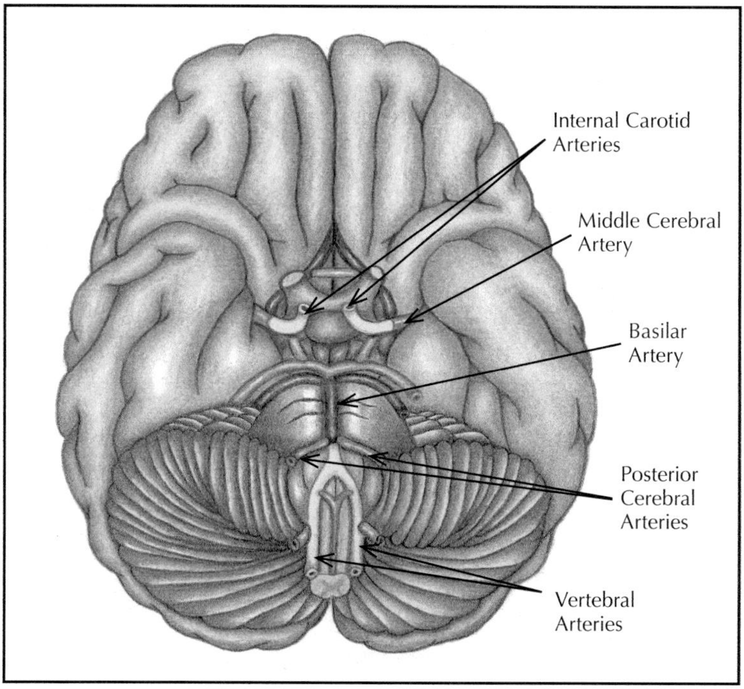

Figure 9-3. Blood supply to the brain. (Reprinted with permission from Gutman SA. *Quick Reference Neuroscience for Rehabilitation Professionals. The Essential Neurologic Principles Underlying Rehabilitation Practice*. Thorofare, NJ: SLACK Incorporated; 2001:197.)

posterior cerebral arteries, which serve as the primary blood supply to the midbrain.[2,11] Complete occlusion of this artery may be fatal. In general, basilar artery strokes may cause the following signs and symptoms[2,9]:

- Disturbances of consciousness (often coma)
- Bilateral cerebellar ataxia
- Decreased strength in facial, tongue, and pharyngeal muscles
- **Locked-in syndrome**, which is characterized by the patient being alert and awake but completely paralyzed. The only functions spared are the ability to move eyes vertically and blink.
- Paralysis
- Diplopia, paralysis of conjugate lateral and/or vertical gaze, ophthalmicmoplegia (paralysis of ocular musculature), and/or nystagmus

AICA stroke, also known as **lateral inferior pontine syndrome**, may cause the following signs and symptoms[2,9-11]:

- Ipsilateral paresis of lateral conjugate gaze and or nystagmus
- Ipsilateral **Horner's syndrome**
- Ipsilateral limb ataxia
- Vertigo, nausea, and/or **oscillopsia** (illusory sensation of the oscillation or swinging of the visual field)

- Impaired hearing and/or tinnitus
- Contralateral impaired pain and temperature sensation in the trunk, limbs, and face

The **ICAs** originate from the common carotid artery, and bifurcate into the external carotid artery and ICAs. These arteries are responsible for the **anterior circulation**. The external carotid arteries divide into extracranial branches, while the ICAs enter the skull through the temporal bones.[3,6] Branches of the internal carotid artery become the **posterior communicating arteries**, which join the ICAs to the posterior cerebral artery.[6] Near the optic chiasm, the ICAs divides into anterior and middle cerebral arteries. ICA stroke may cause the following signs and symptoms[2,9,10]:

- Paralysis and sensory impairments of the contralateral face, UEs, and LEs
- Aphasia if the dominant hemisphere is affected
- Apraxia, agnosia, and unilateral neglect if the non-dominant hemisphere is affected
- **Homonymous hemianopsia**, which involves similar visual loss in both eyes involving half of each visual field

The **circle of Willis** (Figure 9-4) is an anastomotic ring of 9 arteries: the anterior communicating, left anterior cerebral, left internal carotid, left posterior cerebral, basilar, right posterior cerebral, right posterior communicating, right internal carotid, and right anterior cerebral artery (ACA).[6,12] Because of its communicative design, the circle of Willis serves as a potential vascular shunt. This mechanism may assist in the development of collateral circulation to the brain should one of the proximal vessels, such as the carotid or basilar, become occluded.

The 3 major **cerebral arteries** (anterior, middle, and posterior) have cortical branches that supply the cortex and outer white matter and deep branches that supply the central gray matter and adjacent white matter.[6,8] The ACA supplies the medial surfaces of the frontal and parietal lobes as well as the anterior head of the caudate nucleus, which is part of the basal ganglia.[3,6] The ACA is the least likely vessel to become occluded. The **middle cerebral artery** (MCA) divides into branches that ultimately supply the lateral surface of the frontal, parietal, temporal, and occipital lobes.[6] The branches that supply these regions, also known as **lateral striate arteries**, are frequently the site of rupture or occlusion.[6] The **posterior cerebral artery** (PCA) supplies the midbrain, thalamus, occipital lobe, and sections of the medial and inferior temporal lobe.[3]

The **watershed** area represents an area of marginal blood flow on the surface of the lateral hemispheres, where small anastomoses link the distal ends of the cerebral arteries.[13] Hypotension, or hypoperfusion, may cause decreased blood flow to this area and may cause upper limb paresis and paresthesia.[8] The most common watershed cerebral infarct is between the ACAs and MCAs.[13]

Health Conditions

Stroke

A **stroke** or brain attack is currently the third leading cause of mortality and the leading cause of disability in the United States.[14-16] This disease process manifests as a sudden neurologic deficit, with a duration greater than 24 hours, due to a disruption of blood supply to the brain.[17]

A **transient ischemic attack** (TIA) is described as a temporary focal brain or brainstem ischemia with symptoms lasting less than 24 hours. TIAs often preclude stroke.[15] There are approximately 700,000 strokes per year in which more than 300,000 individuals sustain significant disability. Stroke can be linked to the following risk factors[16-19]:

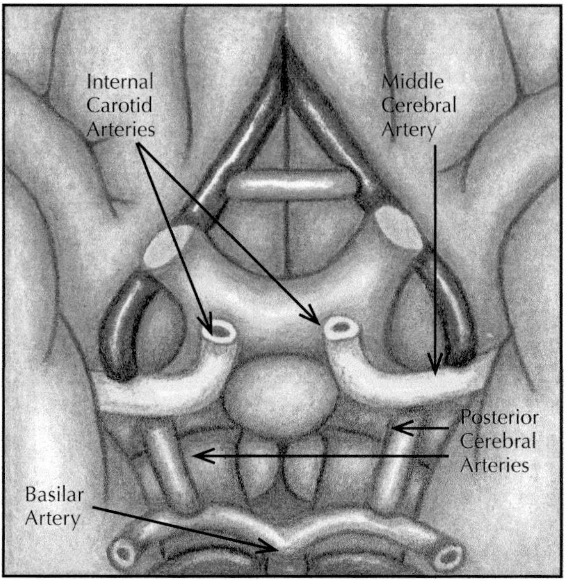

Figure 9-4. Circle of Willis. (Reprinted with permission from Gutman SA. *Quick Reference Neuroscience for Rehabilitation Professionals. The Essential Neurologic Principles Underlying Rehabilitation Practice*. Thorofare, NJ: SLACK Incorporated; 2001:199.)

- Atherosclerosis
- Hypertension (HTN)
- Vascular insufficiency
- Diabetes
- Cardiac disease
- Advanced age

Table 9-1 provides general descriptions of the impairments that may result from damage to regions of the brain.

The pathological processes causing strokes are classified as ischemia or hemorrhage. Cerebral damage occurs secondary to reduced oxygenation of brain tissue, which leads to cell damage and/or death.[14,16] The location and severity of the lesion, coupled with the quality of collateral blood flow, influence the severity of neurologic deficits that evolve following a stroke.[14,15]

Ischemic strokes are more common than hemorrhagic strokes and account for approximately 80% of the strokes in the United States.[17] Ischemic strokes are characterized by cerebral hypoperfusion, which causes tissue injury secondary to a reduced oxygen and glucose supply.[14,17] The most common cause of ischemic stroke is thromboembolic atherosclerotic disease with emboli traveling from the cervical vessels (ie, carotid arteries or vertebrobasilar system) and/or the heart.[19] Additional causes include thrombosis, hemodynamic compromise, and vessel stenosis.[16,18]

Symptoms of ischemic stroke develop and worsen over time. Ischemic strokes occur most often in the early morning or the evening. Warning symptoms, such as visual changes, cognitive impairment, slurred speech, motor dysfunction, and impaired ambulation, usually precede an ischemic stroke.

Hemorrhagic strokes are characterized by abnormal bleeding of cerebral vessels. This type of stroke may occur within the brain parenchyma (intracerebral hemorrhage [ICH]) or within the meninges (subdural hemorrhage [SDH] or subarachnoid hemorrhage [SAH]).[15] Cellular destruction is caused by ischemia secondary to reduced

Table 9-1

Cerebrovascular Accident Impairments Based on Central Nervous System Region

Region	*Impairment*
Right cerebral hemisphere	Left-sided paresis, decreased attention span, decreased awareness and judgment, memory deficits, left hemianopsia, left inattention, decreased abstract reasoning, emotional lability, impulsivity, and/or decreased spatial orientation
Left cerebral hemisphere	Right-sided paresis, right hemianopsia aphasia, apraxia, decreased right and left discrimination, dysphagia, decreased initiation of tasks, increased frustration, and/or compulsive behavior
Brainstem	Bilateral paresis, unstable vital signs, decreased consciousness, and/or dysphagia
Cerebellum	Bilateral decreased coordination, ataxia, nystagmus, nausea, and/or decreased postural control

Adapted from Umphred DA. *Neurological Rehabilitation*. 3rd ed. St. Louis, MO: Mosby-Year Book, Inc; 1995.

blood flow beyond the damaged portion of the vessel and mechanical injury caused by edema and the pressure of blood collection.[17] Causes of hemorrhagic strokes include advanced age, HTN, arteriovenous malformation (AVM), closed head injury, coagulopathy, ruptured aneurysms, and drug abuse.[14,19,20]

Unlike ischemic strokes, the area of infarction association with hemorrhagic strokes does not follow vascular territories, but instead may travel deep into brain structures and extend into several vascular territories causing unique clinical symptoms.[20] Vomiting, a severe headache, and/or impaired consciousness are symptoms that typically occur with hemorrhagic strokes. The sudden onset of these symptoms may help differentiate hemorrhagic strokes from ischemic strokes.[18,19]

Acute diagnosis for a stroke typically involves a thorough systems review, past medical history, physical examination, and diagnostic testing to determine the origin and the extent of the stroke.[21] The signs and symptoms manifested by the stroke often enable the medical team to determine whether it is affecting the anterior or posterior circulation, which is useful in determining which tests are indicated. Lab values, electrocardiogram (ECG), and imaging are performed prior to the initiation of a treatment plan. Computed tomography (CT) scan, magnetic resonance imaging (MRI), and magnetic resonance angiography (MRA) to examine blood flow and vascular integrity in the neck, brain, and intracranial arteries are also typically performed. Transcranial Doppler (TCD) is the use of ultrasound waves to measure blood velocity through the major intracranial arteries as well as the collateral circulation.[18] Increased TCDs may signify ischemic stroke. Acute ischemic strokes may be treated with intravenous tissue plasminogen activator (tPA) if the onset of symptoms is known to be less than 3 hours and specific criteria, including brain imaging, confirms a nonhemorrhagic event.[17] tPA is a thrombolytic agent known to be effective in reducing impairments and/or disability caused by ischemic strokes by reducing or eliminating the presence of a blood clot within the brain.[17]

When managing patients with acute stroke, coordinated care is essential to optimizing outcomes.[22,23] Please refer to Table 9-2 for impairment classifications. There is considerable evidence that care of persons after stroke in a dedicated, specialized stroke unit reduces mortality and improves overall functional outcome.[24-26] The Joint Commission, in conjunction with the American Heart Association and American

Table 9-2

MODIFIED NATIONAL INSTITUTES OF HEALTH STROKE SCALE

#	*Item Name*	*Response*
1A	Level of consciousness	0 = Alert 2 = Not alert, obtunded 3 = Unresponsive
1B	Questions	0 = Answers both correctly 1 = Answers one correctly 2 = Answers neither correctly
1C	Commands	0 = Performs both tasks correctly 1 = Performs one task correctly 2 = Performs neither task correctly
2	Gaze	0 = Normal 1 = Partial gaze palsy 2 = Total gaze palsy
3	Visual fields	0 = No visual field loss 1 = Partial hemianopsia 2 = Complete hemianopsia 3 = Bilateral hemianopsia
4	Facial palsy	0 = Normal 1 = Minor paralysis 2 = Partial paralysis 3 = Complete paralysis
5	Motor arm	0 = No drift 1 = Drift before 5 seconds 2 = Falls before 10 seconds 3 = No effort against gravity 4 = No movement
6	Motor leg	0 = No drift 1 = Drift before 5 seconds 2 = Falls before 5 seconds 3 = No effort against gravity 4 = No movement

(continued)

Stroke Association, has specific guidelines to certify dedicated stroke centers. Comprehensive stroke centers are typically academic medical centers with tertiary care and offer the most services, including a dedicated neurocritical care unit and constant access to neurosurgery. Primary stroke centers offer standard stroke care, including tPA, and must have a dedicated stroke unit.[27]

Earlier mobilization of persons with stroke is one component of care noted as being different in these specialized settings. Evidence indicates that early mobilization and functional training post-stroke are important to foster neuroplasticity, which improves recovery and prevents complications.[24,25] Currently, the literature lacks consensus for the exact timing of mobilization. Often, a person with stroke

Table 9-2 (continued)

Modified National Institutes of Health Stroke Scale

#	*Item Name*	*Response*
7	Ataxia	0 = Absent 1 = One limb 2 = Two limbs
8	Sensory	0 = Normal 1 = Mild loss 2 = Severe loss
9	Language	0 = Normal 1 = Mild aphasia 2 = Severe aphasia 3 = Mute or global aphasia
10	Dysarthria	0 = Normal 1 = Mild 2 = Severe
11	Extinction and inattention	0 = Normal 1 = Mild 2 = Severe

Adapted from Kasner SE, Cucchiara BL, McGarvey ML, et al. Modified National Institutes of Health Stroke Scale can be estimated from medical records. *Stroke*. 2003;34:568-570.

is on bed rest for the first 24 hours following stroke, especially when tPA is used. One study examining mobilization in less than 24 hours following stroke identified a trend toward increased poor outcomes, death rate, and dependency.[25] In another study, better outcomes in neurological functioning was found in patients mobilized between 24 and 48 hours post-stroke.[28] Additional research is needed in this area to identify best practice for the timing of mobilization.

Neuromuscular Diseases

Parkinsonism syndrome is characterized by clinical features of tremor, rigidity, bradykinesia, changes in handwriting (micrographia), reduction in speech volume, and gait disorders.[14] Medical conditions that cause Parkinsonism syndrome include toxic exposures, hypothyroidism, hypoparathyroidism, and other neurologic conditions. One of the main causes of Parkinsonism is **Parkinson's disease**.[15] Parkinson's disease is an idiopathic neurodegenerative disorder that affects approximately 1/100 people over the age of 75 years old, and 1/1,000 people over the age of 65.[9,29,30] The etiology is unknown; slightly more males than females are affected by the disease. Management of Parkinson's disease typically involves pharmacologic therapy with antidyskinetic agents.[13]

Clinical features include tremor at rest, rigidity, bradykinesia, and gait impairments. Tremor is characterized by "pill rolling" of the fingertips and hands. Tremor is exacerbated by conditions of stress, fatigue, or by the beginning or end of movement. **Dyskinesia**, over activity of muscles, can cause rigidity of movement patterns. Rigidity in the extremities is a "cogwheel" phenomenon, which is resistance to passive movement in a jerking fashion throughout the range of motion (ROM) or "leadpipe" phenomenon, which is resistance to passive movement throughout the

Table 9-3 HOEHN AND YAHR CLASSIFICATION	
Stage I	Unilateral involvement only with minimal or no functional impairment
Stage II	Bilateral or axial involvement without balance impairment
Stage III	Impaired righting reflexes; functional impairments exist, but patient remains independent
Stage IV	Able to walk but severe disability
Stage V	Confined to bed or chair and requires assistance for all tasks
Adapted from Morris ME. Movement disorders in people with Parkinson's disease: a model for physical therapy. *Phys Ther.* 2000;80:578-596.	

entire motion. Facial rigidity, fixed trunk flexion, and loss of trunk rotation may occur as the syndrome/disease progresses. **Bradykinesia** is slowness in initiating movement or completion of tasks. Persons with Parkinsonism syndrome/Parkinson's disease demonstrate decreased ability to initiate movement and change directions (mild hypokinesia). Associated gait disorders can vary in presentation and severity. **Festinating gait** (small shuffling gait pattern), **akinesia** (decreased initiation of motion), and **severe hypokinesia** (reduction in movement) can result in instability and falls.[30] Recent studies have shown that patients with Parkinsonism syndrome/ Parkinson's disease have difficulty when trying to self-initiate a task. In gait, for instance, the patient would have a more difficult time when walking across a floor because he or she has to choose the path and the sequence of the task. If presented the same task with external cueing by music or verbal commands, then the patient would be motivated by external stimulus and have less difficulty in initiation and completion of the motor task.[31]

The pathophysiology of Parkinson's disease is related to decreased amounts of the neurotransmitter dopamine. **Dopamine** is produced by nerve cells in the substantia nigra and is responsible for smooth and balanced movement. Parkinson's disease causes nerve cell death that impacts the production of dopamine. Changes of dopamine receptors result in decreased binding of dopamine within the basal ganglia.[14,15] Diagnosis is often delayed because symptoms can initially mirror other neurologic conditions. There is no specific diagnostic test for Parkinson's disease. Rather, diagnosis of the disease is made by the physical examination, comprehensive history, activity level, and elimination of other neurologic causes for the symptom manifestation. Use of the Hoehn and Yahr classification allows for a clinical representation and staging progression of the disease process (Table 9-3).

Multiple sclerosis (MS) is an upper motor neuron disease characterized by an inflammatory process that results in the destruction of the myelin sheath within the white matter of the central nervous system (CNS).[9,32] This process disrupts neurotransmission and leaves patches of sclerotic tissue or scarring that contributes to the destruction of axons.[14] With prolonged scarring produced by damaged glial cells, called **gliosis**, the nerve fibers in that region degenerate and cause permanent disability.[5,15] Initially, neurologic symptoms typically correspond to the affected region of the CNS and disappear completely during remission.[15]

The signs and symptoms of MS are widely varied because the disease affects multiple regions within the CNS. Typical impairments include fatigue, sensory dysfunction, motor symptoms, spasticity, ataxia, visual disturbances, and/or decreased coordination.[33] When the brainstem is involved, **Charcot triad** may emerge, which includes nystagmus, intentional tremors, and staccato speech scanning.[34]

Table 9-4

CLINICAL COURSE OF MULTIPLE SCLEROSIS

Type	*Incidence*	*Description*
Benign	20%	Abrupt onset with mild symptoms and few exacerbations. Remissions are near complete with minimal or no disability.
Exacerbating-remitting	20% to 30%	Increased frequency of attacks with sudden onset of symptoms; partial or complete remission of symptoms after exacerbations. Patients often go for long periods between attacks, but may be left with permanent disabilities.
Remitting-progressive	40%	Similar to exacerbating-remitting except the remissions are fewer with decreased resolution of symptoms. The disease becomes cumulative and disability increases.
Progressive	10% to 20%	Insidious onset without remission, leads to progressive loss of function and severe disability.

Adapted from Hickey JV. *Clinical Practice of Neurological and Neurosurgical Nursing*. Philadelphia, PA: JB Lippincott; 1992; O'Sullivan, Schmitz TJ. *Physical Rehabilitation, Assessment and Treatment*. 3rd ed. Philadelphia, PA: FA Davis; 1994; and Umphred DA. *Neurological Rehabilitation*. 3rd ed. St. Louis, MO: Mosby-Year Book, Inc; 1995.

MS is the most common cause of severe physical disability in young adults; the highest rate of incidence is between 20 and 40 years of age.[2,35] The majority of persons with MS report the onset of symptoms to occur in their 30s, with women being slightly more affected than men, and White people being more affected than Black people.[15] The etiology of MS is unknown. There is no specific diagnostic test for MS. Diagnosis is primarily clinical diagnosis and supportive evidence from MRI, spinal tap, electromyogram (EMG), and laboratory studies.[33]

The clinical description of MS can be roughly divided into 4 patterns as described in Table 9-4. MS is often managed pharmacologically with the use of interferons, immunosuppressive agents, and hormones; steroids are commonly administered during exacerbations (see Pharmacological Information in Chapters 7, 10, and 14).[33]

The most common cause of acute neuromuscular paralysis is **Guillain-Barré syndrome** (GBS), also called **acute idiopathic polyneuritis**.[15] GBS occurs in approximately 1/100,000 people annually with a 10% mortality rate.[36]

GBS is a lower motor neuron disease that involves rapid demyelination causing motor weakness, areflexia, and sensory abnormalities.[37] Symptoms typically begin distally with fine paresthesias in toes and/or hands and develop into acute motor weaknesses and sensory disturbances that ascend symmetrically to the upper body. Weakness may also involve respiratory, bulbar, and/or autonomic failure.[9,15]

The etiology of GBS is unknown. Approximately 40% to 60% of patients with GBS report a preceding bacterial or viral infection.[37] The predominant pathological finding is an immune-mediated inflammation of the cranial and spinal nerve roots with lymphocytic and macrophage infiltration and demyelination.[36,37] Damage to the myelin sheath reduces and/or blocks saltatory nerve conduction, causing paresis.[6] In addition, axonal degeneration has been noted in many cases in which conduction velocity is within normal limits, but the total number of motor units is decreased.[38]

At the peak of its course, which is typically 7 to 14 days, 20% to 30% of persons with GBS will require mechanical ventilation.[38] The recovery phase typically begins

2 weeks to 1 month following onset and involves remyelination that usually begins proximally and spreads distally.[37,38] Weakness that progresses chronically (longer than 4 weeks) or relapses may be considered **chronic idiopathic demyelinating polyradiculoneuropathy** (CIDP).[37] The recovery phase for GBS may continue for many months. Approximately 80% of patients become ambulatory within 6 months following onset, with 70% to 80% of individual making a full recovery.[15] Medical treatment of GBS typically includes plasmapherisis and high-dose immunoglobulin therapy.[9]

The most common primary disorder of neuromuscular transmission is **myasthenia gravis** with an incidence of 14 out of every 100,000 people in the United States.[39,40] Myasthenia gravis is a chronic, progressive autoimmune disease that is characterized by weakness of the voluntary muscles, particularly those of chewing, swallowing, and speaking, as well as the facial and extraocular muscles.[41] The onset of symptoms is typically gradual, with symptoms progressing over a period of 5 to 7 years.[39] The ocular, facial, and oropharyngeal muscles are most often affected first with weakness eventually extending to the extremities and diaphragm.[39] A sudden exacerbation of symptoms that involves respiratory failure is known as a **myasthenic crises** and often requires mechanical ventilation.[40,41]

The pathophysiology of myasthenia gravis is related to antibodies that bind and degrade acetylcholine (Ach) receptors located within the neuromuscular junction.[35] This process reduces the number of receptor sites interfering with the transmission of nerve impulses to the muscle and inhibiting muscle contraction.[39,40] There is currently no cure for myasthenia gravis. Treatment options include cholinesterase inhibitors, immunosuppressive medications, plasmapheresis, thymectomy, and intravenous immunoglobulin.[39-41]

Amyotrophic lateral sclerosis (ALS), also known as **Lou Gehrig's disease**, is a rapidly progressive, fatal, degenerative disease that affects both upper and lower motor neurons.[15] In the United States, the incidence of ALS is 1.4/100,000 people with a ratio of 3 men to every woman.[2] It is characterized by an insidious onset of asymmetrical weakness. Additional symptoms include muscle cramping and fasciculations, hyperreflexia, and cranial nerve dysfunction with intact sensation and cognition.[2,39]

The etiology of ALS is unknown; however, numerous theories, including viral, toxic, defective DNA, and/or hormonal malfunction, have been proposed.[2,15] ALS is characterized by massive destruction of anterior horn cells and motor cranial nerve nuclei, along with demyelination and gliosis of the pyramidal tracts.[15] ALS progresses rapidly; researchers estimate that by the time patient identifies his or her first symptom, 80% of the motor neurons in the affected region have already been destroyed.[15] Patients with an initial onset of bulbar and respiratory weakness tend to have a more rapid progression than patients who report their initial symptoms in the distal extremities.[9] The median survival time is approximately 4 years after onset of symptoms.[15] Currently, there is no cure for ALS.

Traumatic Brain Injury

According to Davies,[42] 1.5 to 2 million traumatic brain injuries (TBIs) occur annually in the United States and up to 90,000 of these persons will experience long-term functional impairments, cognitive impairments, and emotional changes. TBI is currently the number 1 killer and disabler of children and young adults, with child abuse accounting for 64% of infant brain injuries.[15] The most common age group for TBI is 15 to 24 years old, with the incidence in males 2 to 3 times greater than females.[2,15,42]

Motor vehicles accidents are the most common cause of TBI, accounting for 50%, falls account for 20%, violence accounts for 12%, and sports-related injuries account for 12%.[42] According to Yanko and Mitcho,[43] there has been gradual decline of

TBIs in the past 20 years, which is attributed to improvements in automobile safety standards.

The pathophysiology of TBI involves primary and secondary injuries. The **primary** mechanism of injury occurs at the moment of impact and involves extracranial injury (open head injury), including skull fractures and/or intracranial injury (closed head injury).[43] **Secondary** brain injuries are related to the pathophysiologic changes that occur after the primary insult to the brain. These changes include systemic hypotension, edema, respiratory complications, hypoxia, autodestructive cellular phenomena, which involves neurochemical changes that ultimately cause the destruction of neurons, and increased **intracranial pressure** (ICP), which may result in **herniation** of brain tissue.[15,43,44]

Intracranial injury often includes local brain damage caused by contusions and/or lacerations along the surface of the brain. These may occur at the location of impact (coup), directly opposite the site of impact (contrecoup), or in both regions (coup-contrecoup).[13] **Diffuse axonal injury** (DAI) is characterized by diffuse white matter degeneration, global neurologic dysfunction, and diffuse cerebral edema.[43] DAI occurs secondary to a widely scattered shearing of subcortical axons within their myelin sheaths in the presence of impact forces.[39,40] DAI remains a diagnosis of exclusion because imaging technology often fails to detect changes in the brain tissue despite clinical presentation of cognitive impairment or conscious changes.[44,45] If damage is widespread and extends into the midbrain and brainstem, it may cause cumulative effects such as coma and/or autonomic dysfunction.[44,46]

Late-occurring intracranial hematomas and/or ICHs are additional sources of secondary brain injury. Hematomas are named for the location in which they occur (ie, epidural, subdural, intracerebral) and by the time in which they develop (ie, acute, subacute, chronic).[46]

TBIs can be classified based on the location, extent, severity, and/or the mechanism of injury.[13] In addition, several clinical rating scales have been developed to standardize the descriptions of patients who have sustained brain injury. The **Glasgow Coma Scale** (GCS), as described in Table 9-5, rates the level of consciousness from 3 to 15 using the following 3 parameters: eye opening, motor response, and verbal response.[14] Jennett and Teasdale are the researchers who developed the GSC, and patients who score 8 or less are classified as having severe head injuries. Scores between 9 and 12 are indicative of moderate head injuries, and those classified as mild head injuries score 13 and above. The minimum GCS score is 3, and the maximum is 15.[5,15]

The **Rancho Los Amigos Level of Cognitive Functioning** (LOCF), as featured in Table 9-6, was also designed to assess arousal by describing a predictable sequence of cognitive and behavioral recovery seen in patients with TBI.[14] A patient may plateau at any level but will typically progress through the described stages. By referring to the appropriate stage, therapists are able to complete a uniform assessment, documentation, and prediction of behavior.[14,15]

Physical Therapist Management

Neurologic Evaluation

One of the most important aspects of completing a thorough neurologic examination (Table 9-7) is to first complete a comprehensive chart review. After the chart review, approach the patient with an observant eye. Many functional and cognitive behaviors are apparent with a brief period of observation at the start of the examination and intervention.[47]

To assess **tone**, ask the patient to relax and allow the examiner to do the work of moving the patient's muscles. The examiner begins by passively moving each limb

Table 9-5

Glasgow Coma Scale

Activity	*Score*
Eye opening (E):	
Spontaneously	4
To verbal command	3
To pain	2
No response	1
Best motor response (M):	
To verbal command:	
Obeys	6
To painful stimulus:	
Localizes pain	5
Flexion-withdrawl	4
Flexion-abnormal	3
Extension	2
No response	1
Verbal response (V):	
Oriented and converses	5
Disoriented and converses	4
Inappropriate words	3
Incomprehensible sounds	2
No response	1
Coma score (E + M + V) = 3 to 15	
Adapted from O'Sullivan, Schmitz TJ. *Physical Rehabilitation, Assessment and Treatment.* 3rd ed. Philadelphia, PA: FA Davis; 1994.	

through all available planes of motion at a constant speed while providing support to the joints in motion.[14,48,49] Next, the examiner completes the same movements with an increased and then decreased speed to assess the effects of velocity. The characteristics of movement should be described according to the muscle groups tested and include a bilateral comparison along with a description of how velocity affected the movements.[48,49]

Flaccidity refers to hypotonia or decreased/absent muscular tone. Resistance to passive range of motion (PROM) is decreased, causing the limbs to feel heavy and/or floppy to the examiner. This state can be caused by upper motor neuron lesions affecting the cerebellum or pyramidal tracts, as a temporary state following injury to the CNS, or secondary to a lower motor neuron lesion affecting the peripheral nervous system (PNS).[49]

Rigidity refers to non-velocity dependent resistance that is felt in both the agonist and antagonist muscles with PROM. Two types of rigidity are typically described:

Table 9-6

RANCHO LOS AMIGOS LEVELS OF COGNITIVE FUNCTIONING

#	*Level*	*Description*
I	No response	The patient does not demonstrate any response to stimuli.
II	Generalized response	The patient reacts in a nonspecific and nonpurposeful way to stimuli. Responses are inconsistent and may be physiologic changes, gross movements, and/or vocalization.
III	Localized response	The patient reacts specifically but inconsistently to stimuli. Simple commands such as closing eyes or squeezing hand may be followed in a delayed inconsistent manner.
IV	Confused, agitated	The patient demonstrates increased activity with bizarre nonpurposeful behavior in relation to his or her surroundings. Decreased attention, short-, and long-term recall, and often with incoherent and/or inappropriate verbalization. Not able to directly cooperate with treatment efforts.
V	Confused, inappropriate	The patient can follow simple commands but demonstrates nonpurposeful, random, or fragmented responses to complex commands. Highly distractible with an inability to focus on a specific task. May perform previously learned tasks with structure, but does not demonstrate ability to learn new information. Verbalization is often inappropriate and/or confabulatory.
VI	Confused, appropriate	The patient is able to demonstrate goal-directed behavior but is dependent on external input or direction. Demonstrates carryover for relearned tasks, such as self-care. Past memories more intact than recent. Responses may by incorrect secondary to memory problems, but they are appropriate to the situation.
VII	Automatic, appropriate	Patient demonstrates appropriate behavior within the hospital and home settings, is oriented, and, with structure, is able to initiate social or recreational activities. There is carryover for new learning but at a decreased rate; affect is robot-like and automatic. Judgment remains impaired.
VIII	Purposeful, appropriate	The patient is aware of and responds to his or her surroundings, demonstrates carryover, and is able to demonstrate new learning as well as recall and integrate past and recent events. The patient may still have difficulty when faced with stress, abstract reasoning, emergencies, and/or unusual circumstances.

Adapted from O'Sullivan SB, Schmitz TJ. *Physical Rehabilitation, Assessment and Treatment*. 3rd ed. Philadelphia, PA: FA Davis; 1994 and Umphred DA. *Neurological Rehabilitation*. 3rd ed. St. Louis, MO: Mosby-Year Book, Inc; 1995.

leadpipe, which refers to constant hypertonia (increased tone), and **cogwheel**, which describes a rachet-like response to passive movement in which the tone increases and then decreases.[15] Rigidity is a characteristic of disorders within the extrapyramidal system, such as Parkinson's disease.[14]

Table 9-7

Acute Neurologic Physical Therapy Examination

Examination Feature	*Documentation*	*Clinical Tips*
History	Prior neurological events, smoking, other stroke risk factors; social history; employment history; medical and/or surgical history	This may guide your education strategy for the patient Include set-up at discharge if known.
Chief complaint	A subjective statement from the patient	Often taken as the first statement made by the patient.
Prior level of function		Include use of assistive devices and the need for orthotics/prosthetics; any adaptive equipment at home
Medications	All medications including over-the-counter	Include adherence to medications in the past
Observation of the patient	Notice the self-selected positioning of the patient prior to mobilization	Neglect/inattention to hemiparetic side often apparent
Arousal, attention, and cognition	Use Rancho Los Amigos LOCF, GCS, Mini-Mental State Examination (MMSE), motivation, memory, and ability to follow commands	Sitting upright may stimulate the reticular activating system (RAS) and increase patient arousal[36]
ROM and tone assessment	Consider any hypo- or hypertonicity	Consider grading a muscle with neurologic impairment means isolation movement. If increased tone is present, alternate methods of grading need to be considered. See text for full description. *(continued)*

Dystonia refers to a condition in which tone fluctuates unpredictably from low to high with sustained and twisting involuntary movements. Dystonia results from a central deficit and may be inherited (primary idiopathic dystonia), related to neurodegenerative disorders such as Parkinson's disease or Wilson's disease, or secondary to metabolic disorders.[2,15]

Spasticity refers to a velocity dependent (ie, the quicker the stretch, the stronger the resistance of the spastic muscle) increase in tonic stretch reflexes. Spasticity is felt within the muscles on one side of the joint that is being stretched and is indicative of upper motor neuron damage.[14,44] The **Modified Ashworth Scale for Grading Spasticity**, as described in Table 9-8, may be used to objectively describe the muscles demonstrating increased spasticity.[14,50]

Table 9-7 (continued)

ACUTE NEUROLOGIC PHYSICAL THERAPY EXAMINATION

Examination Feature	*Documentation*	*Clinical Tips*
Integumentary system	Inspect the skin for edema, discoloration, and breakdown	Ensure inspection is completed for redness. Blanching check for any redness is indicated. Consider using Braden scale when skin breakdown is present
Gait and balance	Describe characteristics of gait and use of assistive devices and/or orthotics	Consider the Functional Independence Measure (FIM), Barthel Index, Berg Balance Test, Timed Up and Go (TUG) Test, Functional Reach Test, and Dynamic Gait Index
Pain	Use 0 to 10 pain scale	Consider using the Brief Pain Inventory; when language is impaired consider using Faces Pain Scale
Sensation	Deep touch, light touch, vibration, proprioception	Deficits can also cause impaired motor response[11]
Medical interventions in patient care	Peripheral or central lines, catheter, drains, supplemental oxygen, mechanical ventilation	Origin and implication for treatment of lines should be known prior to movement of the patient
Physiologic readings	Blood pressure (BP), heart rate (HR), ECG, respiratory rate (RR)	May need to use mean arterial pressure (MAP)[43]; record with each session and more than one time within a session. See text for full details.

Clinical Tips

- Position patients with low tone in positions that will preserve the correct anatomical position of their joints.[48]
- To facilitate a muscular contraction, attempt a quick stretch or light strokes in the desired motion, tapping the muscle belly, high-intensity vibration, and/or functional electrical stimulation.
- To reduce spasticity, complete active assistive range of motion (AAROM), PROM, and stretching with slow gradual motions; avoid sudden quick movements.
- Deep pressure applied to the muscle belly and/or tendons, prolonged ice, low-intensity vibration, heat, and maintained touch may inhibit muscle tone.
- Gentle rocking and rhythmic stabilization and the addition of a rotational component to the desired motion may help reduce rigidity.

Table 9-8

MODIFIED ASHWORTH SCALE FOR GRADING SPASTICITY

Grade	*Description*
0	No increase in muscle tone
1	Slight increase in muscle tone, detectable by a catch and release or by minimal resistance at the end range of flexion or extension.
2	Slight increase in muscle tone, detected by a catch, followed by minimal resistance throughout the remainder (less than half) of the ROM. The affected parts are easily moved.
3	More marked increase in muscle tone through most of the ROM, but affected musculature easily moved.
4	Considerable increase in muscle tone; PROM difficult.
5	Affected musculature rigid in flexion or extension.

Adapted from Howe T. Measuring muscle tone and movement. *Nursing Standard.* 1995;9:25-29.

- Positioning the patient in side-lying helps to reduce rigidity; complete ROM from this position when possible.[48]
- MAP may serve as a parameter for BP limits as indicated by the medical team.
- Normal MAP values range between 70 and 110 mm Hg (see Table 3-1).[51] The parameters for patients with decreased perfusion, such as following an ischemic stroke, may involve MAP up to 130 mm Hg. Be sure to note BP parameters in the patient's chart and confer with the patient's nurse and/or doctor if BP measurements are outside of the specified parameters.

Treatment Strategies

Focusing the activity of the patient to functional tasks that have meaning is important in any setting. Task specificity, quantity of practice, and environmental set-up enable success in the presence of neurologic injury. Common treatment strategies for the neurologic patient are provided in Tables 9-9 through 9-11.

Secondary medical conditions must be considered. Coordinating interventions with medication dosing is helpful; however, the physical therapist/physical therapist assistant should not neglect teaching the patient and family strategies during periods when medication is not at peak levels.[45] Due to the chronic and progressive nature of many neurologic conditions, durable medical equipment will likely be needed to maximize the patient's functional level. Consideration should be given to rental equipment if change in the neuromuscular condition may warrant different equipment within a year.

From the acute care environment, many patients will require another level of care post-discharge. This may include inpatient rehabilitation, outpatient, home, or long-term care services. Continuation of the rehabilitation process should be considered in the plan of care for the patient.

Table 9-9

ACUTE CARE PHYSICAL THERAPY AND STROKE

Impairments	*Interventions*	*Clinical Tips*	*Goals*
Shoulder subluxation	• Positioning • Functional electrical stimulation (FES)[33,35]; taping techniques • Strength training • Preserve ROM especially for external rotation[52]	• Facilitate anatomic positioning to avoid stretch of the brachial plexus.[53,54] • FES protocol for shoulder subluxation can be initiated in acute care.[52,55] • ROM preservation is preventative for painful shoulder syndrome.[52]	• Promote stability in affected musculature to prevent pain • Maintain ROM • Facilitate motor return to involved area
Sensory changes	• Tactile input to stimulate affected region • Patient and family education to draw visual attention to affected regions and forced use of extremity[17]	• Sling may be indicated for hemiparetic arm if there is decreased awareness and potential for injury.[54] • Protect affected side from injury while moving.	• Improve motor control of affected region • Prevent injury to affected area
Altered communication	• Determine which method of communication works best for your patient[47] • Use short, simple commands	• Coordinate with speech therapy. • Use the same commands with a consistent voice tone.	• Participate in therapy session • Decrease frustration
Decreased endurance	• Cardiovascular exercise, such as a restorator, kinetron, upper body ergometer (UBE), or treadmill[16,56,57] • Monitor physiologic response to all exercise[16,58]	• Consider use of the Borg scale. • Consider strengthening of the uninvolved side as weakness is present.[59] • Consider pre-existing cardiac deconditioning of the patient.[16]	• Improve patient's cardiovascular condition • Initiate a lifestyle change for personal fitness program

(continued)

Table 9-9 (continued)

ACUTE CARE PHYSICAL THERAPY AND STROKE

Impairments	*Interventions*	*Clinical Tips*	*Goals*
Gait deficits	• Body weight support[60,61] • Early mobilization is beneficial[62] • Repetition of practice[63]	• Consider using the TUG test or Lite Gait. • Mass practice is more beneficial for learning of the motor task.	• Early mobilization • Gait will be crucial to assist with discharge to another level of care
Cognitive changes	• Use MMSE • Ensure arousal level is optimized	• Consider subtle cognitive deficits and referral to neuropsychology for future interventions.	• Upright position stimulates RAS and ensures successful intervention
Neglect and/or inattention	• Draw attention to hemiparetic side[58,59]	• Position patient to attend to affected side in room and when talking with visitors.	• Prevent learned disuse
Lack of knowledge related to healthy lifestyle	• Patient and family education[16,58]	• Consider use of the American Heart Association guidelines for stroke.[16,58]	• Facilitate lifestyle change for daily exercise

Table 9-10

Acute Care Physical Therapy and Parkinsonism

Impairments	*Interventions*	*Clinical Tips*	*Goals*
Postural instability	• Transfer training • Bed mobility training, turning and reaching activities	• Emphasize whole body movements and speed of action; increase the height of the chair and use of armrests.[30] • Mental rehearsal and a night light[30]	• Facilitate functional mobility that requires spinal ROM[64]; prevent falls
Bradykinesia	• External cueing,[32,65,66] energy conservation compensation, muscle strengthening	• Focus attention to task to avoid degradation.	• Refocus attention of the task to decrease the slowed movement pattern[65]
ROM deficits	• Flexibility and ROM exercises, yoga, t'ai chi techniques	• Axial rotation loss is present especially as trunk flexion progresses.[64]	• Preserve biomechanical alignment, preserve motion for functional tasks
Muscle strength	• Therapeutic exercise[67]	• Loss may be from insufficient neural activation and/or disuse.[30]	• Prevent deconditioning and focus strengthening for targeted muscle groups
Cardiopulmonary deconditioning	• Bicycle (recumbent vs upright), kinetron, treadmill, boxing	• Encouragement of conditioning should occur with the first and every subsequent session.[30,67,68]	• Prevent deconditioning and increase aerobic capacity
Gait dysfunction	• Use of treadmill training, enhanced gait training with external cueing,[30,65,66] timed walks over ground	• Consider the 6 Minute Walk Test (6MWT), TUG test,[68] bimanual tasks.	• Encourage mobility for aerobic conditioning • Maintain ambulation for functional tasks
Depression	• Use Beck Depression Inventory[69,70]	• More prevalent in patients with akinetic rigidity than tremor dominance.	• Monitor affective mood on ability to perform tasks and participate in therapy

(continued)

Table 9-10 (continued)

ACUTE CARE PHYSICAL THERAPY AND PARKINSONISM

Impairments	*Interventions*	*Clinical Tips*	*Goals*
Quality of life issues	• Use of Parkinson's disease quality of life (QoL) questionnaire (PDQoL 39) • Unified Parkinson's Disease Rating Scale (UPDRS) motor part/part III	• UPDRS scale correlates to QoL,[69,70] depression important predictor of QoL[69,70]	• Enables therapist to ensure patient-centered goals
Cueing	• External cueing assists with improved motor performance (ie, verbal, visual, proprioceptive)[30,65,66]	• Cues of "take longer steps" will assist to correct gait deficits.[65] • Use of auditory cues successful for akinesia • Use of visual cues for hypokinesia	• Enables enhanced performance of tasks and process of the motor program
Cognitive impairment	• Use MMSE	• Score below 24 of 30[30]	• Monitor to maintain safe functional ability
Balance deficits	• Structure activity for avoidance of dual tasks, environmental set-up, balance exercises for single limb stance, rotation of the trunk, and reaching[30,71]	• Consider using Berg Balance Test, 1-leg stance, step test, and external perturbation to assist in prediction of falls and tailor program accordingly.[71]	• Prevention of falls • Promote functional independence in the safest environment

Table 9-11

Acute Care Physical Therapy and Neuromuscular Disease and Disorders

Impairments	*Interventions*	*Clinical Tips*	*Goals*
Changes in muscle tone	• Medications[72] • Baclofen pump[73] • Orthotics[15] • Positioning[74,75]	• See previously described tone assessment.	• Prevent tonal changes from interfering with functional ability[74,75]
Altered sensation	• Tactile input, prevent injury to affected area with positioning and possible splinting[14,76]	• Visual compensation	• Prevention of injury • Increase awareness of affected area[74]
Decreased endurance	• Short bouts of therapeutic exercise with monitoring for fatigue[41,76]	• Use of assistive device may conserve energy[2,40] • Prioritization of tasks for importance to the patient[41] • Consider use of Borg scale.	• Preserve cardiovascular conditioning
Fatigue	• Strengthen large muscle groups to maximize compensation strategies	• Do not overexert; this may exacerbate the medical condition.[15,36,41]	• Maintain balance of strengthening and precautions to enable full benefit of exercise session
Pain management	• Limitation of sensory input • Positioning and turning schedule • Maintain ROM[37,39]	• Coordination of medications[33] • Consider use of complimentary alternative medicines (CAMs) and modalities.	• Recognize and remediate pain for patient comfort[37]
Decreased ROM	• Gentle stretching, splinting, bracing, and casting[37,39,76]	• Decreased ROM can increase tonal changes or cause pain syndromes.[37,39]	• Preserve biomechanical alignment for best functional outcome[39]

(continued)

Table 9-11 (continued)

ACUTE CARE PHYSICAL THERAPY AND NEUROMUSCULAR DISEASE AND DISORDERS

Impairments	*Interventions*	*Clinical Tips*	*Goals*
Visual impairments	• Patch may assist with diplopia • Teach scanning techniques[15]	• Check for vestibular component by examination of nystagmus and vestibulo-ocular reflex (VOR).[14,15]	• Decrease symptoms that can cause nausea or impair safety[15]
Decreased balance	• Clinical Test of Sensory Interaction and Balance (CTSIB) to identify specific area of deficit[15]	• Consider affect of proprioception as deficit may cause further balance impairment.[15]	• Prevention of falls • Promote functional independence in safest environment
Gait deficits	• Gradual increase of gait distance • Consider use or change of assistive device[2,40] • Consider use or change of orthotic device[14,15]	• When fatigue occurs at the end distance of gait, patients have little reserve and require immediate rest. • Planning should include wheelchair follow, immediate stand-by assistance, or chairs for rests along the path.	• Encourage mobility for aerobic conditioning • Maintain ambulation for functional tasks

Summary

The clinical signs and symptoms resulting from neurologic dysfunction vary greatly depending on the region of the nervous system affected. By first gaining an understanding of the anatomy and physiology of an intact system, a clinician may better understand the mechanisms underlying pathology and, thereby, provide appropriate interventions for the resulting impairments and activity limitations.

The 2 general categories of stroke are ischemia and hemorrhage; ischemic strokes are more common. In both instances, cerebral damage is caused by reduced oxygenation of brain tissue, which leads to cell damage and/or death. The location and severity of the lesion coupled with the quality of collateral blood flow influence the severity of neurologic deficits that evolve following a stroke.

Similar to strokes, TBIs also involve cerebral damage; however, the pathophysiology of head injury involves primary and secondary injuries. TBI may also involve local brain damage caused by contusions and/or lacerations along the surface of the brain and/or DAI. If cellular damage is widespread and extends into the midbrain and brainstem, it may cause a dramatic cumulative effect, such as coma and/or autonomic dysfunction. TBIs can be classified based on the location, extent, severity, and/or the mechanism of injury.

Neuromuscular diseases, such as Parkinson's disease, MS, GBS, and ALS, involve both upper and lower motor neuron dysfunction, which results in various impairments, such as muscle weakness, fluctuations in muscle tone, impaired balance, and decreased coordination leading to impaired functional mobility.

In the acute care setting, a thorough chart review and understanding of the source of physiologic pathology are essential prior to mobilization of the patient. In addition, a description of the patient's prior level of function should be ascertained prior to the functional examination in order to best understand the acuity of impairment.

When examining patients with neurologic impairment, assess level of arousal, cognition, and ability to communicate first to determine the most appropriate techniques for conducting the functional assessment. When establishing the patient's plan of care, the therapist should consider the estimated length of stay, the social support available for the patient, and the recommendations for the next level of care.

In treating patients with neurologic impairment, it is important to focus treatment activities to functional context. The task specification in the acute care setting is typically transfers, bed mobility, and gait training. These activities provide the patients with practice as well as the justification for continued therapy services.

Many patients and families need to cope with significant change in function and role within the family unit after neurologic impairment. Some acute care institutions offer specific support groups for patients and family members, while additional support groups and disease/disorder information can be found on the internet.

Case Study

Mr. Bryant is a 68-year-old male with a past medical history (PMHx) including HTN, coronary artery disease (CAD), atrial fibrillation, and increased cholesterol. After dinner one evening, he was having difficulty moving his left arm and leg. He thought after a good night sleep, his symptoms would resolve. His wife noticed a left-sided facial droop and garbled speech. She could not convince her husband that he required medical attention. After several hours passed, Mrs. Bryant called 911. Mr. Bryant was transported to the local hospital where he was evaluated for stroke. His MRI revealed an infarct in the distribution of the right MCA. The attending neurologist ordered that Mr. Bryant be positioned with his bed flat, intravenous (IV) fluids be administered, and that neurological checks be completed every 2 hours along with a recording of the patient's vital signs (VS). Mr. Bryant was declared NPO (nil per os, nothing by mouth) until the speech therapist assessed his ability to swallow. After spending 48 hours flat in bed, Mr. Bryant's doctor consulted physical therapy to complete an examination.

Patient/Client History

General Demographics, Social History, and Living Environment

Mr. Bryant lives with his wife in a 2-story home with the bathroom on the second floor. There are 6 steps to enter.

General Health Status, Social, Health Habits, and Family History

Mr. and Mrs. Bryant are both retired. They walk 1 mile every other day during nice weather.

Medical/Surgical History

Mr. Bryant has HTN, CAD, atrial fibrillation, and increased cholesterol. He had been diagnosed with HTN and atrial fibrillation 5 years ago and has been taking medication prescribed by his family physician. His cholesterol was being managed through diet only. His surgical history is not significant.

Current Conditions

Mr. Bryant presented with a right-sided ischemic stroke of duration >12 hours. He has no active movement in the left upper extremity (LUE) or left lower extremity (LLE) except for trace left hip flexion and extension. He has left-sided neglect as well as dysarthria. There is increased extensor tone in the LLE and the LUE is flaccid

Activities and Participation

Mrs. Bryant was present during the initial examination and provided the therapist with a description of the patient's prior level of function and the home setting. Prior to this event, Mr. Bryant was independent with all of his activities of daily living (ADLs) and instrumental activities of daily living (IADLs). As noted previously, Mr. and Mrs. Bryant walk 1 mile every other day, weather permitting.

Medications

Mr. Bryant's medications included Tenormin (atenolol), Vasotec (enalapril maleate), and Crestor (rosuvastatin) for the HTN and CAD and aspirin as an anti-platelet due to atrial fibrillation. There is a question that Mr. Bryant might be allergic to other anticoagulants according to the family.

Other Clinical Tests

Laboratory results revealed hyperglycemia with a blood glucose of 190 mg/dL, and elevated white blood cells (WBCs) at 16,000. Arterial blood gas (ABG) examination revealed a respiratory acidosis with pH 7.32, $PaCO_2$ 50, PaO_2 90, HCO_3^- 24.

Systems Review

Cardiovascular and Pulmonary

Resting VS supine in bed are HR 96 beats per minute (bpm), pulse irregularly irregular, BP 160/86, and RR 18 breaths/minute.

Integumentary

Skin intact with IV line in right upper extremity (RUE) and a Foley catheter was present.

Musculoskeletal

Manual Muscle Test (MMT) results for LUE and LLE revealed no active movement except trace left hip flexion and extension. ROM was within normal limits (WNL) for bilateral upper extremity (BUE)/bilateral lower extremity (BLE).

Neuromuscular

There is increased extensor tone in the LLE and flaccidity in the LUE. Mr. Bryant's LUE was placed in a sling to protect the shoulder joint. Sensation not evaluated. Mr. Bryant required assistance to transfer from supine to sit and his balance is poor in static sitting.

Communication, Affect, Cognition, Language, and Learning Style

Mr. Bryant's speech is dysarthric. His wife explains that Spanish is his primary language, but he is fluent in English.

Tests and Measures

Aerobic Capacity and Endurance

Mr. Bryant demonstrated a blunted VS response during the examination. There were minor changes in HR, BP, and RR. It is hypothesized that these blunted responses could be a side effect of many of his prescribed medications or possibly reflect his active lifestyle prior to the stroke.

Assistive and Adaptive Devices

Left knee immobilizer is recommended for gait training. His left ankle should be ACE wrapped to provide passive dorsiflexion, and a sling should be used for his LUE for standing activities. A hemi-walker is recommended for gait training with progression to a smaller based support device when his mobility status is improved.

Balance, Gait, and Mobility (Including Locomotion)

Mr. Bryant required moderate assistance to transfer from supine to sit (FIM 3) and his balance is poor in static sitting requiring moderate assistance at the edge of the bed (FIM 3). He required maximal assistance to stand and transfer onto the commode (FIM 2). Following use of the commode, maximal assistance of 1 and moderate assistance of 1 was required to ambulate 4 steps with a left knee immobilizer donned and a supportive ACE wrap on the left ankle (FIM 1). Moderate assistance was required to advance the LLE. His Activity Measure for Post Acute Care (AM-PAC) "6 Clicks" Basic Mobility score is 6/24.

Circulation (Arterial, Venous, Lymphatic) and Ventilation and Respiration

Following ROM, MMT, bed mobility, transfers, and neurologic examination, his VS ranges were HR 96-104 bpm, BP 160/86-154/84 mm Hg, RR 18-22 breaths/minute and SpO_2 94% to 96% on 3 liters per minute. HTN is noted at rest and with activity and the breathing pattern was rapid (RR 22) and shallow.

Mental Function

Mr. Bryant was initially sleeping but became alert and awake. Orientation was not assessed. He followed commands easily but appeared fatigued.

Muscle Performance

MMT results for LUE and LLE revealed no active movement except trace left hip flexion and extension. ROM was WNL for BUE/BLE. As noted previously, there is increased extensor tone in the LLE and flaccidity in the LUE. The RUE/right LE strength was 5/5.

Pain

Pain is difficult to measure due to communication challenges. Pain was assessed by observation of facial expressions/grimaces during therapy session to qualify pain. Mr. Bryant did not appear to be in pain.

Sensory Integrity

Due to the history of cerebrovascular accident (CVA), an examination of sensation was indicated but was not performed during the initial examination.

Diagnosis

In Mr. Bryant's examination, the therapist described his diagnosis as a right ischemic stroke resulting in left-sided hemiplegia. He presents with multiple impairments consistent with this medical diagnosis, including left-sided hemiplegia, balance deficits, and dysarthria. These impairments have led to activity limitations with transfers and gait, and, currently, an inability to return home. The prescribed medications and persistent atrial fibrillation may blunt the HR and BP responses with functional activities. The respiratory acidosis is most likely related to an altered breathing pattern and diaphragm weakness.

Prognosis

The physical therapist estimated that Mr. Bryant would require daily physical therapy services until his predicted discharge in 5 days. The recommended goals were that the patient be able to roll onto his involved side and transfer from supine to a sitting position with moderate assistance. The patient will maintain static sitting balance on the edge of bed for 10 minutes with minimal assistance and BUEs supported on the bed. The patient will transfer onto a commode toward his strong side with moderate assistance. The patient will stand and ambulate 25 to 50 feet with moderate assistance, a left knee immobilizer, left ankle dorsiflexion wrap, and a single-point cane. In the acute setting, trial bracing provides stability; however, definitive bracing orders typically occur in rehabilitation. With supervision from the therapist, the patient's family will demonstrate proper positioning and ROM for the patient's LUE and LLE, as well as the proper techniques for assisting the patient with his bedside therapeutic exercise routine. He is at risk for aspiration pneumonia due to potential swallowing dysfunction and limited mobility. He is NPO.

Intervention

In order to accomplish these goals and, thereby, decrease Mr. Bryant's activity limitations, the physical therapist incorporated the following interventions into Mr. Bryant's plan of care: strength, coordination, balance, gait and perceptual training, and neuromuscular education, including FES to the supraspinatus and deltoid muscles to stabilize the humeral head in the glenoid fossa. Patient/family education regarding the intervention techniques, as well as long-term health and social concerns for a stroke survivor, were incorporated into each treatment session. The communication and documentation of Mr. Bryant's plan of care to the interdisciplinary team members was completed following evaluation.

Outcomes

Mr. Bryant requires minimal assistance to mobilize from supine to the edge of the bed (FIM 4) and he is ambulating with left knee immobilizer 20 feet x 2 with moderate assistance of 2 (FIM 1). He still requires a sling for protection of his LUE. He is able to transfer with moderate assistance of one from a chair with arms and a mat table with maximal assistance of 1 (FIM 2). His speech is still dysarthric, and he is progressing with swallowing exercises with speech therapy. Mr. Bryant continues to be unaware of his left side and must receive continued cues for safety. His AM-PAC "6 Clicks" basic mobility score improved from 6 to 11/24.

Mr. Bryant has been accepted to transfer to the inpatient rehabilitation hospital.

ICF Clinical Reasoning Tool Case Study Summary

Health Condition

HPI: Right MCA CVA; left-sided neglect, dysarthria, extensor tone LLE, flaccid LUE; respiratory acidosis
PMHx: HTN, CAD, atrial fibrillation, increased cholesterol; leisurely activity level prior to admission.

Precautions/Contraindications

Orthostatic hypotension, safety/fall risk, universal precautions, mild hypoxia with examination
RF for CAD (minimally active prior to admission, +CVA, elevated cholesterol, HTN), RF for DVT related to tone/flaccidity in extremities, atrial fibrillation may limit BP responses to OOB functional activities

Body Structure and Function			*Activity/Task Limitations*			*Participation*		
Impairment/ Problem	*Tests and Measures*	*Intervention*	*Activity*	*Tests and Measures*	*Intervention*	*Participation*	*Tests and Measures*	*Intervention*
• Impaired respiratory status • Impaired endurance • Decreased responsiveness to stimuli • Impaired communication • Impaired nutrition intake • Abnormal tone and weakness UE/LE • Pain	• Chest assessment • VS including ECG and SpO_2 • ROM/MMT • Modified Ashworth • Deep tendon reflexes • Wong-Baker Faces Scale • mNIHSS	• Breathing exercises • Bedside ROM, PNF & Progressive resistance exercises • FES • Donning/doffing sling • Consult speech pathologist, registered dietician, diabetes team	• ADLs/IADLs • Bed mobility • Transfers • Gait • Balance	• Functional task analysis • FIM • AM-PAC "6 Clicks" • mFRT/FIST as able • RPE	• Progressive/interval functional retraining • Education on risk for falls	• Unable to live independently • Unable to walk community distances	• SS-QoL	• Continue physical therapy services • Family meeting to discuss discharge plans

(continued)

ICF Clinical Reasoning Tool Case Study Summary (continued)

Personal Factors	*Other Considerations*	*Environmental Factors*
• Age: 68 y/o male • Primary language: Spanish, but fluent in English • Retired, married • IADL, ADL independent prior to admission • Grimace instead of verbalizing pain with movement		Home: • 2 story house, 6 steps to enter, bathroom on 2nd floor • Hospital: • IV RUE, sling, L knee immobilizer, L ankle ACE wrapped, hemi-walker, NPO

FES = functional electrical stimulation; FIST = Function in Sitting Test; HPI = history of present illness; L = left; mFRT = Modified Functional Reach Test; mNIHSS = Modified National Institutes of Health Stroke Scale; PMHx = past medical history; PNF = proprioceptive neuromuscular facilitation; RF = risk factors; RPE = rate of perceived exertion; SS-QoL = Stroke Specific Quality of Life Scale; y/o = year old.

Adapted from American Physical Therapy Association. *Guide to Physical Therapist Practice*. 3rd ed. http://www.apta.org/Guide/. Updated October 21, 2015. Accessed October 5, 2018 and *Towards a Common Language for Functioning, Disability and Health*. World Health Organization. www.who.int/classifications/icf/icfbeginnersguide.pdf. Published 2002. Accessed April 29, 2019.

PART II: NEUROSURGERY

Intervention by the physical therapist in cases involving neurosurgery has not been well documented in the acute care literature. While patients often demonstrate functional deficits that are similar in nature to the patient with neurologic deficit, there are certain unique characteristics to this patient population. As hospital length of stay decreases, interventions are often requested for discharge planning purposes, initial functional retraining, and patient/family education. Therapists need to consider the medical stability of the patient as well as the consequence of intervention in lieu of the surgical procedures performed.

ANATOMY AND PHYSIOLOGY

Spinal Region

The spinal region is responsible for carrying impulses for sensations, such as pain and temperature, and for the signals that command voluntary movements in the limbs, trunk, and neck.[2,8] This region includes the spinal cord, dorsal and ventral roots, spinal nerves, and the meninges.[8] Damage to the spinal region may cause paralysis and/or the loss of general sensations.

The adult **spinal cord** forms a cylindrical column approximately 0.5 m long with an estimated diameter between 1 and 1.5 cm and is located within the vertebral canal.[48] It begins as the inferior continuation of the medulla and extends from the foramen magnum to the intervertebral disc between the first and second lumbar vertebrae (Figure 9-5).[4,8] The internal structure of the spinal cord consists of white matter that surrounds a distinctive H-shaped pattern of gray matter located centrally. The **white matter** contains a large number of myelinated fibers (accounting for its white appearance) that transmit impulses superiorly or inferiorly.[3,6] The **gray matter** within the spinal cord consists largely of nerve cell bodies and interneurons; its lateral sections are divided into the dorsal, lateral, and ventral horns.[8,48] The **dorsal horns** contain groups of neurons that are largely responsible for carrying sensory information.[8] Many neurons within this region communicate with axons that enter the white matter and contribute to the **ascending tracts**.[4,8] The nuclei within the **anterior horns**, which are located between the anterior and lateral funiculi, are related to voluntary movement and are hence referred to as the **motor part** within the spinal gray matter.[4] The **lateral horns** contain cell bodies of preganglionic neurons of the sympathetic nervous system and are largely responsible for processing autonomic information.[4,8] The **ascending tracts** carry sensory information from nerve endings and joint receptors to the cerebrum or cerebellum.[4,6] Table 9-12 provides descriptions of the ascending spinal tracts commonly assessed.

The **descending pathways** originate in the cerebrum, cerebellum, midbrain, and brainstem and carry information responsible for voluntary motor activity, posture, tone, and coordination.[6,8] Table 9-13 provides descriptions of the descending spinal tracts commonly assessed.

Axons relaying efferent information to the periphery exit the anterolateral cord in small groups termed **rootlets**. Ventral rootlets from a single spinal cord segment coalesce to form a single ventral root.[6,8] The **dorsal root** is composed of sensory axons carrying afferent information. Each dorsal root corresponds to a dorsal root ganglion located outside the spinal cord that contains the cell bodies of sensory neurons. The dorsal and ventral roots from each segment merge to form a **spinal nerve**, which contains all of the sensory and motor axons that correspond to a single segment of the spinal cord.[3,6,8] There are 31 pairs of spinal nerves with the following distribution: cervical, 8; thoracic, 12; lumbar, 5; sacral, 5; coccygeal, 1 (Figure 9-6).[8,77]

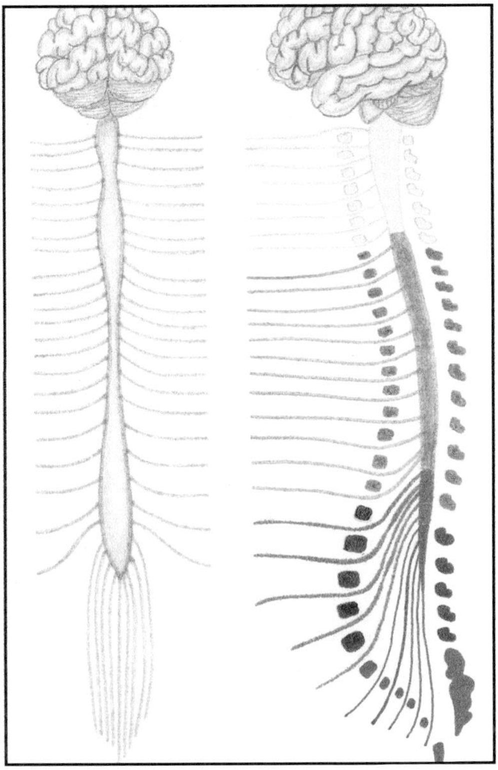

Figure 9-5. Spinal cord. (Reprinted with permission from Gutman SA. *Quick Reference Neuroscience for Rehabilitation Professionals. The Essential Neurologic Principles Underlying Rehabilitation Practice.* Thorofare, NJ: SLACK Incorporated; 2001:35.)

The peripheral distribution of each spinal nerve represents an original segmental organization that relates to a specific region of skin, muscle, and connective tissue.[8] The region of skin supplied by the sensory fibers from an individual spinal nerve is referred to as a **dermatome**.[14] Clinical diagnosis may be aided by tracing regions with impaired sensory signals to its respective spinal cord segment (Figure 9-7).

Reflex contraction of muscles may also be used in clinical diagnosis of specific spinal segments. Hyper- or hypoactivity at a specific segment is often useful in forming a clinical picture of a disease process. Segmental organization for motor innervation is represented by myotomes. The term **myotome** refers to a group of muscles innervated by the same segmental spinal nerve.[14] Refer to Tables 9-14 and 9-15 for descriptions of spinal nerves, corresponding dermatome distribution, and the muscles that correspond to each motion. **Bolded** muscles and/or sensory levels within the table indicate key muscles and/or sensory levels used to identify the neurologic level of injury as defined by the American Spinal Cord Injury Association (ASIA) (Table 9-16).[55]

Table 9-12

ASCENDING SPINAL TRACTS

Spinal Tract	*Pathway*	*Function*	*Symptoms of Dysfunction*
Dorsal columns (fasciculus gracilis and fasciculus cuneatus) Also called medial lemniscus or the posterior columns	Originates in receptors located in skin, muscle, and joints. Cell bodies are located in dorsal root ganglion. **Crosses in the lower medulla**, and travels to the primary somatosensory area within the post-central gyrus.	Tactile discrimination, vibration, **stereognosis**, joint and muscle sensation. Also responsible for conscious and unconscious proprioception, integrating sensory information and spatial discrimination.	Dysfunction of the fasciculus gracilis may cause **astereognosis**, loss of vibration sense, loss of 2-point discrimination, and/or impaired proprioception in the lower extremity (LE) on the contralateral side.
Lateral spinothalamic	Originates in free nerve ending receptors. Cell bodies are located in dorsal root ganglion. The impulse ascends 1 to 2 segments, **crosses**, and travels to the thalamus and somatosensory area.	Detection of pain, temperature, and touch.	Decreased ability to detect pain and temperature sensations on the contralateral side below the level of the lesion; bilateral sensory loss at the level of the lesion.
Anterior spinothalamic	Originates in light touch receptors, such as Merkel's discs. Cell bodies located in dorsal root ganglion. **Crosses at level of entry** and travels to the thalamus and somatosensory area.	Detection of light touch. Also responsible for detecting pressure and crude touch from the extremities and trunk.	Bilateral destruction of this tract may result in general tactile impairment as well as reduced tickling and sexual sensations.
Posterior spinocerebellar	Originates in muscle spindles and golgi tendon organs, travels to the posterior horn and then to the cerebellum **without crossing**.	Enables the precision and smoothness of movement; provides the coordination of muscle movement and position sense, subconscious proprioception, and kinesthetic sense.	Damage to this tract causes uncoordinated postural movements on the ipsilateral side of the lesion.

Adapted from Parent[1]; Hickey[2]; Adams et al[10]; and Gutman.[81]

Table 9-13

Descending Spinal Tracts

Spinal Tract	*Pathway*	*Function*	*Symptoms of Dysfunction*
Lateral corticospinal (pyramidal)	Originates in the precentral gyrus, premotor cortex and/or the post-central gyrus. **Crosses in the lower medulla**; travels to the anterior and/or posterior horn.	Controls voluntary skilled motor activity with an influence predominantly over the limbs.	Voluntary muscle paresis/paralysis on the contralateral side, hyperactive reflexes and spasticity of muscles distal to the lesion.
Anterior (ventral) corticospinal (pyramidal)	Originates in the precentral gyrus, premotor cortex, and/or the post-central gyrus; travels to the anterior and/or posterior horn. **Does not cross until level of termination.**	Controls voluntary skilled motor activity with an influence predominantly over the trunk and axial muscles.	Voluntary muscle paresis/paralysis on the contralateral side, hyperactive reflexes and spasticity of muscles distal to the lesion.
Vestibulospinal (extrapyramidal)	Originates in the brainstem and travels to the anterior horn; interneurons play a role in this pathway. **This tract does not cross.**	Controls the antigravity muscles, by facilitating extensor alpha motor neurons and inhibiting the flexors. Responsible for involuntary movements of balance and coordination. Also influences sweating, pupillary dilation, and circulation.	**Decerebrate posture** (continuous extensor rigidity) which results secondary to a lack of inhibition of vestibulospinal impulses and is indicative of a poor prognosis.
Rubrospinal (extrapyramidal)	Originates in the red nucleus within the midbrain. **Crosses in the midbrain** and travels to anterior horn cells ending in the thoracic region. Interneurons play a role in this pathway.	Facilitates flexor alpha and gamma motor neurons and inhibits the extensors. Also influences muscle tone and posture, especially in the upper extremities (UEs)	Altered muscle tone and posture, with increased extensor tone; may result in decerebrate posture (described previously).

(continued)

Table 9-13 (continued)

Descending Spinal Tracts

Spinal Tract	*Pathway*	*Function*	*Symptoms of Dysfunction*
Tectospinal (extrapyramidal)	Originates in the superior colliculus of the midbrain. **Crosses in the midbrain** and travels to anterior horn cells located within the cervical region. Interneurons play a role in this pathway.	Integrates visual and auditory reflexes with postural reflexes (ie, causes one to turn head toward a visual and/or auditory stimulus).	Impaired integration of visual, auditory, and/or postural reflexes.
Reticulo-spinal (extrapyramidal)	Two divisions, the pons and medulla, that originate in the brainstem; both divisions synapse on the same interneurons with antagonistic effects and project to alpha and gamma motor neurons. **This tract does not cross.**	Facilitates or inhibits voluntary movement, muscle tone, and reflex activity. Also influences respiratory and circulatory systems. Pons division increases blood pressure (BP) and heart rate (HR) and facilitates tone. Medulla division decreases BP and HR and inhibits tone.	Altered muscle tone and posture, with increased extensor tone; may result in decerebrate posture. May also result in an altered cardiovascular response.

Adapted from Parent[1]; Hickey[2]; Adams et al[10]; and Gutman.[81]

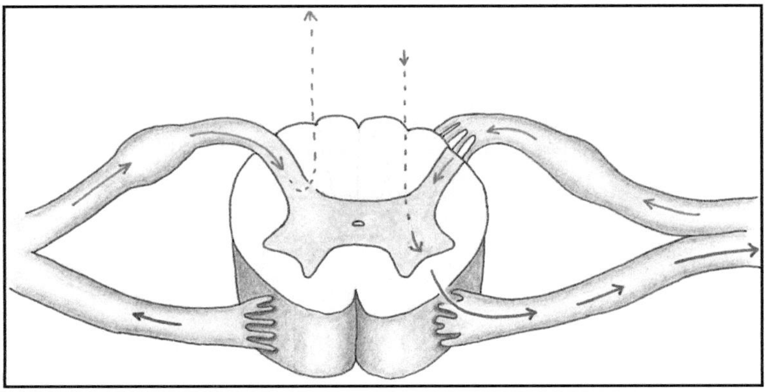

Figure 9-6. Ventral horn of spinal cord, rootlets, and root. (Reprinted with permission from Gutman SA. *Quick Reference Neuroscience for Rehabilitation Professionals. The Essential Neurologic Principles Underlying Rehabilitation Practice*. Thorofare, NJ: SLACK Incorporated; 2001:35.)

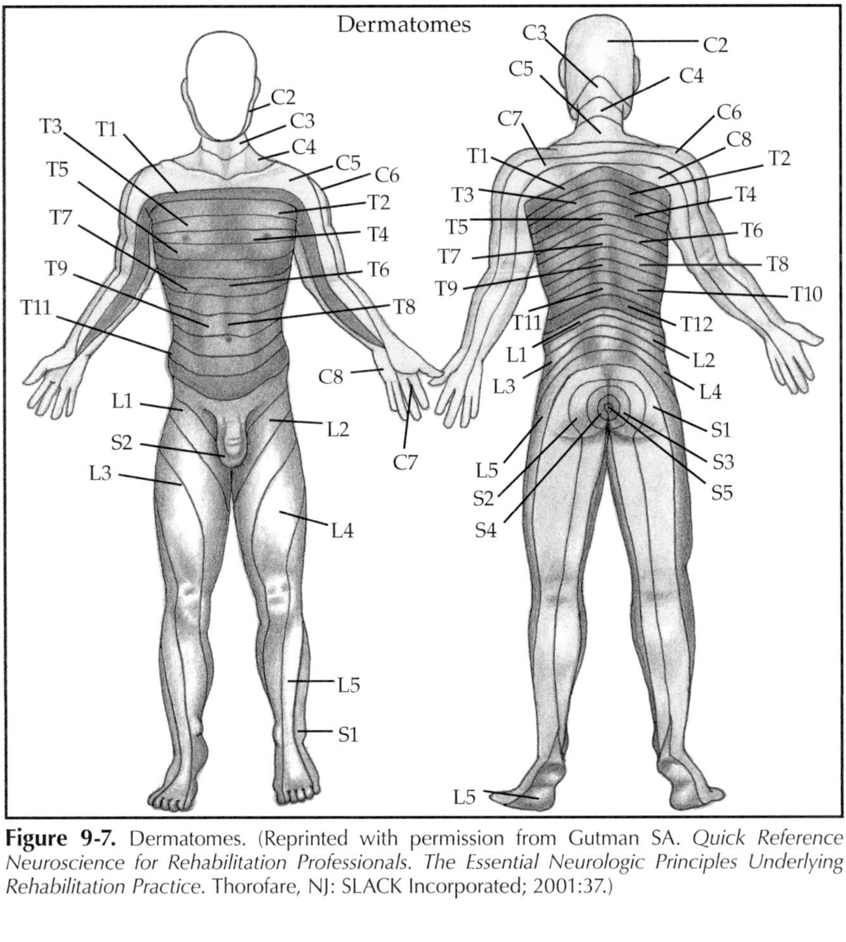

Figure 9-7. Dermatomes. (Reprinted with permission from Gutman SA. *Quick Reference Neuroscience for Rehabilitation Professionals. The Essential Neurologic Principles Underlying Rehabilitation Practice*. Thorofare, NJ: SLACK Incorporated; 2001:37.)

Table 9-14

UPPER EXTREMITY SPINAL NERVE ROOT DISTRIBUTION

Nerves	*Dermatome Distribution*	*Motions*	*Muscles*
C1	Vertex of the skull (top of head)	None	None
C2	Superior region of neck, posterior cheek, superior temporal region, and posterior skull	Weak cervical flexion, lateral flexion, rotation, and extension	Longus colli, partial sternocleidomastoid, and rectus capitis
C3	Anterior and posterior neck region and inferior temporal region	Weak shoulder elevation and extension of head; accessory muscles of respiration	Partial trapezius, sternocleidomastoid and splenius capitis
C4	Upper clavicular region and superior region of shoulders	Respiration and full shoulder elevation	**Diaphragm** and **trapezius**
C5	Delton region of shoulder extending inferiorly down the arm to the base of the thumb	Partial elbow flexion and supination, scapular elevation and external rotation, partial shoulder abduction, internal and external rotation	Partial innervation of **biceps**, **brachialis**, and **brachioradialis**; supraspinatus, infraspinatus, rhomboid, and deltoid
C6	Anterior region of arm extending to and including the thumb	Adduction, protraction, and full rotation of shoulder; strong elbow flexion and supination; wrist extension	Clavicular portion of pectoralis major, serratus anterior and full rotator cuff musculature; full biceps, brachialis, supinator, and brachioradialis; **extensor carpi radialis** and **brevis**
C7	Posterior lateral region of arm extending to and including the second and third digits	Shoulder depression, adduction, internal rotation, and horizontal adduction; elbow extension; pronation of forearm; wrist flexion; thumb and finger extension	Latissimus dorsi, sternal portion pectoralis major, **triceps**, pronator teres, flexor carpi radialis, extensor pollicus longus and brevis; finger extensors

(continued)

Table 9-14 (continued)

UPPER EXTREMITY SPINAL NERVE ROOT DISTRIBUTION

Nerves	*Dermatome Distribution*	*Motions*	*Muscles*
C8–T1	Medial region of arm and forearm extending to and including the fourth and fifth digits	Finger flexion, full movement of thumb, normal grasp and finger dexterity	**Flexor digitorum profundus** (C8), finger flexors, flexor carpi ulnaris, flexor pollicus longus and brevis; **interossei** (T1); intrinsic finger flexors
T1–T6	Anterior and posterior upper thorax region (T4 corresponds to the level of the chest)	Extension of thoracic spine, control of inspiration and forced expiration	Sacrospinalis and semispinalis, partial intercostal musculature
T1–T12	Inferior thorax region extending inferiorly to superior pelvic region(T10 corresponds to the level of the umbilicus); **T2–L1 sensory level** for ASIA	Trunk flexion and rotation; partial pelvic elevation	Full innervation of abdominal musculature; partial quadratus lumborum

Adapted from Rohan et al[7]; Lundy-Ekman[8]; Nette[12]; and O'Sullivan and Schmitz.[14]

Table 9-15

LOWER EXTREMITY SPINAL NERVE ROOT DISTRIBUTION

Nerves	*Dermatome Distribution*	*Motions*	*Muscles*
L1–L2	Groin region extending anteriorly and inferiorly to the mid-thigh region	Hip flexion and full pelvic elevation	**Iliopsoas** and full innervation of quadratus lumborum
L3–L4	Anterior and posterior region of thigh extending medially to include medial ankle and dorsum of great toe	Lumbar extension, hip adduction, knee extension, and partial knee flexion	Lower erector spinae, **quadriceps** (L3), adductor longus, brevis, and longus; partial hamstrings (semi-tendinosus, semi-membranosus, biceps femoris), and **anterior tibialis** (L4)
L5	Posterior and lateral region of thigh extending down lateral leg to the dorsum and plantar regions of the foot, including the first 3 digits	Partial hip extension and abduction, ankle dorsiflexion and extension of great toe	Partial gluteus medius and maximus; anterior tibialis and **extensor hallicus longus**
S1	Buttock region extending down posterior region of thigh to the lateral region of the ankle and fifth digit	Hip internal rotation, partial plantarflexion, flexion; extension of great toe, ankle inversion, and eversion	Gluteus minimus and tensor fasciae latae; partial **gastrocnemius**, and soleus; flexor hallucis longus; flexor digitorum and tibialis posterior
S2–S4	S2 extends down the medial region of the posterior thigh terminating within the plantar aspect of the foot; S3–S4 correspond to the perineal area; **S2–S5 sensory levels** for ASIA	Full hip extension, abduction, and external rotation; full plantarflexion and knee flexion, extension, internal and external rotation	Full innervation of hamstrings and plantarflexors, gluteus maximus, obturator internus, piriformis, and gracili; **sphincter tone** for ASIA

Adapted from Rohan et al[7]; Lundy-Ekman[8]; Netter[12]; and O'Sullivan and Schmitz.[14]

Table 9-16

AMERICAN SPINAL CORD ASSOCIATION IMPAIRMENT SCALE

Letter	*Classification*	*Description*
A	Complete	No sensory or motor function is preserved in the sacral segments S4–S5.
B	Incomplete	Sensory, but not motor, function is preserved below the neurological level and includes the sacral segments S4–S5.
C	Incomplete	Motor function is preserved below the neurological level, and more than half of the key muscles below the neurological level have a muscle grade less than 3.
D	Incomplete	Motor function is preserved below the neurological level, and at least half of the key muscles below the neurological level have a muscle grade greater than or equal to 3.
E	Normal	Sensory and motor function are normal.

Adapted from Somers MF. *Spinal Cord Injury Functional Rehabilitation*. East Norwalk, CT: Appleton & Lange; 1992.

Meninges

Three layers of meninges cover and protect the central nervous system (CNS). They include the external **dura mater**, the delicate **arachnoid membrane** that lines the dura, and the innermost **pia mater** that adheres to the brain and spinal cord.[3,6] The space between the arachnoid membrane and pia mater, the **subarachnoid space**, is filled with **cerebrospinal fluid** (CSF). The CSF, coupled with the dura mater, serves as a protective cushion between the brain and the skull, as noted in Figure 9-8.[54] The **dura mater** is a dense, firm layer of connective tissue that surrounds the spinal column and the brain. The innermost layer of the dura lies superior to the arachnoid membrane and is in close contact with this region.[54]

A **subdural hematoma** (SDH) refers to bleeding within the subdural space, and may be caused by the rupture of small vessels, bleeding from damaged areas of the brain, and/or a contusion of brain tissue.[2] The hemorrhage caused by a SDH is often venous blood, which does not flow as rapidly as arterial blood. Therefore, the signs and symptoms may worsen over a prolonged period, as the hematoma causes compression of the underlying brain tissue.[52] The manifestation of a SDH is classified as either acute (within 48 hours), subacute (from 2 days to 2 weeks), or chronic (from 2 weeks to several months) depending on the interval between injury and the appearance of symptoms.[2]

SDHs may be treated without surgical intervention if small in size because the blood may be reabsorbed. If the SDH is large, surgical evacuation is often necessary to prevent secondary damage from brain herniation and/or increased **intracranial pressure** (ICP).[2,8,13] Burr holes and a gentle irrigation technique can be used to drain the SDH if the hemorrhage does not coagulate. Once the SDH has solidified, a craniotomy with evacuation may be indicated.[52,56,57]

Skull fractures that lacerate the meningeal arteries supplying the dura may result in an **epidural hematoma** (EDH), also called an **extradural hematoma**.[2] EDH typically occurs in a younger population because the dura is more likely to rip from underlying skull in this population.[51] Symptoms develop rapidly, and include a worsening headache, vomiting, altered consciousness, and/or hemiparesis.[13] Lateralizing of

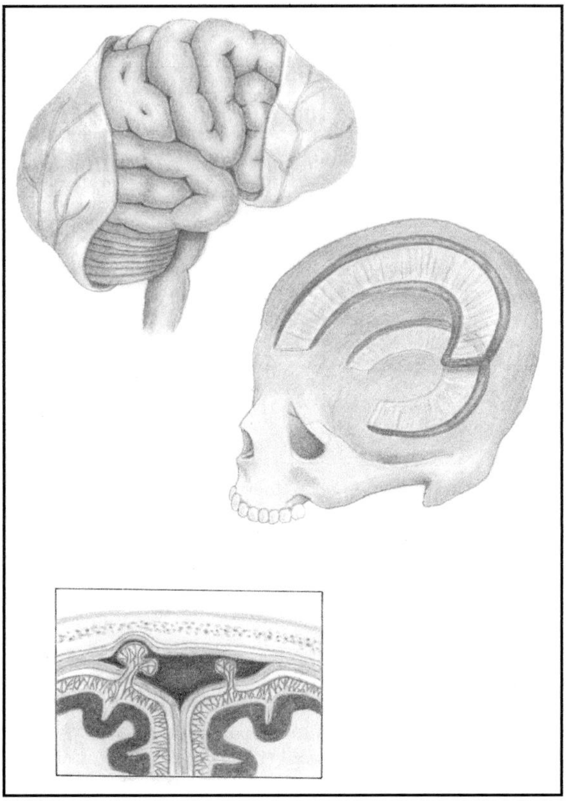

Figure 9-8. Meninges. (Reprinted with permission from Gutman SA. *Quick Reference Neuroscience for Rehabilitation Professionals. The Essential Neurologic Principles Underlying Rehabilitation Practice.* Thorofare, NJ: SLACK Incorporated; 2001:33.)

cranial nerve III (dilation of pupil), progressive hemiparesis, a change in mental status, and/or and decreased consciousness indicate emergent surgical evacuation.[8,13,52]

The **arachnoid mater** is a nonvascular membrane located between the dura and pia mater, with loose attachments to the dura. It serves as the principal physiologic barrier that separates the CNS from the surrounding connective tissue.[54] Projections of arachnoid from the arachnoid villi allow CSF to flow into the sinuses, enabling CSF to flow into the venous system.[8]

The **subarachnoid space** surrounds the brain and conforms to its shape by forming a narrow passage in convex regions and deeper areas within the sulci.[54] At the base of the brain, the space between the pia and arachnoid layer enlarges, creating a subarachnoid cisternae.[6] The **lumbar cistern** extends from the conus medullaris to S2. It contains the **filum terminale** and nerve roots of the **cauda equine** and is the site most often used for a spinal tap.[2]

The **pia mater** is a highly vascular, loose connective tissue that is tightly apposed to the surfaces of the brain and spinal cord.[1,3] It is also located within the roof of the third ventricle and contributes to the formation of the **choroid plexuses** of the lateral, third, and fourth ventricles. The **denticulate ligaments**, which are extensions of the pia mater, anchor the spinal cord to the dura mater.[6]

Ventricular System

CSF, a watery, clear, and colorless substance, fills the ventricular system and the subarachnoid space (Figure 9-9). It protects the brain by serving as a cushion and

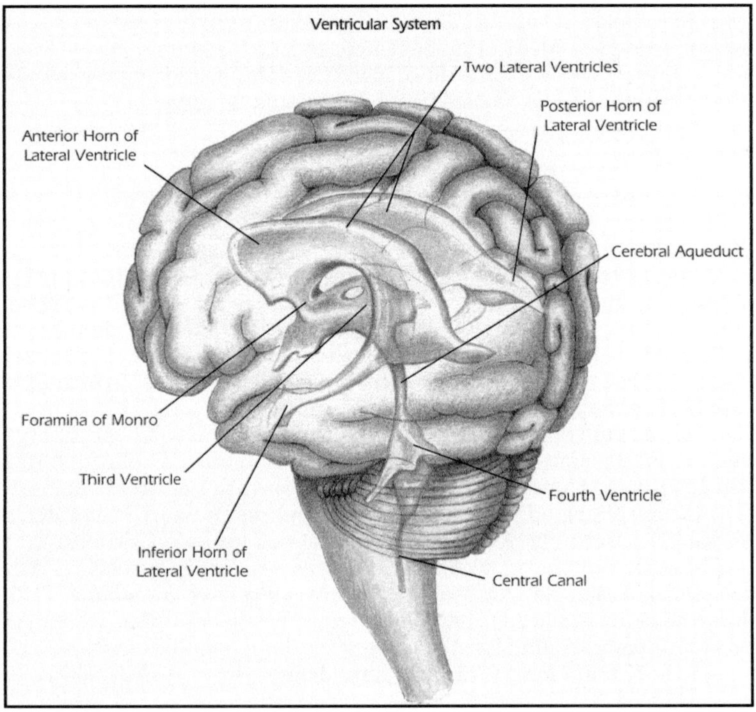

Figure 9-9. CSF within ventricular system. (Reprinted with permission from Gutman SA. *Quick Reference Neuroscience for Rehabilitation Professionals. The Essential Neurologic Principles Underlying Rehabilitation Practice*. Thorofare, NJ: SLACK Incorporated; 2001:27.)

provides a suitable environment for nervous tissue. It is produced by the **choroid plexuses**, which are located primarily within the lateral ventricles.[3]

CSF flows from the lateral ventricles, into the third ventricle through the interventricular foramina. Next, it passes through the cerebral aqueduct into the fourth ventricle.[3] CSF exits the ventricular system through the median and the 2 lateral apertures of the fourth ventricle.[3] CSF then travels within the subarachnoid space superiorly over the medial and lateral surfaces of the cerebral hemispheres and inferiorly around the spinal cord.[3] Finally, CSF is absorbed through the arachnoid villi, which project into the dural venous sinuses and direct the flow into venous blood.[3,6,8]

Damage or dysfunction within the ventricular system may cause a CSF leak and/or hydrocephalous. **Hydrocephalous** is related to the blockage of CSF circulation or secondary to excessive production of the fluid.[13] Hydrocephalous often causes the following symptoms[13]:

- Increased ICP
- Gait and balance impairments
- Frontal lobe dysfunction
- Headaches

A CSF leak occurs when CSF is discharged from a body orifice and/or wound secondary to a meningeal tear. A CSF leak may occur following a lumbar puncture, neurosurgical procedure, or skull fracture. Signs of a CSF leak include the presence of a clear fluid leaking from a wound site or body orifice and is often accompanied by a posturally related severe headache (worse with upright), and/or a salty taste in the patient's mouth.[13] Medical management of a CSF leak may involve use of an epidural blood patch, repairing the dura, inserting a shunt, and/or prophylactic antibiotics.[10,43,57] Until the leak is repaired, mobility should be limited.

Venous System

The capillary bed of the brain stem and the cerebellum drain into the dural venous sinuses adjacent to the posterior cranial fossa. The cerebral veins are divided into external and internal veins that both drain into dural venous sinuses.[3] The internal veins drain the cortex and the adjacent white matter and empty into the superior sagittal sinus. The internal cerebral veins drain the basal ganglia, diencephalon, and nearby white matter and drain into the straight sinus. The superior sagittal sinus and the straight sinus merge at the confluence, which forms the transverse sinus.[6] The transverse sinus then travels anterior to become the sigmoid sinus, which ultimately drains into the internal jugular vein.[3]

Damage or dysfunction within the venous system may be secondary to an **arteriovenous malformation** (AVM), which is a disorganized collection of abnormally thin and dilated blood vessels that directly shunt arterial blood into the venous system.[2,13] As a result, blood flow is accelerated and the pressure is elevated within the malformed vessels of the AVM. The AVM is at risk for leaks or ruptures.[2]

The signs and symptoms of AVMs include seizures, severe headaches, dizziness, syncope, aphasia, motor and/or sensory deficits; subjective complaints of hearing a "swishing noise in the head" may also occur.[2] Treatment options for managing AVMs include surgery to embolize the vessels, irradiation to thicken the vessel walls, and/or radiation therapy for nonsurgical candidates.[2]

Health Conditions

Upper Motor Neuron Disease

Upper motor neuron diseases involve lesions within the descending motor tracts, within the cerebral motor cortex, internal capsule, brainstem, or spinal cord.[10,55] Typical symptoms of upper motor neuron dysfunction include weakness of the involved muscles, hypertonicity, hyperreflexia, disuse atrophy, and abnormal reflexes. [10,54] Strokes, birth injuries, multiple sclerosis (MS, brain tumors, hydrocephalous, and cerebral palsy are examples of upper motor neuron disease.[10,54]

Lower Motor Neuron Disease

Lower motor neuron diseases involve lesions that affect nerves or their axons at or below the level of the brainstem.[10,54] Typical symptoms of lower motor neuron dysfunction include flaccidity or weakness of the involved muscles, decreased tone, fasciculations, muscle atrophy, and decreased or absent reflexes.[10,54] Muscular dystrophy, poliomyelitis, amyotrophic lateral sclerosis (ALS), tumors involving the spinal cord, trauma, and infection are all examples of lower motor neuron disease.[10,54]

Spinal Cord Injury

Approximately 250,000 to 400,000 individuals in the United Stated are currently affected by spinal cord injury (SCI), with an average of 10,000 new cases annually.[58,60] According to statistics from the National Spinal Cord Injury Data Research Center, 50% of SCIs occur between the ages of 16 and 30 years; 82% of this population is male.[14,60] SCIs can be divided into 2 broad categories: traumatic and nontraumatic; traumatic SCIs account for roughly 80% of all cases.[14,60]

The most common cause of traumatic SCI is motor vehicle accidents. Acts of violence rank second and falls are third.[14,58,59] Nontraumatic injuries are typically the result of a disease or pathologic process that compromises the integrity of the spinal cord. Some examples include transverse myelitis, syringomyelia, arterial venous malformation, spinal tumors, thrombosis, embolus, and vertebral subluxations secondary to arthritis.[14,61]

The mechanism of SCI is often acceleration—deceleration events such as hyperflexion, hyperextension, deformation, axial loading, compression, and/or rotation that produce excessive forces within the spinal column.[55,59] While the spinal cord is usually not severed at the time of injury, the damage typically occurs secondary to the inflammatory process that follows the injury.[13,55]

An overview of the sequence of physiologic events that precede SCI include hyperemia, edema, decreased BP, ischemia, hemorrhagic areas within the center of the cord, increased norepinephrine, serotonin, and histamine levels, and decreased dopamine within the injured tissue.[2,11] This response causes the formation of glial and fibrotic scar tissue that may result in permanent neurologic damage.[2]

The 2 broad classifications of SCI include tetraplegia (quadriplegia) and paraplegia. **Tetraplegia** results from injury to the cervical spinal cord region and involves partial or complete paralysis of all 4 extremities and the trunk.[14,33,55] Paraplegia results from lesions of the thoracic or lumbar spinal cord or sacral roots and involves partial or complete paralysis of all or part of the trunk and both LEs.[14,39,55] Paraplegia does not apply to lumbosacral plexus lesions.[14,49]

The severity of SCI is classified based on motor function according to spinal level. The examiner indicates the most distal uninvolved segment with motor function (3/5 strength) at the intact skeletal level.[59] The ASIA Impairment Scale is used to classify the extent of the damage (see Table 9-16).

In addition to classifying SCIs by the level and degree of impairment, some incomplete lesions have distinct clinical signs and symptoms that enable further classification. Refer to Table 9-17 for a description of incomplete spinal cord syndromes.

Brain Tumors

Brain tumors account for approximately 2% of all cancer-related deaths in the United States. They are the leading cause of solid tumor deaths in children under the age of 20, the leading cause of cancer-related deaths in males from 20 to 39 years old, and the fifth leading cause of cancer-related deaths in women ages 20 to 39 years.[63] The general incidence in the United States is 14 to 15 per 100,000 persons.[62]

Classification of tumors is difficult because there are at least 100 different types of brain tumors. The current system of classification, developed by the World Health Organization (WHO), describes tumors according to the origin of the cell type.[52,63]

Clinical presentation of a person with a brain tumor varies greatly depending on the type, size, and duration of tumor. Elevated ICP symptoms, such as headache, drowsiness, nausea and vomiting, seizure activity, personality change, eye weakness, speech disturbance, memory loss, and/or focal neurologic deficits, may occur in the presence of a brain mass.[63] Medical work-up includes imaging scans, such as a computed tomography (CT), magnetic resonance imaging (MRI) with or without contrast, and cerebral angiography.

Surgery is considered when a definitive diagnosis, alleviation of symptoms, and/or reduction/elimination of the tumor is possible. Nonsurgical interventions include radiation therapy, chemotherapy, and steroid medications (see Chapter 13).[63]

Table 9-17

INCOMPLETE SPINAL CORD SYNDROMES

Syndrome	*Mechanisms of Injury*	*Clinical Description*
Anterior cord	Flexion injury; damage to the anterior third of spinal cord	Motor function, pain, temperature, and sensation are lost bilaterally below the injured segment; poor prognosis for return of bowel and bladder function, hand function, and ambulation
Central cord	Hyperextension injury; damage to the central gray matter; most common syndrome	More neurologic involvement of UEs than LEs; sensory deficits less than motor; ambulation, bowel, and bladder functions typically preserved with distal UE weakness; proprioception, stereognosis, 2-point discrimination and vibration sense are lost below the lesion; with preservation of motor function, pain, and light touch; a wide-based steppage gait pattern is common
Posterior cord	Compression or infarction of the posterior spinal artery (very rare)	Impairment varies but typically includes bilateral loss of proprioception, fine touch, pressure, and vibration below the level of the lesion; deep tendon areflexia; severe cases may also cause complete paralysis below the level of the lesion
Brown-Séquard	Penetrating injuries (eg, gunshot, stab wound); damage to half of the spinal cord	Ipsilateral loss of motor function and position sense; contralateral loss of light touch pain and temperature sensation several levels below the lesion; good prognosis for ambulation, bowel and bladder function, and hand function
Cauda equina/conus medullaris	Damage at L1 vertebral level and below; **lower motor neuron** lesion	Flaccid paralysis below level of lesion without the presence of reflex activity; loss of bowel, bladder, and sexual function

Adapted from Adams RD, Victor M, Ropper AH. *Principles of Neurology*. 6th ed. New York, NY: McGraw Hill; 1998; Rohan JW, Yokichi C, Lutjen-Drecoll. *Color Atlas of Anatomy*. 4th ed. Media, PA: Lippincott Williams & Wilkins; 1998; and Tyedin K, Cumming TB, Bernhardt J. Quality of life: An important outcome measure in a trial of very early mobilisation after stroke. *Disabil Rehabil*. 2010;32(11):875-884.

Intracranial Surgery

Intracranial surgery may be necessary to decrease ICP, obtain a brain biopsy, evacuate a hemorrhage, embolize an aneurysm, excise a brain tumor, repair an AVM, and/or to repair damage to the cerebrum.[13,64] Table 9-18 provides descriptions of the most common intracranial neurosurgical procedures.

Table 9-18

Intracranial Neurosurgical Procedures

Procedure	*Description*
Burr hole	A small hole is made in the cranium with a specialized drill. This procedure may be used to evacuate an extracerebral clot, such as an SDH or EDH, access brain tissue for a brain biopsy, access the brain for placement of ICP monitoring systems, or to place stereotactic devices. A series of burr holes may be used to perform a craniectomy.
Craniotomy	Involves surgically opening the skull to provide access to the brain. This procedure may be used to remove a tumor, clip an aneurysm, and/or to repair damage to the cerebrum. A craniotomy is named according to the area of bone that is affected (ie, frontal, occipital, or tempoparietal craniotomy).
Craniectomy	This surgical procedure is similar to a craniotomy except that a bone flap is removed. This procedure is often done to decompress brain tissue and/or to fight infection. The excised bone may be stored in a bone bank, or placed within the subcutaneous tissue of the abdomen in order to maintain blood supply. Note: Patients without a bone flap should wear a helmet whenever OOB to protect the exposed area after a craniectomy.
Cranioplasty	Involves replacing the bone flap excised during a craniectomy. The replacement flap may be the original bone removed, a graft, or acrylic material. This procedure typically takes place 3 to 6 months after a craniectomy and is indicated in order to restore the protective properties of the skull and for cosmesis.

Adapted from Adams RD, Victor M, Ropper AH. *Principles of Neurology*. 6th ed. New York, NY: McGraw-Hill; 1998; Parent A. *Carpenter's Human Neuroanatomy*. 9th ed. Media, PA: Lippincott Williams & Wilkins; 199; and Scandalis TO, Bosak A, Berliner JC, Helman LL, Wells MR. Resistance training and gait function in patients with Parkinson's disease. *Am J Med Rehabil*. 2001;80:38-61.

Spinal Surgery

Spinal surgery is indicated to provide stability to a fractured region, correct a disc abnormality, correct a dislocation, correct spondylolisthesis or scoliosis, correct neural compression, remove osteophytes, repair a dural tear, remove a tumor, for emergent treatment of acute cauda equine syndrome, and/or to correct spinal stenosis.[55,65-68]

Table 9-19 provides descriptions of the various spinal neurosurgical procedures.

Physical Therapist Management

Neurosurgical Examination and Treatment

Prior to the initiation of intervention strategies, a thorough chart review is essential. The chart review should include the following factors: the patient's symptoms prior to surgery, the nature of the surgical procedure, any complications related to the surgery, and the postoperative instructions and/or precautions. In addition, it is important to gain an understanding of the patient's social history and functional abilities prior to admission.

Table 9-19 SPINAL NEUROSURGICAL PROCEDURES	
Procedure	*Description*
Discectomy	Refers to the decompression of nerve root material accomplished by removing intervertebral nuclear disc material, which is often indicated to treat chronic disc herniation and/or nerve root impingement. This procedure may be accomplished via a laminectomy or microdiscectomy.
Laminectomy	Involves the excision of the laminae, or posterior vertebral arch, via an anterior or posterior approach (posterior is most common). May be performed independently to excise disc material or as part of a spinal fusion procedure.
Microdiscectomy	Less invasive than a laminectomy, this procedure involves the decompression of nerve roots and excision of extruded disc material through an incision made in the inferior aspect of the lamina.
Foraminotomy	This procedure involves the surgical enlargement of the intervertebral foramen to increase the exit space surrounding a spinal nerve in order to decompress spinal nerve root impingement. This procedure is most commonly performed in the cervical region secondary to reduced anatomical size of the foramina in this region.
Spinal fusion	Refers to the union, or arthrodesis, of 2 or more vertebrae in order to immobilize specific vertebrae and strengthen the integrity of a compromised vertebral column. This procedure involves the insertion of bone graft segments between the involved vertebrae. It may or may not include instrumentation, also referred to as fixation, which may include pedicle screws, rods, and/or plates. Graft material may by autologous bone from the anterior or posterior iliac spine, nonautolgous bone, typically from a cadaver, or manufactured substitutes, such as hydroxylapatite.
Posterolateral lumbar fusion (PLF)	This procedure typically involves a midline posterior incision with the potential decortication (excision) of the laminae, as well as additional structures, in order to reach the desired region and accomplish the objectives of surgery. A bone graft is implanted over the decorticated surfaces, forming a contiguous region that includes all surfaces to be fused. Instrumentation may or may not be included. *(continued)*

Care of the patient with neurosurgical involvement should begin in the intensive care unit (ICU). Knowledge of the medical management and equipment is vital to successful interventions. Often, patients will have numerous lines and monitors, but this should not deter the interventions (see Chapter 3).[68] Safety and efficacy of

Table 9-19 (continued)

Spinal Neurosurgical Procedures

Procedure	Description
Posterior lumbar interbody fusion (PLIF)	This procedure is similar to the procedures described for PLF, except it also involves the excision of the disc in between the involved vertebrae with subsequent placement of instrumentation (interbody cage device) within the evacuated disc space. The available area for bone union is increased with the creation of the interbody space.
Anterior lumbar interbody fusion (ALIF)	This procedure involves an anterior retroperitoneal approach with disc excision and interbody bone grafting. Because ALIFs are typically not as secure as PLIFs, many surgeons protect this type of graft by adding posterior instrumentation as well. The anterior approach is also used for cervical levels C3–C7, called anterior cervical discectomy with fusion (ACDF).
Vertebroplasty	This procedure involves injection of cement to repair a compression fracture. Complications can include cement extravasation and, rarely, complications related to anesthesia. This is a relatively new procedure, started in the United States in 1993. The primary purpose of the procedure is to relieve back pain, which is reported in 84% of cases, and to decrease the duration of the immobility associated with compression fracture of the spine.

Adapted from Parent[1]; Broderick et al[20]; Schmidt and Lee[31]; Diamond et al[82]; and Maxey and Magnusson.[83]

interventions for physical therapy have been studied.[68,69] Careful progression of the patient from supine to out of bed (OOB) can occur with coordination from the medical team. Family education and teaching regarding the patient's plan of care should begin from the onset of therapy and include discharge planning discussions, therapeutic exercise, and cognitive considerations.

Clinical Tips

- Elevating the head of the bed to 30 degrees will reduce ICP by promoting venous return from the head; this position is often required for postoperative intracranial surgery.[68-70]
- Cognitive arousal is typically best in upright positions.[5]
- Families are often seeking ways to assist with care. Consider teaching passive range of motion (PROM), therapeutic exercise, and positioning techniques.

Comprehensive therapy should begin early and often involves coordination with respiratory and speech therapists, nursing, orthotists/prosthetists, and occupational therapists.

If the patient's activity is restricted following surgery and/or if the patient requires assistance for a certain postoperative brace, this information must be gathered at the onset to incorporate these factors into the patient's plan of care. Based on the type of brace, the interventions must incorporate the precautions for movement and donning and doffing the brace. Consultation with the physician and the orthotist for mobility concerns is essential. Table 9-20 provides descriptions of common orthotics used for stabilization following spinal surgery.

Table 9-20

COMMON ORTHOTICS FOLLOWING SPINAL SURGERY

Name of Brace	*Precautions*	*Indication*
Soft cervical collar	No sudden movement of the cervical spine; driving may be difficult	Pain relief; reduce muscular demand to hold head upright
Hard cervical collar (eg, Philadelphia, Miami J)	No sudden rotation of the cervical spine is possible; no driving; heat builds up under the collar	Pain relief; reduce muscular demand to hold head upright; restrict cervical flexion and extension[15]
Halo	Pin care; maintain range of motion (ROM) of the shoulders especially for end range; monitor for swallowing dysfunction	Maximum stability to prevent flexion, extension, or rotation of the cervical spine[15]
Thoracic lumbar sacral orthosis (TLSO)	No trunk flexion beyond 90 degrees to avoid compression of the femoral nerve	Limits trunk flexion and rotation; positions in neutral or extension for postural control or spinal stabilization
Lumbar sacral orthosis (LSO) or corset	No trunk flexion beyond 90 degrees to avoid compression of the femoral nerve	Pain relief; proprioceptive retraining; positions in neutral or slight extension for postural control or spinal stabilization
All orthotics mentioned generally require the patient to limit lifting and to wear the brace, at a minimum, while out of bed.		

The therapist should assess the patient's strength, muscular tone, coordination, and overall quality of movement. To the extent that the patient is able, examine the patient's ability to complete functional tasks, such as rolling side to side and transferring from supine to sit, sit to stand, and wheelchair to mat. Document the patient's balance, postural stability, quality of movement, the impairments limiting mobility, and the types of compensatory strategies used when the patient attempts to complete the aforementioned tasks. Finally, assess and describe the patient's standing balance and gait, when applicable.

- If the patient has specific postoperative lifting and activity precautions, the therapist should not break test the patient to determine his or her strength.
- If the patient demonstrates unusually decreased arousal, check with the patient's nurse to determine whether it is related to a pharmacologic response; if so, coordinate activity with medication schedules.
- Pain management is essential following surgery in order to promote early mobilization of the patient. Coordination with nursing to ensure proper management of pain often results in more efficient therapy sessions.

An orthopedic surgeon and/or a neurosurgeon can perform spinal surgery. Pain management should be a consideration regardless of the surgical procedure. Good outcome measures for adequate pain control include the ability to participate in the therapy session, deep breathe, and cough. Use of the Oswestry Pain Questionnaire can provide evidence-based data related to patients' subjective pain complaints.[71]

Patient education should include postoperative precautions, procedure to don/doff brace, and lifestyle changes, such as quitting smoking.[72]

Table 9-21 describes general information regarding the typical clinical presentation of a patient following spinal surgery along with a general plan of care.

SCI therapy starts with the first interaction with the patient and the family. Often, this is in the ICU, but may be delayed until medical and spinal stability is certain. Much of the rehabilitation for the SCI patient will occur at a post-acute level of care; however, early intervention can enhance functional outcomes. Patients should be encouraged to continue to attempt movement of muscle groups that have been reported nonfunctional. The plan of care will need to include extensive education for the long-term deficits that may occur with the SCI. Skin integrity is a major concern for all patients with SCI and a goal of intact skin should be the gold standard throughout the course of the care.[73] Table 9-22 provides general descriptions of the physical therapy plan of care following SCI based on the level of injury.

When evaluating and treating a patient following neurosurgery, it is essential to first gain an understanding of the operative technique and the location and indications for surgery, as well as any intraoperative tissue injury that may have occurred.

In addition to careful monitoring of the patient for complications following surgery, such as increased ICP, mental status changes, and seizure activity, early mobilization of the patient is essential.[75] Patients and family members should be informed of the postoperative precautions following surgery and instructed on positions to avoid during the initial mobilization process. Individual treatment plans should also address impairments specific to the location of surgery, cognitive involvement, and consider the prognosis and expected course of the disease process.

For patients with a poor prognosis, careful consideration must be given to psychosocial care. Goals for this patient population may include family training for positioning and comfort, as well education to understand the support resources available, such as palliative and hospice care.[15]

For patients who have intracranial surgery to remove a malignant brain tumor, it is essential to consider the additional treatment techniques that may accompany intracranial surgery and their effects on rehabilitation. Gliomas are typically located in the cerebral hemispheres and are the most common type of cancerous brain tumors in adults.[15,75] The standard treatment for this type of tumor consists of surgery, chemotherapy, including a localized form called **Gliadel wafers**, which is implanted into the surgical site, radiation therapy, and/or biologic therapy.[76] The side effects of radiation therapy and chemotherapy, which include fatigue, anemia, nausea, difficulty eating, skin irritation, edema, and neuropathy, must be considered during the rehabilitation process (refer to Chapter 13).[78]

Acoustic neuromas, also called **vestibular schwannomas**, account for approximately 8% to 10% of all intracranial tumors and usually occur in the third or fourth decade of life.[75,79] This nerve sheath tumor is typically benign, slow growing, and is often located on the vestibular portion of the eighth cranial nerve (vestibulocochlear nerve).[75] The most common intervention for this type of tumor is surgical removal.[75,79]

Because of the vestibular involvement, patients with this form of tumor often have balance and visual impairments both pre- and postoperatively.[79] Additionally, the vestibulocochlear nerve is located within close proximity to the facial and auditory nerves; patients often have permanent or transient postoperative facial paralysis and/or hearing impairment. The most favorable outcomes for patients with this type of tumor are associated with participation in vestibular rehabilitation.[80]

The goals for vestibular rehabilitation following surgical excision of an acoustic neuroma include improved functional balance, especially during ambulation,

Table 9-21

ACUTE CARE PHYSICAL THERAPY AND SPINAL SURGERY

Type of Surgery	*Impairments*	*Interventions*	*Goals*
Spinal fusion, decompression, and spinal stenosis	Muscle weakness; decreased functional mobility; dependence to don/doff brace; maintenance of precautions in functional tasks and IADLs	Limited strength training in functional tasks, abdominal strengthening, and stabilization; neural mobilization is controversial; patient education for brace care and maintenance	Independent transfers and gait for household distances; independent bed mobility; able to instruct or apply the orthotic device; independence in application of precautions in functional mobility
Discectomy and laminectomy	Muscle weakness; decreased functional mobility; maintenance of precautions in functional tasks and IADLs; sitting tolerance may be limited to 30 to 60 minutes	Early mobilization and gentle therapeutic exercise; a soft corset may be indicated for comfort; functional retraining, which may include initiation of "back school"	Independence in all functional tasks; independent with home exercise program; referral to outpatient therapy after follow up with physician

Adapted from Fritz et al[67]; Danielsen et al[84]; Kjellby-Wendt and Styf[85]; Philleps and Cunningham[86]; Scrimshaw and Maher[87]; and Wilner.[88]

Table 9-22

Acute Care Physical Therapy and Spinal Cord Injury

Level of Injury	*Impairments*	*Interventions*	*Goals*
High cervical injury (C2–C3)	Ventilator dependent; dependent mobility; dependence in weight shifts; no active ROM; potential for contractures, skin breakdown, spasticity, and autonomic dysreflexia[15]	Breathing exercises, inspiratory muscle training, and pulmonary toilet[15]; PROM and positioning; monitor for autonomic dysreflexia; patient/family education and strengthening exercises	Sitting tolerance for 1 to 2 hours per day at 30- to 60-degree angle; suctioning less than every 4 hours; assistance with pulmonary techniques; initiate education for weight shifts, pulmonary hygiene, ROM, and positioning
High cervical injury (C4)	Pulmonary compromise, may have resulted in ventilator use and/or tracheostomy; dependent mobility and weight shifts; potential for contractures, skin breakdown, spasticity, and autonomic dysreflexia	Breathing exercises, inspiratory muscle training, and pulmonary toilet; PROM and positioning; monitor for autonomic dysreflexia; patient and family education and strengthening exercises	Sitting for 1 to 2 hours at 60 to 90 degrees; independent with respiratory exercises and in requesting weight shift in all positions; able to identify symptoms associated with need for airway/secretion clearance
C5–T1	Dependent in mobility and weight shift; respiratory compromise; potential for contracture, spasticity, and autonomic dysreflexia	Functional mobility training, positioning, weight shift training, patient and family education, and strengthening exercises, including respiratory muscles; monitor for autonomic dysreflexia	Strength training, including respiratory musculature (may be independent with secretion clearance); ROM but avoid stretch of finger flexors if tenodysis grip will be required; full day sitting tolerance at 60- to 90-degree angle; assists in pushing wheelchair; independent in requests for weight shifts in all positions

(continued)

Table 9-22 (continued)
Acute Care Physical Therapy and Spinal Cord Injury

Level of Injury	*Impairments*	*Interventions*	*Goals*
High thoracic injury (T2–T6)	Dependent mobility; decreased sitting tolerance and angle; respiratory compromise; potential for contracture and autonomic dysreflexia	Functional mobility training may include standing program; respiratory exercise and pulmonary toilet, positioning; weight shift training; patient and family education; monitor for autonomic dysreflexia	Assist with functional mobility; full day sitting at a 60- to 90-degree angle; independently able to clear secretions; assist with weight shifts in all positions; improve strength and PROM with avoidance of overstretch of the back extensors; able to identify symptoms associated with autonomic dysreflexia
Low thoracic injury (T7–T12)	Decreased mobility and sitting tolerance and angle; respiratory compromise	Functional mobility training, including standing program; respiratory exercise and pulmonary toilet; weight shift training; patient and family education	Assist with all functional mobility; full day sitting at 90-degree angle; independent clearance of secretions and deep breathing
Lumber injury (L1–L5)	Decreased mobility, sitting tolerance, and aerobic conditioning; dependent for weight shifts	Functional mobility training, including gait training, weight shift training; patient and family education	Assist with some functional mobility; gait for short distances with assistive devices and bracing for LEs; full day sitting at 90-degree angle; aerobic training on upper body ergometer (UBE), and/or kinetron.
Lumbar and sacral plexus	Decreased mobility, sitting tolerance and aerobic conditioning	Functional mobility training, including gait training; weight shift training; patient and family education	Assist with all functional mobility; gait for short distances with assistive devices and bracing for LEs; full day sitting at 90-degree angle; aerobic training on UBE, kinetron, and/or bicycle.

Adapted from Consortium for Spinal Cord Medicine. *Autonomic Dysreflexia: What You Should Know.* Washington, DC: Paralyzed Veterans of America; 1997; Fujiwara T, Hara Y, Chino N. Expiratory function in complete tetraplegics. Study of spirometry, maximal expiratory pressure, and muscle activity of pectoralis major and latissimus dorsi muscles. *Am J Phys Med Rhabil.* 1999;78(5):464-469; and Massery M. What's positioning got to do with it? *Neurology Report.* 1994;18(3):11-14.

improved visual acuity during head movements, and decreased sense of disequilibrium.[79] Specific treatment strategies include standing balance exercises with the eyes open and closed with changes in the base of support and support surface, vestibulo-ocular reflex (VOR) x1 and VOR x2 viewing paradigms, and gait training with progression to the incorporation of head turns and changes in direction.[79,80]

- Instruct the patient to avoid any activities that may involve the valsalva maneuver, this tends to increase ICP, which is contraindicated following intracranial surgery.
- A CSF leak may present as clear fluid draining from the patient's incision and/or body orifice. If detected, halt any physical activity and report findings to the physician for evaluation.[13]
- If the intracranial surgery involved removal of a portion of the patient's skull, also called a **bone flap removal** or **craniectomy**, use of a helmet or other protective measures is indicated.
- Following intracranial surgery, patients are at risk for developing deep vein thrombosis (DVT) and/or a pulmonary embolism because of immobility and the contraindication of anticoagulation following surgery. Patients must be monitored carefully for any signs or symptoms of these complications.[15]

Summary

When treating a patient who has recently undergone neurosurgery, the therapist should first understand the pathology of the underlying disorder that required surgery. Next, it is important to understand the nature of the surgery, any postoperative complications, and the postoperative precautions associated with activity. Prior to mobilizing the patient, it is also essential to have a clear understanding of the wearing schedule and donning/doffing technique for any braces and/or orthotics required.

The clinical presentation of a person with a brain tumor varies greatly depending on the type, size, and amount of tumor excised and/or the residual growth that could not be surgically removed. When treating a patient with a brain tumor it is important to understand the clinical effects with respect to the specific area of the brain that is affected. This may enable a therapist to identify subtle changes in a patient that may have otherwise gone unnoticed.

Spinal surgery may be indicated to provide stability, correct a disc abnormality, correct a spinal stenosis, spondylolisthesis or scoliosis, relieve neural compression, remove osteophytes, correct a dural tear, remove a tumor, or for emergent treatment of acute cauda equine syndrome.

Spinal surgery may also be indicated to stabilize a patient's spine following an SCI. When evaluating a patient with an SCI it is important to understand the ASIA impairment scale in order to correctly classify and, thereby, describe the amount of motor and sensory impairment.

When evaluating and treating a neurosurgical patient in the acute care setting, the therapist must understand the postoperative surgical protocol in order to educate the patient and family. During the first interaction with the patient postoperatively, all of the precautions and activity guidelines must be incorporated into the plan of care. Family education is essential to ensure the patient consistently follows the postoperative instructions and is provided with the assistance required to continue implementing the required protocol within the home setting. Additionally, the postoperative precautions, estimated length of stay in acute care, social support available for the patient following discharge, and any activity restrictions may affect the discharge recommendation for the next level of care.

Case Study

Ms. Cook, a 76-year-old female, presents to her primary care physician (PCP) with progressive weakness in the UEs and difficulty walking over the past 4 months. She had 1 fall, which did not result in injury. Her PCP refers her to a neurosurgeon for further work-up. MRI reveals degenerative disc disease throughout the spine with a herniation at C6–C7. Following multiple consultations, Ms. Cook elects to have surgery. The neurosurgeon performs an ACDF of levels C6–C7. A physical therapy evaluation was ordered the day of the surgery.

Patient/Client History

General Demographics, Social History, and Living Environment

Ms. Cook's social history reveals she was living with her daughter who works during the day. They live in a 2-story house with the bedroom and bathroom on the second floor. There are 6 steps to enter. Both sets of stairs have a railing on the right side.

General Health Status, Social/Health Habits, and Family History

Ms. Cook has survived her husband by 8 years. She states her mother had some heart problems but cannot remember what they were. Other than the recent fall and weakness, she reports feeling fine.

Medical/Surgical History

Ms. Cook is 1 day post ACDF of levels C6–C7. The chart review reveals a previous medical history of hypertension (HTN), diabetes, laminectomy 10 years ago, and a history of chest pain. Her medical conditions are managed with medications. The surgeon has ordered a Philadelphia collar to be worn at all times for 6 weeks following surgery.

Current Condition

Ms. Cook is complaining of some neck soreness and difficulty swallowing. She is also complaining of a sore throat. She is seen in her room for the initial examination.

Activities and Participation

Ms. Cook has been limited to household ambulation recently due to a fall last month. She states that she walks to the mailbox only when her daughter is home from work. Otherwise, she stays in the house most of the day. She reports using a straight cane when needed. Prior to the onset of weakness, she could walk outside the house and throughout the community to perform chores without difficulty.

Other Clinical Tests

Laboratory findings reveal troponin 0.9 ng/mL (elevated), glucose 240 mg/dL (elevated), and white blood cells 11,500 (WBCs; slightly elevated).

Systems Review

Cardiovascular and Pulmonary

Resting vital signs (VS) in bed (head of bed >30 degrees) HR 96 bpm, BP 136/84 mm Hg, pulse regular, respiratory rate (RR)18 breaths/minute and oxygen saturation (SpO_2) on room air was 95%. Edema is noted distally in both UEs/LEs.

Integumentary

Ms. Cook is wearing a Philadelphia collar. She has an anterior surgical bandage on her neck. There is no drainage noted. She does have moderate edema (2+) distal UEs and LEs.

Musculoskeletal

Ms. Cook had decreased AROM bilateral upper extremities (BUEs) at the end range. Instrumental activities of daily living (IADLs) were assessed and she was unable to reach above her head. Her BUE/ bilateral lower extremities (BLE) strength is 4/5 throughout the available ROM. Her trunk strength was limited as demonstrated by decreased sitting and standing tolerance.

Neuromuscular

Ms. Cook reports that her arms and legs feel clumsy and heavy. A quick check of proprioception reveals deficits. Ms. Cook also has mild dysphagia.

Communication, Affect, Cognition, Language, and Learning Style

Ms. Cook was able to speak slowly but complained of the collar bothering her chin. Her speech was hypophonic, and she was unable to complete a sentence without taking a rest.

Tests and Measures

Aerobic Capacity and Endurance

Ms. Cook may be deconditioned as demonstrated by her HR and RR response to activity as noted later. However, the increased pain may also be contributing to these VS responses.

Assistive and Adaptive Devices

A Philadelphia collar must be worn at all times for 6 weeks. Difficulty swallowing and decreased neck ROM for functional mobility may impact wearing the collar.

Balance, Gait, and Mobility (Including Locomotion)

Ms. Cook is dependent for bed mobility and transfers (Functional Indepependence Measure [FIM] 1). Gait was not assessed due to her drop in BP with supine-to-sit transfer (FIM 0). Her Activity Measure for Post Acute Care (AM-PAC) "6 Clicks" Basic Mobility Score is 6/24. Postoperative cervical precautions include no lifting >5 pounds with the UEs and no rotation of the cervical spine. Increased time was required to complete functional tasks and activities of daily living (ADLs). Her balance was poor in sitting. She had an inability to maintain balance without visual cues.

Circulation (Arterial, Venous, Lymphatic) and Ventilation/Respiration

Pulse oximetry reading are normal at rest and with activity. Her breath sounds are diminished but clear. Her cough is weak and nonproductive. Following ROM, Manual Muscle Test (MMT), bed mobility, and transfers her VS were HR 114 and a regular pulse, RR 28 breaths/minute, BP 146/84 mm Hg, SpO_2 96%, and pain 8/10. She complained of lightheadedness with sitting.

Pain

Ms. Cook's pain increases when sitting upright from 2-8/10 using a numeric pain scale.

Sensory Integrity

Ms. Cook had impaired proprioception distal BUEs and BLEs. She had an inability to maintain balance without visual cues. More thorough examination of sensation is warranted.

Diagnosis

Ms. Cook has impairments of sensation and strength resulting in activity limitation related to her degenerative disc disease with neurologic involvement. Her postoperative course is complicated by pain control, possible myocardial infarction, and delayed healing related to poorly controlled diabetes.

Prognosis

Based on the assessment of the patient's impairments and activity limitations, the physical therapist anticipates that Ms. Cook would require another level of care after discharge from the hospital. Her plan of care included daily physical therapy services until she was medically ready to be transferred to the next level of care. Short-term goals to be achieved by discharge from the acute setting include independently demonstrate neutral spine with the log roll technique for bed mobility and transfer from supine to sit with minimal assistance; will maintain static sitting balance on the edge of bed for 10 minutes with supervision and BUEs supported on the bed; will verbalize understanding of postoperative cervical precautions; and instruct others for the procedure to don/doff her Philadelphia collar. Ms. Cook will stand and ambulate 25 to 50 feet with minimal assistance and a rolling walker. The patient's family will demonstrate the proper technique to don/doff the patient's Philadelphia collar.

Ms. Cook may have had a perioperative myocardial infarction as demonstrated by the elevation in troponin and slightly elevated WBCs. The poor diabetes control, age, and sedentary lifestyle are independent risk factors for cardiovascular disease and may delay healing.

Intervention

The care plan includes strength training for the LEs and compensatory techniques for proprioception deficits, such as visual cues. Additionally, the plan of care will include balance, gait, and endurance training. The patient and family education will include the importance of maintaining postoperative surgical precautions, the wearing schedule for the brace, and lifestyle changes that incorporate a neutral spine and proper body mechanics into daily living. VS and subjective complaints are closely monitored due to the possible perioperative myocardial infarction (elevated troponins). The principles of a phase 1 cardiac rehabilitation program are followed (see Chapter 6). The communication and documentation of Ms. Cook's plan of care to the interdisciplinary team members was completed. Speech therapy was consulted, and the physician was informed that she was having difficulty swallowing. Social work was consulted to arrange for the next level of care.

Outcomes

On postoperative day 4, Ms. Cook is able to mobilize from supine to sit with moderate assistance (FIM 3). She requires moderate assistance of 1 (FIM 3) to stand for 3 minutes. Her balance with visual cues is fair and a mirror is being used during therapy. She is using a huff technique instead of a cough and has no pulmonary complications. She is using a rolling walker with moderate assistance of 1 for 25 feet x 2 (FIM 2). Her pain is now rated a 3/10 with activity. Her AM-PAC 6 clicks basic mobility score increased from 6 to 10/24.

Ms. Cook was transferred to an inpatient rehabilitation unit. Recommend outpatient physical therapy or cardiac rehabilitation following discharge from the rehabilitation unit.

ICF Clinical Reasoning Tool Case Study Summary

Health Condition

HPI: s/p ACDF levels C6–C7, DDD throughout spine with herniation C6–C7
PMHx: Progressive weakness in UE and difficulty walking; one fall past month without injury; diabetes, HTN, laminectomy x 10 years, sedentary lifestyle, h/o CP and distant family history of heart disease.

Precautions/Contraindications

Orthostatic hypotension, safety/fall risk, poorly managed diabetes, positive cardiac enzymes, r/o perioperative myocardial infarction, orthostatic hypotension, leukocytosis, universal precautions

Body Structure and Function			*Activity/Task Limitations*			*Participation*		
Impairment/ Problem	*Tests and Measures*	*Intervention*	*Activity*	*Tests and Measures*	*Intervention*	*Participation*	*Tests and Measures*	*Intervention*
• Ineffective cough • Impaired endurance • Impaired ROM and strength • Impaired proprioception • Impaired swallowing • Abnormal lab values • Pain	• Chest assessment • VS including ECG • ROM/MMT • Grade pitting edema • Sensation testing • Lab values • Pain/ numeric scale	• Breathing exercises: huffing • Bedside ROM and progressive resistance exercises • Education on risk for falls/safety; donning/ doffing collar • Consult registered dietician and speech pathologist	• ADLs • IADLs • Bed mobility • Transfers • Gait	• Functional task analysis • AM-PAC "6 Clicks" • RPE • 10 meter walk; TUG • LEFS	• Progressive functional retraining following Phase 1 cardiac rehab guidelines • Mirror training	• Unable to live independently • Unable to community walking	• HRQoL (SF-12) • Quick-DASH • LEFS	• Continue physical therapy services • Consult social worker and occupational therapist • Family meeting to discuss discharge plans

(continued)

ICF Clinical Reasoning Tool Case Study Summary (continued)		
Personal Factors	*Other Considerations*	*Environmental Factors*
• Age: 76 y/o female • Widowed x 8 years • Lives with daughter who works during day • Household ambulation prior to admission • Walks to mailbox with cane and only with daughter • Fear of falling limits activity level • Speech hypophonic		Home: • 2 story house, 6 steps to enter, bedroom/bathroom on 2nd floor, railing on right Hospital: • Philadelphia collar, anterior surgical bandage at neck

ACDF = anterior cervical discectomy and fusion; ADL = activity of daily living; AM-PAC = Activity Measure for Post Acute Care; CP = chest pain; DASH = Disabilities of the Arm, Shoulder, and Hand; DDD = degenerative disc disease; h/o = history of; HPI = history of present illness; HRQoL = Health Related Quality of Life; HTN = hypertension; IADL = instrumental activity of daily living; LEFS = Lower Extremity Functional Scale; MMT = Manual Muscle Test; PMHx = past medical history; QoL = quality of life; r/o = rule out; ROM = range of motion; RPE = rate of perceived exertion; SF = Short Form; s/p = status post; TUG = Timed Up and Go; UE = upper extremity; y/o = year old.

Adapted from American Physical Therapy Association. *Guide to Physical Therapist Practice*. 3rd ed. http://www.apta.org/Guide/. Updated October 21, 2015. Accessed October 5, 2018 and *Towards a Common Language for Functioning, Disability and Health*. World Health Organization. www.who.int/classifications/icf/icfbeginnersguide.pdf. Published 2002. Accessed April 29, 2019.

Chapter Review Questions

Part I

1. The following are typical findings associated with Parkinson's disease:
   a. Impaired righting reflexes, balance, and gait
   b. Impaired eating, swallowing, and increased initiation of motion
   c. Impaired wound healing, airway clearance, and gait
   d. Impaired cognition, safety, and orthostatic hypotensive
2. What are the mechanisms for ischemic stroke in contrast to a hemorrhagic stroke?
   a. Abnormal bleeding of cerebral vessels due to vascular spasm
   b. Subdural meningeal bleed with coagulopathy
   c. Thromboembolic atherosclerotic disease and vessel stenosis
   d. Cerebral hyperperfusion and HTN
3. Which of the following clinical manifestations best represent an ischemic stroke?
   a. Vomiting, severe headache, impaired consciousness
   b. Sudden onset of vertigo, failure to fix gaze on objects, loss of consciousness
   c. Facial droop, arm drift, difficulty speaking, without vomiting or headache
   d. Loss of balance, urinary incontinence, autonomic dysreflexia, aphony
4. Which components of a neurologic examination should be completed prior to mobilizing a patient?
   a. Rancho Los Amigos LCOF, rigidity, and skin inspection
   b. Comprehensive chart review, resting vital signs, reflexes, and cognition
   c. Modified National Institutes of Health Stroke Scale and Modified Ashworth Scale for Grading Spasticity
   d. Medications, ROM, Hoehn and Yahr classification, and Glasgow Coma Scale
5. Which of the following best represent reasons to complete a thorough assessment of cognition and communication as part of an acute neurologic evaluation?
   a. May stimulate reticular activating system to increase patient arousal to allow for OOB functional progression
   b. May provide information for grading muscle tone by allowing for more objective measurements of functional outcomes
   c. May stimulate spasticity and allow use of the Ashworth grading scale to facilitate appropriate medication dosing for improved function
   d. May provide information for safety, information processing, and need for including other rehabilitation professionals in treatment plan

Part II

1. What are the clinical implications when the lateral spinal thalamic tract is damaged?
   a. Impaired vibratory sense and loss of 2-point discrimination on contralateral side
   b. Impaired bilateral sensory loss above the lesion and impaired postural movements bilaterally
   c. Impaired postural movements on contralateral side of lesion and impaired movement precision
   d. Impaired ability to detect pain and temperature on contralateral side below level of lesion
2. What are the clinical implications when the posterior spinocerebellar spinal tract is damaged?
   a. Impaired 2-point discrimination on contralateral side of lesion
   b. Impaired bilateral sensory loss above the lesion on ipsilateral side of lesion
   c. Impaired coordinated postural movements on ipsilateral side of lesion
   d. Impaired ability to detect temperature on contralateral side below level of lesion
3. Which of the following bests describes a myotome?
   a. Represents region of skin supplied by sensory nerve fibers
   b. Group of spinal nerves that supply sensation to a body region
   c. Individual spinal nerve supplies peripheral distribution
   d. Group of muscles innervated by the same segmental spinal nerve
4. What precautions should be considered during the initial examination of a patient following intracranial surgery for excision of a brain tumor?
   a. Maintain head of bed less than 30 degrees and initiate cognitive arousal in supine
   b. Perform an isometric manual muscle break test to determine strength and evaluate 2 step commands
   c. Encourage valsalva maneuver to stimulate trunk stability with transfers
   d. Understand underlying pathology, type of surgery, and clinical presentation to identify subtle changes
5. Which of the following best describe impairments and activity limitations that typically accompany an acoustic neuroma excision?
   a. Balance and visual changes
   b. Hearing and swallowing changes
   c. Endurance and transfer limitations
   d. Prolonged wound healing and gait limitations

Answers: Part I: 1a, 2c, 3c, 4b, 5d
Part II: 1d, 2c, 3d, 4d, 5a

References

1. Parent A. *Carpenter's Human Neuroanatomy.* 9th ed. Media, PA: Lippincott Williams & Wilkins; 1996.
2. Hickey JV. *Clinical Practice of Neurological and Neurosurgical Nursing.* Philadelphia, PA: Lippincott Williams & Wilkins; 1992.
3. Barr ML, Kiernan JA. *The Human Nervous System.* 6th ed. Philadelphia, PA: Lippincott Williams & Wilkins; 1993.
4. Young PA, Young PH. *Basic Clinical Neuroanatomy.* Media, PA: Lippincott Williams & Wilkins; 1997.
5. Clark DL, Boutros NN. *The Brain and Behavior: An Introduction to Behavioral Neuroanatomy.* Malden, MA: Blackwell Science Inc; 1999.
6. Diamond MC, Scheibel AB, Elson LM. *The Human Brain Coloring Book.* New York, NY: Harper Collins Publishers Inc; 1985.
7. Rohan JW, Yokichi C, Lutjen-Drecoll. *Color Atlas of Anatomy.* 4th ed. Media, PA: Lippincott Williams & Wilkins; 1998.
8. Lundy-Ekman L. *Neuroscience Fundamentals for Rehabilitation.* Philadelphia, PA: WB Saunders Co; 1998.
9. Greenwood R, Barnes MB, McMillan TM, Ward CD. *Neurological Rehabilitation.* New York, NY: Churchill Livingstone; 1993.
10. Adams RD, Victor M, Ropper AH. *Principles of Neurology.* 6th ed. New York, NY: McGraw-Hill; 1998.
11. Thomas CL. *Taber's Cyclopedic Medical Dictionary.* 17th ed. Philadelphia, PA: FA Davis; 1993.
12. Netter FH. *Atlas of Human Anatomy.* 2nd ed. East Hanover, NJ: Novartis; 1997.
13. Paz JC, Panik M. *Acute Care Handbook for Physical Therapists.* Newton, MA: Butterworth-Heinemann; 1997.
14. O'Sullivan SB, Schmitz TJ. *Physical Rehabilitation, Assessment and Treatment.* 3rd ed. Philadelphia, PA: FA Davis; 1994.
15. Umphred DA. *Neurological Rehabilitation.* 3rd ed. St. Louis, MO: Mosby-Year Book, Inc; 1995.
16. Gordon NF, Gulanick M, Costa F, et al. Physical activity and exercise recommendations for stroke survivors: an American Heart Association scientific statement from the Council on Clinical Cardiology, Subcommittee on Exercise, Cardiac Rehabilitation, and Prevention; the Council on Cardiovascular Nursing; the Council on Nutrition, Physical Activity, and Metabolism; and the Stroke Council. *Stroke.* 2004;35(5):1230-1240.
17. Lewandowski C, Barsan B. Treatment of acute ischemic Stroke. *Ann Emerg Med.* 2001;37:202-216.
18. Gillen G, Burkhardt A. *Stroke Rehabilitation: A Function Based Approach.* St. Louis, MO: Mosby-Year Book, Inc; 1995.
19. Jamieson DG. Acute management of the stroke patient. *Phys Med Rehabil Clin North Am.* 1991;2:437-454.
20. Broderick JP, Adams HP Jr, Barsan W, et al. Guidelines for management of spontaneous intracerebral hemorrhage: a statement for healthcare professionals from a special writing group of the Stroke Council, American Heart Association. *Stroke.* 1999;30:905-915.
21. Gilroy J, Holliday PL. *Basic Neurology.* New York, NY: Macmillan; 1982.
22. Kasner SE, Cucchiara BL, McGarvey ML, et al. Modified National Institutes of Health Stroke Scale can be estimated from medical records. *Stroke.* 2003;34(2):568-570.
23. Appelros P, Terent A. Characteristics of the National Institutes of Health Stroke Scale: results from a population-based stroke cohort at baseline and after one year. *Cerebrovascu Dis.* 2004;17:(1):21-27.
24. Tyedin K, Cumming TB, Bernhardt J. Quality of life: An important outcome measure in a trial of very early mobilisation after stroke. *Disabil Rehabil.* 2010;32(11):875-884.
25. Sundseth A, Thommessen B, Rønning OM. Outcome after mobilization within 24 hours of acute stroke: a randomized controlled trial. *Stroke.* 2012;43:2389-2394.
26. Indredavik B, Bakke F, Slørdahl SA, Rokseth R, Håheim LL. Stroke unit treatment: 10-year follow-up. *Stroke.* 1999;30(8):1524-1527.
27. Higashida R, Alberts MJ, Alexander DN, et al. Interactions within stroke systems of care: a policy statement from the American Heart Association/American Stroke Association. *Stroke.* 2013;44:2961-2984.

28. Ovbiagele B, Goldstein LB, Higashida RT, et al. Forecasting the future of stroke in the united states. a policy statement from the American Heart Association and American Stroke Association. *Stroke*. 2013;44(8):2361-2375.
29. Scandalis TO, Bosak A, Berliner JC, Helman LL, Wells MR. Resistance training and gait function in patients with Parkinson's disease. *Am J Med Rehabil*. 2001;80:38-61.
30. Morris ME. Movement disorders in people with Parkinson's disease: a model for physical therapy. *Phys Ther*. 2000;80:578-596.
31. Schmidt RA, Lee TD. *Motor Control and Learning, A Behavior Emphasis*. Champaign, IL: Human Kinetics; 1999.
32. Chiara T, Carlos J, Martin D, Miller R, Nadeau S. Cold effect on oxygen uptake, perceived exertion, and spasticity in patients with multiple sclerosis. *Arch Phys Med Rehabil*. 1998;79:523-527.
33. Confavreux C, Vukusic S, Moreau AP. Relapses and progression of disability in multiple sclerosis. *N Engl J Med*. 2000;343(20):1430-1438.
34. Goldstein LB, Samsa GP. Reliability of the National Institutes of Health Stroke Scale. *Stroke*. 1997;28:307-310.
35. LaBan MM, Martin T, Pechur J, Sarnacki S. Physical and occupational therapy in treatment of patients with multiple sclerosis. *Phys Med Rehabil Clin North Am*. 1998;3:603-614.
36. Meythaler JM. Rehabilitation of Guillain-Barré syndrome. *Arch Phys Med Rehabil*. 1997;78:872-879.
37. Ensrud ERT, Krivickas LS. Acquired inflammatory demyelinating neuropathies. *Phys Med Rehabil Clin North Am*. 2001;12(2):321-334.
38. Worsham TL. Easing the course of Guillain Barre syndrome. *RN*. 2000;63(3):46-50.
39. Mills VM, Cassidy JW, Katz DI. *Neurologic Rehabilitation: A Guide to Diagnosis, Prognosis, and Treatment Planning*. Malden, MA: Blackwell Science; 1997.
40. Cunning S. When the DX is myasthenia gravis. *RN*. 2000;63(4):26-30.
41. Lee CA. Gettting a grip on myasthenia gravis. *Nursing*. 2002;32:32-34.
42. Davies AE. Cognitive impairments following traumatic brain injury. *Crit Care Nurs Clin North Am*. 2000;12:447-455.
43. Yanko JR, Mitcho K. Acute care management of severe traumatic brain injuries. *Crit Care Nurs Q*. 2001;23:1-23.
44. Smith DH, Meaney DF, Shull WH. Diffuse axonal injury in head trauma. *J Head Trauma Rehabil*. 2003;18(4):307-316.
45. Andrews BT. Initial management of head injury. *Phys Med Rehabil Clin North Am*. 1992;3:249-258.
46. Roth P, Farls K. Pathophysiology of traumatic brain injury. *Crit Care Nurs Q*. 2001;23:14-25.
47. Maher L. A quick neurologic examination. *Patient Care*. 1999;1:19-33.
48. Davies PM. *Steps to Follow*. 2nd ed. New York, NY: Springer; 2000.
49. Howe T. Measuring muscle tone and movement. *Nurs Standard*. 1995;9:25-29.
50. Williams LE, Yilmaz EY, Lopez-Yunez AM. Retrospective assessment of initial stroke severity with the NIH Stroke Scale. *Stroke*. 2000;31(4):858-862.
51. Hillegass EA, Sadowsky HS. *Essentials of Cardiopulmonary Physical Therapy*. Philadelphia, PA: WB Saunders; 1994.
52. Kaye A. *Essential Neurosurgery*. New York, NY: Churchill Livingstone; 1991.
53. American Physical Therapy Association. Guide to Physical Therapist Practice. 2nd ed. *Physical Therapy*. 2001;81(1):9-746.
54. Greenberg MS. *Handbook of Neurosurgery*. 5th ed. New York, NY: Thieme Medical Publishers; 2001.
55. Somers MF. *Spinal Cord Injury Functional Rehabilitation*. East Norwalk, CT: Appleton & Lange; 1992.
56. Weigel R, Krauss JK, Schmiedek P. Concepts of neurosurgical management of chronic subdural hematoma: historical perspectives. *Brit J Neurosurg*. 2004;18(1):8-18.
57. Cousins MJ, Brazier D, Cook R. Intracranial hypotension caused by cervical cerebrospinal fluid leak: treatment with epidural blood patch. *Anesthia Analog*. 2004;98(6):1794-1797.
58. DeVivo MJ. Causes and costs of spinal cord injury in the United States. *Spinal Cord*. 1997;35(12):809-813.
59. Behrman AL, Harkema SJ. Locomotor training after human spinal cord injury. *Phys Ther*. 2000;80(7):688-700.

60. McCutcheon EP, Selassie AW, Gu JK, Pickelsimer EE. Acute traumatic spinal cord injury, 1993-2000. A population based assessment of methylprednisolone administration and hospitalization. *J Trauma.* 2004;56(5):1076-1083.
61. DeVivo MJ. Causes and costs of spinal cord injury in the United States. *J Spinal Cord Med.* 2002;25(4):335-338.
62. American Brain Tumor Association. http://www.abta.org/. Accessed April 2, 2006.
63. Reis LG, Eisner MP, Kosary CL, et al, eds. *SEER Cancer Statistics Review, 1973–1996.* Bethesda, MD: National Cancer Institute; 1999.
64. Wick R, Wade J, Rohrer D, O'Neil O. Use of decompressive craniectomy after severe head trauma. *AORN Journal.* 1999;69(3):517-529.
65. Wang JC, McDonough PW, Kanim LE, Endow KK, Delamarter RB. Increased fusion rates with cervical plating for three-level anterior cervical discectomy and fusion. *Spine.* 2001;26:643-646.
66. Beattie P. The relationship between symptoms and abnormal magnetic resonance images of lumbar intervertebral disks. *Phys Ther.* 1996;76:601-608.
67. Fritz JM, Delitto A, Welch WC, Erhard RE. Lumbar spinal stenosis: a review of current concepts in evaluation, management, and outcome measures. *Arch Phys Med Rehabil.* 1998;79:700-707.
68. Murdocke KR. Physical therapy in the neurologic intensive care unit. *Neurology Report.* 1994;16(3):17-24.
69. Brimioulle S, Moraine JJ, Norrenberg D, Kalin RJ. Effects of positioning and exercise on intracranial pressure in a neurosurgical intensive care unit. *Phys Ther.* 1997;77(12):1682-1689.
70. Cold GE, Holdgaard HO. Treatment of intracranial hypertension in acute injury with social reference to the role of hyperventiliation and sedation with barbiturates; a review. *Intensive Care World.* 1992;9:172-178.
71. Niskanen RO. The Oswestry Low Back Pain Disability Questionnaire. A two-year follow-up of spine surgery patients. *Scand J Surg.* 2002;91(2):208-211.
72. Anderson T, Christensen FB, Laursen M, et al. Smoking as a predictor of negative outcome in lumbar spinal fusion. *Spine.* 2001;26(23):2623-2628.
73. Goldstein B, Sanders JE, Benson E. Pressure ulcers in SCI: does tension stimulate wound healing? *Am J Phys Med Rehabil.* 1996;75:130-133.
74. Block G, Liss C, Reines S, et al. Comparison of immediate release and controlled release carbidopa/levodopa in Parkinson's disease. A multicenter 5-year study. *Eur Neurol.* 1997;37(1):23-27.
75. Hill CI, Nixon CS, Ruemeier JL. Brain tumors. *Phys Ther.* 2002;82(5):496-502.
76. Cancerconsultants.com. Oncology resource center. http://www.cancerconsultants.com. Accessed April 2, 2006.
77. Sawauchi S, Marmarou A, Beaumont A, Signoretti S, Fukui S. Acute subdural hematoma associated with diffuse brain injury and hypoxemia in the rat: effect of surgical evacuation of the hematoma. *J Neurotrauma.* 2004;21(5):563-573.
78. RadiologyInfo - the radiology information resource for patients. http://www.radiologyinfo.org. Accessed April 2, 2006.
79. Herdman S. *Vestibular Rehabilitation.* Philadelphia, PA: FA Davis; 1994.
80. El-Kashlan HK, Shepard NT, Arts HA, Telian SA. Disability from vestibular symptoms after acoustic neuroma resection. *Am J Otol.* 1998;19(1):104-111.
81. Gutman SA. *Quick Reference Neuroscience for Rehabilitation Professionals: The Essential Neurologic Principles Underlying Rehabilitation Practice.* Thorofare, NJ: SLACK Incorporated; 2001.
82. Diamond TH, Champion B, Clark WA. Management of acute osteoporotic vertebral fractures: a nonrandomized trial comparing percutaneous vertebroplasty with conservative therapy. *Am J Med.* 2003;114(4):257-265.
83. Maxey L, Magnusson J. *Rehabilitation for the Postsurgical Orthopedic Patient.* 3rd ed. St. Louis, MO: Elsevier; 2013.
84. Danielsen JM, Johnson R, Kibsgaard SK, et al. Early aggressive exercise for postoperative rehabilitation following discectomy. *Spine.* 2000;25(8):1015-1020.
85. Kjellby-Wendt G, Styf J. Early active training after lumbar discectomy. A prospective, randomized and controlled study. *Spine.* 1998;23(21):2345-2352.

86. Philleps FM, Cunningham B. Managing chronic pain of spinal origin after lumbar surgery: the role of decompressive surgery. *Spine*. 2001;27(22):2547-2553.
87. Scrimshaw SV, Maher CG. Randomized controlled trial of neural mobilization after spinal surgery. *Spine*. 2001;26(24):2647-2652.
88. Wilner S. Effects of a rigid brace on back pain. *Acta Orthop Scand*. 1985;56:40-42.

Appendix

Pharmacological Information: Neurologic and Neurosurgical Diseases and Disorders Pharmacology

Anti-Alzheimer Agents

Action

Anti-alzheimer medications inhibit cholinesterase, an enzyme that metabolizes Ach, thereby increasing the amount of Ach within the CNS, to temporarily lessen dementia.

Side Effects

CNS: Headache, depression, drowsiness, fatigue, insomnia
CV: HTN, hypotension, syncope, atrial fibrillation
GI: Diarrhea, nausea, vomiting, anorexia/weight loss, flatulence
Miscellaneous: Muscle cramps, arthritis, hot flashes

Common Medications

Aricept (donepezil), Reminyl (galantamine), Exelon (rivastigmine), Cognex (tacrine)

Anxiolytics/Sedatives/Benzodiazepines

Action

Benzodiazepines are the most common group of anxiolytics and sedative hypnotics. Benzodiazepines potentiate the effect of GABA, an inhibitory neurotransmitter, within the CNS. These agents lead to hyperpolarization of cells, resulting in reduced synaptic transmission.

Side Effects

CNS: Dizziness, drowsiness, lethargy, depression
CV: Hypotension, bradycardia
GI: Constipation, diarrhea, nausea, vomiting
Miscellaneous: Dependence, drug tolerance, blurred vision
Pulmonary: Respiratory depression, apnea, bronchospasm

Common Medications

Xanax (alprazolam), Librium (chlordiazepoxide), Valium (diazepam), Ativan (lorazepam), Versed (midazolam), Serax (oxazepam)

Anticonvulsants

Action

Anticonvulsants inhibit sodium channels of neurons decreasing excitability and action potential propagation, enhance the effects of GABA, a CNS inhibitory neurotransmitter, or block calcium channels. These agents attempt to raise the seizure threshold, decrease the spread of seizure activity, or depress the motor cortex.

Side Effects

CNS: Drowsiness, lethargy, delirium, incoordination
CV: Hypotension
GI: Constipation, nausea, vomiting, GI discomfort
Miscellaneous: Arthralgias, myalgias, neuralgias, allergic reactions
Pulmonary: Bronchospasm, respiratory depression

Common Medications
Sodium channel blocking agents: Dilantin (phenytoin), Tegretol (carbamazepine), oxcaraepine, Lamictal (lamotrigine)
GABA agonists: Neurotonin (gabapentin)
Calcium channel blockade: Zarontin (ethosuximide), trimethadione
Combined effects: Benzodiazepines (eg, Klonopin [clonazepam], Luminal [phenobarbital], Myosoline [primdone])

Antidepressants

Action
Antidepressants potentiate the effect of serotonin and norepinephrine in the CNS. Depression is characterized by diminished interest in normal activities, anorexia and weight loss, fatigue, insomnia, and an inability to concentrate. Mania is characterized by inflated self-esteem, poverty of sleep, and expansive mood.

Side Effects
CNS: Lethargy, sedation, reduced seizure threshold
CV: Dysrhythmias, orthostatic hypotension
GI: Constipation, diarrhea, nausea
Miscellaneous: Blurred vision, weight gain, increased appetite, tremor

Common Medications
Tricyclic antidepressants: Elavil (amitriptyline); Pamelor (nortriptyline); Imprin, Tofranil (imipramine)
Selective seotonin reuptake inhibitors (SSRI): Prozac (fluozetine Hcl), Zoloft (sertaline Hcl)
Monoamine oxidase (MAO) inhibitors (block metabolism of norepinephrine and serotonin): Nardil (phenelzine), Parnate (tranylcypromine), Marplan (isocarboxazid)
Miscellaneous: Wellbutrin (buprion), Desyrel (trazadone), Effexor (venlafaxine)

Antiparkinson (Antidyskinetic) Agents

Action
Antiparkinson agents attempt to either increase CNS concentrations of dopamine (eg, levodopa), potentiate dopamines actions (eg, amantadine, bromocriptine), or limit its breakdown (eg, catechol-o-methyl transferase (COMT) inhibitors, MAO inhibitors, Selegiline), reduce cholinergic activity (eg, benztropine, beperiden), or diminish neuronal outlflow from the basal ganglia.

Side Effects
CNS: Involuntary movements, ataxia, anxiety, dizziness, hallucinations
CV: Orthostatic hypotension, tachycardia, palpitations
GI: Anorexia, nausea, vomiting
Miscellaneous: Dry mouth, blurred vision, leukopenia, anemia

Common Medications
Dopaminergic: Symmetrel (amantadine); Parlodel (bromocriptine); L-Dopa, Larodopa (levodopa)
COMT inhibitors: Comtan (entacapone)
MAO inhibitors: Eldepryl (selegiline)
Anticholinergics: Cogentin (benztropine), Akineton (biperiden)

Antipsychotics

Action

Antipsychotics are used in the treatment of psychosis and schizophrenia. Psychosis refers to mental disorders characterized by diminished capacity to process information, hallucinations, delusions, incoherence, aggression, or violence. Schizophrenia is a mental disorder associated with disturbances of thinking and affect. Antipsychotic drugs primarily block dopamine receptors but may additionally impact histamine, serotonin, and alpha adrenergic receptors.

Side Effects

CNS: Tardive dyskinesia, Parkinsonism, dystonia, drowsiness, lethargy, neuroleptic syndrome
CV: Orthostatic hypotension, tachycardia
GI: Dry mouth, constipation
Miscellaneous: Impotence, infertility, blurred vision

Common Medications

Clozaril (clozapine), Chlorpromazine, Haldol (haloperidol), Mellaril (thioridazine), lithium

CV = cardiovascular; GI = gastrointestinal.

Chapter 10

Endocrine Diseases and Disorders

Christine F. Ehlers, PT, CWS, CLWT and Daniel J. Malone, PT, PhD, CCS

The endocrine system is a complex arrangement of glands that regulate multiple body systems through the synthesis and secretion of hormones. The endocrine glands secrete their products directly into the circulatory system to communicate with their effector tissues. The major glands include the hypothalamus, pituitary, thyroid, parathyroid, adrenals, pancreas, ovaries, and testes (Figure 10-1). This chapter will briefly review each gland, define the actions of its hormones, and discuss the impact of common health conditions. Particular attention will be directed at diabetes mellitus, the most common endocrine disease.

Anatomy and Physiology

Hormones

Hormones are specialized blood-borne substances that regulate and coordinate a variety of body functions. They are produced by the endocrine cells of glands and other tissues in response to specific stimuli and exert their actions on specific target tissues. Hormone cell structure can be an amine, peptide (protein), or steroid. The specific hormone structure permits binding to different cell receptors with high affinity and specificity. Peptides and amines, including the catecholamines (ie, epinephrine, norepinephrine) and dopamine, bind to cell membrane receptors and initiate signaling cascades within the cell to initiate the desired responses. Steroids, which are synthesized from cholesterol, are able to penetrate the cell membrane and bind to specific receptors in the cell nucleus influencing gene transcription to direct the physiologic responses.

Hormone secretion is regulated by the following:

- **Feedback mechanisms**: Chemical signals or other hormones are released into the bloodstream resulting in hormone release or suppression. Responses can be positive (ie, high levels of substance increases hormone secretion and low levels suppress), negative (ie, high levels of substance suppress hormone secretion and

Malone DJ, Bishop KL, eds. *Acute Care Physical Therapy: A Clinician's Guide, Second Edition* (pp 421-458).

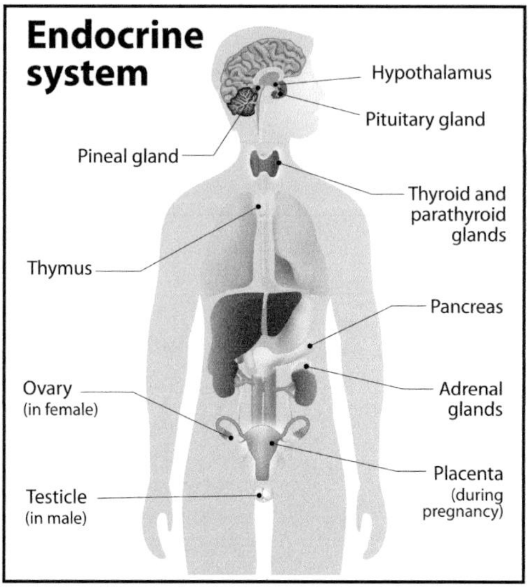

Figure 10-1. Anatomical location of the endocrine glands. (Designua/Shutterstock.com)

low levels stimulate), or complex, when multiple substances can stimulate or suppress the same hormone. A common example of a negative feedback loop is insulin and glucagon regulation. Insulin release is stimulated by high levels of circulating glucose, amino acids, and fats, and glucagon is depressed. As nutrients are taken up by cells, insulin secretion declines and glucagon release is increased.

- **Direct signaling**: Implies that endocrine glands are directly stimulated by other structures to secrete or suppress hormone secretion. An example is dehydration. The increased blood osmolarity and low blood pressure (BP) stimulate osmoreceptors in the brain and baroreceptors in the aorta that signal the pituitary and hypothalamus to produce more antidiuretic hormone (ADH). ADH circulates to the kidneys promoting increased renal reabsorption of water. Renal conservation of body water expands the blood volume decreasing the osmolarity of the blood and increasing BP. As blood osmolarity falls, secretion of ADH decreases.
- **Circadian rhythm**: Levels rise and fall predictably during a 24-hour period. Examples include cortisol and thyroid hormones. Cortisol levels rise early in the day, decline as the day progresses, and begin rising during sleep to peak levels upon awakening. Thyroid-stimulating hormone (TSH) releases periodically throughout the day and, therefore, experiences little fluctuation.
- **Cycling**: Hormones are released at periodic times, but it is unsure how this is controlled. Examples include luteinizing hormone (LH) and follicle-stimulating hormone (FSH), which control reproductive functions and the menstrual cycle.

The nervous and endocrine systems are mutually dependent on each other. Autonomic nerves control endocrine gland blood flow and hormone secretion, and hormones have a regulatory effect on nervous tissue.[1] Hormones can influence behavior and stress, while emotional states (eg, anxiety, fear) can influence hormone production. Dependent on the origin of secretion, substances can be hormones or neurotransmitters. For example, catecholamines (ie, epinephrine, norepinephrine) are hormones when they are secreted by the adrenal medulla and neurotransmitters when they are secreted by the post-synaptic cells of the sympathetic nervous system.

Specific Endocrine Organs and Their Health Conditions

Hypothalamus

The **hypothalamus** is part of the diencephalon, surrounded by the cerebrum of the brain, and functions as a regulator of the autonomic nervous system and the majority of endocrine glands. The hypothalamus is described in Table 10-1. Neurotransmitters and hormones are used to carry out hypothalamic regulatory functions on body temperature, sexual behavior, appetite control, fluid balance, levels of arousal, and emotional expression. The hypothalamus primarily impacts the pituitary gland. Hypothalamic hormones may be stored in the pituitary (ADH/oxytocin) or act as stimulators or inhibitors of hormones released by the pituitary. Table 10-2 lists the major hypothalamic hormones and how each functions.

Pituitary Gland

The **pituitary gland**, also termed the **hypophysis**, is surrounded by a bony structure, the sella turcica, and is divided into 2 parts. The anterior lobe, which is approximately 80% of the pituitary's weight, connects to the hypothalamus by the infundibular/pituitary stalk. Through this stalk runs a vein called the **hypophyseal portal vascular system**. The hypothalamus secretes its hormones into the hypophyseal portal vascular system for direct delivery to the pituitary. The posterior lobe, which is approximately 20% of the gland's total weight, is considered an extension of the hypothalamus. The posterior lobe consists of unmyelinated nerve fibers and terminals of axons that transport and store ADH, also termed **vasopressin**, and oxytocin, which are produced by the hypothalamus. Although pituitary hormone secretion is regulated by hypothalamic function, the pituitary is called the **master gland** because it produces 6 hormones and stores 2 additional ones. The pituitary has 3 specific targets: the reproductive organs (ovaries and testes), adrenal cortex, and thyroid. Details regarding pituitary gland functions are found in Table 10-3. Table 10-4 describes the major hormones and their impact on the body.

Disorders that occur in the hypothalamus and the pituitary are difficult to discuss separately because the 2 glands are interrelated. Damage to the hypothalamus impairs stimulating or inhibiting factors from reaching the pituitary, which alters pituitary function.

Most common disorders involving the hypothalamus and pituitary are due to tumors, increased intracranial pressures (as seen in severe hypertension [HTN] and traumatic brain injuries), inflammatory diseases, infection, surgical excision of either gland, autoimmune disease, or ischemia from blood clots or severe bleeding. Hypopituitarism is underproduction of hormones, while hyperpituitarism is overproduction of hormones. Primary disorders result from direct damage to the pituitary, while secondary disorders are due to damage to the hypothalamus or to the adjoining pituitary stalk. Specific signs and symptoms related to malproduction of pituitary hormones can be found in Table 10-5.

Diagnostic testing for hypothalamus and pituitary disorders includes blood testing for specific hormone concentrations in conjunction with stimulation or suppression tests. Computed tomography (CT) and magnetic resonance imaging (MRI) scans provide anatomic descriptions of possible gland damage or disease.

Table 10-1 **HYPOTHALAMUS AT A GLANCE**	
Location	• Below the thalamus and cerebral hemisphere • Anterior and superior to the pituitary gland • Behind the optic chiasm and between the optic tracts
Special Features	• Connects to the pituitary gland by the infundibular or pituitary stalk • Communication with the anterior lobe is by hormone and chemical release • Communication with the posterior lobe is via neurotransmission • Utilizes the posterior lobe for storage of oxytocin and ADH also termed vasopressin. ¤ Regulates body temperature, sweating, appetite, thirst, gastrointestional (GI) secretion and motility, BP, sleep, sexual behavior, defensive reactions (eg, rage, fear), and body rhythms
Functions	• Integrates communication between the endocrine and nervous systems in conjunction with the pituitary gland • Mediates central nervous system (CNS) control input with hypothalamic hormones and neurotransmitters • Influences fluid and electrolyte balance and cell metabolism by hormone production (eg, ADH) and hormone-releasing hormones
Secretes	• Hormones: ¤ ADH and oxytocin (both stored in posterior pituitary) • Releasing hormones: ¤ Corticotropin-releasing hormone (CRH) ¤ Thyrotropin-releasing hormone (TRH) ¤ Growth hormone (GH)–releasing factor or somatotropin-releasing hormone ¤ Gonadotropin-releasing hormone ¤ Prolactin-releasing factor • Inhibiting hormones: ¤ Prolactin release inhibiting factor (PIF) ¤ Somatostatin or GH inhibiting hormone
Major Target	• Pituitary gland

Thyroid Gland

The **thyroid gland** is described in Table 10-6. **Thyroid hormone** (TH) strongly influences growth, development, and metabolism. Its production is dependent on the dietary intake and circulating concentrations of iodine to convert TH into a usable form. The kidney metabolizes TH, the iodine is cleaved from the hormone and returned to the thyroid gland. TH production begins in the hypothalamus with release of TRH. TRH travels to the anterior pituitary promoting release of TSH. TSH

Table 10-2

HYPOTHALAMIC HORMONES AND THEIR FUNCTIONS

Hormone/Chemical Substance	*Cell Structure*	*Target Area*	*Function/Action*
CRH	Peptide	Anterior pituitary	• Stimulates release of adrenocorticotropin hormone (ACTH)
TRH	Peptide	Anterior pituitary	• Stimulates the release of TSH and prolactin • Can stimulate the release of GH
GH releasing factor or somatotropin releasing hormone	Peptide	Anterior pituitary	• Stimulates the release of GH
Gonadotropin releasing hormone	Peptide	Anterior pituitary	• Stimulate the release of LH and FSH
Prolactin releasing factor	Peptide	Anterior pituitary	• Stimulates the release of prolactin
PIF	Peptide	Anterior pituitary	• Suppresses the release of prolactin
GH inhibiting hormone or somatostatin	Peptide	Anterior pituitary	• Suppresses the release of GH
Dopamine	Amine	Anterior pituitary	• Prolactin inhibition

Table 10-3

PITUITARY AT A GLANCE

Location	• Base of the brain in the sella turcica ("Turkish saddle") above the sphenoid bone
Special Features	• Referred to as the master gland • Anterior and posterior lobes
Functions	• Controls the functions of most of the other endocrine glands • Anterior lobe primarily functions to control metabolism, reproductive organ growth, body growth, and secretion of steroid hormones • Posterior lobe functions for reproduction (eg, milk secretion/uterine contraction) and fluid balance (eg, reabsorption of sodium and water by kidneys)
Secretes	• GH, TSH, ACTH, prolactin, FSH, LH, ADH or vasopressin, oxytocin
Major Target	• Reproductive organs (ovaries and testes), thyroid, adrenal glands and kidneys

Table 10-4

PITUITARY HORMONES AND THEIR FUNCTIONS

Hormone	*Cell Structure*	*Target Area*	*Function/Action*
GH	Peptide	Muscles and bones	• Regulates growth • Influences intermediary metabolism
Prolactin	Peptide	Mammary glands	• Lactation
LH	Peptide	Gonads (ovaries and testes)	• Reproductive control • Regulates ovarian and testicular function • Controls testosterone production in males • Stimulates production of androgen, which converts to estrogen and progesterone in females
FSH	Peptide	Gonads (ovaries and testes)	• Reproductive control in males and females • Helps stimulate the production of sperm in males • Stimulates maturation of the ovarian follicles in females
TSH	Peptide	Thyroid or thyrotropin	• Regulates thyroid function
ACTH	Peptide	Adrenal cortex	• Controls glucocorticoid function of the adrenal cortex
ADH or vasopressin	Peptide	Kidney	• Controls water conservation by the kidneys • Potent vasoconstrictor • Potentiates the effect of corticotropin releasing hormone • Controls BP along with aldosterone
Oxytocin	Amine	Uterus and mammary glands	• Stimulates milk ejection or "let down" for mammary glands • Contraction of smooth uterine muscle • Possibly stimulates prolactin release • Establish maternal behavior

travels to the thyroid gland promoting release of TH as illustrated in Figure 10-2. This action is termed the **hypothalamus-pituitary-thyroid axis** and TH release is an example of a negative feedback loop. High levels of TH decrease pituitary secretion of TSH. Low concentrations of TH increase pituitary secretion of TSH. Thyroid stimulation results in secretion of both **thyroxine** (T_4) and **triiodothyronine** (T_3). Specific information on thyroid hormones can be found in Table 10-7. T_4 has few effects on the body's metabolism; however, T_4 can be converted to T_3 and T_4 conversion accounts for approximately 80% of T_3 in the body. T_4 binding and conversion help extend the life of the hormone and maintain a metabolic steady state. T_4 half-life in the bloodstream is 6.7 days; T_3 half-life is about 30 hours. Only 0.04% of T_4 and 0.4% of T_3 are free in the bloodstream at any given time, with the majority bound to plasma

Table 10-5

SIGNS AND SYMPTOMS OF HYPOTHALAMIC AND PITUITARY DYSFUNCTION

Hormone	*Overproduction*	*Underproduction*
GH	• Gigantism (children) • Acromegaly (adults) • Bony and soft tissue overgrowth • Enlarged hands, feet, and head • Enlarged tongue • Laryngeal hypertrophy • Sinus enlargement • Muscle weakness • Amenorrhea • Goiter	• Few symptoms in adults • Slow growth or dwarfism in children
Prolactin	• Amenorrhea • Galactorrhea • Hypogonadism • Decreased sex drive • Decreased sperm production and impotence in men • Breast enlargement and decreased fertility in women	• Fatigue • Loss of pubic and axillary hair • Inability to produce breast milk
LH	• Essentially no biological effect	• Hypogonadism • Decreased sex drive • Decreased sperm production (men) • Impotence • Amenorrhea (in women)
FSH	• Essentially no biological effect	• Hypogonadism • Decreased sex drive • Decreased sperm production • Impotence • Amenorrhea
TSH or thyrotropin	• See Table 10-8	• See Table 10-8
ACTH	• See Table 10-14	• See Table 10-14
ADH or vasopressin	• Syndrome of inappropriate ADH: ¤ Increased water retention with hyponatremia ¤ Muscle aches and weakness; myoclonus and ataxia; lethargy and delirium	• Diabetes insipidus • Excessive dilute urine • Polydipsia (excessive thirst)

(continued)

Table 10-5 (continued) SIGNS AND SYMPTOMS OF HYPOTHALAMIC AND PITUITARY DYSFUNCTION		
Hormone	*Overproduction*	*Underproduction*
Oxytocin	• Erectile dysfunction and decreased libido • Irregular or absent menstrual periods, infertility, menopausal symptoms, production of breast milk	• Decreased milk ejection • Decreased uterine contraction during birth

Table 10-6 THYROID AT A GLANCE	
Location	• The butterfly-shaped thyroid consists of 2 lateral lobes connected by a narrow section called the isthmus and is located in the neck, in close approximation to the first part of the trachea, just below the larynx.
Special Features	• Right lobe is larger and more vascular than the left. • Needs iodine to produce thyroid hormones • Innervated by the sympathetic nervous system via the cervical ganglia and by the parasympathetic nervous system via the vagus nerve • Able to store large amounts of hormone (up to 30-day supply) • Stimulated by the hypothalamus-pituitary-thyroid axis
Functions	• Secretes thyroid hormones that control the body's chemical functions by influencing protein production and oxygen consumption. • Thyroid hormones increase the basal metabolic rate.
Secretes	• T_4 • T_3 • Thyrocalcitonin (calcitonin)
Major Target	• All major body systems (see Tables 10-7 and 10-8)

proteins.[2] Adequate levels of thyroid hormone are dependent on proper functioning of the hypothalamus-pituitary-thyroid axis and the protein binding and release of T_3 and T_4. **Calcitonin** is also secreted by the thyroid gland and is involved in calcium homeostasis. Calcitonin is released when serum calcium levels are high and acts to lower blood calcium by inhibiting calcium absorption in the intestines and decreasing bone degradation. Calcitonin is suppressed by decreased serum calcium levels. Calcitonin counteracts parathyroid hormone (PTH).

Thyroid function is altered by multiple factors, including gender and sex hormones, pregnancy, age, glucocorticoids, environmental temperature, nutrition and non-thyroid illness, such as liver cirrhosis and chronic renal failure.[1] Signs and symptoms

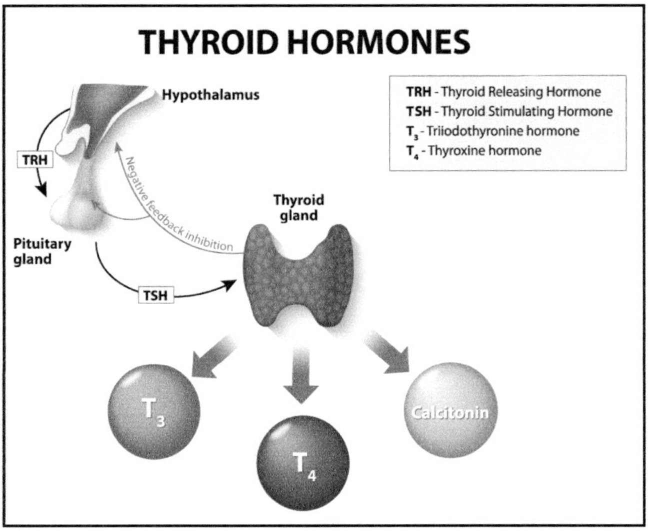

Figure 10-2. Hypothalamus-pituitary-thyroid axis. (Designua/Shutterstock.com)

Table 10-7

THYROID HORMONES AND THEIR FUNCTIONS

Hormone	*Cell Structure*	*Target Area*	*Function/Action*
T_4	Peptide	All body tissues	• Energy metabolism • Growth and development • Metabolism speed • Control of body temperature • Maturation
T_3	Peptide	All body tissues	• Energy metabolism • Growth and development • Metabolism speed • Control of body temperature • Maturation
Calcitonin	Peptide	Plasma	• Regulation of calcium and phosphate blood levels • Stimulation of bone demineralization

of hyper- and hypothyroidism can be found in Table 10-8. **Hyperthyroidism**, overproduction of TH, is associated with Grave's disease (an autoimmune disease), toxic nodular goiter, and secondary hyperthyroidism. **Thyroid storm**, an acute disproportionate production of TH, is caused by inadequately treated hyperthyroidism. The individual will develop fever, extreme weakness, restlessness, mood swings, confusion, altered mental status, and, eventually, coma. Thyroid storm is life threatening and requires immediate medical attention.[3] **Hypothyroidism**, underproduction of

Table 10-8

SIGNS AND SYMPTOMS OF THYROID DYSFUNCTION

System Affected	Hyperthyroidism	Hypothyroidism
Cardiovascular	• Increased heart rate (HR), palpitations • Increased cardiac output • Systolic HTN • Cardiac hypertrophy • Angina • Dyspnea with mild exertion • Increased respiratory rate (RR)	• Slowed HR • Decreased cardiac output • Varied changes in BP • Tendency to develop congestive heart failure, angina, and myocardial infarction • Dyspnea with decreased breathing capacity
Neurological	• Shakiness, tremors • Nervousness • Lability of mood • Restlessness • Personality changes of irritability and agitation • Confusion • Rapid speech	• Slowed, slurred speech • Slow movements • Decreased hearing • Carpel tunnel syndrome • Paresthesias • Confusion, forgetfulness • Depression • Lethargy • Anxiety • Dementia • Hoarse voice
GI	• Frequent bowel movements with diarrhea • Weight loss with increased appetite • Splenomegaly	• Constipation • Distended abdomen • Weight gain with decreased appetite

(continued)

TH, is associated with deficiency in dietary iodine, and thyroid cancers, including papillary, follicular, anaplastic, and medullary cancer. Hypothyroidism is also associated with 3 types of thyroiditis:

1. Hashimoto's thyroiditis (autoimmune thyroiditis)
2. Subacute granulomatous thyroiditis (usually occurs after viral illness)
3. Silent lymphocytic thyroiditis (occurs most often in women after childbirth)

Euthyroid sick syndrome occurs when the thyroid is functioning normally, but T_4 does not convert to T_3. This may result from malnutrition, acute illness, or surgery. Euthyroid sick syndrome typically resolves with resolution of the initiating event.

Thyroid function can be evaluated by blood tests measuring TSH (TSH is high when the thyroid is underactive and low when it is overactive) and free T_4. Blood tests may also be performed in conjunction with stimulation agents. Ultrasound, CT scans, MRI, and nuclear imaging determine the presence of anatomic anomalies. Nuclear imaging using radioactive iodine can demonstrate deficiencies in iodine uptake and thyroid hormone production.

Table 10-8 (continued)

SIGNS AND SYMPTOMS OF THYROID DYSFUNCTION

System Affected	*Hyperthyroidism*	*Hypothyroidism*
Musculoskeletal	• Weakness with proximal muscle wasting	• Muscle aches and pains
Reproductive	• Decreased libido • Impotence in men • Menstrual irregularities	• Infertility • Decreased libido • Prolonged menstrual periods
General appearance	• Swollen, reddened, bulging eyes • Hair loss • Thin, brittle nails detached from beds • Raised, thickened skin over shins • Premature graying • Palmar erythema • Moist, warm skin • Goiter	• Drooping eyelids • Loss of eyebrows • Sparse, course, dry hair • Dry, scaly, thick coarse skin; raised and thickened over shins • Decreased sweating • Puffy face
Other	• Intolerance to heat • Increased basal temperature • Increased sensitivity to stimulant drugs • Fatigue, exhaustion • Insomnia • Eyes with increased sensitivity to light	• Intolerance to cold • Increased susceptibility to infections • Anemia • Enlarged coarse tongue

Parathyroid

The **parathyroid glands** are 4 small glands located behind the thyroid that regulate calcium and phosphate metabolism through the production and secretion of **PTH**. The parathyroid gland is described in Tables 10-9 and 10-10. Parathyroid regulation is a negative feedback loop responding to serum calcium levels. Increased serum calcium inhibits PTH secretion, and decreased serum calcium stimulates PTH secretion. PTH has 3 main targets: bone, kidney, and intestinal mucosa. PTH stimulates osteoclasts and inhibits osteoblasts in the bone, resulting in decreased bone mineral density and increased serum calcium levels. PTH stimulates renal reabsorption of calcium and increases the excretion of phosphate to provide equilibration of calcium to phosphate by limiting renal losses of calcium. In the intestinal mucosa, PTH stimulates Vitamin D, which increases calcium absorption in the small intestine. PTH and calcitonin are antagonistic, allowing for precise maintenance of calcium homeostasis. As noted in Chapter 2, calcium is vital for bone formation, cell division and growth, blood coagulation, muscle contraction, and release of neurotransmitters by exocytosis. Profound hypoparathyroidism and resultant hypocalcemia can lead to tetany and death.

Parathyroid gland disorders are **hyperparathyroidism** causing hypercalcemia and **hypoparathyroidism** causing hypocalcemia. Primary causes of hyperparathyroidism

Table 10-9 **PARATHYROID AT A GLANCE**	
Location	• Posterior surface of the thyroid gland • Sometimes in the mediastinum within the thyroid gland or behind the esophagus
Special Features	• Usually there are 2 pairs of glands. There may be as few as 3 or as many as 6.
Functions	• Calcium and phosphate homeostasis • Production and secretion of PTH stimulates the body to reserve its serum calcium by inhibiting formation of bone, equalizing calcium and phosphate levels, and increasing calcium absorption in the intestines.
Secretes	• PTH
Major Target	• Bone, kidney, and intestinal mucosa

Table 10-10 **PARATHYROID HORMONE AND ITS FUNCTIONS**			
Hormone	*Cell Structure*	*Target Area*	*Function/Action*
PTH	Peptide	Bone, kidney, and intestinal mucosa	• Regulates calcium, phosphate, and bone metabolism • Maintains serum/calcium concentration • Regulates Vitamin D synthesis

are adenomas, carcinomas, and hereditary diseases. Secondary causes are related to diseases that stimulate excessive secretion of PTH, including renal disease and nutrition deficiencies of calcium or Vitamin D. Clinical signs and symptoms of parathyroid dysfunction are noted in Table 10-11.

Diagnostic testing is accomplished with PTH blood studies. Additionally, evaluation of nutritional history emphasizing intake of Vitamin D and calcium is important.[4]

Adrenal Glands

The **adrenal glands** sit atop the kidneys and are detailed in Table 10-12. Each adrenal is composed of an outer cortex surrounding the inner medulla. The **adrenal cortex** is separated into 3 zones producing the glucocorticoids (ie, cortisol, corticosterone), mineralocorticoids (ie, aldosterone), and androgens (ie, androstenedione [the precursor to testosterone]); from outter to inner zon: the zona glomerulosa (produces aldosterone), zona fasiculata (produces cortisol and androgens), and zona reticularis (produces cortisol and androgens). The zona fasiculata and zona reticularis are regulated by adrenocorticotropin hormone (ACTH) from the pituitary. CRH from the hypothalamus stimulates the secretion of ACTH from the anterior pituitary gland regulating androgens and glucocorticoid production.

The **adrenal medulla** (the innermost tissue of the adrenal glands) consists of chromaffin cells that can be considered modified sympathetic ganglia synthesizing

Table 10-11

SIGNS AND SYMPTOMS OF PARATHYROID DYSFUNCTION

Hyperparathyroidism	*Hypoparathyroidism*
• GI: ¤ Constipation ¤ Indigestion, nausea, vomiting ¤ Peptic ulcers ¤ Pancreatitis ¤ Anorexia • Kidney: ¤ Renal stones ¤ Nephrocalcinosis ¤ Polyuria (increased urine) ¤ Polydipsia (increased thirst) ¤ Uremia • Bones: ¤ Osteitis fibrosa with bone cysts, osteoclastomas, subperiosteal resorption ¤ Radiologic osteoporosis ¤ Osteomalacia or rickets ¤ Arthritis • Mental: ¤ Lethargy, fatigue ¤ Depression ¤ Memory loss ¤ Psychotic paranoia ¤ Confusion, stupor, coma • Other: ¤ Proximal muscle weakness ¤ Itching	• Neurological: ¤ Paresthesias, seizures ¤ Organic brain syndrome ¤ Cataracts ¤ Calcification of basal ganglia ¤ Tetany • Cardiac: ¤ Prolonged QT interval ¤ Congestive heart failure • Bones: ¤ Shortened digits, especially fourth and fifth fingers • Reproductive: ¤ Infertility in males ¤ Oligomenorrhea in females • Skin: ¤ Dry and flaky ¤ Brittle nails

and storing dopamine and the 2 catecholamines, epinephrine and norepinephrine. Sympathetic nervous system stimulation releases the catecholamines into the bloodstream. Like other hormones, catecholamines exert their effects by binding to specific receptors and activating signaling pathways in their target cells.[2] The cellular responses associated with catecholamines depend upon the receptors activated (eg, the alpha [α] and beta [β] receptors). Specific hormone targets and functions are outlined in Table 10-13.

Adrenal gland disorders also involve over- and underproduction of the various hormones. A deficiency of corticosteroids causes **Addison's disease**, while corticosteroid overproduction or overexposure can result in **Cushing's syndrome**. Excessive amounts of androgen can cause virilization, an exaggeration of masculine features in men and women. **Hyperaldosteronism** is a condition that affects the blood levels of sodium, potassium, bicarbonate, and chloride. **Pheochromocytoma** is a tumor that arises from the chromaffin cells and causes an overproduction of catecholamines.[3] Specific signs and symptoms for each of these disorders can be found in Table 10-14.

Table 10-12 ADRENAL GLANDS AT A GLANCE	
Location	• Superior or medial to the upper poles of the kidneys
Special Features	• Composed of the adrenal cortex and adrenal medulla • Influenced by the hypothalamic-pituitary and autonomic nervous systems
Functions	• Impacts multiple organ systems • Metabolic (carbohydrate, protein, and fat metabolism) • Cardiovascular (HR, BP) • Renal (sodium and potassium levels)
Secretes	• Aldosterone (mineralocorticoid) • Cortisol (glucocorticoid) • Catecholamines (epinephrine, norepinephrine, and dopamine) • Androgens
Major Target	• Kidneys, GI, cardiovascular, and reproductive organs

Diagnostic testing is done with blood and urine samples depending on the hormone. CT or MRI scans can help discover anatomic abnormalities. Exploratory surgery and biopsy are also used for accurate diagnosis.

Reproductive System (Ovaries and Testes)

The endocrine glands of the reproductive system are the gonads, ovaries, or testes. This system is mainly regulated by the gonadotrophins (LH and FSH) released from the anterior pituitary and the androgens (testosterone, progesterone, estrogen) released from the ovaries and testes. Gonadotrophin release is regulated by the hypothalamic delivery of gonadotropin-releasing hormone (GnRH). LH and FSH stimulate the production of the steroid-based androgens. In men, testosterone is synthesized in the Leydig's cells of the testes. In women, LH and FSH stimulate maturation of the ovarian follicles where the primary female sex hormone, estradiol, is produced. The follicle also contains the oocyte, the egg cell. The corpus luteum is formed from the evacuated follicle and is a temporary endocrine structure. The corpus luteum primarily secretes progesterone, which is essential during the first trimester of pregnancy. LH and FSH secretion follows a cycling rhythm to bring about the menstrual cycle. Specific functions of the gonadotrophic hormones are outlined in Table 10-15.

Disorders involving the gonads will interfere with puberty and normal growth and development in children. In adults, problems often lead to infertility.

Diagnostic testing of the gonad system involves physical examination and serum levels of the specific hormone. Reproductive hormones are typically measured repeatedly due to the cyclic pattern of release.

Pancreas

The **pancreas** is located within the left upper abdominal quadrant, and has both endocrine and exocrine functions. The exocrine portion secretes digestive enzymes while the endocrine portion participates in glucose, fat, and protein homeostasis through the production of insulin and glucagon. The islets of Langerhans are responsible for the endocrine functions as outlined in Table 10-16. The islets contain 4 cell types. The alpha cells secrete glucagon, beta cells secrete insulin, delta cells secrete

Table 10-13

ADRENAL HORMONES AND THEIR FUNCTIONS

Hormone	*Cell Structure*	*Target Area*	*Function/Action*
Aldosterone (mineralocorticoid)	Steroid	Kidneys	• Regulates sodium and potassium levels by promoting renal sodium conservation and potassium secretion • Controls BP by maintenance of extracellular volume
Cortisol (glucocorticoid)	Steroid	GI	• Affects excretion of digestive enzymes • Catabolic effect on cellular proteins • Regulates carbohydrate, fat, and protein metabolism • Maintenance of normal excitability of the myocardium and catecholamine action • Anti-inflammatory agent • Decreases capillary permeability • Maintenance of emotional well-being
Androgen	Steroid	Testes and ovaries	• Increase masculinization, axillary and pubic hairs in females and pubic hair in males
Catecholamines (epinephrine/ norepinephrine)	Amine	Cardiovascular and metabolic system	• Stress response (ie, fight or flight) • Increase rate and force of cardiac contraction • Constricts blood vessels • Dilates airways/bronchioles • Increases metabolic rate • Blocks insulin secretion and stimulates glucagon release • Activates glycogen breakdown (glycogenolysis)

somatostatin, and the gamma cells secrete gastrin. Elevated blood glucose levels are the primary stimulus for insulin release, resulting in increased cellular uptake of blood glucose. Insulin, an anabolic hormone, stimulates the liver and skeletal muscle to store glucose in the form of glycogen and increases amino acid transport into liver, muscle, and adipose tissues. Insulin also stimulates protein and fatty acid (lipogenesis) synthesis in the liver and adipose tissues. Blood glucose is a readily

Table 10-14

Signs and Symptoms of Adrenal Hormonal Dysfunction

Hormone	*Overproduction*	*Underproduction*
Androgen	• Adrenogenital syndrome: ¤ Hairiness of the face and body ¤ Baldness ¤ Acne ¤ Deepening of the voice/ increased muscularity ¤ Increased sex drive ¤ In women, uterus shrinks, clitoris enlarges, breasts shrink, amenorrhea	• Androgen deficiency: ¤ Lethargy and fatigue ¤ Loss of libido (erectile dysfunction in males) ¤ Decreased muscle mass and weakness ¤ Reduced bone mass
Aldosterone (mineralocorticoid)	• Hyperaldosteronism: ¤ Weakness ¤ Tingling muscle spasms ¤ Paralysis ¤ Polydipsia (increased thirst) ¤ Increased urination	• Hypoaldosteronism: ¤ Hypotension ¤ Cardiac failure ¤ Low blood glucose levels ¤ Fatigue ¤ Decreased tolerance to stress
Cortisol (glucocorticoid)	• Cushing's syndrome: ¤ Altered distribution of body fat ¤ Large round face ("moon face") ¤ Obesity ¤ Increased fat of torso ("buffalo hump") ¤ Muscle wasting/weakness ¤ Thinned skin ¤ Increased bruising ¤ Poor wound healing ¤ Increased BP ¤ Osteoporosis ¤ Decreased resistance to infection ¤ Diabetes ¤ Kidney stones	• Addison's disease: ¤ Weak, tired, dizzy on standing ¤ Skin darkens overall ¤ Black freckles over face and shoulders ¤ Lethargy ¤ Weight loss ¤ Dehydration ¤ Loss of appetite ¤ Muscle aches ¤ Nausea, vomiting, and diarrhea ¤ Decreased blood glucose levels ¤ Untreated: Profound weakness, extremely low BP, kidney failure, shock

(continued)

available energy source, but without insulin, a number of the body's cells are unable to absorb glucose. These cells can also use fatty acids as an alternative energy source. The brain, however, does not require insulin for glucose uptake but solely relies upon blood glucose for metabolism, which is why the central nervous system (CNS) is extremely sensitive to low blood glucose levels.

Table 10-14 (continued)

Signs and Symptoms of Adrenal Hormonal Dysfunction

Hormone	*Overproduction*	*Underproduction*
Catecholamines (epinephrine/ norepinephrine)	• High BP • Fast, pounding HR • Excessive sweating • Lightheaded on standing • Increased RR • Severe headaches • Nausea and vomiting • Visual disturbances • Tingling fingers • Cold and clammy skin • Chest and stomach pain	• May be present in autonomic neuropathy (eg, diabetes), adrenal gland destruction or congenital adrenal medulla maldevelopment. • Orthostatic hypotension • Fatigue/lethargy • Ptosis • Nasal stuffiness • Hyperextensible joints • Retrograde ejaculation

Table 10-15

Reproductive Hormones and Their Functions

Hormone	*Cell Structure*	*Target Area*	*Function/Action*
Testosterone	Steroid	Pituitary	• Regulation of gonadotropic secretions • Spermatogenesis • Maintains muscle mass and bone tissue in the adult male
Estrogen	Steroid	Uterus	• Affects uterine growth • Causes thickening of the vaginal mucosa • Thinning of cervical mucus • Develops ductile system of breasts • Alter lipid profiles and exert vascular effects to help prevent cardiovascular disease (CVD)
Progesterone	Steroid	Uterus	• Affects uterine growth • Causes thickening of the vaginal mucosa • Thinning of cervical mucus • Develops ductile system of breasts • Alter lipid profiles and exert vascular effects to help prevent CVD • Induction of secretory activity in the endometrium preparing for egg implant in the uterus • Inhibits uterine contraction • Increases viscosity of cervical mucus • Glandular development of breasts • Increases basal body temperature

Table 10-16 **Pancreas at a Glance**	
Location	• In the abdomen, behind the stomach, and anterior to the first and second lumbar vertebrae
Special Features	• Performs both endocrine (hormones) and exocrine (digestive) functions • Attached to duodenum by the pancreatic ducts • Islets of Langerhans are discrete clusters of cells scattered throughout the pancreas • Linked to autonomic nervous system
Functions	• Glucose homeostasis • Secreting its hormones into the bloodstream that diffuse to neighboring and distal cells to exert its actions
Secretes	• Insulin • Glucagon • Somatostatin
Major Targets	• Liver, duodenum, and all major body systems

Glucagon is a catabolic hormone and functions in opposition to insulin. Low blood glucose levels stimulate the secretion of glucagon from the pancreas. Glucagon promotes the breakdown of glycogen (glycogenolysis) and amino acids resulting in glucose formation (gluconeogenesis). The major hormones secreted by the pancreas and their actions are summarized in Table 10-17.

The most common pancreatic disease is diabetes mellitus. However, the acute care therapist may also encounter other hormonal abnormalities of pancreatic origin. Hyperinsulinemia is caused by an insulin-secreting tumor, an insulinoma, or an overdose of exogenous insulin. Hypoglycemia, or low blood glucose, develops when blood glucose levels fall resulting from excess insulin or a meal or snack not ingested in a timely manner after an insulin dose. This will be covered further in the section on diabetes. Glucagon abnormalities are rare and typically develop from cancers of the alpha cells, called **glucagonomas**.

Diagnostic testing for pancreatic abnormalities includes blood testing to determine specific levels of hormones or blood glucose. CT and MRI are performed to identify abnormal growth or lesions. Specific testing for diabetes is discussed later in this chapter and in Chapter 2.

Diabetes Mellitus

Diabetes mellitus is the most common endocrine disorder, affecting an estimated 29% of the US population with approximately 1/3 undiagnosed. Diabetes is the seventh leading cause of death.[5] Diabetes results in impaired carbohydrate metabolism because of deficient insulin secretion, increased peripheral insulin resistance, or both. Diabetes is classified as type 1, type 2, and gestational diabetes mellitus (GDM). Pancreatic disease, hormonal abnormalities, drug side effects, and genetic syndromes can precipitate diabetes. GDM is the most common medical complication of pregnancy. The etiology of GDM is poorly understood but possibly involves increased secretion of cortisol and estrogen interfering with the insulin receptor leading to increased peripheral insulin resistance. GDM is typically diagnosed during the second or third trimester of pregnancy. Identification and treatment of GDM is important because of

Table 10-17

PANCREATIC HORMONES AND THEIR FUNCTIONS

Hormone	*Cell Structure*	*Target Area*	*Function/Action*
Glucagon	Peptide	Liver	• Enhances adipose tissue lipolysis • Raises blood glucose levels • Stimulates hepatic glycogenolysis and gluconeogenesis • Raises serum glucose levels
Insulin	Peptide	All body systems	• Promotes cellular uptake and storage of ingested carbohydrates (glucose), fats, and amino acids • Reduces serum glucose levels
Somatostatin	Peptide	Pancreas	• Inhibition of insulin and glucagon

increased fetal risks (eg, mortality, jaundice, obesity, diabetes) and maternal complications (eg, preeclampsia, caesarean section). GDM usually resolves after delivery of the baby[6]; however, 5% to 10% of women with GDM continue to have high blood glucose levels and are diagnosed as having diabetes, usually type 2.[5]

Type 1 diabetes, also termed **insulin-dependent** or **juvenile diabetes**, accounts for approximately 5% of the diabetes population. It is theorized to be an autoimmune reaction triggered by an environmental factor, such as a virus or nutritional deficiency.[5] The immune system attacks the pancreatic beta cells of the islets of Langerhans and insulin production is substantially reduced. Type 1 diabetes onset is typically before the age of 30 and progresses rapidly. Clinical features of an acute diabetic exacerbation include metabolic acidosis, increased appetite (**polyphagia**) with weight loss, fatigue, frequent urination (**polyuria**), excessive thirst (**polydipsia**), and dehydration.

Missed injections, poor glucose control, and concurrent illness can lead to **diabetic ketoacidosis** (DKA). In DKA, fatty acids and proteins are the predominate fuel source resulting in increased ketone formation. Normally, ketones are produced in small quantities and are completely metabolized by extrahepatic tissues, so negligible amounts enter the blood or urine. However, when glucose can no longer be used as a fuel source, ketone formation increases and excess ketones enter the blood (**ketonemia**) and urine (**ketonuria**) leading to ketoacidosis. Patients present with hypotension and tachycardia due to dehydration. Severe dehydration can lead to mental confusion, drowsiness, seizures, and eventually coma. Patients may present with malaise, weakness and abdominal complaints including nausea, vomiting, and pain.[7]

Type 2 diabetes is also referred to as **adult onset** or **non–insulin dependent diabetes mellitus** (NIDDM), although individuals may require exogenous insulin as the disease progresses. Type 2 diabetes is the most common form of diabetes accounting for 90% to 95% of all cases.[5] Type 2 diabetes has been found in children but usually occurs after the age of 30. Obesity is an important risk factor. Race and ethnicity influence the prevalence of type 2 diabetes. Native Americans and Alaskan Natives account for 15.9%, Hispanic-Americans account for 12.8%, non-Hispanic Black people account for 13.2%, Asian-Americans account for 9.0%, and non-Hispanic White account for 7.6% of type 2 diabetes.[5] Type 2 diabetes is associated with failure of the beta cells to meet an increased demand for insulin due to peripheral insulin resistance. Peripheral cells are unable to respond to circulating insulin and blood glucose levels remain elevated. The signs and symptoms may take several years to be expressed. Clinical features of an acute exacerbation are similar to type 1 diabetes. Patients with type 2 diabetes are less likely to develop DKA due to the continued production of insulin; however, the type 2 diabetes patient can develop a similar complication called **hyperosmolar hyperglycemic state** (HHS). Patients with HHS present similarly to patients with DKA, exhibiting dehydration, hypotension, tachycardia, and altered mental status.[7]

Prediabetes is defined as a condition in which blood glucose or hemoglobin A1C levels are elevated but not high enough to be classified as diabetes. It is estimated that 86 million, or 1 in 3, Americans have prediabetes, and upwards of 90% of these individuals do not know they have it. People with prediabetes have an increased risk of developing type 2 diabetes, heart disease, and stroke.[5] The Diabetes Prevention Program, a large prevention study of people at high risk for diabetes, showed that lifestyle intervention that resulted in weight loss and increased physical activity in this population can prevent or delay type 2 diabetes and in some cases return blood glucose levels to within the normal range.[5,8]

Complications of Diabetes Mellitus

Exogenous insulin has greatly improved long-term survival and reduced complications of diabetes. The common complications of diabetes include neuropathy, cardiovascular disease (CVD), nephropathy, retinopathy, impaired wound healing, and increased infection risk. These complications are generally related to the severity and duration of the hyperglycemia.

Diabetic neuropathy is classified as **peripheral neuropathy** or **diabetic autonomic neuropathy** (DAN). **Peripheral neuropathy** is characterized by pain and impaired sensation with eventual progression to motor dysfunction in the extremities. Peripheral neuropathy impairs protective sensation and increases the risk of ignoring trauma to the distal extremities, leading to wounds, and may play a role in the development of joint deformities, such as Charcot foot (Figure 10-3). Charcot foot is described as a "rocker-bottom" foot where the midfoot collapses.[9] DAN may cause difficulty with swallowing, delayed gastric emptying, constipation, and diarrhea. DAN is associated with orthostatic hypotension, syncope, cardiac arrest, and sudden death.[4,10]

Heart disease is the leading cause of death in persons with diabetes and the mortality rate for adults with diabetes is 1.7 times higher than adults without diabetes.[5] Arteriosclerosis of the large- and medium-sized arteries of the heart and peripheral circulation occurs earlier and more extensively, leading to coronary artery disease (CAD) and peripheral vascular disease. DAN in the setting of CAD can lead to the development of silent myocardial infarctions and silent orthostatic hypotension. The person will experience little to no physical warning signs, such as chest pain or dizziness, until cardiac failure or near loss of consciousness.

HTN and stroke is also more prevalent, possibly due to atherosclerotic changes in the large and small vessels. About 71% of adults with diabetes have BP greater than or equal to 140/90 mm Hg or use prescription medications for HTN. Risk for stroke is 1.5 times higher in individuals with diabetes.[5]

Diabetes is the most common cause of end-stage renal disease and is the leading reason for kidney transplantation.[5] **Nephropathy** is associated with glomerular destruction (glomerulosclerosis) and protein in the urine (proteinuria). Progression of renal destruction leads to uremia, nausea, lethargy, acidosis, anemia, and worsening HTN. Diabetes is also a leading cause of blindness in adults over the age of 40. It is estimated that 28.5% of people with diabetes have diabetic retinopathy.[5] **Retinopathy** is related to vascular abnormalities leading to neovascularization, microaneurysms, hemorrhage, and ischemia that may result in vision loss. Additional visual changes include visual blurring, glaucoma, cataracts, and macular degeneration.

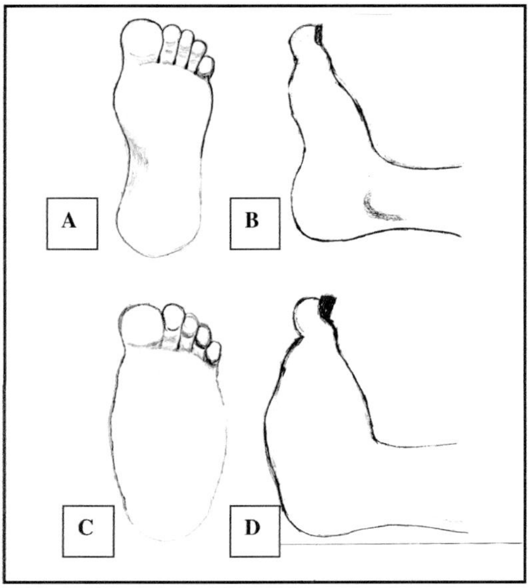

Figure 10-3. (A, B) Plantar and lateral views of a normal foot. (C, D) Plantar and lateral views of a Charcot foot.

Wound Healing and Infection Risk

Vascular changes include atherosclerosis in the larger vessels but also include the microcirculation. Abnormalities of the microcirculation include basement membrane thickening, amyloid deposition (hyalin arteriosclerosis), increased platelet aggregation and clotting, and impaired fibrinolysis. These abnormalities lead to impaired blood flow, impaired oxygen diffusion, and delayed wound healing. These microvascular abnormalities also contribute to the renal and visual changes associated with diabetes.

Poorly controlled blood glucose levels increase the risk of infection. Hyperglycemia leads to immune cell dysfunction, such as a blunted immune response to an infection with impaired leukocyte phagocytosis and chemotaxis. Hyperglycemia is also an optimum environment for proliferation of bacteria. The immune dysfunction, combined with the vascular and sensory changes, increases the incidence of wounds and amputation. In 2010, 73,000 non-traumatic lower-limb amputations, or approximately 60% of all non-traumatic limb amputations, were performed in the diabetes population.[5]

Medical Management

Medical management of diabetes involves pharmacologic, dietary, and exercise therapies. Injectable insulin is indicated for type 1 diabetes and some patients with type 2 diabetes. Insulin is prescribed in multiple forms with each type possessing varying duration and peaks of action (see Appendix at the end of this chapter). Different types of insulin can be combined to provide full-day coverage. Insulin pumps, an implantable delivery system, provide a continuous infusion of insulin for prolonged coverage and avoids repeated injections. Diet and exercise are standard initial medical management for type 2 diabetes. Diabetic diets generally consist of a balanced plan with reduced carbohydrates to meet daily caloric needs. If blood glucose levels continue to remain high, oral medications can be prescribed. Oral medications stimulate the pancreas to release insulin or enhance insulin sensitivity and include glipizide, glyburide, tolbutamide, and chlorpropamide. Glucophage (metformin) helps increase the body's response to its own insulin.[3] The oral medications can be given alone or when greater glucose control is needed combined with injectable insulin.

Physical Therapist Management and Diabetes Mellitus

The physical therapist/physical therapist assistant must remember that CVD is the leading cause of mortality in the diabetic population. Patients may present with atypical symptoms (eg, silent myocardial infarction) secondary to DAN and the therapist should be aware of angina equivalents, including nausea, vomiting, dizziness, and shortness of breath (SOB). These symptoms may represent ongoing ischemia. Patients with diabetes have an increased incidence of dysrhythmias after a myocardial infarction. Therapists should monitor the hemodynamic status frequently and should include measures of perceived exertion, as this may relate to angina equivalents (see Table 1-2). Additionally, **postural/orthostatic hypotension** may be encountered in diabetic patients. The therapist needs to assess orthostatic vital signs and to instruct the patient in adequate warm-up and cooling down exercises.

Peripheral neuropathic pain usually comes and goes and can last for months or even years. Sensation loss occurs more often in the feet than hands. Individuals may not lose complete sensation, and deep pressure tends to be preserved the longest. **Protective sensation** alerts the individual to problems such as tight-fitting shoes, pebbles in shoes, or hot water temperature, and is generally absent first. The fact that not all elements of sensation are lost confuses many patients to believe that they have no problems. Injury can be sustained with little forewarning because of a lack of protective sensation. Peripheral neuropathies in diabetes are believed to be the largest contributor to excessive callous, foot wounds, impaired wound healing, and lower extremity (LE) amputation.[5] Assessment should include sensation testing by monofilament followed by foot inspections for areas of callous and skin breakdown. Protective sensation can be assessed using a 5.07 monofilament that applies 10 grams of pressure when used correctly. Shoes should be assessed for proper fit and the patient educated in proper foot care with daily inspections, proper shoe fit, and utilization of shoes anytime the feet are on or near the ground. If the individual is wheelchair bound, shoes are imperative to provide protection to the feet while trying to maneuver in tight spaces.

Muscle weakness occurs in peripheral neuropathy and is usually preceded by loss of sensation. This weakness can be assessed in mobility and gait activities and may be the cause for clumsiness or observed foot drop or foot slap.

Visual acuity needs to be closely assessed because proper foot inspections can reduce the incidence of wounds and LE amputations. Can the patient see small areas of trauma, like blisters or subtle shades of erythema as seen in the initial phases of wounding? If not, alternative solutions will need to be explored to provide adequate care. For example, teaching a spouse or friend with adequate vision to inspect the feet. Assistive devices for gait might be helpful in increasing safety with ambulation by helping identify barriers before falling over them or providing extra support for surprise changes in terrain. Patients with **retinopathy** are instructed to avoid isometric exercise, valsalva maneuvers, and head down/Trendelenburg positioning as excessive BP may increase the risk of hemorrhage of fragile blood vessels.[11] Activities that increase systolic BP >180 mm Hg are typically avoided.[12]

Peripheral vascular disease, especially small vessel diseases, is one speculative cause for peripheral nerve damage. Atherosclerotic changes in the small vessels may limit the information obtained from blood flow studies unless toe cuff pressures are also obtained to assess if adequate distal blood flow exists. **Ankle Brachial Index** (ABI) is often performed to assess peripheral circulation. The systolic pressure of the brachium is divided into the systolic pressure of the ankle obtained by using a Doppler ultrasound and BP cuff. ABIs of 1.0 or greater are considered normal, while lower values indicate blood flow obstruction.

Wound infections are common in patients with diabetes. The macrophage is one of the key cells in wound debridement and repair (see Chapter 15) and leukocyte dysfunction occurs in diabetes. The physical therapist must be vigilant and educate the patient on wound and infection prevention.

Charcot foot (Charcot arthropathy/rocker bottom foot; see Figure 10-3) develops as blood is shunted away from bones of the foot causing the bone to soften and, due to repeated trauma, the bones will fracture and crumble. The tarsal bones of the foot and the calcaneus collapse leading to severely misshapen feet at higher risk for further skin breakdown. The only clinical signs of Charcot foot may be diffuse foot pain, mild edema, possibly erythema, and, eventually, foot deformity.

Poor wound healing results from small vessel disease, elevated blood glucose, and peripheral neuropathies. Wound contraction is vital to wound closure, and loss of protective sensation eliminates normal protection of the wounded area. The individual will continue to bear weight regardless of the wound. Wounded areas need to be removed from weightbearing or off loaded. Total contact casting is the optimal choice to alleviate pressure in the wound area and promote weightbearing at intact areas. Total contact casting combined with assist devices can further encourage decreased weightbearing and increase ambulation safety and stability. Other offloading options exist in the form of total contact cast boots, modified cast walking boots, and, as a temporary option, modified shoes. Educating the individual in nonweightbearing or hopping should be closely assessed. Diabetes is a systemic disease, and problems encountered in one limb can easily occur in the other. Improper care of LE wounds can easily lead to LE amputation. Sixty percent of non-traumatic lower-limb amputations in the United States occur among people with diabetes according to the Centers for Disease Control and Prevention National Diabetes Fact Sheet.[5]

Hypoglycemia, blood glucose levels less than 70 mg/dL, is a condition that can occur in both types 1 and 2 diabetes. Hypoglycemia can occur when a meal is late or missed, especially if timed insulin or oral medications have been taken or with health conditions impacting the GI tract. The therapist must also consider the insulin-like effect of exercise. Hypoglycemia activates the sympathetic nervous system and adrenal medulla and common symptoms include sweating, nervousness, quivering, faintness, palpitations, and sometimes hunger. Severe hypoglycemia causes dizziness, confusion, fatigue, weakness, headaches, abnormal behavior mistaken for inebriation, inability to concentrate, vision abnormalities, seizures, and coma. Prolonged hypoglycemia can lead to permanent brain damage.[3] People with diabetes are recommended to keep high carbohydrate snacks (eg, hard candies), glucose tablets, or glucagon, available to counteract episodes of hypoglycemia. Fifteen grams of carbohydrate can remedy symptoms for approximately 15 minutes until an appropriate meal can be ingested.

Diagnostic testing includes blood tests. Two methods are recommended to make a diagnosis of diabetes[4]:

1. After overnight fasting, venous plasma glucose levels ≥7.8 mmol/L or 140 mg/dL on 2 separate occasions
2. After ingestion of 75 grams of glucose, venous plasma glucose is ≥11.1 mmol/L or 200 mg/dL at 2 hours and on at least 1 other occasion with the same test

Normal blood glucose range is 70 to 110 mg/dL with an increased risk for complications at >126 mg/dL. Individuals with diabetes are also recommended to have quarterly blood testing of their HbA1c. This gives an average range of the individual's blood glucose over approximately a 3-month period. Normal range HbA1c is considered 4% to 6.7%, which corresponds to 70 to 110 mg/dL (see Table 2-18). Therapists should remember that **prediabetes** is present when blood glucose is abnormally high but does not reach the threshold for diagnosis of diabetes. These patients are at an increased risk of developing diabetes, heart disease, and stroke within the next 5 to 10 years but intensive lifestyle managements, including diet and exercise, can reduce the risk of developing diabetes by 50%.[8,12] The acute care environment is an appropriate place and time to begin and reinforce patient education regarding healthy lifestyle choices.

SUMMARY

The endocrine system is a very complex network of glands that utilizes hormones, the CNS, and the immune system to perform and alter its functions. These small glands can secrete hormones that can impact most every tissue in the body. Endocrine diseases and disorders are commonly caused by the immune system, and damage can be permanent. Although many of these processes are treated pharmacologically, rehabilitation may be oriented to managing the enduring functional limitations and disabilities.

CASE STUDY

Mr. Casey is a 56-year-old male admitted to the hospital because of SOB with minor exertion and a non-healing ulcer of his first metatarsal head. He has type 2 diabetes and uses oral medication. He is diagnosed with a non–ST segment elevated myocardial infarction (NSTEMI) and undergoes coronary artery bypass graft (CABG) surgery.

PATIENT/CLIENT HISTORY

General Demographics, Social History, and Living Environment

He lives with his wife and 3 children in a 2-story home with 12 steps to enter from the outside and a bathroom on each level. He is employed as a manager of a grocery store.

General Health Status, Social/Health Habits, and Family History

Mr. Casey's father and brother died at age 46 and 52, respectively, from heart disease (presumed myocardial infarction). He states he walks around the store all day at work, but does not participate in a formal exercise program

Medical/Surgical History

The patient has been diagnosed with type 2 diabetes for 10 years. He also has a history of HTN, obesity, elevated cholesterol, and hypothyroidism and quit smoking last week prior to admission to the hospital. He has a 60-pack/year history. Blood glucose levels on admission reveal hyperglycemia as noted. Blood flow studies revealed decreased flow just below the popliteal fossa with an ABI of 0.6. A resting electrocardiogram (ECG) in the emergency room revealed a NSTEMI. A cardiac catheterization was performed revealing >75% blockages of 3 coronary arteries. CABG surgery was performed and the patient returned to the floor after a 3-day stay in the intensive care unit (ICU). Bypass grafting of the LE is postponed until full recovery is achieved from the CABG. Physical therapy is consulted to evaluate and treat.

Current Conditions

Mr. Casey is seen at bedside complaining of pain in his right foot and in the middle of his chest. He states that he is ready to begin physical therapy.

Activities and Participation

Prior to admission, Mr. Casey was using a cane and rocker shoe to ambulate. He was staying on the first floor of his house because the climb to the second-floor master bedroom made him "winded."

Other Clinical Tests

Laboratory results revealed a normal electrolyte panel and complete blood cell count. Abnormalities included blood glucose of 240 mg/dL, HbA1c was 9.6, and ABI of 0.6. Arterial blood gases in the ICU prior to extubation were pH 7.34/PCO_2 38/PO_2 94/HCO_3^- 20.

Systems Review

Cardiovascular and Pulmonary

Resting vital signs (VS) sitting at the edge of the bed were HR 88 bpm, pulse regular, BP 106/86 mm Hg, RR 18 breaths/minute and pulse oximetry (SpO2) 96% on 2 liters nasal cannula oxygen.

Integumentary

Mr. Casey has a surgical dressing in the middle of his thorax and left upper extremity (LUE) peripheral intravenous (IV) line. He has a dressing around his right foot and one on the inside of his left lower extremity (LLE) with some red-brownish drainage on the edges. He has mild edema of the LLE > right lower extremity (RLE).

Musculoskeletal

Mr. Casey's range of motion (ROM) is normal but he did complain of feeling weak. He could easily move bilateral upper extremity (BUEs)/bilateral lower extremity (BLEs) against gravity.

Neuromuscular

Mr. Casey presented with a non-healing and non-painful ulcer, implying altered sensation. His dynamic balance was normal in sitting but decreased in standing. He required the rolling walker to stand. Proprioception was also decreased in distal BLE. He needs minimal assistance of the bedrail for bed mobility (Functional Independence Measure (Functional Indepence Measure [FIM] 4) and minimal assistance of 1 for transfer sit to/from standing from an elevated surface without handrails (FIM 4).

Communication, Affect, Cognition, Language, and Learning Style

Mr. Casey uses English as his primary language. Sternal precautions were reviewed with him due to his high risk for falling. He was able to repeat the precautions and the rationale.

Tests and Measures

Aerobic Capacity and Endurance

Mr. Casey demonstrated an expected BP/HR response to position change and ambulation. It should be remembered that he did not have the classic symptoms associated with angina but instead complained of SOB. This may reflect diabetic autonomic neuropathy. This atypical presentation should be considered as the intensity of interventions increases as a precaution.

Assistive and Adaptive Devices

Mr. Casey will need to continue to use a rocker shoe to lessen weightbearing on his non-healing ulcer. He will benefit from a rolling walker instead of a standard walker to decrease the lifting with sternal precautions.

Balance, Gait, and Mobility (Including Locomotion)

Gait and balance are both impacted by his poor endurance, possible peripheral and diabetic autonomic neuropathy, and pain following surgery. Gait required minimal assistance of 1 with rolling walker for 50 feet (FIM 2). He was able to stand independently using a rolling walker (FIM 6). The Activity Measure for Post Acute Care (AM-PAC) basic mobility score was 16/24.

Circulation (Arterial, Venous, Lymphatic) and Ventilation/Respiration

Following examination of ROM, Manual Muscle Test (MMT), bed mobility, transfers, and gait his VS ranges were HR 88-90 bpm, BP 106/86-88/84 mm Hg. The ECG remained with sinus rhythm with infrequent premature ventricular contractions noted. Heart sounds at rest were normal with an audible S1 and S2 only.

Pulse oximetry was stable with the SpO_2 > 94% on 2 L/minute. He did demonstrate tachypnea with a RR increasing 18 to 26 breaths/minute. Auscultation of breath sounds revealed crackles at bilateral bases and are probably related to postoperative atelectasis. His cough was nonproductive and strong while splinting the sternotomy incision.

Mental Function

Mr. Casey was alert, awake and oriented x4 and he followed commands easily.

Muscle Performance

MMT revealed that his strength was grossly 4–/5 in the UEs and 4/5 in the LEs.

Pain

Mr. Casey reported pain of 2/10 on a numerical pain scale at rest. His complaints of pain increased during the examination from 2-4/10 and will benefit from pain medication prior to therapy sessions.

Sensory Integrity

Sensation testing by 5.07 monofilament demonstrated diminished sensation in RLE > LLE consistent with diabetic peripheral neuropathy.

Diagnosis

Mr. Casey presents with vascular and neurological complications from diabetes. His laboratory and diagnostic testing revealed poorly controlled diabetes with large vessel involvement, and also an uncompensated metabolic acidosis possibly representing impaired renal function. Additionally, Mr. Casey has mobility deficits and currently requires minimal assistance for transfers and ambulation of short distances. His presentation suggests a silent myocardial infarction with angina equivalents (ie, SOB).

Prognosis

The physical therapist estimated that Mr. Casey would require daily physical therapy services until discharge at day 4 post ICU transfer. The recommended goals are to be independent with transfers, bed mobility, and gait with rolling walker a minimum of 100 feet x 3 and modified independent ascending/descending a flight of stairs. He also needs to be independent with monitoring his blood glucose and his sternal precautions.

Intervention

Mr. Casey was seen daily with a focus on progressing muscle performance, mobility (including locomotion), and airway clearance. A phase I cardiac rehabilitation program (see Chapter 6) was initiated with interventions that included bed mobility, transfers, gait on level surfaces and stairs, incentive spirometry hourly with splinted coughing, and sitting exercises progressing to standing exercises to increase muscular strength and endurance. Wound care was also delivered to promote healing of RLE. Patient and family education emphasized home glucose monitoring and management in conjunction with the diabetes team and frequent foot inspections.

Outcomes

After 4 days, Mr. Casey continued using a rolling walker for balance and was able to walk 100 feet x 2 (FIM 2), required standby assistance for transfers (FIM 5), bed mobility was independent (FIM 7), but he required minimal assistance with activities of daily living (ADLs), especially lower body dressing and bathing (FIM 4). Mr. Casey was not able to climb up 6 steps without increasing discomfort in his RLE and chest. Also, the vascular consultants recommend limiting stair climbing due to excessive pressure on the RLE as the longstanding diabetes had compromised the vascular bed resulting in a chronic wound. The AM-PAC score increased from 16 to 20/24. He can independently recall his sternal precautions.

Mr. Casey was transferred to an inpatient rehabilitation facility to continue his progress towards independence with his activity limitations, specifically ADLs and stair climbing. He should continue to progress to independence/modified independence in his home and ultimately return to work. He will be scheduled for vascular surgery to restore adequate blood flow to his ischemic RLE at a later date.

ICF Clinical Reasoning Tool Case Study Summary								
Health Condition								
HPI: CAD, s/p CABG x 3; postoperative c/o pain right foot and middle of chest and metabolic acidosis; atelectasis BLLs; elevated BG; HbA1C, PMHx: HTN, type 2 diabetes x 10 years, obese, CAD, PAD								
Precautions/Contraindications								
Poorly controlled diabetes; safety/fall risk due to sensation loss and orthostatic hypotension; pain, RF for CAD (family history, limited exercise besides work, HTN, obesity, recently quit smoking, elevated cholesterol, diabetes), sternal precaution; risk for poor or delayed wound healing (diabetes and poor BG control), at risk for postoperative pneumonia, universal precautions								
Body Structure and Function			*Activity/Task Limitations*			*Participation*		
Impairment/ Problem	*Tests and Measures*	*Intervention*	*Activity*	*Tests and Measures*	*Intervention*	*Participation*	*Tests and Measures*	*Intervention*
• Abnormal breath sounds • Impaired strength • Impaired endurance • Impaired sensation and proprioception • Edema • Pain • Abnormal lab values	• Chest Assessment • ROM/MMT • Grade pitting edema • Sensation/ monofilament testing • Proprioception testing • Review ABI • Wound examination • Lab values • Pain/VAS	• Breathing exercises: huffing, splinted coughing, incentive spirometry • Bedside ROM • Progressive resistance exercises • Wound care • Education: sternal precautions, donning/doffing rocker shoe • Consult registered dietician	• ADLs • Bed mobility • Transfers • Gait • Balance	• Functional task analysis • AM-PAC "6 Clicks" • 2- or 6MWT • TUG	• Progressive functional retraining following Phase 1 Cardiac Rehab guidelines • Pain control strategies	• Unable to return work	• MMSE • ADDQoL • DHP-1	• Continue physical therapy services • Consult social worker • Family meeting to discuss discharge plans

(continued)

ICF Clinical Reasoning Tool Case Study Summary (continued)		
Personal Factors	*Other Considerations*	*Environmental Factors*
• Age: 56 y/o male • Primary language: English • Lives with wife and 3 children • Sleeping on 1st floor of house because of symptoms • Employed as manager of grocery store • 60 pk/yr history; quit smoking x 1 week		Home: • 2 story house, 12 steps to enter, bathroom each level • Uses cane and rocker shoe for ambulation Hospital: • 2 L NP, bandage (R foot, R forearm, inside LLE), rolling walker

ABI = Ankle Brachial Index; ADDQoL = Audit of Diabetes-Dependent Quality of Life; BG = blood glucose; BLLs = bilateral lower lobes; c/o = complain of; DHP-1 = Diabetes Health Profile; Hb = hemoglobin; HPI = history of present illness; MMSE = Mini-Mental State Examination; MMT = Manual Muscle Test; MWT = Minute Walk Test; NP = nasal prongs; PAD = peripheral arterial disease; pk/yr = pack per year; PMHx = past medical history; R = right; RF = risk factors; RPE = rate of perceived exertion; s/p = status post; VAS = visual analog scale; y/o year old.

Adapted from American Physical Therapy Association. *Guide to Physical Therapist Practice*. 3rd ed. http://www.apta.org/Guide/. Updated October 21, 2015. Accessed October 5, 2018 and *Towards a Common Language for Functioning, Disability and Health*. World Health Organization. www.who.int/classifications/icf/icfbeginnersguide.pdf. Published 2002. Accessed April 29, 2019.

Chapter Review Questions

1. Which of the following best represents type 1 diabetes?
   a. Earlier age of onset, requires exogenous insulin, prone to ketoacidosis
   b. Medication induced, autorecessive genetic defect, nutritional deficiency
   c. Later age of onset, coinciding metabolic syndrome, family history
   d. Viral exposure, environmental trigger, dependent on diet and exercise to manage
2. What is the most common endocrine disorder?
   a. Corticosteroids
   b. Pancreatitis
   c. Hypopituitarism
   d. Diabetes mellitus
3. The examination tool used to evaluate peripheral arterial circulation is:
   a. Doppler ultrasound
   b. Two-point discrimination
   c. ABI
   d. Pitting edema scale
4. The clinical features of an acute diabetic exacerbation include:
   a. Polyphagia, polyuria, and polydipsia
   b. Fatigue, weight gain, and ketones in the urine
   c. Increased appetite, dehydration, and metabolic alkalosis
   d. Irritability, confusion, and metabolic alkalosis
5. The following should be primary safety considerations while treating patients with diabetes:
   a. CVD is the leading cause of mortality and a physical therapist should recognize anginal equivalents
   b. Peripheral neuropathic pain can be a sign of poor blood glucose management
   c. Muscle weakness occurs with autonomic neuropathy and can lead to balance impairments
   d. Visual acuity decline can be an indication of poor renal and vascular function

Answers: 1a, 2d, 3c, 4a, 5a

References

1. Haas LB. Endocrine system. In: Lewis SM, Collier IC, eds. *Medical-Surgical Nursing, Assessment and Management of Clinical Problems*. 9th ed. St. Louis, MO: Elsevier Mosby; 2014.
2. Gardner DG, Shoback D. *Greenspan's Basic & Clinical Endocrinology*. 9th ed. New York, NY: McGraw-Hill; 2011.
3. Berkow R, Beers MH, eds. Hormonal disorders. In: *The Merck Manual of Medical Information, Second Home Edition*. New York, NY: Pocket Books; 2004.
4. Jameson JL. Endocrinology and metabolism. In: Longo DL, Fauci AS, Kasper DL, et al., eds. *Harrison's Principles of Internal Medicine*. 18th ed. New York, NY: McGraw-Hill; 2012.
5. Centers for Disease Control and Prevention. *National diabetes statistics report: estimates of diabetes and its burden in the United States, 2014*. Atlanta, GA: US Department of Health and Human Services; 2014.
6. Mumtaz M. Gestational diabetes mellitus. *Malays J Med Sci*. 2000;7(1):4-9.
7. Kitabchi AE, Umpierrez GE, Murphy MB, et al. Hyperglycemic crises in diabetes. *Diabetes Care*. 2004;27(suppl 1):S94-S102.
8. Knowler WC, Barrett-Connor E, Fowler SE, et al; Diabetes Prevention Program Research Group. Reduction in the incidence of type 2 diabetes with lifestyle intervention or metformin. *N Engl J Med*. 2002;346:393-403.
9. Rogers LC, Frykberg RG, Armstron DG ,et al. The Charcot foot in diabetes. *Diabetes Care*. 2011;34(9):2123-2129.
10. Vinik AI, Maser RE, Mitchell BD, Freeman R. Diabetic autonomic neuropathy. *Diabetes Care*. 2003;26(5):1553-1579.
11. Colberg SR, Sigal RJ, Fernhall B, et al; American Diabetes Association. Exercise and type 2 diabetes: the American College of Sports Medicine and the American Diabetes Association: joint position statement. *Diabetes Care*. 2010;33(12):e147-e167. doi: 10.2337/dc10-9990
12. Nichols GA, Hillier TA, Brown JB. Progression from newly acquired impaired fasting glusose to type 2 diabetes. *Diabetes Care*. 2007;30(2):228-233

Bibliography

Barrat Solomon BL, Choate Loriaux T, Drass JA. Endocrine and metabolic systems. In: McFarland GK, Hirsch JE, Tucker SM, Thompson JM, eds. *Clinical Nursing*. St. Louis, MO: Mosby; 1986.

Craig CR, Stitzel RE. *Modern Pharmacology with Clinical Applications*. New York, NY: Little, Brown, and Co; 1997.

Deglin JH, Vallerand AH. *Davis's Drug Guide for Nurses*. 8th ed. Philadelphia, PA: FA Davis; 2003.

Greenspan FS, Gardner DG. *Basic & Clinical Endocrinology*. 6th ed. New York, NY: Lange Medical Books/McGraw-Hill; 2001.

Karch AM. *Lippincott's Nursing Drug Guide*. Springhouse, PA: Lippincott Williams & Wilkins; 2004.

Ritter JM, Lewis LD, Mant TG. *Textbook of Clinical Pharmacology*. London, United Kingdom: Edward Arnold Co; 1995

West JB. The hypothalamic-pituitary control system. In: Brobeck JR, Taylor NB, Best CH, eds. *Best and Taylor's Physiological Basis of Medical Practice*. 12th ed. Baltimore, MD: Lippincott Williams & Wilkins; 1991.

Appendix

Pharmacological Information: Endocrine Diseases and Disorders Pharmacology

Antidiabetics: Oral Hypoglycemics

Sulfonylureas and Meglitinides

Action

Sulfonylureas and meglitinides stimulate release of insulin from functioning beta cells in the islets of Langerhans. These agents increase the influx of calcium leading to enhanced insulin secretion.

Side Effects

CNS: Confusion, dizziness, flushing, headache
CV: Palpitations, tachycardia
GI: Nausea, vomiting, constipation, dry mouth
Miscellaenous: Hypoglycemia, allergic reactions

Common Medications

Suflonylureas: Amaryl (glymepride), Glucotrol (glipizide), glyburide
Meglitinides: Starlix (nateglinidine), Prandin (repaglinide)
Combination of meglitinide/biguanide: Prandin (repaglinide), Glucophage (metformin)

Alpha-Glucosidase Inhibitors

Action

Alpha-glucosidase inhibitors reduce the GI absorption of mono-saccharides and glucose by inhibition of the intestinal enzyme alphaglucosidase (alpha glucoside hydrolases).

Side Effects

GI: Abdominal pain, diarrhea, flatulence
Miscellaneous: Hypoglycemia

Common Medications

Precose (acarbose), Glyset (miglitol)

Biguanides

Action

Biguanides decrease glucose production in the liver, decrease glucose absorption from the GI tract, and improve peripheral insulin sensitivity.

Side Effects

GI: Abdominal discomfort, diarrhea, nausea, vomiting
Miscellaneous: Hypoglycemia, metallic taste, lactic acidosis

Common Medications

Glucophage (metformin)

Table 10-18

INSULIN PREPARATIONS AND ACTIVITY CHARACTERISTICS

Type	*Onset (Hr)*	*Peak (Hr)*	*Duration (Hr)*
Rapid acting (regular)	0.5 to 1	2 to 4	6 to 8
Intermediate acting (Lente; NPH)	1 to 3	6 to 12	18 to 26
Long acting (Ultralente; human)	4 to 8	12 to 18	24 to 28

Insulin Therapy (Table 10-18)

Insulin Preparations

Action

Insulin increases the cellular uptake of serum glucose, promotes the conversion of glucose to glycogen and amino acids to proteins, while inhibiting the release of fatty acids. Formulations of insulin are available in ratios of short and longer lasting preparations (eg, humulin 70/30). Insulin may be conjugated with protamine and zinc to prolong its duration of action. Insulin can be extracted from ox or pig or be created by recombinant technology (rDNA).

Side Effects

Miscellaneous: Hypoglycemia, rebound hyperglycemia (Somogyi effect), allergic reactions, lipidystrophy (disappearance of subcutaneous fat at injection sites), redness/swelling at injection site

Common Medications

Insulin rDNA: Humalog (insulin lispro), Novolog (insulin aspart)
NPH (isophane)/regular insulin: Humulin, Novolin
Insulin zinc suspension: Lente insulin, Humulin L, Novolin L
Insulin zinc suspension, extended: Ultralente, Humulin U, Novolin U

Thiazolidinediones

Action

Thiazolidinediones (glitazones) increase insulin sensitivity by promoting greater uptake of blood glucose by muscle, fat, and hepatic cells and decreasing hepatic glucose production.

Side Effects

CV: Edema
Miscellaenous: Hypoglycemia, weight gain, hypercholesterolemia, anemia

Common Medications

Actos (pioglitazone), Avandia (rosiglitazone)

Sodium-Glucose Transport Protein 2 Inhibitors

Action

Sodium-glucose transport protein 2 (SGLT2) inhibitors decrease reabsorption of glucose in the proximal tubule of the kidney leading to increase glucose excretion in the urine.

Side Effects

CV: Hypotension
Miscellaneous: Hypoglycemia, ketoacidosis, urinary tract infection, polyuria, increase low-density lipoprotein (LDL) cholesterol, kidney dysfunction

Common Medications

Invokana (canagliflozin)

Thyroid Hormones

Thyroid Preparations

Action

Thyroid preparations are medications that resemble the hormones T_4 and T_3. These medications are prescribed for patients with hypothyroidism.

Side Effects

CNS: Insomnia, irritability, headache
CV: Tachycardia, dysrhythmias, HTN
GI: Abdominal discomfort, diarrhea, vomiting
Miscellaneous: Weight loss, heat intolerance

Common Medications

Levothroid (levothyroxine sodium), Synthroid (levothyroxine sodium), Levoxine (levothyroxine sodium)

Thyroid Hormone Inhibitors

Action

Thyroid hormone inhibitors are indicated for the treatment of hyperthyroidism/thyrotoxicosis (eg, Graves' disease, toxic adenoma, thyroiditis). Medications may inhibit thyroid hormone production and secretion (eg, thiourea, iodides), reduce the amount of functional thyroid tissue by ablation (eg, radioiodine), or control symptoms of hyperthyroidism (eg, beta blockers).

Side Effects

CV: Dysrhythmias
GI: Diarrhea
Miscellaneous: Skin rash, arthralgia, myalgia, drug fever, hypothyroidism, goiter, hyperkalemia

Common Medications

Thioureas: Propylthiouracil, Tapazole (methimazole)
Iodides: Pima, Lodopen (amlodipine)
Radioiodine: Iodine 131 [131I]

Parathyroid

Parathyroid Hormone

Action

PTH is primarily regulated by plasma calcium concentration (↓ Ca^{++}/↑ PTH). PTH influences bone health through its stimulatory effect on osteoclasts and bone resorption, renal reabsorption of Ca++, and enhanced intestinal Ca^{++} absorption.

Side Effects

CV: Edema
GI: Nausea
Miscellaneous: Tenderness at injection site, allergic reactions

Common Medications

Paroidin (repaglinide)

Calcitonin

Action

Calcitonin secretion is regulated by plasma calcium concentration (↑ Ca++/↑ calctonin). These medications are primarily indicated for the treatment of hypercalcemia, osteoporosis/osteopenia, and Paget's disease.

Side Effects

CNS: Headache
CV: Edema
GI: Nausea, vomiting
Miscellaneous: Tenderness at injection site, allergic reactions

Common Medications

Calcimar, Cibacalcin

Biphosphonates

Action

Biphosphonates are indicated for the treatment and prevention of osteoporosis and to reduce bone pain and risk of fracture in patients with bone metastases and Paget's disease. These medications reduce the resorption of bone by inhibiting the activity and recruitment of osteoclasts. Additionally, biphosphonates stimulate the production of osteoblasts.

Side Effects

CNS: Headache
CV: Dysrhythmia (atrial fibrillation), HTN
GI: Abdominal discomfort, constipation, dyspepsia, esophageal irritation
Miscellaneous: Hypocalemia, muscle weakness, musculoskeletal pain (osteonecrosis of the jaw), fatigue

Common Medications

Fosamax (alendronate), Didronel (etidronate), Aredia (pamidronate)

Adrenocortical Hormones

The adrenal cortex is divided into 3 functional zones producing several hormones: zona glomerulosa (mineralcorticoid: adlosterone, fludrocortisone), zona fasciculata (corticosteroids: cortisol [hydrocortisone]), and zona reticularis (androgens). Corticosteroids are indicated in the treatment of adrenal insufficiency, inflammatory processes, leukemia, and for immunosuppression (see Pharmacological Information in Chapters 7 and 14).

Hypothalamus and Pituitary Hormones

Growth Hormone/Somatotroponin; Somatostatin

Action

GH, or somatotroponin, is inhibited or released from the anterior pituitary secondary to hypothalamic production of GH releasing hormone and GH release inhibiting hormone (somatostatin). GH stimulates lipolysis and release of free fatty acids, increases blood glucose levels, and promotes protein synthesis. A deficiency of GH leads to dwarfism, while excessive secretion results in gigantism and acromegaly.

GH/Somatotroponin

Side Effects

CV: Edema
Miscellaneous: Hyperglycemia, insulin resistance, hypothyroidism

Common Medications

Genotropin, Humatrope, Norditropin, Nutropin, Protropin

Somatostatin

Side Effects

CNS: Dizziness, drowsiness, fatigue
CV: Edema, orthostatic hypotension, palpitations
GI: Anorexia, nausea, vomiting, abdominal pain, gallstones
Miscellaneous: Reduced insulin secretion, impaired glucose tolerance

Common Medications

Sandostatin (octreotide)

Antidiuretic Hormone/Vasopressin

Action

ADH, also called vasopressin, is released from the posterior pituitary in response to increases in plasma osmolarity or a decrease in BP. ADH acts on the kidneys to increase water retention, which increases blood volume and reduces plasma osmolarity. ADH also stimulates vasoconstriction leading to increased BP.

Side Effects

CNS: Dizziness, headache
CV: Myocardial infarction, angina
GI: Abdominal cramps, nausea, vomiting, heartburn
Miscellaneous: Fever, allergic reactions

Common Medications

Pitressin (vasopressin)

Reproductive Hormones

Estrogens and Progestin

Action

Common estrogens and progestins include estradiol, estrone, estriol, and progesterone. These steroid hormones are produced in the ovaries of nonpregnant, premenopausal women. During pregnancy, the fetal-placental unit produces these hormones. The testes in men produce small amounts of progesterone. These hormones are under the influence of hypothalamic secretion of GnRH that stimulates the anterior pituitary to release leutinizing hormone and follicle-stimulating hormone. Estrogens and progestins are primarily prescribed for oral contraception, as replacement hormones for menopause, hypogonadal disorders, osteoporosis, and, less commonly, as neoplastic agents.

Side Effects

CNS: Headaches, lethargy
CV: Thromboembolic disease, congestive heart failure, edema, HTN
GI: Nausea, vomiting, increased appetite
GU: Endometrial cancer
Miscellaneous: Weight gain, gynecomastia (men)

Common Medications

Estropipate (Ogen, Estrone sulfate), ethinyl estradiol/desogestrel/ drospirenone/ ethynodiol/levonorgestrel/norgestrel/norethindrone (Allesse, CyclessaDesogen, Levlen, Mircette, Nelova, Nortrel, Ovrette, Ortho-cept, Ortho Evra, Ovral, Norplant, Preven), Progesterone (Crinone, Prometrium)

Testosterone and Androgens

Action

Testosterone, produced by the testes, is the principal circulating androgen in men. Additional androgens include androstenedione, produced by the adrenal cortex and testes, and dehydroepiandrosterone, produced by the adrenal glands. Testicular androgen synthesis is primarily influenced by hypothalamic production of GnRH and anterior pituitary release of leutinizing hormone. Testosterone and androgens are prescribed for hypogonadism, delayed puberty, and androgen-responsive breast cancer.

Side Effects

CV: Edema
GI: Nausea, vomiting
Miscellaneous: Deepening of voice, decreased breast size (women), gynecomastia (men), acne, facial hair

Common Medications

Testosterone: Andro, Andronate, Testamone, Depotest, Testex

Antiandrogens

Action

Antiandrogens inhibit the production of testosterone (finasteride) or the uptake of testosterone (flutamide). Antiandrogens are often prescribed for prostate cancer, benign prostatic hypertrophy, and hair loss.

Side Effects

CNS: Fatigue, lethargy, depression
GI: Nausea, vomiting, abdominal discomfort
Miscellaneous: Leukopenia, thrombocyopenia, gynecomastia, impotence, reduced libido

Common Medications

Cyproterone; Propecia, Proscar (finasteride); Eulexin (flutamide)

CV = cardiovascular; GU = genitourinary.

Chapter 11

Gastrointestinal Diseases and Disorders

Daniel J. Malone, PT, PhD, CCS

The Gastrointestinal System

The gastrointestinal (GI) system is a complex set of organs and glands that provide the many nutrients, electrolytes, vitamins, minerals, and fluids necessary for cellular, organ, and whole body function (Figure 11-1). The normal GI tract provides the optimal environment for nutrient absorption through the coordination of motor, neural, and secretory functions.[1] The GI system is more than simple absorption of nutrient and has both exocrine and endocrine functions. Exocrine function aids digestion through the secretion of a variety of substances from the salivary glands (eg, amylase), stomach (eg, hydrochloric acid, pepsin), pancreas (eg, trypsin, amylase, lipase), liver, and gallbladder (eg, bile).[2,3] Endocrine functions of the gut involve the release of over 30 hormones, and these hormones control the release of digestive enzymes from the duodenum, pancreas, and liver. The GI tract is considered the largest endocrine organ in the body.[4,5] Digestion begins in the mouth and continues through the alimentary canal, terminating in the anus.[6] This chapter will introduce the complex processes involving hormonal, mechanical, and neurologic inputs that enable normal digestion and will introduce how dysfunction in select components leads to impaired GI function.

GI dysfunction may be difficult to manage medically and surgically leading to alterations in body structure and function (muscular weakness), activity limitations (limited ambulation post-surgery), and participation limitations (loss of job due to advanced liver disease). GI issues may also be a secondary diagnosis that the acute care practitioner needs to consider as the physical therapist creates the plan of care. The underlying GI process may complicate a patient's ability to perform specific interventions (eg, bed mobility and out of bed [OOB] activities following abdominal surgery) leading to challenging rehabilitation management.

For this chapter, the GI system is separated into the upper GI tract, lower GI tract, and glands/organs (Table 11-1).

Malone DJ, Bishop KL, eds. *Acute Care Physical Therapy: A Clinician's Guide, Second Edition* (pp 459-509).

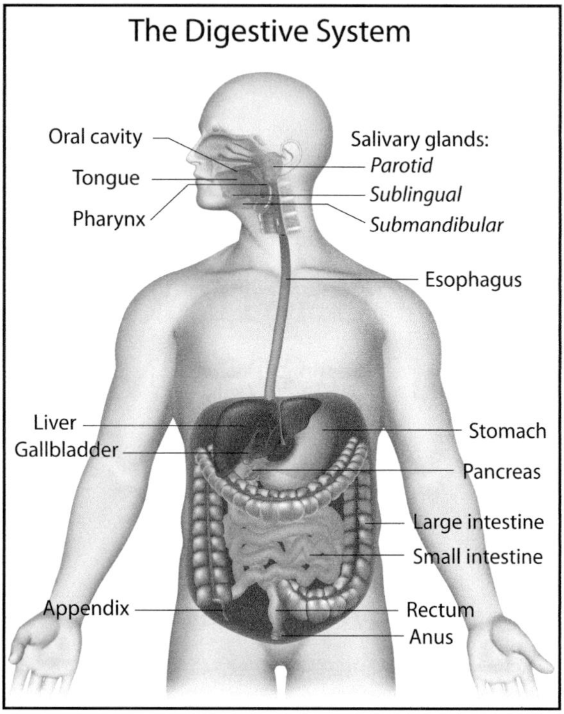

Figure 11-1. Anatomy of the digestive system. (Alila Medical Media/Shutterstock.com)

Table 11-1
GASTROINTESTINAL ANATOMY

Upper Gastrointestinal Tract	*Lower Gastrointestinal Tract*	*Glands/Organs*
• Mouth (including tongue and salivary glands) • Esophagus • Stomach	• Small intestine: ¤ Duodenum ¤ Jejunum ¤ Ileum • Large intestine/colon: ¤ Ascending colon ¤ Transverse colon ¤ Descending colon ¤ Sigmoid ¤ Rectum	• Salivary glands • Pancreas • Liver • Gallbladder • Kidneys • Spleen

THE UPPER GASTROINTESTINAL TRACT

Anatomy and Physiology

The upper GI tract contains all parts of the alimentary canal from the mouth through the esophagus to the pyloric valve of the stomach. The most common set of disorders affecting the upper GI tract are hyperacidity diseases. The extent and

Table 11-2

SIGNS AND SYMPTOMS OF GASTROESOPHAGEAL REFLUX DISEASE

• Heartburn	• Pain (substernal [non-cardiac], mid-thoracic)
• Regurgitation	• Hoarseness, sore throat
• Esophagitis	• Occult anemia
• Dysphagia	• Hematemesis

location of the disease is usually dependent upon the direction, intensity, and duration of acid flow, most commonly involving the stomach and esophagus.[7]

The **esophagus** is a long hollow muscular tube that originates at the distal pharynx and ends at the lower esophageal sphincter (LES) of the stomach, about the level of T1 and runs parallel and posterior to the trachea.[7,8] The esophagus transports material by muscular contraction from the oral cavity to the stomach while preventing material from entering the trachea by contraction of the upper esophageal sphincter (UES), and prevents the reflux of gastric contents back into the esophagus by the contraction of the LES.[3,7]

The **stomach** begins at the LES and terminates at the pyloric valve, which controls the entry of food into the duodenum. Anatomical landmarks include the greater and lesser curvatures, as well as the cardia, fundus, body, pylorus, and pyloric canal. The stomach stores liquids and solid foods prior to passage into the duodenum, continues the digestive process through the secretion of acids and gastric enzymes, and mixes and grinds the ingested meal (trituration). Exocrine functions of the stomach include secretion of hydrochloric acids, pepsin, bicarbonate, and mucous, as well as producing intrinsic factor that is necessary for the absorption of Vitamin B_{12}.[3,4] Endocrine functions of the stomach include the release of the hormone gastrin that initiates the release of various digestive enzymes from the duodenum, pancreas, and liver.

HEALTH CONDITIONS OF THE UPPER GASTROINTESTINAL TRACT

Gastroesophageal Reflux Disease/Reflux Esophagitis

Gastroesophageal reflux disease (GERD) is the reflux of gastric contents (acid, pepsin) or bile from duodenum into the esophagus and is the most common form of esophagitis.[8-10] GERD is the most common inpatient GI-related discharge diagnosis and accounted for approximately 4.5 million hospitalization in 2009.[8,9] GERD often goes untreated or is self-managed by over-the-counter medications. It is related to weakness, inappropriate relaxation, or damage to the muscular ring of the LES. Other causes include disruption of the normal gastric defense mechanisms by non-steroidal anti-inflammatory drugs (NSAIDs), alcohol, infectious agents (eg, *Helicobacter pylori, Salmonella*), smoking, decreased mucous production, as well as excessive amounts of peptic acids at the esophagogastric junction.[8,10-13] Common signs and symptoms of GERD are listed in Table 11-2.

The diagnosis is suggested by patient symptoms, but diagnostic testing may include endoscopy with biopsy, barium swallow, or pH monitoring.[13] Treatment is dependent on the extent of damage and dysfunction. Symptom control is often accomplished with lifestyle modifications as listed in Table 11-3.[4,10,11] Therapists should add these lifestyle modifications into their patient instructions. If lifestyle modifications fail, medications include antacids and anti-ulcer agents (see Appendix B).[9]

Table 11-3

LIFESTYLE MODIFICATIONS TO REDUCE GASTROESOPHAGEAL REFLUX DISEASE

- Elevating the head of the bed
- Reducing weight for obese people
- Avoiding fatty foods that promote reflux
- Avoiding bedtime snacks
- Eliminating alcohol and tobacco use
- Avoiding chocolate
- Using thickened liquids

Barrett's Esophagus and Esophageal Cancer

Barrett's esophagus is the metaplastic transformation of the normal esophageal squamous epithelium to intestine-like columnar epithelium in response to chronic GERD.[4,13] Barrett's esophagus increases the risk of developing esophageal adenocarcinoma.[4] Barrett's esophagus affects nearly 700,000 people yearly in the United States, occurs most frequently over the age of 60, and affects men and women equally. It is associated with regular alcohol consumption and smoking.[13] Diagnosis is confirmed by endoscopy with biopsy.[9] Initial treatment consists of lifestyle modifications and medications similar to those for GERD. If the dysplasia or metaplastic changes are severe, or if adenocarcinoma is present, surgical intervention becomes an option.

Esophageal cancers are most often a squamous cell carcinoma that is associated with alcohol consumption; smoking; diets lacking fresh fruits, vegetables, and animal protein; **achalasia** (impaired esophageal peristalsis with failure of LES to relax during swallowing); and esophageal stricture. Adenocarcinoma arising from Barrett's esophagus is increasing.[7,13] Additional information regarding cancer can be found in Chapter 13.

Surgery of the Esophagus

Thoracoscopy and **mediastinoscopy**, the introduction of an endoscope into the thorax, allow visualization of the thoracic cavity (esophagus, trachea, azygos vein, aorta, pericardium, lungs, and diaphragm) and permits tissue sampling or excision. **Laparoscopy** is useful in evaluation and biopsy of the peritoneal cavity and abdominal organs and may be performed in conjunction with thoracoscopy. Stents may be applied to bridge esophageal obstructions. Endoscopic ablation by thermal, chemical, or mechanical methods have been used for abnormal and cancerous tissue. After tissue removal, regeneration of squamous epithelium allows healing of the surgical site. **Esophagectomy**, either partial or complete excision, involve multiple surgical approaches depending on surgeon preference and anatomic location of the lesion. Common approaches include a left-sided thoracoabdominal incision, posterior lateral thoracotomy, and upper-midline abdominal and cervical incisions. After a portion of the esophagus is removed, a conduit must be established. The stomach, colon, and jejunum have all been used as esophageal substitutes and these structures are mobilized from their usual anatomic location and pulled-through the diaphragm into the thorax. Common complications post–esophageal surgery include incisional pain, respiratory insufficiency, sepsis, and anastomotic leak.[14-16]

Table 11-4

RISK FACTORS FOR THE DEVELOPMENT OF STRESS GASTRITIS

• Mechanical ventilation >48 hours	• Trauma
• Coagulopathy	• Renal failure
• Increased intracranial pressure	• Liver failure
• Sepsis	• Multiple organ system failure

Table 11-5

SIGNS AND SYMPTOMS OF GASTRITIS

• Epigastric pain	• Nausea
• Hematemesis	• Bleeding
• Temperature	• Anorexia

Dyspepsia

Dyspepsia, also known as **indigestion**, is defined as impaired or painful digestion and is usually a symptom of other GI disorders. It is characterized by vague abdominal discomfort, a sense of fullness after eating, heartburn, nausea, vomiting, flatulence, and loss of appetite.[11]

Gastritis

Gastritis is inflammation of the inner layer of the stomach, the mucosa. **Acute gastritis**, also termed **acute erosive gastritis**, **acute stress erosion**, or **acute gastric ulcer**, occurs in the setting of severe trauma, surgery, or medical illness (Table 11-4).[13,17] While similar in presentation to GERD, the symptoms of gastritis tend to be more intense.[5] Gastritis is often caused by direct parasitic infection (eg, *Salmonella*), gastric ischemia (eg, trauma), excessive acid production (eg, alcohol), or impaired mucosal lining of the stomach (eg, aspirin). The most common symptoms are listed in Table 11-5.

Clinically, symptoms and medical history determine diagnosis and, if necessary, endoscopy can determine disease severity. Treatment is similar to that of GERD. Additional measures include prevention of the spread of infections, hydration, and allowing the stomach to rest. Gastric rest is accomplished by placement of a nasogastric (NG) tube to relieve pressure, maintaining the patient NPO (nil per os; nothing by mouth) while providing parenteral nutrition and intravenous (IV) hydration. Medications commonly include antacids, antiulcer agents, antiemetics, and antibiotics.[2,18]

Peptic Ulcer Disease

Peptic ulcers are disruptions of the gastric or duodenal mucosa. They occur in approximately 10% of the population and are responsible for significant morbidity, frequent hospitalization, and significant health care costs.[8,19] Peptic ulcers result from an imbalance between the protective mechanism of the stomach and the hypersecretion of stomach acids and pepsin. Stomach protection is accomplished by mucus barrier, bicarbonate to buffer acids and gastric blood flow. Mucosal breakdown is associated with the presence of the bacteria *H Pylori* and medications such as aspirin and NSAIDs (eg, ibuprofen, naproxen). Additional irritants include excessive alcohol

Table 11-6

Signs and Symptoms of Ulcer Disease

• Burning or gnawing pain • Reduction of pain with eating (reduction lasts 2 to 3 hours) • Burping • Nausea and/or vomiting	• In severe cases: ¤ Bleeding ¤ Perforation ¤ Obstruction ¤ Malignancy

intake, certain foods, and stress.[11,17,19] Common signs and symptoms are listed in Table 11-6.

Diagnosis is usually based off symptoms. Endoscopy with biopsy can determine disease severity and rule out carcinoma. Patients may present with anemia or bloody emesis or stool warranting assessment of the complete blood count (CBC) and fecal blood content.[2,10] A breath test is used to measure carbon dioxide and halitosis produced from *H pylori* metabolism.[13]

Medical treatments of peptic ulcer disease (PUD), like many other esophageal and stomach disorders, involves antiulcer agents to decrease acid production and antibiotics to counter infections in order to promote symptom relief and allow the stomach to heal.

The Lower Gastrointestinal Tract

Anatomy and Physiology

The lower GI tract consists of the intestine from the duodenum to the anus and includes the **small** and **large intestines**. The small intestine consists of 3 segments, the duodenum, jejunum, and ileum, and is approximately 5 meters long. The **large intestine** includes the cecum, ascending colon, transverse colon, descending colon, sigmoid colon, and rectum.

Motility, or movements of foods through the intestinal tract, occurs via segmentation and peristalsis. **Segmentation** is contraction of intestinal circular smooth muscle into parts, or segments, that mix the food bolus (chyme) with intestinal secretions to aide absorption. **Peristalsis** is the coordinated smooth muscular contractions creating the forward flow of chyme through the lower GI tract.[2,3,7]

The intestines are the primary location for digestion and absorption of nutrients with assistance from the liver and pancreas. Additional functions include the movement of intestinal contents (motility), feedback regulation of gastric and hepatobiliary function, and immune defense. Each intestinal division plays specific roles in the absorption and excretory function of the GI tract. The processes of digestion are completed in the small intestine, where the nutrients are absorbed by finger-like projections of the epithelial lining, the villi.[4] The large intestine is a primary site of water absorption and produces and stores solid wastes.

Health Conditions of the Lower Gastrointestinal Tract

Irritable Bowel Syndrome

Irritable bowel syndrome (IBS) is a disorder that interferes with normal digestion, resulting in abdominal discomfort along with changes in bowel habits. It is

Table 11-7

SIGNS AND SYMPTOMS OF IRRITABLE BOWEL SYNDROME

• Alternating loose stools and constipation • Bloating • Abdominal pain • Cramping • Mucous and/or blood in stool	• The criteria to test positive for IBS includes[24]: ¤ Abdominal pain for greater than 12 weeks over the past 12 months ¤ Pain that is relieved by bowel movement ¤ A change in the frequency of bowel movements ¤ A change in the appearance of stool

estimated that 20% of Americans have IBS, with women being affected most often and onset typically during the second decade of life.[12,20,21] While the cause for IBS remains elusive, it is suggested to develop from an interplay between susceptibility genes, impaired gut barrier functions, immunological dysregulation, bacterial and viral infections, and environmental factors, including colonic sensitivity to stress, anxiety, and specific foods (food allergy).[22,23] Although mental health disorders (eg, generalized anxiety disorder, depression) do not cause IBS, they often coexist. IBS presents with a spasmodic motility pattern and decreased absorption resulting in nutritional deficiencies and loose stool. Common signs and symptoms are listed in Table 11-7.

IBS is diagnosed when a person has abdominal discomfort at least 3 times per month for the last 3 months without other disease or injury. Other diseases with similar presentations that are ruled out include Crohn's disease, diverticulosis, and ulcerative colitis (UC). Diagnostic testing includes blood work, computed tomography (CT) scan with contrast, and colonoscopy. Treatment for IBS is multifactorial. Lifestyle modifications include stress reduction, increased exercise, restriction diets, and adequate sleep.[23] Medications to stabilize the motility pattern of the colon and increase absorption include Lotronex (alosetron hydrochloride) and Zelnorm (tegaserod maleate). Additional medications include Lomotil (atropine/diphenoxylate; antidiarrhea) and, possibly, steroids to decrease inflammation.[7,10] A common diet change is the BRAT diet. BRAT stands for non-irritating foods, including banana, rice, apple, and tea or toast. Patients with IBS are told to avoid large meals, wheat, rye, barley, milk, alcohol, and caffeine. Other treatments for symptom reduction include fiber supplementation, laxatives, antidiarrheal medications, tranquilizers, and antidepressants.

Crohn's Disease (Ileitis, Enteritis)

Crohn's disease is a progressive, discontinuous inflammatory process of unknown etiology involving all layers of the intestinal wall (transmural) (Figure 11-2 and Table 11-8).13 Crohn's disease may result from a hypersensitive immune reaction to certain viruses or bacteria resulting in extensive inflammation. Crohn's disease can occur in any location from the mouth to the anus but most commonly occurs in the terminal ileum and colon.[25] The inflammatory process results in rigidity, loss of peristalsis, and ulcerations causing right lower quadrant pain, fever, malaise, and diarrhea.[13,25] Intestinal obstruction, fistulas, and bleeding may develop.[10] Crohn's disease occurs equally in men and women and is not age discriminate. Younger patients often have worse occurrences.[8,21,26]

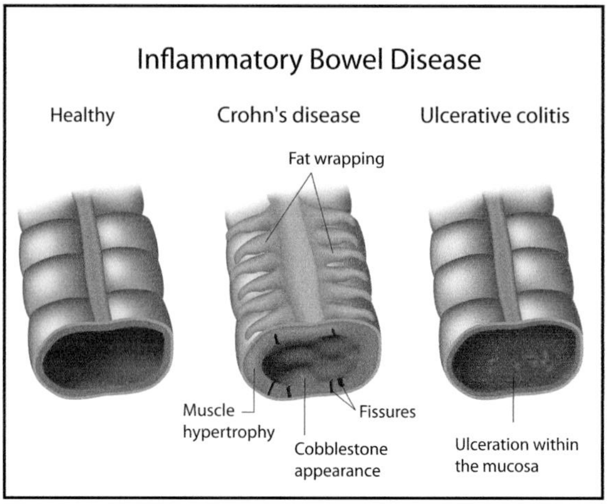

Figure 11-2. Examples of inflammatory bowel disease. Crohn's disease involves the entire bowel wall while ulcerative colitis only involves the inner lining, the mucosa. (Alila Medical Media/Shutterstock.com)

Table 11-8 SIGNS AND SYMPTOMS OF CROHN'S DISEASE	
• Abdominal pain • Diarrhea • Occasional rectal bleeding • Weight loss	• Small bowel obstruction • Fistula formation (especially bladder, vagina, rectum, and skin) • Nutritional deficiencies

Diagnosis is difficult because it is hard to differentiate Crohn's disease from other disorders, such as UC and IBS. Testing includes blood work, fecal blood testing, upper GI series (x-rays with barium), and colonoscopy.[8,13,18] Treatment goals include inflammation control, symptom relief, and elimination of nutritional deficiencies. Treatment may include long-term use of drugs, nutritional supplements, diet modification, and surgery. Medications include anti-inflammatory agents, immunosuppressives, antidiarrheal agents, and antibiotics. Surgery is palliative due to the progressive nature of Crohn's and includes surgical resection of diseased portions with colostomy.[15,25] Crohn's disease is variable in its presentation, intensity, and frequency of occurrence. The variable pattern of disease may result in inconsistent treatment effectiveness over time.[12]

Ulcerative Colitis (Colitis, Proctitis)

UC is a diffuse inflammatory disease of the colon and rectum. The difference between UC and Crohn's disease is that UC affects only the mucosa layer (inner region) of the intestinal lining, resulting in intestinal pain, recurrent diarrhea, bleeding, and increased mucus in stool.[13,25] UC generally occurs equally in men and women between the ages of 15 and 40 years old. There is no known cause for UC, but autoimmune and hypersensitivity reactions to viral or bacterial infections are considered. Common signs and symptoms are listed in Table 11-9. Diagnostic testing includes blood tests, colonoscopy or sigmoidoscopy, and lower GI series (barium enema with x-ray). Medications include anti-inflammatory agents, immunosuppressive drugs, antibiotics, and antidiarrheal agents.[10,14] Medications can manage the symptoms for many patients; however, surgery can lead to a cure for UC. Surgery is required in

Table 11-9

SIGNS AND SYMPTOMS OF ULCERATIVE COLITIS

• Abdominal pain	• Rectal bleeding
• Bloody diarrhea	• Loss of nutrients
• Fatigue	• Electrolyte deficiencies
• Weight loss	• Depression

25% to 50% of patients. Common surgical procedures include proctocolectomy, the removal of the rectum and colon, with the formation of an ileal reservoir (ileum is sewn to the upper anal canal and a pouch is created), colon resection with ileostomy, and ileo-anal pull through (Figure 11-3).[15,24,25]

Malabsorption Disorders

Malabsorption is a general term used to describe multiple disorders where essential nutrients are inadequately absorbed. Malabsorption can be caused by disorders of the stomach (eg, gastritis, gastric resection), small bowel (eg, Crohn's disease, HIV, celiac/tropical sprue, lactose intolerance), pancreas (eg, pancreatitis, cystic fibrosis), liver (eg, liver cirrhosis), and biliary tract (eg, biliary tumors, primary sclerosing cholangitis [PSC], primary biliary cirrhosis [PBC]).[27]

Whipple's Disease

Whipple's disease is caused by the bacterium *Tropheryma whippelii* leading to lesions and scar tissue along the mucosal lining, blocking the villi's ability to absorb nutrients. This disease primarily affects 30- to 40-year-old men, and common signs and symptoms are listed in Table 11-10. Diagnosis is accomplished by review of symptoms and endoscopy with biopsy. Treatment consists of antibiotics and nutritional supplementation, including iron, folate, Vitamin D, calcium, and magnesium.[8]

Short Bowel Syndrome

Short bowel syndrome (SBS) is a secondary disorder that occurs in patients who have had abdominal surgery with removal of greater than 50% of their small intestines (eg, Crohn's, IBS, UC, trauma). The lack of available intestinal surface area for absorption causes malabsorption. Common signs and symptoms are listed in Table 11-11. Medical treatment includes total parenteral nutrition (TPN) and hydration and small bowel transplant in select individuals.[7]

Diverticulosis and Diverticulitis

Diverticulosis is outpouchings or herniations of the inner intestinal lining (mucosa and submucosa) through the intestinal wall (Figure 11-4).[11,17] Diverticulum affect 30% of adults in the US population and the incidence increases with age, starting from about 40 years.[27] Infection or inflammation due to retained fecal material within diverticuli leads to **diverticulitis**. Diverticulitis can cause intestinal necrosis and perforation. Diverticulitis occurs in 10% to 25% of people with diverticulosis.[13] Common signs and symptoms of diverticulitis are listed in Table 11-12. Physical examination is suggestive and confirmed by endoscopy, blood analysis for infection, and CT with contrast.

Medical management focuses on the underlying cause. Important factors for treatment include diet modification, infection control, intestinal rest, and minimizing

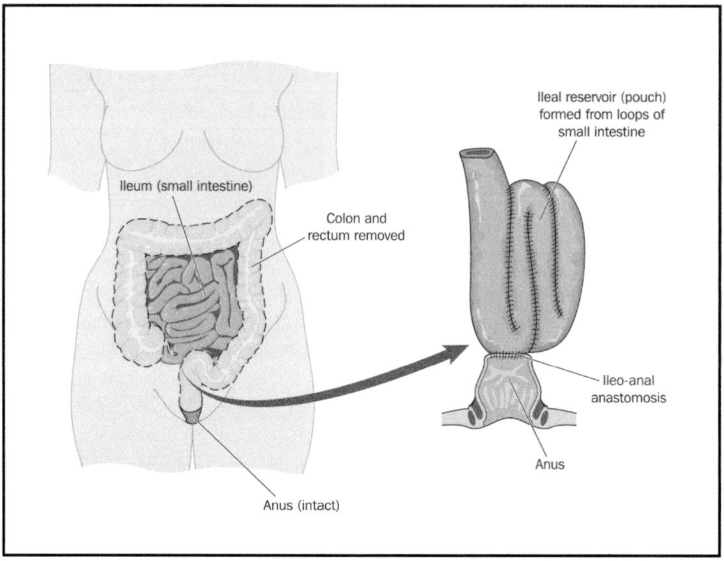

Figure 11-3. Drawing of a proctocolectomy, the removal of the rectum and colon, with the formation of an ileo-rectal pouch. (Blamb/Shutterstock.com)

Table 11-10
Signs and Symptoms of Whipple's Disease

• Abdominal pain	• Diarrhea
• Weight loss	• Intestinal bleeding
• Incomplete breakdown of intestinal materials	• Fatigue and weakness

Table 11-11
Signs and Symptoms of Short Bowel Syndrome

• Malnourishment and dehydration	• Diarrhea
• Weakness	• Cramping
• Fatigue	• Bloating
• Depression	• Heartburn
• Weight loss	

further complications. Diet modification includes increasing fiber intake. Fiber keeps stool soft and lowers the internal colonic pressure. Additionally, patients are discouraged from eating nuts, popcorn, and seeds that are small enough to get lodged within the diverticulum.[21,27] Intestinal rest is promoted by reducing patient activity, insertion of an NG tube, initiating a liquid diet, and management of pain. Surgical intervention (eg, CT-guided drainage, laparotomy, bowel resection) is necessary with severe obstruction, intestinal necrosis, perforation, and abscess formation.[8,21]

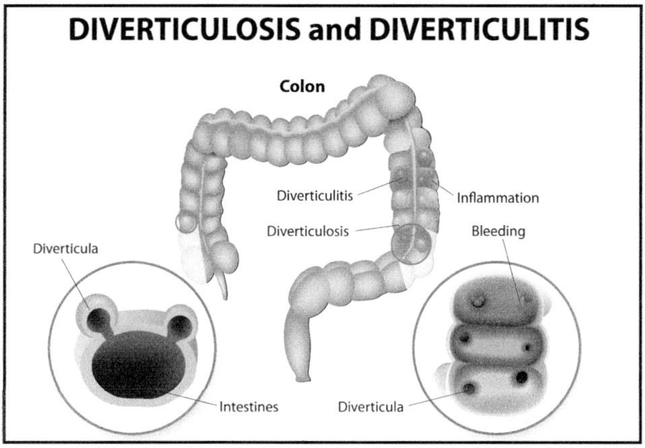

Figure 11-4. Diverticulosis and diverticulitis in colon wall. (Designua/Shutterstock.com)

Table 11-12

SIGNS AND SYMPTOMS OF DIVERTICULITIS

• Abdominal pain (often classified as dull and in the left lower quadrant) • Fever and chills • Nausea and vomiting	• Cramping • Constipation • Fistula formation

Colon Cancer

Colon cancer is the second leading cause of cancer related deaths in the United States and colorectal cancers are the primary cause of GI-related mortality.[9] Colorectal polyps are masses of tissue that project into the lumen (Figure 11-5). Polyps are often an adenoma (adenomatous polyps, tubular adenoma, villous adenoma, adenomatous polyposis coli, Gardner syndrome) and most colon cancers arise from preexisting polyps.[13] Risk factors for colon cancer include modifiable and non-modifiable factors:

Non-modifiable factors:

- Age: Greater than 50
- History of polyps or family members with cancer
- Inflammatory bowel disease, including Crohn's Disease and UC
- Ethnicity: Increased risk in African-Americans and Jewish people of Eastern European descent (Ashkenazi)

Modifiable factors:

- Physical inactivity
- Obesity
- Smoking and alcohol abuse
- Diet: High fat, low fiber, high red and processed meats
- Type 2 diabetes mellitus

Common signs and symptoms of colon cancer are listed in Table 11-13 and staging of the disease is found in Table 11-14. Diagnosis includes a thorough history and physical examination. Diagnostic testing includes digital rectal exam and palpation

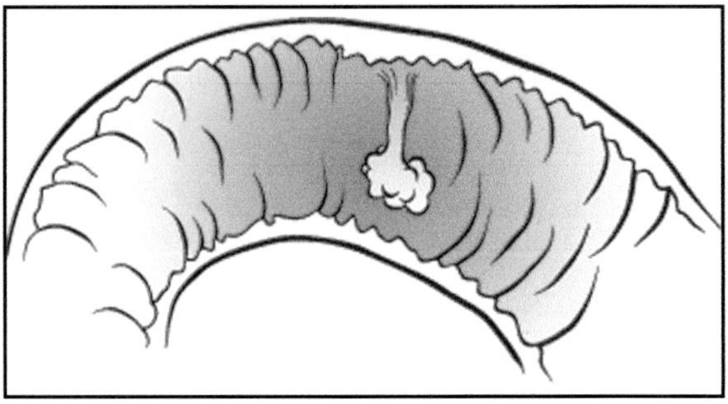

Figure 11-5. Adenomatous polyp and adenocarcinoma of the colon. (Reprinted with permission from Crutchlow E, Dudac P, MacAvoy S, Madara B. *Pathophysiology.* Sudbury, MA: Jones and Bartlett; 2002.)

of abdominal masses, fecal blood testing, radiologic studies, and proctosigmoidoscopy/colonoscopy. Medical treatment includes chemotherapy, radiation therapy, and immunotherapy (see Chapter 13). Surgical interventions vary depending on the resectability and site of the lesion and distribution of lymphatic tissue. Anastomosis of remaining bowel or colostomy may be performed following resection. Surgical approaches involve abdominal or perineal incisions.[24]

Ostomies and Stomas

Ostomies are surgically created openings linking the intestines to the abdominal wall for discharge of body wastes. The **stoma** is the end of the small or large intestine that is visible on the surface of the abdomen. Stomas can be permanent or temporary/reversible and the location will vary depending on the underlying condition. Stoma placement is above the waistline and should not limit dressing or other activities of daily living (ADLs). Common patient questions include the following: Can I exercise? Can I swim? Can I have sex? The answer to all of these is yes, but timing of these activities should be discussed with an ostomy/stoma expert (eg, enterostomal nurse).[21] Therapists should be familiar with emptying an ostomy pouch (sometimes called **appliance** or **bag**). The pouch is typically a heavy plastic bag attached to the skin covering the stoma with an adhesive ring and a clip at the distal end for drainage without pouch removal. The pouch should form an airtight seal so the wearer can remain active.

Ileostomy, externalization of the ileum, is common after removal of colon and rectum (proctocolectomy). Ileostomies drain fairly continuously, and an appliance is worn at all times. **Continent ileostomy** involves the creation of a reservoir or pouch that must be evacuated periodically.

With a **colostomy**, the rectum is removed and distal colon is attached to the abdominal wall. The **ileo-anal reservoir surgery** (**ileo-anal pull through** [IAPT]) is a 2-stage process where (1) the colon and rectum are removed except for the outer muscles of the rectum, an ileostomy is placed, and (2) an ileostomy is closed and the distal small intestine is attached to the remaining rectal muscle. This creates an internal pouch that allows for normal elimination (see Figure 11-3).

Hernia

Hernias are abnormal protrusions of intra-abdominal tissue through an opening, and most often involve a fascial defect in the abdominal wall.[11,24] Hernias are **reducible** when the protruding contents can be returned to the abdomen. Irreducible, or incarcerated, hernias cannot be returned to their anatomic position. A hernia is **strangulated** when the vascular supply of the protruding organ is compromised, resulting in ischemia and potentially necrosis. Incarcerated hernias are surgically repaired

Table 11-13

Signs and Symptoms of Colon Cancer

• Changes in bowel habits	• Narrow stools (ribbon like)
• Diarrhea	• Constant fatigue
• Blood in the stool	• Weight loss

Table 11-14

Staging of Colon Cancer

0 = Present in the innermost lining only
1 = Present on the inner wall of the colon
2 = Present outside the colon, but not the liver
3 = Metastasis to the liver
4 = Metastasis to other parts of the body (usually liver and/or lungs)

because there is danger of strangulation. Because of difficulty determining whether a hernia is incarcerated or strangulated, incarcerated hernias are considered urgent and require immediate medical attention.[28]

Common hernias include inguinal, femoral, umbilical, ventral, and incisional. Groin hernias account for the majority of all hernias and include **inguinal hernias**, the bulging of intestine or fat through a weakened area of the lower abdominal wall in the area of the inguinal canal, and a **femoral hernia**, a protrusion into the femoral canal.[9,10,21] Risk factors for hernias include obesity, heavy lifting, straining during bowel movements, ascites, pregnancy, postoperative infection and pulmonary complications, delayed wound healing, impaired nutrition, placement of drains, and general debility.[21] Symptoms of inguinal hernias include groin pain, palpable or pulsatile lump in the groin, and bowel obstruction at the point of herniation (strangulated bowel). If the physical examination is inconclusive, additional studies may include radiology with contrast. Surgery to reduce herniations include:

- **Herniorrhaphy**: After the hernia is reduced, the abdominal or inguinal wall is reinforced.
- **Hernioplasty**: A herniorrhaphy with the reinforcement of mesh or steel wire.
- **Bowel resection** is necessary if the loop of intestine becomes strangulated or obstructed.

Hemorrhoids

Hemorrhoids are swelling and stretching of veins in and around the anal canal and are a normal part of aging. Hemorrhoids occur in greater than 50% of people over the age of 50 and develop because of increased anal pressure (eg, straining during bowel movements, chronic constipation, pregnancy/childbirth). Hemorrhoids cause pain, discomfort in sitting, itching, and bleeding. There are two types of hemorrhoids: internal, within the anal canal, and external, which are outside the rectum.[3] Diagnosis is confirmed by physical examination or endoscopy as needed. Medical treatment goals include elimination of constipation (if present), creams (eg, Preparation H [Pfizer], Anusol [hydrocortisone], witch hazel pads), a Sitz bath (a seated bathing tool to irrigate and cleanse the perianal region and promote muscular relaxation) and stool softeners. Diet modifications include increasing fluid and fiber

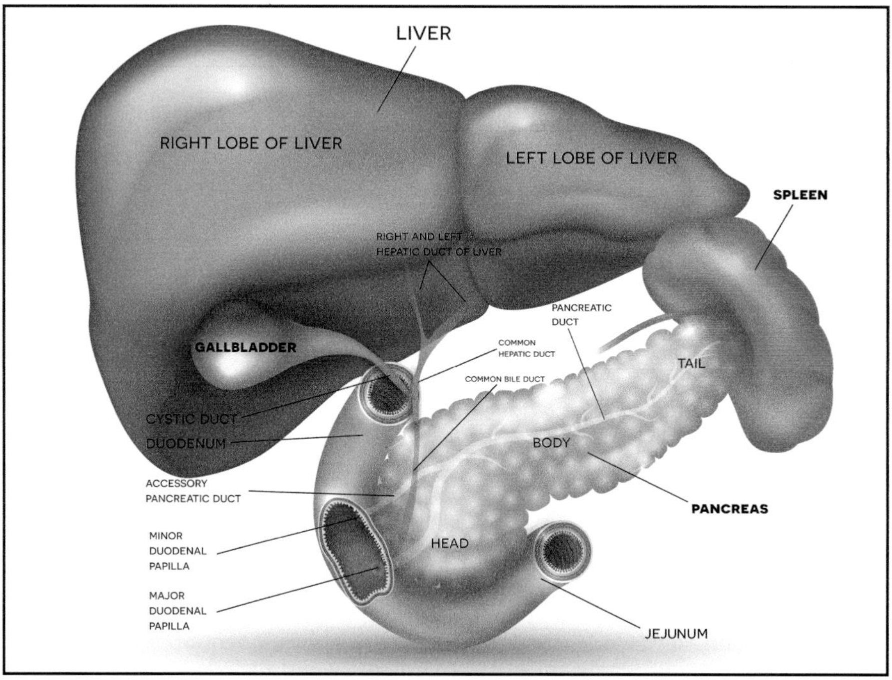

Figure 11-6. Anatomy of the liver, gallbladder, bile duct, and pancreas. (Tefi/Shutterstock.com)

intake. The use of rubber, inflatable donuts are not recommended because the donut increases the vascular pressure around external hemorrhoids by compression and promotes venous stasis.[3,4] Surgical interventions include:

- **Sclerotherapy**: Injection of inflammatory agent leading to fibrosis and scarring
- **Banding**: Placement of rubber bands leading to ischemic necrosis
- **Hemorrhoidectomy**: Surgical cauterization and removal of involved veins and tissue

The Liver and Gallbladder

The liver is the largest organ in the body (Figure 11-6).[7] It has important metabolic and digestive functions that are essential and hepatic abnormalities impact multiple organ systems (see Table 11-17 later in the chapter). The liver possesses tremendous resilience and regenerative ability if resected or traumatized.[28] In contrast, the gallbladder, located underneath the liver, is very susceptible to damage or injury.

Anatomy and Physiology

The liver is located in the right upper quadrant (RUQ) of the abdomen, under the diaphragm and within part of the lower rib cage. The liver has 2 lobes, right and left, which can be subdivided into lobules, each of which has their own arterial, venous, and biliary supply. Hepatic blood supply arises from 2 sources, the hepatic artery, branching from aorta, and the hepatic portal vein, arising from mesenteric and splenic veins. On the posterior inferior surface of the liver lies the gallbladder. The gallbladder lies within a groove separating the right and left hepatic lobes and has direct connections to each of the liver lobes (biliary ducts) as well as to the duodenum and the pancreas (ampulla of Vater).[2,28]

Hepatic function can be clinically defined into 4 categories:

1. **Synthetic**: Production of plasma proteins, including albumin and the coagulation factors
2. **Excretory**: Production of bile (plus bilirubin, cholesterol, urobilogen, and bile salts)
3. **Metabolism**
   a. **Fat metabolism**: Triglycerides, cholesterol, and phospholipids are synthesized in the liver
   b. **Carbohydrate metabolism**: Blood glucose is converted to glycogen (glycogenesis) for storage when blood glucose levels increase; glycogen is broken down (glycogenolysis) and glucose is synthesized (gluconeogenesis) when blood glucose level decrease
   c. **Protein metabolism**: The liver is the primary organ for protein catabolism and removal of ammonia by synthesizing urea that is transported to the kidney for excretion
4. **Detoxification**: The liver detoxifies many noxious compounds found in chemicals and drugs, making them less harmful[1,3]

The **gallbladder** stores and concentrates bile synthesized in the liver. Bile is delivered to the duodenum via contraction of the gallbladder passing through the common bile duct and the sphincter of Oddi. Bile is an emulsifier that facilitates the digestion of fats and stimulates intestinal peristalsis.[1,3]

Health Conditions of the Liver

Jaundice

Jaundice develops from excessive deposition of bile pigments resulting from **hyperbilirubinemia**, an increase in plasma bilirubin (>0.8 mg/dL). The bile pigments create the yellow discoloration of the skin, eyes, and fingernails and account for dark, foul-smelling urine. Jaundice may result from excessive destruction of red blood cells as seen in hemolytic anemia (**prehepatic jaundice**), hepatic dysfunction, as in cirrhosis of the liver (**hepatic jaundice**), or from obstruction of the bile passageways, such as the common bile duct by a gall stone (**obstructive jaundice, posthepatic jaundice**). Bilirubin is a byproduct of hemoglobin catabolism. Under normal circumstances, the liver conjugates bilirubin as part of bile where it is ultimately excreted in the feces or reabsorbed in the intestines, transported to the kidneys, and excreted in the urine.[1,3]

Hepatic Encephalopathy

Hepatic encephalopathy is a reversible decrease in neurologic function due to shunting of blood away from the portal circulation or hepatic failure resulting in accumulation of noxious metabolic byproducts, especially ammonia.[23] Hyperammonemia (high blood ammonia) and other toxic substances in the blood alter cerebrovascular permeability, interfere with normal cerebral energy metabolism, disrupt cell integrity, and alter the normal balance of neurotransmitters, creating the typical signs and symptoms of hepatic encephalopathy listed in Table 11-15.[11,29] It is important to recognize that the presentation of the patient with hepatic encephalopathy is variable and the findings listed in Table 11-15 may not be consistently reproducible.

Table 11-15

SIGNS AND SYMPTOMS OF HEPATIC ENCEPHALOPATHY

Grade	*Cognition and Behavior*	*Neuromuscular Function*
0	• Asymptomatic loss of cognitive abilities	• None—difficulty to detect
Minimal	• Alterations in tests of psychomotor speed/executive functions	• None—difficulty to detect
1	• Impaired concentration • Shortened attention span • Sleep disturbances • Impaired simple addition/ subtraction	• Monotone voice • Tremor • Poor handwriting • Apraxia
2	• Lethargy or apathy • Disorientation for time • Short attention span • Personality change	• Dyspraxia • Dysarthria • Asterixis
3	• Somnolence to semi-stupor but responsive to stimuli • Gross disorientation (eg, time, place) • Confusion • Bizarre behaviors (eg, anger, paranoia)	• Nystagmus • Muscular rigidity • Ataxia • Hyper- or hyporeflexia
4	• Coma • No response to pain	• Unconscious

Adapted from Vilstrup H, Amodio P, Bajaj J, et al. Hepatic encephalopathy in chronic liver disease: 2014 Practice Guideline by the American Association for the Study of Liver Diseases and the European Association for the Study of the Liver. *Hepatology*. 2014;60(2):715-735.

Ascites and Peripheral Edema

Ascites is the presence of fluid in the peritoneum or swelling of the abdomen. The mechanisms for causing both peripheral edema and ascites are the same, an alteration in the Starling forces that regulate fluid balance. Fluid balance is a function of osmotic, arterial, venous, and tissue pressures. Ascites results from the synergistic relationship between an elevated portal venous pressure and low serum osmotic pressure due to hypoalbuminemia. Albumin, synthesized in the liver, is the most common protein of the body. Albumin maintains the osmotic pressure of the blood and facilitates absorption of fluid into the vasculature.[1,3] If albumin concentrations decrease (**hypoalbuminemia**), as seen in hepatic disease, osmotic pressures are low and fluid is poorly reabsorbed into the vasculature. In addition, portal hypertension creates excessive pressure in the venous system, favoring capillary leakage. The sum of these forces results in the movement of fluid across the peritoneal membrane into the abdomen.

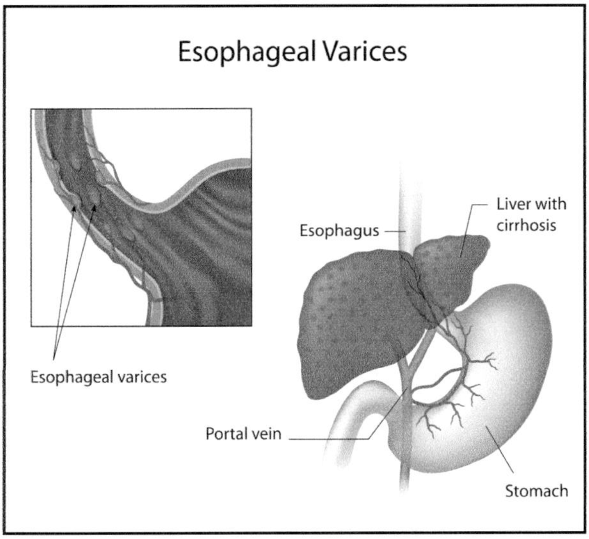

Figure 11-7. Esophageal varices. The portal vein carries blood from the spleen, pancreas, gallbladder, and GI tract to the liver. With cirrhosis, the portal circulation can become obstructed leading to congestion and varices. (Alila Medical Media/Shutterstock.com)

Portal hypertension is caused by elevated venous pressure in the portal vein (>12 mm Hg). The underlying cause may be multifactorial, including portal vein thrombosis, neoplasm, or other form of obstruction (eg, PBC Cirrhosis causes fibrosis of liver tissue and restriction of the portal circulation). Long-term portal hypertension may lead to other disorders, such as variceal bleeding, ascites, splenomegaly, right heart dysfunction, and pulmonary edema.[13,28]

Esophageal Varices

The portal veins carry blood from the upper GI tract, spleen pancreas, and gallbladder to the liver. Portal hypertension, a sustained increase in portal venous pressures, results in elevated venous pressure and congestion in the spleen, stomach, and esophagus. Collateral vessels develop that become distended and varicosities develop, especially in the stomach and esophagus (Figure 11-7). In advanced liver disease, varices may burst, leading to upper GI bleeding and **hematemesis** (coffee ground vomitus).[30]

Hepatomegaly and Splenomegaly

Hepatomegaly, enlargement of the liver, is a common finding in hepatic disease. The usual lower border of the liver is slightly below the right costal margin and extension below the rib cage is consistent with hepatomegaly. **Splenomegaly**, enlargement of the spleen, results from passive venous congestion and is often associated with portal hypertension.[13,28]

Cirrhosis

Cirrhosis is the replacement of normal liver tissue with fibrotic tissue and nodules and is the end result of hepatic injury (see Figure 11-7).[13] This alteration in liver architecture blocks normal blood flow throughout the liver, causing many of the symptoms listed in Table 11-16. Cirrhosis is the 12th leading cause of death in the United States, resulting in over 30,000 deaths annually.[9,31]

Table 11-16 CLINICAL FEATURES OF HEPATIC DYSFUNCTION	
System	*Signs and Symptoms*
Hematology	Anemia, coagulopathy
Cardiovascular	Tachycardia, hypotension/hypertension (HTN), peripheral edema, portal hypertension
Pulmonary	Hepatopulmonary syndrome leading to hypoxemia
Neurological	Encephalopathy
GI	Varices (especially of the esophagus/stomach), risk for bleeding, ascites
Musculoskeletal	General weakness and muscular atrophy, overstretched abdominal muscles (may have associated back pain)
Metabolic	Poor drug and toxin excretion, electrolyte abnormalities
Integumentary	Poor wound healing, brittle skin/hair
Other	Malnutrition/anorexia, hypoalbuminemia, electrolyte abnormalities

Adapted from Bishop Lindsay KL, Galantino ML, Huber F, Wells CL. *Handout: Management of Medically Complex Patient.* American Physical Therapy Association Combined Sections Meeting: Pre-Conference Program. October 1997.

Cirrhosis is a secondary complication of multiple liver diseases including:

- Alcoholic liver disease
- Chronic viral hepatitis (most commonly hepatitis B virus [HBV] and hepatitis C virus [HCV])
- Non-alcoholic fatty liver disease (NAFLD; fatty deposition without inflammation)
- Non-alcoholic steatohepatitis (NASH; fatty deposition with inflammation)
- Obesity, diabetes, metabolic syndrome (increases risk of developing NAFLD)
- Autoimmune hepatitis
- Wilson's disease
- Biliary duct obstruction (eg, gall stones, inflammation, pancreatitis, tumor)
- Drug toxicity (eg, Tylenol [acetaminophen] poisoning, amiodarone, methotrexate, antibiotics [macrolides, sulfonamides])

Patient presentation is variable depending upon inciting cause, but encephalopathy, ascites, and jaundice are common. Patients frequently experience exhaustion, fatigue, and weakness.

After establishing the cause of the underlying disease, the extent of liver scarring can be assessed through the combination of CT scan, ultrasound, and/or biopsy. Treatment is dependent on the underlying disease process, but there is no cure or reversibility of cirrhosis except liver transplantation. Many of the symptoms of cirrhosis are managed with lifestyle changes and with medications such as lactulose. Lactulose increases the acidity of the intestinal lumen, which prevents ammonia absorption decreasing the risk of encephalopathy; however, this often leads to diarrhea and flatulence.

Hepatitis

Hepatitis is inflammation of the liver. Symptoms vary from a minor flu-like illness to fulminant, fatal liver failure. The major causes of hepatitis are viral infections (common: hepatitis A virus [HAV], HBV, HCV, hepatitis D virus; rare: cytomegalovirus [CMV], yellow fever), alcohol, drugs (eg, Isoniazid, statins, NSAIDs), and other toxic agents. Patients typically present with many of the signs and symptoms listed in Table 11-16, and diagnosis is a combination of a thorough history, physical examination, and laboratory testing (liver function tests [eg, aspartate aminotransferase/alanine aminotransferase (AST/ALT)]). Viral hepatitis is usually self-limiting and complete in 3 to 16 weeks. However, chronic hepatitis, hepatitis lasting greater than 6 months, may develop in non-HAV infections, autoimmune disorders, and as a drug side effect.[8,12]

Acute viral hepatitis will usually resolve and much of the treatment is supportive. Antiviral treatments (eg, HBV: entecavir, lamivudine, interferon, telbivudine; HCV: ribavirin, telaprevir, interferon) and anti-inflammatory agents (eg, corticosteroids) are indicated depending on etiology. Chronic hepatitis may progress to cirrhosis and liver failure. Ultimately, the only cure for advanced stages of the disease is liver transplantation (see Chapter 14).

Primary Sclerosing Cholangitis

PSC is a rare disease process where inflammation, fibrosis, and stricture of the bile duct prevents bile from passing into the gallbladder (obstructive jaundice) resulting in liver damage (**biliary cirrhosis**).[13] More men than women are affected by PSC, usually between the ages of 30 to 60.[28,29] There is an increased incidence of PSC in patients with UC. The cause of PSC is unknown, but sensitivity to bacteria or virus may account for the combined presentation of PSC and UC. The progression of PSC is gradual, and prognosis is poor. Common symptoms include jaundice, pruritus, fatigue, anorexia, and indigestion.

Common diagnostic procedures include[8,10]:

- Cholangiography x-ray with dye injection into the bile ducts
- Endoscopic retrograde cholangiopancreatography (ERCP): An endoscopic evaluation of the bile ducts
- Magnetic resonance imagine (MRI) retrograde cholangiopancreatography (MRCP)
- Liver biopsy

Treatment focuses on symptom management. Specifically, patients are often deficient in fat-soluble vitamins (A, D, E, K) because of bile duct obstruction and limited fat absorption. Surgical management may include balloon dilatation, stent placement, and eventual liver transplantation.

Primary Biliary Cirrhosis

PBC is an insidious chronic disease noted by progressive destruction of the biliary duct wall interfering with bile transport (**cholestasis**) and digestion. It commonly occurs in 40- to 60-year-old women (nearly 90%) and is often found as a secondary diagnosis (eg, thyroiditis, rheumatoid arthritis, scleroderma, Sjögren syndrome, systemic lupus erythematosus).[13] The cause of PBC is unknown but is believed to be an autoimmune disease with hepatic lymphocytes and plasma cells destroying the biliary ducts. Common signs and symptoms include hepatosplenomegaly, jaundice, pruritus, edema, cholesterol deposits on the skin (xanthomas), and dry eyes and/or mouth.

Patients with PBC often develop osteoarthritis, osteoporosis, portal hypertension, xanthomatous neuropathy, and thyroid problems. Diagnostic testing includes:

- Cholangiography x-ray with dye injection into the bile ducts
- ERCP
- MRCP
- Liver biopsy
- Assessment of thyroid function

Treatments for PBC include vitamin and calcium supplementation, medications for symptom management, and hormone therapy (for hypothyroidism and for women who are menopausal). If treatment fails or the disease process continues to progress, a liver transplant is recommended.

Wilson's Disease

Wilson's disease is an autosomal recessive disorder resulting in excess absorption of copper from the small intestine with limited hepatic excretion, leading to copper deposition in the liver, brain, corneas, and kidneys.[10,28] Wilson's disease usually affects children but can be diagnosed between the ages of 3 and 55 years of age due to variations in clinical presentation. If left untreated, Wilson's Disease can be fatal.[28]

The hallmark sign of Wilson's disease is the **Kayser-Fleisher ring**, a brownish ring around the cornea. Other signs are dependent upon which organs are involved, such as hepatomegaly, splenomegaly, portal hypertension, and neurological symptoms, such as dysarthria, ataxia, resting tremors, and rigidity (Parkinsonian symptoms).

The pathognomonic sign, the Kayser-Fleisher ring, is unique to Wilson's disease. Other important diagnostic tools include blood and urine analysis and liver biopsy to determine the concentrations of copper.[10] Neurological testing is important if symptoms are present. Often, CT or MRI in conjunction with electromyography (EMG) is done to assess the neuromuscular component of the disease process. Treatment includes drug therapy along with diet modification. D-Penicillamin, and trientine hydrochloride are chelating agents that bind to copper and help remove copper from the bloodstream. Zinc acetate aids in blocking intestinal absorption of copper, thus promoting increased excretion of copper. Patients take Vitamin B_6 and eat a diet low in copper, which includes avoidance of mushrooms, nuts, chocolate, dried fruit, liver, and shellfish.[8] Treatment for Wilson's disease is life-long and prognosis is good for patients who are successfully diagnosed early and managed before liver or brain damage has occurred.

HEALTH CONDITIONS OF THE GALLBLADDER

Cholelithiasis (Gallstones, Biliary Calculi)

Gallstones are a common event, occurring in nearly 1/12 Americans. Most gallstones are asymptomatic; however, excruciating pain may be experienced. Risk factors for developing stones include sex (females more than males), obesity, diabetes mellitus, and age over 40 years. Ethnically, Native American, Mexican, and South American people are at an increased risk.[8,28]

Gallstones are the most prevalent health condition of the gallbladder and biliary tract. There are 2 different types of gallstones based on their chemical composition: cholesterol and bilirubin stones. Cholesterol stones are due to an increase in cholesterol concentration, decrease in bile salts, or delayed emptying of the gallbladder. Bilirubin stones are rare and generally occur in chronic forms of anemia, such as sickle cell anemia or thalassemia. Obstruction to bile flow into the duodenum causes distension of the bile ducts, impairs digestion, and may result in spillage of bile pigments into the circulation causing obstructive jaundice.[32] Signs and symptoms of gall stones include severe pain in the epigastric region or RUQ, referred pain under the right scapula, indigestion after eating fatty foods, and nausea and/or vomiting.

Gallstones are typically diagnosed through an abdominal ultrasound. Other tests performed include CT scan, MRCP, ERCP, and blood tests. Differential diagnosis for acute cholelithiasis includes myocardial infarction, appendicitis, ulcers, IBS, hiatal hernia, and pancreatitis.

The most common treatment for acute cholelithiasis is a cholecystectomy (excision of the gallbladder), which can often be done laproscopically. Other treatments include medications such as chenodial, monoctanoin, and ursodiol.

The Pancreas

The pancreas is a complex organ, having both endocrine and exocrine functions. Endocrine function involves insulin and glucagon production, and the regulation of lipids, protein, and carbohydrates, which is discussed in Chapter 10. For purposes of this chapter, only the exocrine functions will be presented.[3]

Anatomy and Physiology

Anatomically, the pancreas is a large, flat, finely lobulated gland associated with the duodenum. It is located posterior to the stomach along the posterior abdominal wall in the left upper quadrant (LUQ) (see Figure 11-6). The pancreatic ducts carry the exocrine secretions and connect with the bile duct at the **ampulla of Vater** (hepatopancreatic ampulla) before entering the duodenum. Rings of smooth muscle form the **sphincter of Oddi**, that close the ampulla until stimulated to relax by the intestinal hormone **cholecystokinin** (CCK).[1-3]

The **pancreas** secretes 2 to 2.5 liters per day of a bicarbonate fluid containing digestive enzymes. Regulation of pancreatic secretion of this fluid involves the chemical composition of the meal, hormones released from the small intestine (secretin and CCK) and neural reflex arcs involving the vagus nerve.[1,3,33]

Health Conditions of the Exocrine Pancreas

Pancreatitis

Pancreatitis is an inflammation of the pancreas and presentation is variable from mild symptoms to severe complications with risk of death. Pancreatitis is classified as acute or chronic. The acute form of pancreatitis is usually sudden in onset, of short duration, and self-limited. Chronic pancreatitis results in progressive destruction of pancreatic tissues.

Pancreatitis is often caused by excessive alcohol consumption or by cholelithiasis. Alcohol prematurely activates digestive enzymes and increases ductal permeability while gallstones block the pancreatic ducts. Both allow activated pancreatic enzymes to reach the surrounding tissues damaging the pancreas. Additional causes include hypercalcemia, hyperlipidemia, abdominal trauma, end-stage renal disease (ESRD), bacterial and viral infections, medications (thiazides, sulfonamides), and structural anomalies. Common signs and symptoms are listed in Table 11-17.

Clinical symptoms and laboratory testing are used to determine diagnosis. Laboratory findings may include elevations in serum amylase and lipase, c-reactive protein, white blood cells (WBCs) and hematocrit. Abdominal ultrasound, MRCP, and CT scans assess anatomy of the pancreas and check for the presence of gallstones, tumors, perforated ulcers, or ileus.

Treatment is variable and dependent on the severity and chronicity of the symptoms. Acute pancreatitis will often resolve spontaneously within several days with pancreatic rest. Pancreatic rest includes withholding foods and liquids by mouth, and possibly bed rest and NG suction.

Table 11-17

SIGNS AND SYMPTOMS OF PANCREATITIS

• Abdominal/epigastric pain (worse with eating, walking, supine), often radiating to the back • Abdominal muscle guarding and distention	• Nausea and/or vomiting • Fever • Dehydration • Tachycardia and hypotension

If symptoms are progressive, admission to the intensive care unit (ICU) along with aggressive rehydration and electrolyte replacement, antibiotics for confirmed infections, and NG decompression are instituted. Patients are observed for organ failure and other systemic complications including shock, renal failure, acute respiratory distress syndrome, and, if the underlying cause of pancreatitis is gallstones, surgery is warranted. Long-term treatments include a high-carbohydrate, low-fat diet, as well as digestive enzyme supplementation.[28,33,34]

PHYSICAL THERAPIST MANAGEMENT

Patients with health conditions involving the GI system are not a common source of referral for physical therapy services; however, GI complaints, especially abdominal discomfort, are common patient symptoms, and many hospitals include physical therapy in GI surgery postoperative management. Table 11-18 provides a survey of common examination procedures and findings associated with GI pathology, Table 11-19 reviews the anatomic location of the viscera, and Figure 11-8 reviews referred pain patterns. Therapists should recognize that patients who have health conditions involving the abdominal viscera may present with apparent musculoskeletal complaints due to referred pain.

Generally, there are no contraindications for patients with GI disorders to participate in physical therapy. The examination process will guide therapeutic interventions (see Chapter 1 and Table 11-20). The high prevalence of PUD makes recognition important. Patients may have active bleeding or anemia making close monitoring of lab values and observation of heart rate (HR) and blood pressure (BP) necessary. Peptic ulcers are associated with chest or mid-thoracic back pain that may mimic cardiac disease (see Table 6-9). Additionally, exercise tends to increase acid secretion, which may exacerbate symptoms. Esophageal and stomach disorders in acute care can be limiting but are usually quick to resolve with proper medical and lifestyle interventions.

Patients with GI disorders, especially malabsorptive diseases, can be malnourished, cachectic, and have frequent bouts of diarrhea. These side effects have the potential to leave patients dehydrated and deficient in essential nutrients, vitamins, and minerals. Nutritional deficiencies increase the risk for osteoarthritis, osteoporosis, kidney stones, gallstones, liver dysfunction, and muscular weakness and atrophy.

Medications must also be considered. Patients with Crohn's disease and UC are often prescribed anti-inflammatory agents, such as corticosteroids. The long-term effects of these medications include hyperglycemia and diabetes, fluid retention, muscle wasting, and peripheral neuropathies.

Abdominal surgery, including esophageal procedures, require significant attentiveness by the therapist. Complications after surgery include respiratory insufficiency, incision discomfort, stenosis or intestinal obstruction, odor and leakage with

Table 11-18

CLINICAL FEATURES OF HEPATIC DYSFUNCTION

Examination Technique	*Description of Technique*	*Examination Findings in Common Diseases/Disorders*
Common questions/ history	• Abdominal pain: Note onset, duration, character (eg, sharp, dull, stabbing), location/radiation to other areas • Vomiting: Color, fresh blood, "coffee grounds" • Stool characteristics: Color, consistency, frequency, presence of blood (fresh blood vs black) tarry in appearance, diarrhea, constipation, incontinence • Urine characteristics: Color, amount, frequency, presence of blood; incontinence associated with activity, cough, sneeze (see Table 12-6)	• Pain characteristics: Burning (eg, peptic ulcer), cramping (eg, gastroenteritis), knife-like (eg, pancreatitis), gradual onset (eg, infection) • Anatomic location of pain (see Table 11-19) • GI bleeding: ¤ Hematemesis: Bloody vomitus, may be fresh, bright red blood or dark, grainy digested blood with coffee ground appearance ¤ Melena: Black, tarry, and foul-smelling stools caused by digestion of blood
Inspection of abdomen	• Note general appearance and contour of the abdomen. ¤ Surface motion, pulsations, visible peristalsis ¤ Scars/striae ¤ Rashes/lesions ¤ Ascites (the accumulation of fluid in the peritoneal cavity), organomegaly, visible hernia ¤ Presence of masses • Note tenderness: Deep, superficial, guarding, rebound, or rigidity	• Abdominal distension • Intestinal obstruction: ¤ Ascites: Prominent abdomen or bulging flanks in supine (eg, liver disease, cirrhosis, portal hypertension) ¤ Incisional hernia: Protrusion of abdomen through incisional scar ¤ Umbilical hernia: Protrusion of navel (eg, common during pregnancy, ascites) *(continued)*

Table 11-18 (continued)

Clinical Features of Hepatic Dysfunction

Examination Technique	*Description of Technique*	*Examination Findings in Common Diseases/Disorders*
Palpation of abdomen	• Palpation: Always begin palpation lightly in a region where pain is not suspected and gradually move toward painful regions/quadrants • Rebound: Hold hand at 90-degree angle to abdomen, then press gently followed by a rapid withdrawal	• Local tenderness: Intestinal obstruction, appendicitis, cholecystitis, diverticulitis • Guarding: Voluntary contraction of the abdominal muscles due to tenderness, fear, or anxiety (eg, appendicitis, intestinal torsion [volvulus], fibrous adhesions) • Rebound: Abdominal tenderness that increases when the palpating fingers are quickly removed (eg, peritoneal inflammation, gastric and duodenal ulcers) • Rigidity: Involuntary contraction of the abdominal muscles due to peritoneal inflammation (eg, cholecystitis, gastric ulcer)
Percussion of abdomen	• Percussion should be performed in all 4 quadrants: ¤ Note that the abdomen should have both tympanic regions (eg, stomach, gastric air bubble), gas-filled bowel, and dull areas (eg, fluid-filled bowel, liver). ¤ Percussion can be used to determine the span of the liver (~6 to 12 cm) upper border around the fifth to seventh intercostal spaces and lower border at or slightly below the costal margin.	• Localized percussive tenderness suggests peritoneal inflammation. • Diffusely tympanic abdomen suggests intestinal obstruction. • Upward displacement of liver: Liver atrophy, abdominal fluid, abdominal mass • Downward displacement of liver: Hepatomegaly, chronic obstructive pulmonary disease (COPD), hyperinflation

(continued)

Table 11-18 (continued)

Clinical Features of Hepatic Dysfunction

Examination Technique	*Description of Technique*	*Examination Findings in Common Diseases/Disorders*
Auscultation	• Bowel sounds: ~5 to 34/minute, low pitch and gurgling in nature • Vascular sounds: Listen over aorta (midline/superior to umbilicus), renal (midclavicular line/superior to umbilicus), iliac (midclavicular line/inferior to umbilicus), and femoral arteries • Consider review of clinical laboratory data (see Chapter 2, Tables 2-1, 2-13, 2-14, 2-15): ¤ ALT/AST ¤ Bilirubin ¤ Amylase/lipase ¤ Albumin/prealbumin ¤ Thrombin/prothrombin time ¤ Platelet count	• ↑ bowel sounds: Hunger, gastroenteritis, diarrhea, diverticulitis • ↓ bowel sounds/absent bowel sounds: Peritoneal inflammation, paralytic obstruction, or ileus • High-pitched ("tinkling") bowel sounds: Intestinal (mechanical) obstruction • Abdominal bruit: Aortic aneurysm/dissection; aneurysm or dissection of splenic, renal, or iliac arteries • ↑ AST/ALT: Hepatocyte inflammation/damage (eg, acute and chronic hepatitis, alcoholic cirrhosis, hepatic tumors, drug-induced hepatotoxicity, myocardial infarction) • ↑ bilirubin: Hepatic damage, hemolytic anemia, biliary obstruction • ↓ albumin: Advanced liver disease, cirrhosis • ↑ prothrombin time: Advanced liver disease, Vitamin K deficiency, drugs (eg, warfarin) • ↓ platelets: Advanced liver disease, splemomegaly • ↑ amylase/lipase: Pancreatitis, pancreatic and bile duct obstruction • ↓ amylase/lipase: Chronic pancreatitis, pancreatic cancer, liver disease

Adapted from Seidel et al[40]; Smith and Paterson-Brown[41]; Fischbach and Dunning [66]; Huether and McCance[67]; and Perloff.[68]

Table 11-19

Anatomic Regions and Abdominal Pain

Anatomic Structures	Causes of Pain
Right Upper Quadrant	
• Liver and gallbladder • Duodenum • Head of pancreas • Right adrenal gland • Portion of right kidney	• Hepatitis • Hepatomegaly • Duodenal ulcer • Cholecystitis • Biliary stones • Pneumonia
Left Upper Quadrant	
• Left lobe of liver • Spleen • Stomach • Body of pancreas • Portion of left kidney • Portions of transverse and descending colon	• Splenic injury/rupture • Gastric ulcer • Aortic aneurysm • Perforated colon • Pneumonia
Right Lower Quadrant	
• Lower pole, right kidney/right ureter • Cecum/appendix • Ascending colon	• Appendicitis • Renal/ureteral stone • Meckel diverticulum • Regional ileitis
Left Lower Quadrant	
• Lower pole, left kidney/left ureter • Sigmoid colon • Portion of descending colon	• Sigmoid diverticulitis • Renal/ureteral stone • Perforated colon • UC • Regional ileitis
Umbilical and Epigastric Regions	
• Sigmoid diverticulitis • Renal/ureteral stone • Perforated colon • UC • Regional ileitis	• Intestinal obstruction • Acute pancreatitis • Aortic aneurysm • Diverticulitis • Mesenteric thrombosis • Hiatal hernia

Adapted from: Huether SE, McCance KL. *Understanding Pathophysiology.* St. Louis, MO: Elsevier Mosby Inc; 2012 and Seidel HM, Ball JW, Dains JE, Benedict GW. *Mosby's Guide to Physical Examination.* St. Louis, MO: Mosby, Inc; 2003.

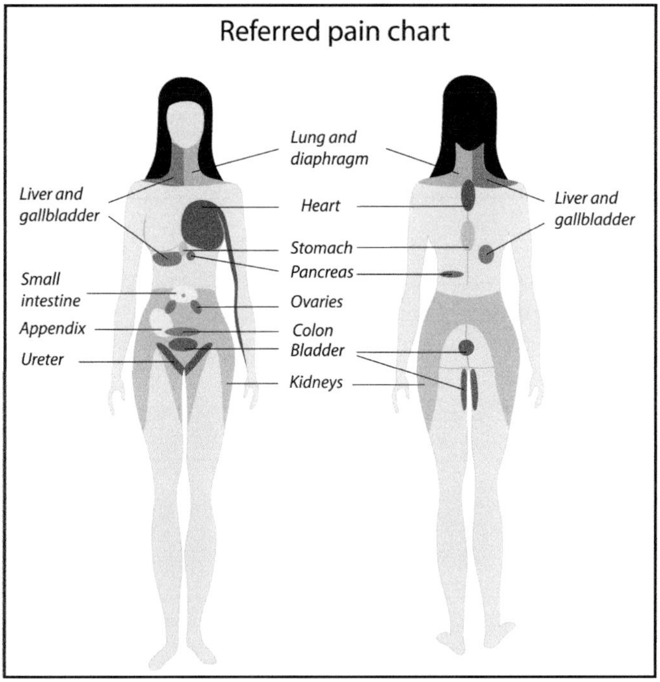

Figure 11-8. Sites of referred pain from abdominal viscera. (Alila Medical Media/Shutterstock.com)

ostomies, postoperative incision and skin irritation, and diarrhea with loss of water and electrolytes due to impaired intestinal absorption. Postoperative pulmonary complications, such as atelectasis and pneumonia, are a major cause of morbidity and mortality after abdominal surgery, resulting in prolonged hospitalization and admission into the ICU.[35] The incidence of postoperative complications ranges from 4.5% to 80% of patients after upper abdominal surgery.[36,37] Postoperative pain, drugs, central nervous system (CNS) suppression due to anesthesia, immobilization, and preexisting lung disease all play a major role in the development of pulmonary complications. It has been shown that physical therapy, including deep breathing exercises, huffing, coughing, and early mobilization, can improve oxygen saturation and reduce the incidence of complications.[38,39]

Early ambulation also stimulates peristalsis, decreases the need for pain control, increases bladder pressures allowing removal of the Foley catheter decreasing urinary tract infection risk, and provides deep vein thrombosis (DVT) prophylaxis. Patients may benefit from a rolling walker to enhance dynamic standing balance and eliminate the need to lift and be unsupported while in transition. Anecdotally, patients frequently report reduced discomfort with a forward leaning posture.

Postoperative pain is difficult to manage, and it is prudent to coordinate pain management with therapy sessions. Splinting of the incision with a pillow or the addition of an abdominal binder for transfers and gait training, and instruction in log rolling for bed mobility tasks may lessen discomfort.

Patient education should include lifestyle and diet modification, proper use of patient-controlled analgesia (PCA), and abdominal protection. Activity restrictions may include limited driving, swimming, active abdominal exercise, and lifting restrictions (< 10 pounds) for 4 to 6 weeks postoperatively. The therapist must collaborate with the surgical team to determine appropriateness of all activity restrictions.

Table 11-20 COMMON THERAPEUTIC INTERVENTIONS FOR THE GASTROINTESTINAL PATIENT
Patient Instruction
• Lifestyle and diet modifications for patients with GERD (see Table 11-3), PUD, IBS, colon cancer • Ostomy appliance management • Wound/incision care • Mobility precautions and restrictions (eg, log rolling, lifting, driving) • Patient to report any increased pain, nausea/vomiting, bloating, change in stools, diarrhea, signs of wound/incision infection • Discharge planning/recommendations
Airway Clearance Techniques (Especially for the Post-Surgical Patient)
• Deep breathing/inspiratory holds • Incentive spirometry • Huffing/directed cough
Assistive Technology
• Rolling walkers to facilitate early mobility and progressive ambulation • Abdominal binders for abdominal support and pain reduction
Functional Training in Self-Care and Motor Function Training
• Log rolling and bracing abdominal incision with pillow • Bed mobility, transfer, and gait training • Progressive ambulation
Therapeutic Exercise
• Aerobic and endurance conditioning and reconditioning (gait and locomotor training) • Breathing exercises

Therapists must consider the psychosocial aspect of GI disorders. The coexistence of mental health disorders and IBS, as well as the acceptance of defecating into an ostomy bag, is often difficult. Always ensure that the colostomy bag is properly attached around the stoma to prevent accidental displacement and spillage. Coordination with an ostomy specialist may allow the performance of ostomy care, providing needed practice for the patient. Many GI conditions are chronic in nature, difficult to diagnose, and present with a perceived social stigma that may challenge the patient psychologically and socially.

Finally, therapists should also recognize the potential risk in hospitalized patients for an acute abdomen, a sudden nontraumatic disorder whose chief manifestation is abdominal pain. Initial physical therapy examination should determine the location, mode of onset, progression, and character of pain.[24,40] This information is critical because an acute abdomen requires rapid recognition, diagnosis, and, potentially, early surgery.[24,40,41] Examination findings may trigger consultation with the patient's nurses and physicians to initiate a more thorough examination.

Case Study

Mr. Taylor is a 52-year-old (y/o) male with a history of (h/o) GERD and Barrett's esophagus for over 25 years. The patient underwent an esophagectomy with gastric pull-up following an annual endoscopy that revealed esophageal cancer. Physical therapy was consulted to initiate ambulation and assist with discharge planning on postoperative day 1.

Patient/Client History

General Demographics, Social History, and Living Environment

Mr. Taylor is married, lives in a second-floor apartment, and has 1 son, who is 10 y/o. He is a manager in an automotive parts store.

General Health Status, Social/Health Habits, and Family History

Mr. Taylor denies smoking and limited alcohol use (1 to 2 drinks on the weekends).

Medical/Surgical History

Mr. Taylor is a 52 y/o male with >25 year h/o GERD and Barrett's esophagus and recent diagnosis of esophageal carcinoma. He underwent am esophageal pull-up and is 1 day post-surgery.

Current Conditions

Mr. Taylor is awake and complaining of pain and soreness in his stomach area and along the incision. The pain is rated a 6 out of 10. He has a nasal cannula running at 3 liters/minute, an NG tube, a right upper extremity (RUE) IV line for fluids and antibiotics, and a Foley catheter.

Activities and Participation

Mr. Taylor was independent in functional activities, ADLs, and instrumental activities of daily living (IADLs) prior to surgery. He states that he has not participated in any type of exercise program since playing spring and summer softball 5 years ago.

Other Clinical Tests

Abnormal laboratory findings: CBC revealed hemoglobin 10.4 g/dL, WBCs >11,500/mm^3, and electrolytes were sodium <130 mEq/L and potassium of 3.3 mEq/L. Laboratory findings are suggestive of either infection or related to cancer history. Hypokalemia and low sodium and edema suggest hypervolemic hyponatremia and may be related to IV fluids, GI loss, diminished intake, or underlying disease. The therapist should monitor the electrocardiogram (ECG) secondary to electrolyte abnormalities.

Systems Review

Cardiovascular and Pulmonary

Resting HR 96 beats per minute (bp)m, BP 110/85 mm Hg, respiratory rate (RR) 20 breaths/minute, and there are +2 edema in both ankles.

Integumentary

Mr. Taylor has an NG tube held in place by adhesive tape, RUE IV line, a Foley catheter, and a large thoracoabdominal surgical dressing with 2 drains. His skin appears to be dry and intact.

Musculoskeletal

Mr. Taylor could move bilateral upper extremities (BUEs) and lower extremities (BLEs) to command against gravity while lying in bed. Range of motion (ROM) was within normal limits (WNL).

Neuromuscular

There was no observed abnormal movement patterns and sensation was intact.

Communication, Affect, Cognition, Language, and Learning Style

Mr. Taylor is awake and alert and his primary language is English, but he can understand Spanish. He is receptive to physical therapy and states "I hope you can help me get home quickly."

Tests and Measures

Aerobic Capacity and Endurance

Mr. Taylor demonstrated expected vital responses for being 1 day following surgery and not being regularly active prior to hospital admission.

Assistive and Adaptive Devices

Recommend Mr. Taylor continue to progress his mobility using a rolling walker that allows him to maintain his forward leaning posture and reduce his abdominal pain.

Balance, Gait, and Mobility (Including Locomotion)

Bed mobility, supine to sit, and transfers sit to stand required minimal assistance of 1 (Functional Independence Measure [FIM] 4) and there was significant complaints of pain. Mr. Taylor was able to ambulate with the rolling walker 50 feet with minimal assistance of 1 (FIM 2). His static and dynamic balance was impaired, and he required the assistive device in standing and during ambulation to prevent loss of balance and falls. The Activity Measure for Post Acute Care (AM-PAC) basic mobility score was 16/24.

Circulation (Arterial, Venous, Lymphatic) and Ventilation/Respiration

Following ROM, MMT, bed mobility, and transfers to a bedside chair, the VS responses were HR increasing from 96 to 102 bpm, BP remained stable at 110/84 to 100/86 mm Hg. There was an initial drop in BP with upright activities that could be related to pain medications or prolonged bed rest and should improve with continued OOB activities. The tachycardia is expected secondary to pain.

Mr. Taylor had a stable RR at 24 breaths/minute and stable oxygen saturation (SpO_2) reading of 95% at rest and with activity. He has a weak cough, diminished breath sounds, and decreased chest wall expansion. These pulmonary findings combined with his complaints of pain increase his risk for pulmonary complications following GI surgery.

Mental Function

Mr. Taylor is awake, alert, and oriented x 4. He follows commands easily.

Muscle Performance)

Mr. Taylor has 5/5 muscle strength of BUE/BLE.

Pain

Mr. Taylor reported pain of 6/10 at rest and had an increase in pain with activity to 8/10. Although he reported a high degree of pain at rest, he fully participated in the therapy session. Recommend coordinating therapy with pain medication delivery.

Integumentary Integrity

Mr. Taylor presents with a large thoracoabdominal incision but no other wounds, redness, or skin breakdown are observed. The incision is closed with Steri-Strips (3M) and will heal by primary intention. There is minimal drainage observed. He presents with an NG tube, drains in incision, Foley catheter, and IV access in his right forearm.

Diagnosis

The patient presents with mild to moderate impairments related to sedentary lifestyle prior to surgery and the effects of a large thoracoabdominal surgical procedure for removal of esophageal cancer. His activity limitations include difficulty with bed mobility, transfers, and ambulation. Monitoring and coordination of pain management will be important. Therapist will also need to assess abdominal function and complaints as liquid and solid food is reintroduced.

Prognosis

Mr. Taylor should progress rapidly with therapy in conjunction with pain management and airway clearance and breathing exercises. He is motivated and participates fully in therapy. Discharge from the hospital to home is expected.

Interventions

The plan of care included breathing exercises (incentive spirometry), airway clearance (huff cough), and instruction to splint incision with coughing. Functional training included frequent transfers OOB and progressive ambulation. Patient instruction included visual inspect of his incision to observe for any redness or drainage. He was instructed to sit OOB for a minimum 6 hours (including meal times) per day and walk with floor staff TID (3 times/day). A rolling walker was left at the bedside. Mr. Taylor was treated 3 times/week to advance his mobility program, determine effectiveness of airway clearance, assess stair climbing prior to discharge home, and continue with patient education.

ICF Clinical Reasoning Tool Case Study Summary								
Health Condition								
HPI: Esophageal carcinoma, s/p esophagectomy with gastric pull-up; c/o nausea and dry heaves; leukocytosis, low Hb, hypernatremia (hypovolemic), and hypokalemia PMHx: GERD and Barrett's esophagus								
Precautions/Contraindications								
Precautions: Pain at rest along incision area and escalated with functional activities (coordinate pain management with RN/medical team); noted tachycardia (probably related to pain), monitor ECG for dysrhythmias related to hypokalemia; noted slight asymptomatic drop in BP with position change; Requires supplemental oxygen and has decreased breath sounds and weak cough, risk for pulmonary complications; universal precautions								
Body Structure and Function			*Activity/Task Limitations*			*Participation*		
Impairment/ Problem	*Tests and Measures*	*Intervention*	*Activity*	*Tests and Measures*	*Intervention*	*Participation*	*Tests and Measures*	*Intervention*
• Ineffective cough • Decreased chest wall movement • Decreased endurance • Pitting edema • Abnormal lab values • Pain	• Chest examination • ROM and MMT • Sensation • Edema/girth • VS including SpO_2 and ECG • Lab values • Pain/ numeric scale	• ACTs and breathing exercises: Huffing, splinted coughing, incentive spirometry • AROM exercises progressing to moderate to higher intensity resistance exercises • Education on ambulation safety with walker, positioning to decrease ankle edema and incision healing	• ADLs • Bed mobility • Transfers • Gait	• Functional task analysis, including stairs • AM-PAC "6 Clicks" • 2- or 6MWT • RPE	• Progressive functional retraining • Pain control	• Unable to return to work	• FACT-E	• Continue physical therapy services • Consult social worker and occupational therapist • Family meeting to discuss discharge plans

(continued)

ICF Clinical Reasoning Tool Case Study Summary (continued)

Personal Factors	*Other Considerations*	*Environmental Factors*
• Age: 56 y/o male • AAO x 4 • Primary language: English • Married, 1 son (10 y/o) • Employed as manager of automotive parts store • I with functional activities prior to surgery, but no regular exercise		Home: • 2nd floor apartment Hospital: • 3 L NC, bandage urinary catheter, NG tube, IV, large thoracoabdominal surgical dressing with drains, rolling walker

AAO = awake, alert, and oriented; ACTs = airway clearance techniques; c/o = complain of; FACT-E = Functional Assessment of Cancer Therapy-Esophagus; Hb = hemoglobin; HPI = history of present illness; I = independent; MWT = Minute Walk Test; NC = nasal cannula; NG = nasogastric; PMHx = past medical history; RN = registered nurse; s/p = status post.

Adapted from American Physical Therapy Association. *Guide to Physical Therapist Practice*. 3rd ed. http://www.apta.org/Guide/. Updated October 21, 2015. Accessed October 5, 2018 and *Towards a Common Language for Functioning, Disability and Health*. World Health Organization. www.who.int/classifications/icf/icfbeginnersguide.pdf. Published 2002. Accessed April 29, 2019.

Outcomes

At the time of the third physical therapy session, the NG tube, drains, Foley, and IV access have been removed and he has started a liquid diet. Mr. Taylor reports decreased abdominal and thoracic discomfort and rates his pain at 2/10. He reports flatulence but has not had a bowel movement. He is independent with bed mobility, transfers, and ambulates > 150 feet TID with supervision and no assistive device (FIM 7). He ascends/descends 12 steps with 1 rail with supervision (FIM 5). The AM-PAC score increased from 16 to 23/24. The plan is to discharge him from the hospital to his home with no additional therapy services.

Chapter Review Questions

1. The primary functions of the GI system include the following:
   a. Immune function and clearance of ketones
   b. Digestion and absorption
   c. Hyperalimentation and excretion
   d. Prevention of aspiration and key mineral preservation
2. Which of the following describes the pathology of GERD?
   a. Weakness of LES and reflux of gastric contents
   b. Damage to upper esophageal sphincter and disruption of muscular ring
   c. Irritation of pharyngeal reflex and aspiration of gastric contents
   d. Inappropriate relaxation of sigmoid sphincter
3. Possible signs and symptoms of GERD include the following:
   a. Hoarseness and pharyngeal spasm
   b. Dysphagia and heartburn
   c. Substernal and lower lumbar pain
   d. Nose bleeds and hematemesis
4. What are 2 possible factors that lead to the development of acute gastritis?
   a. Exposure to *Salmonella*, NSAIDs, ethanol
   b. Exposure to aspirin, pseudomonas, cystic fibrosis
   c. Exposure to parasites, stress, lupus
   d. Exposure to *H pylori*, sepsis, decreased intracranial pressure
5. Which of the following are primary indications for treating a patient with Crohn's disease?
   a. Deconditioning and functional limitations following palliative surgery
   b. Airway clearance following corticosteroid use
   c. Pain assessment and DVT prophylaxis
   d. Balance impairments from antidiarrheal agents

Answers: 1b, 2a, 3b, 4a, 5a

References

1. Guyton AC, Hall JE. *Textbook of Medical Physiology.* Philadelphia, PA: WB Saunders; 2000.
2. Rhoades RA, Tanner GA. *Medical Physiology.* Baltimore, MD: Lippincott Williams & Wilkins; 1995.
3. Junqueira LC, Carneiro J. *Basic Histology Text and Atlas.* 10th ed. New York, NY: McGraw-Hill; 2003.
4. Ahlman H,. Nilsson O. The gut as the largest endocrine organ in the body. *Ann Oncol.* 2001;12(suppl 2):S63-S68.
5. Gunawardene AR, Corfe BM, Staton CA. Classification and functions of enteroendocrine cells of the lower gastrointestinal tract. *Int J Exp Pathol.* 2011;92(4):219-231
6. Moore KL. *Clinically Oriented Anatomy.* Baltimore, MD: Lippincott Williams & Wilkins; 1995.
7. American College of Gastroenterology. *Clinical practice guidelines.* https://gi.org/guidelines. Accessed July 17, 2019.
8. The National Institute of Diabetes and Digestive and Kidney Diseases. www.niddk.nih.gov. Accessed June 2016.
9. Peery AF, Dellon ES, Lund J, et al. Burden of gastrointestinal disease in the United States: 2012 update. *Gastroenterology.* 2012;143(5):1179-1187.
10. Chandrasoma P, Taylor C. *Concise Pathology.* Norwalk, CT: Appleton & Lange; 1999.
11. Papadakis M, Rabow MW, McPhee SJ. *Current Medical Diagnosis and Treatment.* New York, NY: McGraw-Hill; 2016.
12. Friedman SL, McQuaid KR, Grendell JH. *Current Diagnosis and Treatment in Gastroenterology.* 2nd ed. New York, NY: Lange Medical Books; 2003.
13. Rubin E, Reisner HM, eds. The gastrointestinal tract. In: *Essential Pathology.* 6th ed. Philadelphia, PA: Lippincott Williams & Wilkins; 2014.
14. Merahn S. *PDxMD—Gastroenterology.* Philadelphia, PA: Elsevier Science; 2003.
15. Zwischenberger JB, Alpard SK, Orringer MB. Esophagus. In: Townsend CW, ed. *Sabiston Textbook of Surgery. The Biological Basis of Modern Surgical Practice.* 16th ed. Philadelphia, PA: WB Saunders; 2001.
16. Kahrilas PJ, Pandolfino JE. Gastroesophageal reflux disease and its complications, including Barrett's metaplasia. In: Feldman M, Friedman LS, Sleisenger MH, eds. *Sleisenger & Fordtran's Gastrointestinal and Liver Disease Pathophysiology/ Diagnosis/Management.* 7th ed. Philadelphia, PA: WB Saunders Co; 2003.
17. Berkow R. *The Merck Manual of Diagnosis and Therapy.* Rahway, NJ: MerckSharp & Dome Research Laboratories; 1987.
18. Conner CEHS. *The SAGES Manual. Fundamentals of Laparoscopy & GI Endoscopy.* New York, NY: Springer Verlag; 1999.
19. Stotland BR, Ginsber GG. Upper gastrointestinal bleeding. In: Lanken P, ed. *The Intensive Care Unit Manual.* Philadelphia, PA: WB Saunders Co; 2001.
20. Prantera C, Korelitz BI. *Crohn's Disease.* New York, NY: Marcel Dekker Inc; 1996.
21. Becker JM. Surgical therapy for ulcerative colitis and Crohn's disease. *Gastroenterol Clin North Am.* 1999;28:2.
22. Isolauri E, Rautava S, Kalliomäki M. Food allergy in irritable bowel syndrome: new facts and old fallacies. *Gut.* 2004;53(10):1391-1393.
23. Atkinson W, Sheldon TA, Shaath N, et al. Food elimination based on IgG antibodies in irritable bowel syndrome: a randomised controlled trial. *Gut.* 2004;53:1459-1464.
24. Doherty GM. *Current Diagnosis and Treatment: Surgery* New York, NY: McGraw-Hill; 2015.
25. Veronesi J. Inflammatory bowel disease. *RN.* 2003;66:38-46.
26. Kornbluth A, Sachar DB. Ulcerative colitis practice guidelines in adults. *Am J Gastroenterol.* 1997;92:2.
27. McPhee SJ, Hammer GD. *Pathophysiology of Disease. An Introduction to Clinical Medicine.* 6th Ed. New York, NY: McGraw-Hill; 2010.

28. Feldman M, Friedman LS, Sleisenger MS. *Sleisenger & Fordtran's Gastrointestinal and Liver Disease*. 10th ed. Philadelphia, PA: Elsevier; 2016.
29. Arias IM. *The Liver—Biology and Pathobiology*. 4th ed. Philadelphia, PA: Lippincott Williams & Wilkins; 2001.
30. Starr S, Hand H. Nursing care of chronic and acute liver failure. *Nursing Standard*. 2002;16:47-56.
31. Gines P, Cardenas A, Arroyo V, et al. Current concepts: management of cirrhosis and ascites. *N Engl J Med*. 2004;350:1646-1654.
32. Howard DE. Nonsurgical treatment of gallstone disease. *Gastroenterol Clin North Am*. 1999;28(1):133-144.
33. Glazer G, Ranson HC. *Acute Pancreatitis*. London, United Kingdom: Balliere Tindall; 1998.
34. Banks PA. Practice guidelines in acute pancreatitis. *Am J Gastroenterol*. 1997;92(3):377-386.
35. Lawrence VA, Hilsenbeck SG, Mulrow DC. Incidence and hospital stay for cardiac and pulmonary complications after abdominal surgery. *J Gen Intern Med*. 1995;10:671-678.
36. Aldren CP, Barr LC, Leach RD. Hypoxaemia and postoperative pulmonary complications. *Br J Surg*. 1991;78:1307-1308.
37. Schmidt GB. Prophylaxis of pulmonary complications following abdominal surgery, including atelectasis, ARDS, and pulmonary embolism. *Surg Annu*. 1977;9:29-73.
38. Oslen MF, Hahn I, Nordgren S, et al. Randomized controlled trial of prophylactic chest physiotherapy in major abdominal surgery. *Br J Surg*. 1997;84:1535-1538.
39. Thomas JA, McIntosh JM. Are incentive spirometry, intermittent positive pressure breathing, and deep breathing exercises effective in the prevention of postoperative pulmonary complications after upper abdominal surgery? A systematic overview and meta-analysis. *Phys Ther*. 1994;74:3-10.
40. Seidel HM, Ball JW, Dains JE, Benedict GW. *Mosby's Guide to Physical Examination*. St. Louis, MO: Mosby, Inc; 2003
41. Smith GC, Paterson-Brown S. The acute abdomen and intestinal obstruction. In: Garden OJ, Bradbury AW, Forsythe J, eds. *Principles and Practice of Surgery*. 4th ed. New York, NY: Churchill Livingstone; 2002.
42. Preventing obesity and chronic diseases through good nutrition and physical activity. National Center for Chronic Disease Prevention and Health Promotion. http://www.cdc.gov. Published 2003. Accessed June 25, 2004.
43. Ogden CL, Carroll MD, Fryar CD, Flegal KM. Prevalence of obesity among adults and youth: United States, 2011-2014. NCHS data brief, no 219. Hyattsville, MD: National Center for Health Statistics; 2015.
44. Fontaine KR, Barofsky I. Obesity and health-related quality of life. *Obesity Reviews*. 2001;2:173-182.
45. Richards MM, Adams TD, Hunt SC. Functional status and emotional well-being, dietary intake, and physical activity of severely obese subjects. *J Am Diet Assoc*. 2000;100:67-74.
46. Division of Nutrition, Physical Activity and Obesiity. nutrition, physical activity and obesity data, trends and maps. Centers for Disease Control and Prevention. http://www.cdc.gov/nccdphp/DNPAO/index.html. Published 2015. Accessed February 5, 2019.
47. Must A, Spadano J, Coakley EH, et al. The disease burden associated with overweight and obesity. *JAMA*. 1999;282:1523-1529.
48. Mokdad AH, Ford ES, Bowman BA, et al. Prevalence of obesity, diabetes, and obesity-related health risk factors, 2001. *JAMA*. 2003;289:76-79.
49. Finkelstein EA, Trogdon JG, Cohen JW, Dietz W. Annual medical spending attributable to obesity: payer-and service-specific. Estimates. *Health Affairs*. 2009;28(5):w822-w831.
50. Racette SB, Deusinger SS, Deusinger RH. Obesity: overview of prevalence, etiology, and treatment. *Phys Ther*. 2003;83:276-288.
51. *ACSM's Guidelines for Exercise Testing and Prescription*. 8th ed. Philadelphia, PA: Lippincott Williams & Wilkins; 2010.
52. Flegal KM, Carroll MD, Ogden CL, Johnson CL. Prevalence and trends in obesity among US adults, 1999–2000. *JAMA*. 2002;288:1723-1727.
53. Papasavas PK, Hayetian FD, Caushaj PF, et al. Outcome analysis of laparoscopic roux-en-Y gastric bypass for morbid obesity. *Surgical Endoscopy*. 2002;16:653-1657.

54. Postlewait RW, Johnson WD. Complications following surgery for duodenal ulcer in obese patients. *Arch Surg.* 1972;105:438-440.
55. Taylor RR, Kelly TM, Elliott CG, et al. Hypoxemia after gastric bypass surgery for morbid obesity. *Arch Surg.* 1985;120:1298-1302.
56. Livingston EH. Obesity and its surgical management. *Am J Surg.* 2002;184:103-113.
57. Flum DR, Dellinger EP. Impact of gastric bypass operation on survival: a population-based analysis. *J Am Coll Surg.* 2004;199:543-551.
58. Kaminsky J, Gadaleta D. A study of discrimination within the medical community as viewed by obese patients. *Obes Surg.* 2002;12:14-18.
59. Harvey E, Hill A. Health professionals views of overweight people and smokers. *Int J Obes.* 2001;25:1255-1261.
60. Hebl M, Xu J, Mason MF. Weighing the care: patient perceptions of physician care as a function of gender and weight. *Intern J Obesity.* 2003;27:269-275.
61. Sack S, Radler DR, Mairella KK, Touger-Decker R, Khan H. Physical therapists' attitudes, knowledge, and practice approaches regarding people who are obese. *Phys Ther.* 2009;89(8):804-815.
62. Teachman B, Brownaell K. Implicit anti fat bias among health professionals. Is anyone immune? *Intern J Obesity.* 2001;25:1525-1531.
63. National Task Force on the Prevention and Treatment of Obesity. Medical care for obese patients: advice for health care professionals. A*m Fam Physician.* 2002;65:81-88.
64. Abir F, Bell R. Assessment and management of the obese patient. *Crit Care Med.* 2004;32:87-91.
65. Deusinger SS, Deusinger RH, Racette SB. The obesity epidemic: health consequences and implications for physical therapy. *PT Magazine.* 2004;12:82-98.
66. Fischbach FT, Dunning MB. *A Manual of Laboratory and Diagnostic Tests.* Philadelphia, PA: Lippincott Williams & Wilkins; 2004.
67. Huether SE, McCance KL. *Understanding Pathophysiology.* St. Louis, MO: Mosby-Year Book Inc; 1996.
68. Perloff JK. *Physical Examination of the Heart and Circulation.* 3rd ed. Philadelphia, PA: WB Saunders; 2000.

Bibliography

American Physical Therapy *Association. Guide to Physical Therapist Practice.* 3rd ed. http://www.apta.org/Guide/. Updated October 21, 2015. Accessed October 5, 2018.

Deglin JH, Vallerand AH. *Davis's Drug Guide for Nurses.* 8th ed. Philadelphia, PA: FA Davis; 2003.

Karch AM. *Lippincott's Nursing Drug Guide.* Springhouse, PA: Lippincott Williams & Wilkins; 2004.

Marcus DA. Obesity and the impact of chronic pain. *Clin J Pain.* 2004;20: 186-191.

Okoro CA, Hootman JM, Strine TW, et al. Disability, arthritis, and body weight among adults 45 years and older. *Obesity Research.* 2004;12:854-861.

Ritter JM, Lewis LD, Mant TG. *Textbook of Clinical Pharmacology.* London, United Kingdom: Edward Arnold Co; 1995.

Spechler SJ. Peptic ulcer disease and its complications. In: Feldman M, Freidman LS, Sleisenger MH, eds. *Sleisenger & Fordtran's Gastrointestinal and Liver Disease.* 7th ed. Philadelphia, PA: Elsevier Science; 2002.

Thompson D, Edelsberg J, Colditz GA, et al. Lifetime health and economic consequences of obesity. *Arch Intern Med.* 1999;159:2177-2183.

Appendix A

Surgical Information: Obesity and Gastric Bypass Surgeries

Esther H. Bae, PT, DPT and Robin Stott-McNulty, MPT

Prevalence

The prevalence of obesity is increasing every year in the United States with more than 1/3 of adults being obese.[42,43] According to the Centers for Disease Control and Prevention, obesity has increased by more than 60% in the past 10 years, and approximately 93.3 million in 2015–2016 were obese.[42] According to the National Health and Nutrition Examination Survey (NHANES), prevalence of obesity was 39.8% among adults and 18.5% among youth in the United States during 2015–2016. The prevalence of obesity among middle-aged adults aged 40 to 59 was 42.8% and older adults aged 60 and over was 41%, which is higher than young adults aged 20 to 39 at 35.7%.[43] In the United States, about 300,000 deaths a year are attributed to obesity, making it second only to smoking as the most common preventable cause of death.[44] Obesity affects society in many different aspects, such as the cost and quality of health care and risk factors for other diseases.

The World Health Organization (WHO) uses the body mass index (BMI) to classify body weight and levels of obesity as noted in Table 11-21. BMI is defined as weight in kilograms divided by height in meters squared (kg/m^2).

Causes of Obesity/Risk Factors

Obesity is caused by many factors such as genetics, physiology, behavior, environment, culture, and socioeconomic status. Studies have shown that the severely obese population has a significantly higher intake of total fat and report lower activity levels than the normal weight population.[45] In 2014, 23.7% of adults in the United States did not engage in any leisure-time physical activity.[46] Inadequate amounts of physical activity and exercise are associated with requiring more medications, visiting physicians more often, and being hospitalized more frequently. It has been shown that obesity increases the risk of developing various health conditions, including type 2 diabetes, HTN, coronary heart disease, stroke, colon cancer, postmenopausal breast cancer, endometrial cancer, gallbladder disease, osteoarthritis, asthma, and obstructive sleep apnea.[47,48] As weight increases, so does the prevalence of health risks (Table 11-22) and higher BMIs are associated with reduced life expectancies.[44]

Impact on Health Care System

Obesity affects the cost of health care not only in direct medical cost but also in indirect costs. In 2000, the total cost of obesity in the United States was estimated to be $117 billion. Included in the $117 billion were $61 billion for direct medical costs and $56 billion for indirect costs.[42] Direct medical costs include preventive, diagnostic, and treatment services. Indirect costs include value of income lost from decreased productivity, restricted activity, absenteeism, and value of future income lost by premature death. The estimated annual medical cost of obesity in the United States was $147 billion in 2008 U.S. dollars; the medical costs for people who are obese were $1,429 higher than those of normal weight.[49]

Table 11-21

CLASSIFICATION OF WEIGHT USING BODY MASS INDEX

Classification	*Body Mass Index (kg/m^2)*
Underweight	<18.5
Normal range	18.5 to 24.9
Overweight	25.0 to 29.9
Obese Class I	30.0 to 34.9
Obese Class II	35.0 to 39.9
Obese Class III	>40.0

Adapted from Must A, Spadano J, Coakley EH, et al. The disease burden associated with overweight and obesity. *JAMA*. 1999;282:1523-1529

Table 11-22

CLASSIFICATION OF OVERWEIGHT AND OBESITY BY BODY MASS INDEX, WAIST CIRCUMFERENCE, AND ASSOCIATED DISEASE RISK

	Body Mass Index (kg/m^2)	*Obesity Class*	*Disease Risk (Relative to Normal Weight and Waist Circumference*	
			Men: ≤40 in (≤102 cm) **Women**: ≤35 in (≤88 cm)	**Men**: >40 in (≤102 cm) **Women**: >35 in (≤88 cm)
Underweight	<18.5			
Normal	18.5 to 24.9			
Overweight	15.0 to 29.9		Increased	High
Obesity	30.0 to 34.9 35.0 to 39.9	I II	High Very high	Very high Very high
Extreme Obesity	≥40	III	Extremely high	Extremely high

Reprinted from *The Practical Guide Identification, Evaluation, and Treatment of Overweight and Obesity in Adults*. National Heart, Lung, and Blood Institute's (NHLBI) Obesity Education Initiative in cooperation with the National Institute of Diabetes and Digestive and Kidney Diseases (NIDDK). NIH Publication 00-4084. Oct. 2000.

Weight Reduction

Weight reduction is associated with an improved health-related quality of life (HRQoL). Weight loss induced by surgical intervention improves HRQoL as measured by the Short Form 36 (SF-36). Studies have demonstrated that severely obese people who lose weight from surgical interventions tend to begin or return to work. Additionally, modest weight reduction using lifestyle modification of moderately obese people can enhance HRQoL.[44]

The goals for treatment are to achieve and maintain clinically significant weight loss. Weight loss reduces the risk of obesity-related diseases, impairments, and functional limitations, and weight losses of 5% to 10% of initial body weight produce health benefits.[504] There are many different weight management techniques in treating obesity including proper nutrition, regular physical activity and exercise, behavior modification, pharmacological agents, and surgery. The method for losing weight depends on the individual's needs.

Prescribing exercise for the obese individual will be different than for a normal weight individual. The goal for the obese individual is to increase caloric expenditure at the low end of the target HR range for a longer duration. The adult should aim to expend 300 to 500 kcal per session and 1000 to 2000 kcal per week. The exercise program should progress to increasing the intensity to bring the target HR to the higher range. Different modes of exercise can include walking, cycling, and water exercise. Exercise precautions include activities that exacerbate pain, avoiding excess stress on joints, and any restrictions prescribed by the individual's physician.[51]

Bariatrics (Medical Treatment of Obesity)

Clinically severe obesity is defined as an individual with a BMI of 40 kg/m^2 (Obese Class III), which is estimated as 100 pounds overweight (see Table 11-21). An increasing number of people in the United States are falling into this category. Between 2013 and 2016, the prevalence of obesity with BMI greater than 40kg/m^2 was 7.7%, which is a significant increase from 2.9% from 1988 to 1994.[46,52] More people are turning to surgical intervention for long-term weight control. The age of gastric bypass patients range from mid 20s to mid 60s, with about 70% being female.[53]

The National Institutes of Health (NIH) established criteria for bariatric surgery patients in 1991. The criteria states that patients must be selected carefully and must have clinically severe obesity. Clinically severe obesity is defined as a patient with a BMI of 40 or greater (approximately 100 pounds overweight) or 35 or greater with obesity-related comorbidities (eg, diabetes, HTN, sleep apnea). The patient must have failed less invasive weight loss measures and be at risk for obesity-associated illness.

Comprehensive preoperative screening and patient education ensure that appropriate candidates are considered for surgery. The initial consultation with the surgeon includes a complete history and physical examination, nutrition screening, and education regarding the surgical procedure. Other consultants may include a psychologist and nutritionist. In addition, patients must be medically cleared by a combination of internal medicine, cardiology, endocrinology, and pulmonary medicine. Periodically, patients must undergo a physical therapy evaluation prior to surgery. Some patients are also seen by vascular surgery to have an inferior vena cava (IVC) filter placed at the time of surgery to prevent blood clots from traveling to the lungs. The time frame from initial visit until surgery can take up to 2 months.

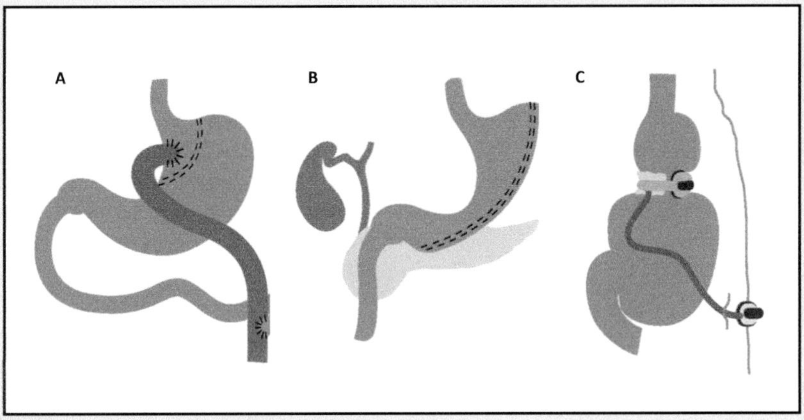

Figure 11-9. Types of bariatric surgical procedures. (A) Roux-en-Y gastric bypass, (B) vertical sleeve gastrectomy, and (C) laparoscopic adjustable gastric band. (Adapted with permission from Arterburn DE, Courcoulas AP. Bariatric surgery for obesity and metabolic conditions in adults. *BMJ*. 2014;349:g3961. doi: 10.1136/bmj.g3961)

Surgical Procedures

The 3 most common bariatric surgical procedures include roux-en-Y gastric bypass, sleeve gastrectomy, and laparoscopic adjustable gastric band (Figure 11-9). These procedures can be performed laparoscopically, hand-assisted, or using an open technique.

The gastric bypass with roux-en-Y anastamosis has become the gold standard for bariatric surgery in the United States. This surgery includes the creation of a small gastric pouch attached to a limb of small intestine. This creates a restrictive component (patients can only consume a small amount of food) and a malabsorbtive component (the duodenum is bypassed). This combination results in excellent weight loss and resolution of comorbidities.

Sleeve gastrectomy involves removing about 75% of the stomach leaving a sleeve. No intestines are removed or bypassed during the sleeve gastrectomy.

The vertical banded gastroplasty is a version of bariatric surgery that is an option for some patients who are not candidates for gastric bypass surgery due to technical complexity or existing medical conditions. This procedure consists of the creation of a small stomach pouch with an inflatable band placed at the proximal part of the stomach. This results in restriction of the amount of food one can consume and, thus, subsequent weight loss.

Postoperative Process

After the procedure, patients remain in the hospital for a short period of time (usually 4 days). This population has unique issues with cardiovascular, pulmonary, and thromboembolic complications postoperatively. Postlewait and Johnson[54] found that the mortality rate in obese patients was 6.6% compared with 2.6% in non-obese patients undergoing GI surgery. Patients with clinically severe obesity have a higher incidence of comorbidities, including diabetes mellitus, HTN, left ventricular hypertrophy, and GERD. They experience an increase in cardiopulmonary complications such as obesity-hypoventilation syndrome, obstructive sleep apnea syndrome, pulmonary hypertension, and right ventricular failure. All of these factors make this patient population high risk.[54]

Table 11-23

COMORBIDITY IMPROVEMENTS FOLLOWING SURGERY

Diabetes	95%
Hypertension	92%
Cardiac function	95%
Osteoarthritis	82%
Sleep apnea	75%
Elevated cholesterol	97%
Gastroesophageal reflux	98%
Stress incontinence	87%

The table lists the percentage of patients whose health problems related to obesity resolve or improve within 5 years of surgery.

Adapted from Wittgrove AC, Clark GW. Laparoscopic gastric bypass Roux-en-Y—500 patients: technique and results with 3–60 month follow-up. *Obesity Surgery.* 2000;10:233-239.

Bariatric patients can experience postoperative complications such as pain, hypoxemia, and atelectasis. In these patients, postoperative pain limits mobility and the ability to breathe deeply. As a result of atelectasis, 75% of patients will exhibit arterial oxygen pressure less than 60 mm Hg after open gastric bypass surgery.[55] For these patients, early mobilization and encouraging deep breathing or the use of the incentive spirometer is vital.

Follow-up visits are scheduled for 1 week, 2 months, 6 months, and annually following surgery. These visits are a combined meeting with the nurse practitioner, surgeon, and nutritionist. Patients are also encouraged to continue attending support groups postoperatively because both they and patients new to the group benefit from this social interaction.

Surgical interventions are effective and safe for weight loss. Not only do patients, on average, lose 70% of their excess body weight 12 to 18 months following surgery, but patients' obesity-related health problems, such as type 2 diabetes, obstructive sleep apnea, asthma, HTN, elevated cholesterol, and degenerative joint disease,[56] are significantly improved or resolved within 1 to 5 years from surgery (Table 11-23). A significant proportion of gastric bypass patients are able to discontinue or decrease medications to treat obesity-related comorbidities.[52] Long-term survival rates are favorable. One study documented a 91% 10-year survival rate after a bariatric procedure.[57]

Patients also experience a significant improvement in their quality of life. Between 3 and 6 months following surgery, patients often describe a sudden increase in energy. With this newfound energy, they are able to participate in family activities and enjoy more productive careers.

Prejudice and Attitude

Clinically obese people often experience discrimination and abuse in society; however, most obese patients do not expect mistreatment by health care professionals.[58] Obese people might believe that health care professionals better understand the factors contributing to obesity and would be more sensitive to their condition; however, studies have shown that attitudes toward obese people by physicians were neutral to negative.[59] Physicians have noted that they spend less time with obese patients and are more likely to attribute medical problems to the patient's obesity as a catch-all etiology.[60] Past studies have also shown that health care professionals associated obese patients with poor hygiene, hostility, and laziness.[56] It should be noted that physical therapists have neutral attitudes toward the obese population.[61]

Hebl and Xu[60] found that a minority of physicians will discuss weight loss and nutrition issues with obese and overweight patients, believing that many could not lose weight. Relatedly, only 20.4% felt competent in providing weight loss interventions to patients who are obese, avoiding this aspect of patient education.[61] Studies have also shown that while many health care professionals are supportive of the conditions of obese patients, the majority do not have appropriately sized gowns, sphygmomanometers, examination tables, or chairs for their obese patients. Despite the fact that the patients in this study were not blatantly discriminated against, the lack of easily attainable equipment for obese patients shows a lack of consideration and may be considered prejudicial.[54] Making simple accommodations may make obese patients feel more comfortable and more likely to seek health care.[662,63]

The negative attitudes of health care professionals may initiate a vicious cycle for obese patients. Health care professionals treat obese patients less favorably causing obese patients to treat themselves poorly. Obese patients may respond negatively toward this unfavorable treatment, in turn reinforcing the negative attitudes of health care professionals. Obese patients may avoid seeking any health care based on their negative experiences contributing to the elevated mortality rate of this population.[60]

If physical therapists realize that they have biases and that they are affecting the quality of care delivered, then they may be able to change the way they act toward obese patients. A method that physical therapists can use to evaluate whether their biases are affecting treatments is the use of patient satisfaction surveys.

The Role of Physical Therapists

Managing and supporting patients who undergo gastric bypass surgery takes a collaborative multidisciplinary team approach starting at the initial examination, continuing throughout the hospital stay and recovery. It is important that a physical therapist is involved in each phase of bariatric care. The evaluation of preoperative functional status is critical for identifying those patients who may require more intensive physical therapy. Patients who are wheelchair dependent, already using assistive devices, limited to household mobility, or have joint problems inhibiting mobility have preoperative safety risks, experience a longer recovery phase, have more postoperative pulmonary complications, less postoperative mobility, and could require further rehabilitation after acute care. A physical therapist who examines and evaluates these patients preoperatively can make immediate recommendations for appropriate assistive devices to improve safety and teach therapeutic exercises to strengthen muscles and improve mobilization in preparation for surgery.

Postoperative examinations by a physical therapist are suggested on all gastric bypass patients. The goal of the physical therapist is to assess patient needs, develop a plan of care, facilitate safe mobilization, and identify discharge recommendations.

The physical therapist collects the following information on the initial evaluation.

Social History

- **Support systems**: Identify who the patient's significant others are and what role they will play in his or her recovery
- **Living environment**: House or apartment, location of stairs inside and outside the home, and other factors, such as presence of stair railings, spiral, width and height, and covering of stairs
- **Personal hygiene**: Location of and ability to use bathrooms or availability of commode. Identify patient's bathing habits at home and ability to use shower, tubs, or sponge bathing.
- **Functional status**: Identify assistive devices used and performance of ADLs preoperatively. Ability to manage outside the home and normal means of transportation.
- **Sleep habits**: Identify where patient slept preoperatively (eg, bed, couch, recliner chair), use of bi-level positive airway pressure machine, hours he or she slept, and use of medications for sleep.

Past Medical History

The physical therapist performs a thorough chart review identifying health history, medication history, and psychosocial factors. This information is used to direct the physical assessment performed, planning and monitoring of interventions, and development of plan for patient education.

Systems Review

- **Cardiovascular/pulmonary assessment**: Measure the resting HR, BP, and RR to obtain a baseline status prior to mobilization. Oscillometric BP cuffs that encircle at least 75% of the arm should be used.[64] Reliable BP readings can also be obtained from the wrist or ankle.[65] This is important because most standardized BP cuffs will not fit properly around the bicep of bariatric patients. Auscultate heart and lung sounds and compare to previously documented assessments. Document and report any changes or concerns.
- **Musculoskeletal**: Assess gross ROM and range of strength. Identify bony or soft tissue restrictions and any abnormal movement patterns.
- **Neuromuscular**: Assess and identify any abnormalities with sensation. Static and dynamic balance should also be assessed in sitting and standing positions. Mobility is assessed as well, including transfers and ambulation. This assessment will be performed over multiple treatment sessions based on patient's ability to mobilize.
- **Integumentary**: The excessive body weight puts this patient population at risk for increased injury to the skin over pressure areas and nerve injuries during the operative and postoperative periods. Brachial plexus and sciatic nerve palsies have been reported. Stretch injuries may be caused by either extreme abduction of the arms or the excessive upright positioning of the patient's outstretched arms, both of which can put stress on the brachial plexus. The sciatic nerve, lateral femoral cutaneous nerve, and ulnar nerve are also susceptible to traction injuries. Ulnar neuropathy has been associated with increased BMI. In a retrospective analysis from the Mayo Clinic, 29% of patients with ulnar neuropathy in their series had a BMI >38 kg/m^2.[60] A neurology consultation

should be obtained when a nerve injury is suspected. Most postoperative nerve injuries will resolve spontaneously. Perform careful inspection of the skin to identify ulcers, tears, and pressure areas. Skin folds need to be inspected for breakdown and infections. Assess drains sites, wounds, and areas of edema. Edema is often mistaken for adipose tissue.

Tests and Measures

Important tests and measures for this population include aerobic capacity and endurance, such as pre- and post-activity vital signs, because the patient will not be able to tolerate a standardized exercise test protocol. The therapist should also observe the patient for cardiovascular and pulmonary signs and symptoms of increased oxygen demand, such as dyspnea, increased RR, patient's perception on exertion scales (eg, Borg scale), and patient reports of lightheadedness, angina, excessive perspiration, or sudden pallor.

Anthropometric characteristics may be helpful in evaluating the patient to compose a plan of care. These measurements include weight and height to obtain a BMI and objective assessments of edema.

Pain should always be assessed at rest and with activity. The pain analog scale (rating pain from 0 to 10) is useful to objectify the patient's pain. Location of the pain should be documented as well to differentiate between incisional pain, referred pain, or any new complaints of pain.

Mobilization

Early mobilization is critical in this patient population, but it can be very challenging and time consuming. It requires a team approach and must include involvement of the patient. Based on the examination and evaluation, the therapist identifies a plan for mobilization and secures the proper resources. The therapist must discuss the treatment plan with the patient, listen to suggestions or concerns of the patient, and modify the plan as appropriate. A key to early mobilization is to develop a trusting relationship with the patient to minimize patient anxiety. Safety for the staff and the patient is a primary concern. Securing the proper number of professional staff and having appropriate equipment is very important. The number of staff and type of equipment needed should be based on the patient's preoperative functional status, weight, BMI, and current clinical condition. The physical therapist acts as the team leader directing the other staff and must be trained in the use of the equipment.

Mobilization and ambulation should begin as early postoperatively as possible, with the goal of having the patient at baseline functional status at time of discharge. Common considerations and suggestions to aide in the mobilization of the obese patient are provided in Tables 11-24 through 11-27.

Monitoring the Patient During the Physical Therapy Session

Vital signs (HR, BP, RR, SpO_2, and perceived exertion) must be monitored throughout the session because it may influence the physical therapist's plan of care. If the patient complains of dyspnea or presents with signs of respiratory compromise, proceed cautiously during physical activities. "Central adiposity may be responsible for mechanical restrictions of breathing particularly in sitting or supine positions, even in the absence of pulmonary disease."[65] The physical therapist should be aware of patterns of pain or postural dysfunction that are consistent with long-term stress on weightbearing joints in these patients.[65]

Table 11-24

Things to Consider Before Getting the Patient out of Bed

- When was the last time the patient was medicated for pain?
- Would an overhead trapeze help the patient to maneuver in bed?
- Is there an air mattress on the bed?
- Do you have the appropriate chair to place the patient into, and will he or she fit?
- Is the chair too low to the ground, making it difficult for the patient to get out of it?
- What if the patient has to go to the bathroom? Could you get the patient to the bathroom or is there a commode in the room?
- How long should the patient be OOB?
- What is the plan for getting the patient back to bed? Who will be available to assist?

Table 11-25

Assisting the Patient From Supine to Sitting Position

Always utilize available equipment. If the patient is in a bed that converts into a chair, place bed in sitting position. Have the patient come forward and make sure the feet can touch the ground.

Minimal assistance: If the patient is able to get to the edge of bed with minimal assistance, then the air mattress should be deflated prior to mobilization to allow the patient to move more easily. Use of cloth under pads or draw sheets is often necessary to assist the patient to get in a sitting position.

Moderate to maximum assistance: When the patient requires this level of assistance, the therapist must utilize good body mechanics to reduce the chance of injury. Encourage the patient to assist with mobility. The therapist must make sure the patient does not attempt to pull on any of the care providers. Place bed in semi-Fowler's position, one person assists in moving legs to side of bed while another person uses a gait belt to bring the patient to a sitting position. Weight of fat and skin around midsection may alter the center of gravity with a forward motion, so the therapist must be positioned in front to support the patient.

Caution: If the patient is brought to a sitting position too far near the foot of the bed, some beds may tip.

Education

Educating the patient on pressure-relieving techniques is important. Patients should be educated on the frequent performance of deep breathing or incentive spirometry and LE exercises. Education should include limiting activities that cause friction and shearing of skin. Patients should be advised to begin an exercise regimen, including a walking program, prior to discharge.

Table 11-26 ASSISTING THE PATIENT FROM SIT TO STAND
Before getting the patient to a standing position, the therapist must assess the height of the patient and the lowest height of the bed. The patient's feet have to completely touch the floor so the patient can successfully return his or her buttocks back on the bed surface. If the patient is too short, the therapist will need to have the patient stand on a stool that can support the body weight. Place gait belt around the lower back or mid buttocks, take up the slack, and secure a tight grip. Follow the 90/90 rule. You must maintain hip/knee/trunk ratio to prevent a potentially dangerous situation. Always have the patient scoot forward at the hip; avoid having the patient slide his or her hips forward. **Minimal assistance:** Place walker in front of patient, therapist and another staff member on either side of patient, each gripping an end of the gait belt. Assist patient to standing position. **Moderate to maximum assistance:** Same as for minimal assistance, except an additional therapist is needed to block the knees to prevent buckling. Perform sit-to-stand transfer 3 times before proceeding to ambulation. If the patient is a total dependent transfer, use a total lift machine designed to support the weight of the patient.

Table 11-27 ASSISTING THE PATIENT WITH TRANSFER/AMBULATION
Have the patient march in place several times using the walker. Have the patient take 2 or 3 steps with the walker while the therapist assesses the gait. Progress to stand pivot transfer. Make sure the patient has a chair to transfer to and avoid chairs that are too low to the ground. Getting the patient out of the chair will often be more challenging than getting him or her out of bed. Be sure to have at minimum the same team/resource available to return the patient to bed. While patient is up, make sure he or she is in upright position have him or her complete therapeutic exercise program (eg, upper extremity D1 and D2 proprioceptive neuromuscular facilitation patterns with breathing exercises incorporated for pulmonary issues).

Conclusion

Obesity is a chronic health condition that is reaching epidemic proportions, especially in the United States. The impact on the individual, the health care system, and society becomes more evident every day. The number of bariatric surgical procedures is increasing, and success depends on a multidisciplinary approach to the care of these patients. Physical therapists are an integral part of this team. Physical therapists must understand that they will be caring for obese patients in every health care setting and must develop multiple strategies for treating this patient population.

Appendix B

Pharmacological Information: Gastrointestinal Disease and Disorders Pharmacology

Antidiarrheals

Action

Antidiarrheals provide control and symptomatic relief from chronic and acute nonspecific diarrhea. These medications slow GI motility, enhance absorption of intestinal fluids, or provide bulk to stools.

Side Effects

CNS: Dizziness, confusion, drowsiness, headache
CV: Tachycardia
GI: Constipation, fullness, urinary retention
Miscellaneous: Allergic reactions

Common Medications

Kaopectate, Immodium, Maalox (loperamide); Logen, Lomotil, Lonox (diphenoxylate/atropine); Pepto-Bismol (bismuth subsalicylate); De-Nol (colloidal bismuth subcitrate); FiberCon, Fiberall (polycarbophil)

Antiemetics

Action

Antiemetics manage nausea and vomiting associated with motion sickness, surgery, anesthesia, chemotherapy, and radiation therapy. Drugs may act by antihistamine, anticholinergic, or serotonin blockage with subsequent CNS depression.

Side Effects

CNS: Sedation, confusion, disorientation, fatigue
CV: Brady- and tachycardia, hyper- and hypotension, palpitations
GI: Constipation, dry mouth
Miscellaneous: Allergic reactions, rash, photosensitivity

Common Medications

Compazine (prochlorperzine); Anergan, Phenazine, Phenergan (promethazine); Dimetabs, Dramamine (dimenhydrinate); Kytril (granisetron); Zofran (ondansetron)

Antacids

Action

Antacids promote healing of gastric ulcers by neutralizing gastric acid. Other proposed benefits include stimulation of mucus and bicarbonate secretion, binding of bile salts, enhanced gastric blood flow, and inhibition of pepsin activity. The treatment of PUD with antacids, generally, is less convenient, palatable, and effective for the long-term control of gastric acidity.

Side Effects

GI: Belching, abdominal fullness or distension, diarrhea (magnesium salts), constipation (aluminum salts)
Miscellaneous: Alkolosis, hypermagnesemia (magnesium salts), hypophosphatemia (aluminum salts)

Common Medications

Magnesium and aluminum hydroxide: Maalox, Mylanta
Calcium carbonate: Tums, Rolaids

Proton Pump Inhibitors

Action

The parietal cells of the gastric mucosa produce gastric acid through the action of the proton pumps on the cell membrane. The proton pump inhibitors are a class of drugs that decrease gastric acid secretion through inhibition of the proton pump.

Side Effects

CNS: Dizziness, drowsiness, fatigue, weakness, headache
CV: Chest pain
GI: Abdominal pain, constipation, diarrhea, nausea, vomiting, flatulence
Miscellaneous: Itching, rash, dry mouth

Common Medications

Prilosec (omeprazole), Nexium (esomeprazole), Prevacid (lansoprazole), Protonix (pantoprazole), Aciphex (rabeprazole)

Histamine-Receptor Blockers

Action

Histamine$_2$ (H_2) receptors are found in the heart, blood vessels, brain, and stomach. Stimulation of stomach H_2 receptors leads to enhanced gastric acid secretion. H_2 antagonists or blockers inhibit the action of histamine at the H_2 receptors of the stomach, inhibiting gastric acid secretion and reducing total pepsin output.

Side Effects

CNS: Dizziness, somnolence, headache, confusion, hallucinations, peripheral neuropathy, symptoms of brain stem dysfunction (eg, dysarthria, ataxia, diplopia)
CV: Cardiac arrhythmias, arrest, hypotension (intravenous use)
GI: Diarrhea
Hematologic: Increases in plasma creatinine, serum transaminase
Miscellaneous: Impotence (reversible with drug withdrawal), gynecomastia (long-term treatment), rash, vasculitis, pain at intramuscular injection site

Common Medications

Tagamet (cimetidine), Pepcid (famotidine), Axid (nizatidine), Zantac (ranitidine)

Prostaglandin Analogs

Action

Inhibit gastric acid secretion, stimulate mucus, and bicarbonate secretion from the GI mucosa, and increase mucosal blood flow.

Side Effects

CNS: Headache
CV: Frequent diarrhea, abortifacient actions
GI: Abdominal pain, diarrhea, dyspepsia, nausea, vomiting

Common Medications

Cytotec (misoprostol)

Laxatives

Action

Laxatives provide short-term relief of constipation and prevent straining; used to evacuate the bowel for diagnostic procedures and to remove ingested poisons from the lower GI tract. These medications increase the water content of stool and increase intestinal peristalsis.

Side Effects

CV: Dizziness
GI: Excessive bowel activity, perianal irritation, abdominal cramps, fullness
Miscellaneous: Weakness, cathartic dependence

Common Medications

Lactulose; FiberCon, Fiberall (polycarbophil); Metamucil (psyllium); Fleet (bisacodyl); Colace, Correctol (docusate); magnesium chloride/citrate

CV = cardiovascular.

Chapter 12

Genitourinary Diseases and Disorders

David Fichandler, MSPT, CLT and Daniel J. Malone, PT, PhD, CCS

The genitourinary (GU) system is not a common source for acute care physical therapy referral, although management of patients with incontinence and pelvic floor issues are becoming a more common population in the outpatient setting. Many of the diseases and conditions associated with GU disorders are curable and often transient. However the acute onset and aggressive nature of symptoms may lead to rapid changes in independence with functional activities and activities of daily living (ADLs) necessitating referral to physical therapy services. The goals of this chapter are to introduce the more common GU disorders, with an emphasis on renal disease, describe the diagnostics and medical management, and illustrate the role of physical therapy services in the management of these patients in the acute care setting.

Overview

The GU system, consisting of the organs for reproduction and the urinary system, are grouped together because of anatomic proximity and embryological origin.[1] The primary components of the GU system include the kidneys, ureters, bladder, and urethra. Secondary components include the prostate, pelvic floor muscles, and genitals.

Anatomy and Physiology of the Genitourinary System

The urinary system is responsible for waste product removal, fluid, electrolyte, and acid-base balance, conservation of nutrients and red blood cell (RBC) production. Blood is constantly filtered at the kidneys and waste products and excess body water are removed to form urine, which is transported out of the kidneys via the **ureter**, a long muscular, contractile tube. The ureters empty the urine into the **bladder** for storage until elimination. The bladder accumulates up to 2 cups of urine in normal

Malone DJ, Bishop KL, eds. *Acute Care Physical Therapy: A Clinician's Guide, Second Edition* (pp 511-538).

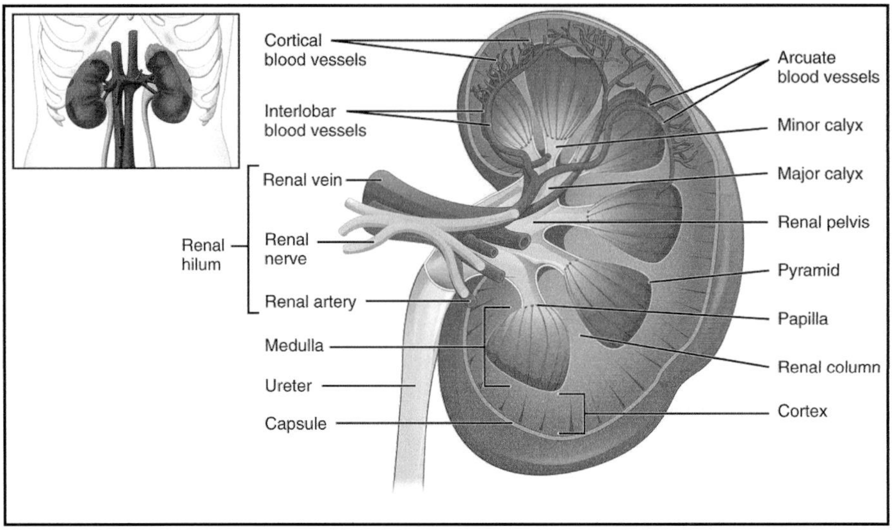

Figure 12-1. Structures of the outer cortex and inner medulla of the kidney.

health before it contracts and releases urine for excretion via the **urethra**. The urethra then excretes urine out of the body via the **genitalia**.[2-4]

Renal System

The kidney is responsible for maintaining the volume and composition of the body's fluids through reabsorption of water, sodium, and other compounds; regulation of electrolytes, acid-base status, and blood pressure (BP); production and secretion of hormones including erythropoietin, activated Vitamin D (calcitriol), renin, and aldosterone; and excretion of metabolic waste products, such as urea and foreign substances, including many medications.[5-7] Anatomically, the kidneys are paired organs located along the posterior wall of the abdomen along either side of the vertebral column. The kidney can be divided into an outer region, the cortex, and an inner region, the medulla (Figure 12-1). The cortex and medulla contain the nephrons, the functional unit of the kidney. Each kidney contains approximately 1.2 million nephrons where the functions of filtration, absorption, secretion, and excretion occur.[7] The kidneys include approximately 10 to 18 conical renal pyramids, which begin at the corticomedullary border and contain the tubules that collect urine for passage to the minor calyx and, eventually, the major calyx and collecting ducts (see Figures 12-1 and 12-2). Renal blood flow is approximately 25% of the cardiac output highlighting the important role of the kidneys in homeostasis, as well as their high metabolic demand. Upwards of 180 L/day of blood is filtered with reabsorption of 99% of the filtrate to maintain homeostasis. The collecting ducts of the nephrons drain into the ureters leading to the bladder.[5-7] Kidney dysfunction impacts many other organ systems in the body as listed in Table 12-1. Common renal disorders are detailed in the following section.

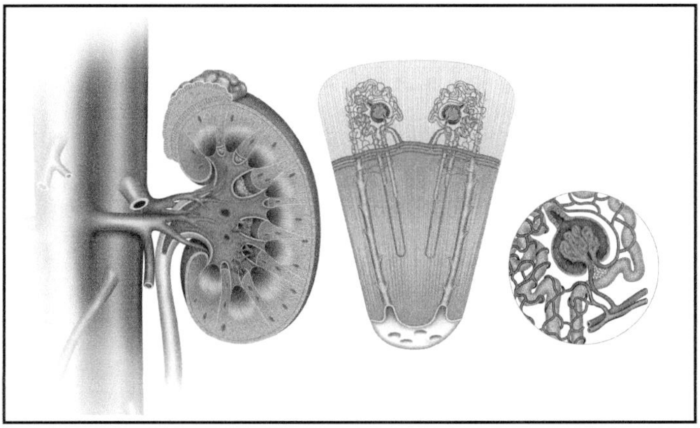

Figure 12-2. Interior structures of the kidney showing a renal pyramid containing the nephron and a close-up of the glomerulus. (Alexilusmedical/Shutterstock.com)

Table 12-1

Clinical Manifestations of Renal Failure

General: Nausea, vomiting, weakness, lethargy, hiccups
Gastrointestinal (GI): Anorexia, nausea/vomiting, gastritis, mucosal ulceration, GI bleeding
Cardiovascular: Hypertension (HTN), coronary artery disease (CAD), pericarditis chest pain, hyperkalemic electrocardiogram (ECG) changes
Respiratory: Pulmonary edema, pleural effusions, pleural rub
Neuromuscular: Fatigue/lethargy, sleep disorders, headache, lethargy, muscular irritability/myoclonus, peripheral neuropathy, seizures, coma
Metabolic and endocrine: Glucose intolerance, hyperlipidemia, sex hormone disturbances causing decreased libido, impotence, amenorrhea
Fluid, electrolyte, and acid-base disturbances: Usually salt and water retention, but may be sodium loss with dehydration, metabolic acidosis, hyperkalemia, hypermagnesemia, hypocalcemia/hypercalcemia, hyperphosphatemia
Dermatologic: Pallor, hyperpigmentation, pruritus, ecchymoses, uremic frost-crystallization of urea on skin
Skeletal abnormalities: Renal osteodystrophy resulting in osteomalacia
Hematologic: Anemia, abnormal platelets, increased bleeding and bruising, white blood cell (WBC) dysfunction/immunocompromise
Psychosocial functions: Personality and behavior changes, alteration in cognition

Health Conditions of the Genitourinary System

Glomerulonephritis

The glomerulus is a specialized tuft of capillaries, leading to the tubules of the nephrons, and is essential for filtering blood passing through the arterioles of the kidney (see Figure 12-2). **Glomerulonephritis** leads to alterations in capillary permeability and renal blood flow modifying glomerular filtration and renal function. Glomerulonephritis is caused by many factors, including immunologic abnormalities (eg, Berger's disease, Goodpasture syndrome), infections (eg, streptococcal organisms, endocarditis), drugs and toxins (eg, cyclosporine), vascular disorders (eg, atherosclerosis, thrombus), and systemic diseases (eg, systemic lupus erythematosus [SLE], hepatitis B).[8] Glomerulonephritis is the most common cause of chronic kidney disease (CKD) and end-stage renal disease (ESRD) and can be categorized in multiple ways, including progression (ie, acute, rapidly progressive, chronic, diffuse) or pathologic lesion (ie, diffuse, focal, segmental, mesangial, membranous, sclerotic, proliferative, crescentic).[8,9] Diagnosis of glomerulonephritis is confirmed by **urinalysis** and renal biopsy. A urinalysis involves checking the appearance, concentration, and content of urine. Urine is composed of water, urea from the degradation of proteins, electrolytes (chloride, sodium, and potassium), creatinine, and small amounts of other organic and inorganic chemicals. Urine output depends upon fluid intake but averages approximately 800 to 2000 mL per day. Urine is generally clear, and color may vary from pale yellow ("straw-colored") to dark amber. Urine color is a general indication of the patient's fluid status with the darker the urine indicating dehydration and a more concentrated urine. Milky or cloudy urine usually indicates abnormal elements, such as RBCs, WBCs, or bacteria. Additionally, a urinalysis will examine odor, turbidity, specific gravity, and concentrations of glucose, ketones, RBC, WBC, bilirubin and urobilinogen, protein, and nitrites. Urinalysis can be performed with a small sample or a 24-hour collection. Therapists should note that a 24-hour collection is dependent upon accurate collection of the entire output volume for the final analysis.

Proteinuria and Nephrotic Syndrome

Proteinuria is excessive amounts of protein ($\geq$3.5 g day) in the urine. **Nephrotic syndrome** is characterized by increased glomerular permeability leading to increased protein movement from the blood into the urine. Trace quantities of protein are normal in the urine, but increasing concentrations are indicative of kidney dysfunction.[2,3,10] Common disorders that cause proteinuria include diabetes mellitus, HTN, kidney failure, and cardiovascular disease. Patients with proteinuria are at increased risk of developing **nephroliathiasis**, kidney stones.

Proteinuria results in foamy urine and with continued protein excretion, peripheral edema will develop due to impaired vascular absorption of fluids that have leaked into the interstitium at the level of the capillaries. The liver compensates for the protein loss by increasing production of albumin and other hepatic proteins, triglycerides, and cholesterol. Unfortunately, this leads to hypercoagulability states and atherosclerosis. Proteinuria is diagnosed by urinalysis, and blood testing will be performed to assess creatinine and blood urea nitrogen (BUN) levels as indicators of kidney function. Treatment for proteinuria is directed at the underlying cause and may include diuretics, steroids, and albumin replacement. Dietary modifications include fat and salt restriction.

Table 12-2

Common Causes of Chronic Kidney Disease

• Diabetes • HTN, prolonged and severe • Glomerulopathies • Interstitial nephritis	• Hereditary renal disease, polycystic disease • Obstructive uropathy • Developmental/congenital disorder

Acute Renal Failure

Acute kidney injury (AKI), also known as **acute renal failure** (ARF), is a sudden decline in renal function over days to weeks and is often associated with an increase in BUN and creatinine (azotemia), hyperkalemia, and fluid overload, which may or may not be associated with oliguria (urine production of less than 200 to 500 mL/day).[11] **Uremia** accompanies renal failure and includes elevated BUN and creatinine levels as well as fatigue, anorexia, nausea, vomiting, pruritis, and neurologic changes (see Table 12-1).[8,12] AKI may present in 2% to 5% of all patients admitted to the general medical/surgical hospital unit and may exceed 20% of patients in the intensive care unit (ICU) following cardiovascular or abdominal vascular surgery.[13-15] AKI is divided into 3 categories:

1. **Prerenal** causes result from conditions that decrease renal blood flow (eg, hypovolemia, shock, hemorrhage, burns, impaired cardiac output, pulmonary emboli, diuretic therapy). This condition typically presents with hypotension, oliguria/anuria (no urine production), dryness of mucous membranes, and decreased tissue turgor.
2. **Postrenal** causes arise from obstruction or disruption to urine flow anywhere along the urinary tract. Obstruction can result from kidney stones, neoplasms (ie, tumors of cervix, prostate, or bladder), benign prostate hypertrophy (BPH), and blood clots.
3. **Intrarenal** causes result from injury to renal tissue and are usually associated with intrarenal ischemia, toxins, immunologic processes, and systemic and vascular disorders.[12,1617]

Common diagnostic testing includes:

- Urinalysis revealing proteinuria, hematuria, casts and urine chemistry analysis to distinguish various forms of ARF
- Blood testing revealing rising serum creatinine and BUN levels. The ratio of creatinine to BUN can help determine the probable site of dysfunction (ie, prerenal, postrenal, intrarenal)
- Renal ultrasonography to estimate renal size and to exclude a treatable obstructive uropathy

Chronic Renal Failure

Chronic renal failure (CRF) is a progressive deterioration of renal function and glomerular filtration due to an irreversible decline in nephron number. CRF arises from multiple causes, but diabetes and HTN account for the majority of cases (Table 12-2). CRF is largely silent due to the kidneys' reserve capabilities. However, when renal function falls to approximately 80% of normal, signs and symptoms of renal insufficiency are evident, and this may be classified as ESRD. Ultimately, CRF ends fatally in uremia with an excess of BUN and other nitrogenous wastes in the blood, altered metabolic and endocrine function and resultant complications (see Table 12-1) unless dialysis or a kidney transplantation is performed. Diagnosis is confirmed through a variety of testing including:

- Blood testing, including the complete blood count (CBC) revealing anemia, elevated serum creatinine, BUN, phosphorus and decreased serum calcium, bicarbonate, and proteins, especially albumin.
- Arterial blood gas analysis may reveal metabolic acidosis, low blood pH, low CO_2, and decreased bicarbonate (HCO_3)
- 24-hour urine analysis is used to determine creatinine clearance, which is an estimate of the Glomerular Filtration Rate (GFR), the amount of blood filtered per minute by the kidneys. The amount of creatinine produced in the body is dependent on muscle mass and is relatively constant for an individual and is usually freely filtered by the kidney and removed in the urine. Renal disorders often lead to a decreased GFR, resulting in less creatinine being removed from the blood and released into the urine; therefore, the serum creatinine increases.

Medical management of CRF aims to conserve renal function as long as possible. Common strategies include:

- Detection and treatment of reversible causes of renal failure (eg, diabetes control, treat HTN)
- Dietary regulation—low-protein diet supplemented with essential amino acids or their keto analogues to minimize uremic toxicity and to prevent wasting and malnutrition
- Treatment of associated conditions to improve renal dynamics:
    - Anemia: Recombinant human erythropoietin (Epogen [epoetin alfa]), a synthetic hormone
    - Acidosis: Replacement of bicarbonate stores by infusion or oral administration of sodium bicarbonate
    - Hyperkalemia: Restriction of dietary potassium, administration of cation exchange resin
    - Phosphate retention: Decrease dietary phosphorus (eg, chicken, milk, legumes, carbonated beverages), administer phosphate-binding agents that bind phosphorus in the intestinal tract
- Maintenance dialysis or kidney transplantation (see Chapter 14) when medical/surgical management fails

Dialysis and Ultrafiltration

Dialysis attempts to perform the normal functions of the kidney by passing blood across a semi-permeable membrane allowing the metabolic waste products to diffuse into a correction fluid, the **dialysate**. Dialysis promotes the correction of fluid and electrolyte abnormalities, removal of toxic materials, and maintenance of acid-base balance. There are 3 modes of dialysis[18]:

1. Intermittent hemodialysis (including slow low efficiency daily dialysis [SLEDD])
2. Peritoneal dialysis
3. Continuous renal replacement therapy (CRRT)

Intermittent Hemodialysis

Hemodialysis circulates the patient's blood in a series of semi-permeable tubes that are bathed in the dialysate in the artificial kidney, or **dialyzer** (Figure 12-3).[19] Hemodialysis may involve a blood flow rate of 200 to 2000 mL/minute through the

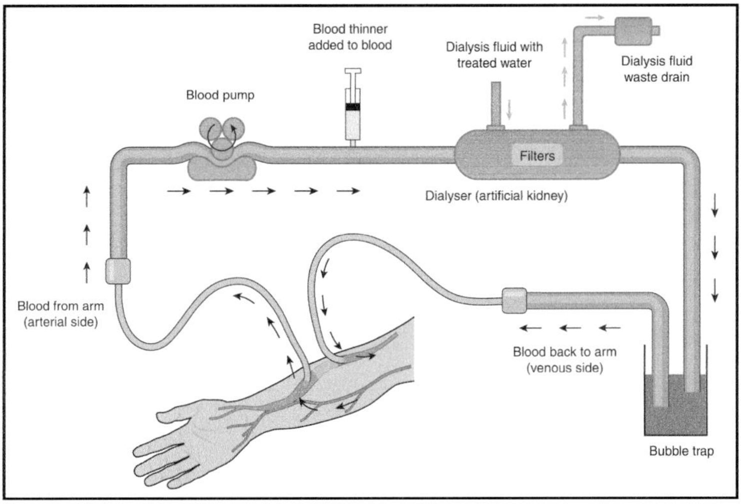

Figure 12-3. Schematic showing blood flow through a kidney dialysis machine after the blood is removed from an arterio-venous fistula. The blood passes through the pump and dialyzer, which includes a filter and the dialysate (dialysis fluid), and returns the blood to the venous circulation. Note the addition of anticoagulants to prevent clot formation and the trap to capture gas bubbles preventing air emboli. (Blamb/Shutterstock.com)

dialyzer, leading to a filtration rate between 300 and 2000 mL/hour. The adequacy of the hemodialysis dose is determined by evaluating urea clearance. A common method, the Kt/V (K: dialyzer clearance of urea; t: dialysis time; V: volume of distribution of urea, approximately equal to patient's total body water), is an analysis of urea clearance, duration of the hemodialysis treatment, and distribution of urea in the body.[4] Blood is accessed through 3 primary approaches: central venous catheters (CVCs), a temporary, direct cannulation of veins (subclavian, internal jugular, or femoral); an **arterial-venous fistula**, the creation of a vascular communication by suturing a vein directly to an artery; or an **arteriovenous graft**, an arteriovenous connection consisting of a tube graft made from autologous saphenous vein or from polytetrafluoroethylene (PTFE). Arteriovenous fistulas and grafts allow repeated access with high flows to the dialyzer, minimize clot formation, and limit recurrent infections. CVCs are usually placed in the femoral or subclavian veins and are usually temporary.[20,21] Many of the complications of intermittent hemodialysis are related to the rapid rate of solute and fluid loss, such as hypovolemia, hypotension, and fatigue (Table 12-3). To limit complications, other options include SLEDD and CRRT. SLEDD involves daily dialysis with treatment times ranging from 6 to 12 hours and lower pump speeds and dialysate flow rates.

Peritoneal Dialysis

Peritoneal dialysis uses the peritoneum as the semipermeable membrane and the dialysate is infused into the abdomen and allowed to remain for several hours prior to drainage. The peritoneum is highly vascularized, allowing waste products and fluids to pass from the blood into the diasylate.[22]

Continuous Renal Replacement Therapy

CRRT consists of **continuous veno-venous hemodialysis** (CVVHD) or **continuous arteriovenous hemodialysis** (CAVHD). These procedures involve the use of an

Table 12-3

PHYSICAL THERAPY PRECAUTIONS WITH HEMODIALYSIS AND CONTINUOUS RENAL REPLACEMENT THERAPY

- Therapeutic exercise, airway clearance, and mobilization activities are applied judiciously during hemodialysis and CRRT and during the inflow or outflow of the dialysate during peritoneal dialysis.
- Monitor hemodynamics and vital signs closely due to potential instability, hypovolemia, and electrolyte disorders.
- Monitor all vascular access for possible bleeding and stability.
- Monitor hemodialysis/CRRT circuit flows, pressures, and possible disconnection or clotting.
- Assess fluid and electrolyte status prior to physical therapy interventions; expect fluid and electrolyte imbalances and modify the plan of care (see Chapter 2).
- Expect dehydration/hypovolemia, hypotension, and patient complaints of fatigue post-hemodialysis.
- Avoid placement of BP cuff over arteriovenous fistula and grafts and maintain patency of all vascular access lines (eg, CVC, Hickmann catheter).

extracorporeal blood circuit that uses a small-volume, low-resistance filter to provide continuous removal of solutes and fluid.[23,24] A related procedure, **slow continuous ultrafiltration** (SCUF), is used for volume control in fluid overloaded patients. CRRT is similar to hemodialysis but the blood flow through the dialyzer is decreased to 100 to 200 mL/minute with a filtration rate of 10 to 20 mL/hour. Patients are critically ill, often hemodynamically tenuous or in shock, and physical therapy may be contraindicated except for careful application of airway clearance techniques, range of motion (ROM) exercise programs, and positioning. The slower rate of solute or fluid removal per unit of time is generally better tolerated than conventional hemodialysis. If patients are hemodynamically stable, mobilization, including ambulation, are appropriate. It is imperative that the physical therapist monitors vital signs and maintains patency of all vascular access and the CRRT circuit.[25,26]

Common precautions associated with hemodialysis and CRRT are listed in Table 12-3.

Urinary Tract Infections

Urinary tract infections (UTIs) are a common infection of adult women and the elderly and account for nearly 10 million infections annually. One in every 5 women is susceptible to UTI, and the prevalence of UTI increases with age. Increased risk of UTI is associated for those with indwelling catheters in the bladder, patients with diabetes, and those with abnormalities of the urinary tract. Recurrence is common and approximately 20% of women with acute infection will experience a repeat UTI.[4,27] UTIs are the most common type of health care–associated infection, accounting for more than 30% of infections reported by hospitals. Almost all hospital-acquired UTIs are due to catheter insertion.[28] Catheter-associated urinary tract infections (CAUTIs) increase morbidity, mortality, hospital costs, and length of stay.[28]

UTIs are most commonly due to infection from bacteria that usually reside in the bowel *(Escherichia coli)*. The entire urinary system, including the urethra, bladder, ureters, and kidney, are at risk for infection. The bacteria may ascend to the bladder resulting in **cystitis**, or to the kidneys resulting in **pyelonephritis**.[27] Sexual

Table 12-4

SIGNS AND SYMPTOMS OF COMMON RENAL DISORDERS

Urinary Tract Infection	
• Frequency of urination/urinary urgency • Painful urination • Burning feeling in the bladder • Milky or cloudy urine	• Reddish or bloody urine (hematuria) • Fever • Back pain
Renal Calculi	
• Severe back/flank pain • Nausea and vomiting • Hematuria	• Burning sensation with urination • Fever or chills

transmission (eg, chlamydia, mycoplasma) is a less common cause of infection.[29,30] Common signs and symptoms of UTI are listed in Table 12-4.

Standard testing for UTI is urinalysis. Urinalysis can detect the presence of bacteria, pus, or other microbes and the urinalysis results are used to direct medical treatment, including antibiotics.[30,31]

UTIs are generally successfully treated and begin to resolve within 1 to 2 days, although the course of antibiotic treatment is commonly 1 to 2 weeks (see Chapter 5, Pharmacological Information). Ancillary treatments include an increased fluid intake, as well as the intake of foods and beverages that act to cleanse the bladder (eg, cranberry juice).

Hematuria

Hematuria is the presence of RBCs in the urine. Often, this is not discernible to the human eye. However, gross hematuria is visible in the urine. Hematuria is usually the symptom of an underlying disease process within the GI or GU systems. Examples include liver and kidney disease, bladder dysfunction, kidney stones, BPH, and GU tumors. Hematuria is diagnosed via urinalysis, **intravenous pyelogram** (IVP), an injection of a radiopaque dye followed by x-ray of the renal pelvis and ureter, or **cystoscopy**, a direct visual of the bladder. Treatment depends on the underlying cause of hematuria.

Nephrolithiasis

Kidney stones are a common GU disorder resulting in pain, obstruction, and secondary infections.[15,29] Over 300,000 people go to the emergency room annually for kidney stones. It is estimated that 8.8% of Americans, or 1 in 11 people, have had a kidney stone. Kidney stones affect men more than women and usually occur between the ages of 20 and 40.[4]

Kidney stones result from crystallization of calcium (80% to 90%), uric acid, magnesium-ammonium acetate, or cysteine in the urine, and can form anywhere along the urinary tract. Microscopic crystal formation is normal, and these crystals easily pass though the urinary tract.

Factors contributing to stone formation include diets high in calcium oxalate, limited fluid intake and low urine volume, genetic factors (cystinuria is an autosomal recessive disorder), hyperparathyroidism, sedentary lifestyle and bed rest, and environmental factors, such as high temperatures and humidity. Additional factors include chronic UTIs, kidney dysfunction, and diabetes. Common signs and symptoms of urinary calculi are noted in Table 12-4. Diagnostic testing includes abdominal x-rays, renal sonogram, IVP, and blood and urine analysis.

Acute medical management includes administration of intravenous (IV) fluids, antibiotics, and pain control. Patients may be asked to strain their urine to determine stone passage. Pharmacologic treatments include allopurinol, diuretics (eg, thiazides), and Thiola (tiopronin). Additional medical and surgical procedures include[4]:

- **Extracorporeal shockwave lithotripsy**: Noninvasive ultrasound is used externally to disrupt stones and allow passage through the ureter.
- **Percutaneous nephrolithotomy**: A surgical technique in which a tunnel is made directly to the kidney and the stone is surgically removed or destroyed via ultrasonic wave.
- **Uteroscopic stone removal**: A uretoscope is fed into the ureter and the stone is removed manually.

Kidney stone recurrence is frequent, and prevention may include diet modifications, increased daily water intake, and prophylactic medications.[31]

Cystocele

Cystocele, or fallen bladder, is defined as the bladder protruding into the vagina. The common causes of cystocele include heavy lifting, straining during bowel movements, decreased estrogen concentrations, and childbirth. The severity of the dropped bladder is graded as follows[4]:

- Grade 1: Bladder drops into the vagina.
- Grade 2: Bladder has sunk into the opening of the vagina.
- Grade 3: Bladder protrudes from the vaginal opening

Diagnosis for grades 2 and 3 cystoceles is confirmed by physical examination. Additional testing may include a cystourethrogram, an x-ray using contrast media that shows the anatomy of the bladder and urethra during bladder contraction and voiding. Treatment for grade 1 cycstoceles includes avoidance of heavy lifting and possibly estrogen replacement therapy in post-menopausal women. Grades 2 and 3 cystoceles may require surgical repositioning and stabilization.

Urinary Incontinence and Neurogenic Bladder

Urinary incontinence is the involuntary loss of urine and may be due to pathologic, anatomical, or physiologic factors affecting the urinary tract. Table 12-5 describes the types of urinary incontinence.

Neurogenic bladder is disruption of the complex interactions of voluntary and involuntary smooth muscle, the autonomic nervous system, and cerebral control that allow controlled micturition. Neurogenic bladder can lead to recurrent infections, urinary frequency, incontinence, or partial or complete urinary retention.

Neurogenic bladder is often due to trauma (eg, SCI, traumatic brain injury [TBI]), demyelinating diseases (eg, multiple sclerosis, amyotrophic lateral sclerosis [ALS]), cerebrovascular accident (CVA), central nervous system (CNS) tumors, lead poisoning, diabetes, and chronic UTIs. Less frequently, neurogenic bladder is a hereditary malformation.

The underlying mechanism is disordered neurologic control of the muscles of the bladder. This lack of impulse coordination often results in reflexive relaxation and discharge of urine.[3,4]

Signs of neurogenic bladder include:

- Urination on exertion
- Urination without sensation
- Chronic UTIs
- Inability to actively control bladder and urination (incontinence)

Table 12-5 **TYPES OF URINARY INCONTINENCE**		
Type	*Description*	*Common Etiologies*
Stress incontinence	Intermittent leakage of urine due to increased abdominal pressure, such as coughing, sneezing, or straining	Weakness of pelvic floor and sphincter muscles in women; damage to the internal sphincter mechanism (usually from prostatic surgery) in men
Urge incontinence	Sensation of the need to urinate followed by sudden, involuntary loss of urine	Neurologic disease affecting the bladder, acute or chronic irritation of the bladder wall, and the effects of prolonged bladder outlet obstruction.
Overflow incontinence	Loss of urine caused by overdistention of the bladder; associated with complete urinary retention	Prostate obstruction, diabetes, spinal cord injury (SCI), multiple sclerosis
Functional incontinence	Loss of urine due to functional impairment that causes difficulty in ambulation or dexterity in getting to the bathroom and positioned to void	Occurs with injury to the sphincteric mechanisms, bladder neck, and urethra
Total incontinence	Continuous leakage of urine from the bladder	May result from a birth defect, SCI, or bladder fistula
Enuresis	Involuntary voiding during sleep	May be physiologic during early childhood; thereafter, may be functional or symptomatic of obstructive or neurogenic disease (usually of lower urinary tract) or dysfunctional voiding

Diagnosis is a 2-phase process involving testing of both the muscular and neurological systems. Testing utilizes an electroencephalogram (EEG) of the brain and an electromyogram (EMG) of the bladder. Additionally, a bladder ultrasound, computed tomography (CT) scan with bladder contrast, and a post-residual void (PRV) test (ie, a catheter is placed into the bladder after the patient has voided to assess residual urine volume) are done.[4]

Treatment for a neurogenic bladder is dependent on the underlying cause. In cases of SCI, TBI, or other traumatic injury to the bladder or brain, a catheter is introduced to evacuate the bladder, or a suprapubic indwelling catheter is inserted through the abdomen. Patients may be taught self-catheterization. If incontinence is due to muscular problems of the bladder, pharmacologic treatments include:

- Bladder relaxants: Propantheline, Urispas (flavoxate), Bentyl (dicyclomine), Ditropan (oxybutynin), Detrol (tolterodine)
- Antidepressants: Tofranil (imipramine)
- Estrogen replacement therapy

Physical therapy interventions include exercise including the pelvic floor muscles, electrical stimulation, biofeedback, timed voiding, and instructed catheterization. Surgery is a final option.[31]

Therapeutic interventions for neurogenic bladder include[4]:

- **Pelvic floor strengthening exercises**: Often referred to as **Kegel exercises,** strengthen and retrain pelvic floor and sphincter muscles. Examples include attempting to contract the urethra, attempting to start and stop urine in mid-stream (see Chapter 13 and Table 13-10). Proper performance of these exercises requires repeated instruction.
- **Electrical stimulation**: Electrodes are placed within the vagina or rectum to stimulate pelvic floor muscles. This aids in stabilizing overactive muscles while stimulating contraction of the urethral muscles.
- **Biofeedback**: Biofeedback uses electronic waves to track the contraction of the bladder and urethral muscles. Visualization of the waveforms facilitates improved coordination of contractile and relaxation activity of the involved muscles.
- **Timed voiding or bladder training**: A chart of voiding and leaking is used to identify patterns and once patterns are identified, scheduled voidings are instituted. This technique works in conjunction with biofeedback and muscle conditioning to slowly increase the time scale for voiding.

Benign Prostate Hypertrophy

The prostate is a small, male reproductive gland located under the bladder, anterior to the rectum, and surrounding the urethra. The prostate begins to enlarge at about 25 years of age. **BPH** can become evident after the age of 40 years and affects nearly 90% of men 70 years or older, requiring almost 400,000 hospital admissions yearly.[4,10,30]

The etiology of BPH is unclear. Hormonal alterations, including diminished testosterone and elevated estrogen concentrations, may stimulate prostate growth.[4] Prostate enlargement exerts pressure on the urethra and this compression stimulates reflexive bladder contraction regardless of urine volume and leads to bladder wall thickening and distension. Interestingly, the amount of hypertrophy does not correlate to the severity of symptoms. Common symptoms of BPH include:

- Hesitancy or a weak stream of urine
- Urinary urgency
- Leaking or dribbling
- Urinary frequency, especially at night

Diagnostic testing attempts to differentiate BPH from prostate cancer. Physical examinations include digital rectal exam allowing palpation of the prostate to determine size and texture. Diagnostic testing may include prostate biopsy or prostate-specific antigens (PSA) testing. PSAs are present in the bloodstream and elevated PSA concentrations are indicative of prostate cancer. Normal values are <4 ng/mL, elevated values are 4 to 10 ng/mL, and abnormal values are 10 to 20+ ng/mL.[3,10,31] Additional testing includes urine flow studies, rectal ultrasound, IVP, and cystoscopy.

Medical treatment for BPH includes medications and surgical management. Medications include the following[6]:

- **Proscar (finasteride)**: Inhibits dihydrotestosterone (DHT), a hormone that promotes prostate enlargement
- **Hytrin (terazosin), Cardura (doxazosin), or Flomax (tamsulosin)**: Relax smooth muscles of bladder and prostate to increase flow

Surgical treatments include:

- **Transurethral microwave thermotherapy** (TUMT): Uses microwaves to heat and destroy excessive prostate tissue while protecting the rest of the urinary system by providing a coolant through the urethra
- **Transurethral needle ablatio**n (TUNA) **system**: Delivers a low-level radio frequency that burns away selected prostate tissues with a shield to protect the urethra
- **Transurethral resection of the prostate** (TURP): Performed through the urethra using a resectoscope. The resectoscope has a light and irrigator and contains an electrical loop to shave away tissue. TURP is the most common surgical intervention and accounts for 90% of all prostate surgeries
- **Transurethral incision of the prostate** (TUIP): Focuses on widening the urethra by making incisions in the bladder neck and prostate
- **Suprapubic** and **retropubic prostatectomy**: More invasive and involve direct resection or excision of prostate tissue
- Newer treatment options include **transurethral laser ablation** and **balloon dilatation**

Postoperative treatment includes continuous bladder irrigation, antibiotics, and pain control with early ambulation.

Genitalia

Male and female genitalia play important roles in both the excretion of wastes and in reproduction; however, these multiple functions leave the human genitalia susceptible to infection and disease (eg, UTI). The genitalia have an extensive vascular tree and robust arteriovenous blood flow. This leaves the external genitalia, specifically the labia and scrotum, vulnerable to edema formation. **Labial edema** is rare and often exclusively caused by liver disease and hypoproteinemia; **scrotal edema** is more common. Scrotal edema is associated with hereditary disease, liver disease and transplantation, inguinal herniation, lymphedema of the lower extremities (LEs), and prostate disease. Scrotal edema secondary to liver diseases and/or transplantation is associated with portal HTN and hypoproteinemia. Inguinal herniation and lymphedema involve obstruction of arterial, venous, or lymphatic flow out of the genitalia. Signs and symptoms of external genitalia edema include the following:

- Large, pitting edema
- Shiny and discolored skin
- Warm to touch
- Difficulty or inability to walk

Edema is identifiable during the physical examination. Additional testing usually consists of blood and urine analysis, CT scan, and/or ultrasound analysis to determine the underlying cause. Interventions are determined by the underlying cause of the genital edema. Lymphedema is responsive to manual lymphatic decompression therapy and referral to a lymphedema specialist can lead to significant reductions in edema.

Physical Therapist Management of Genitourinary System

The physical therapy management of patients with GU disorders present many challenges. The physical therapist/physical therapist assistant may be one of the first health care practitioners who patients confide in and relate GU complaints. Although the GU physical examination is not routinely performed by physical therapists unless they have undergone specialized training (eg, pelvic floor), common questions during the history may allow a more specific description of the patient's complaints and referral to other health care professionals (Table 12-6). For patients with advanced renal disease, the therapists need to consider that these patients are typically physically inactive with reduced exercise capacity prior to hospitalization. Enforced or voluntary bed rest will exacerbate these problems.[32] The reason for the debility of patients with renal disease is far from clear. Anemia, peripheral edema, and the systemic effects of uremia, as well as disuse atrophy, have a significant impact on the physical functioning and quality of life.[32,33] Limited exercise capacity and poor physical functioning has been linked to low quality of life and high mortality. Patients with kidney disease and those receiving dialysis may often demonstrate fluid and electrolyte abnormalities necessitating close observation of laboratory values (see Chapter 2). Renal dysfunction is often associated with diabetes and cardiovascular disease. Patients will present with peripheral neuropathies, intrinsic weakness of the hands and feet, Charcot joint changes, coronary artery disease (CAD), and HTN necessitating close observation of vital signs and the ECG at rest and with activity.

Patients with nephrolithiasis commonly have referred low back and flank pain masquerading as mechanical low back pain. The differential diagnosis of low back pain needs to include kidney inflammation and nephrolithiasis as possible reasons for medical referral.

All patients who have undergone a surgical intervention need to be engaged in an airway clearance and/or mobility program due to the increased incidence of postoperative pulmonary complications. Additionally, the coordination of pain management strategies will optimize physical therapy interventions.

Patients with prostate diseases are generally in the seventh decade, and it is common to encounter premorbid gait, balance, and postural dysfunction.

Pelvic floor strengthening exercises can be prescribed for bladder and pelvic floor dysfunction that can alleviate pain and strengthen those muscles to prevent further incontinence and potential embarrassment (see Table 13-10).

Lymphedema management for genital or lower extremity lymphedema is an effective intervention to start during the hospital stay. Referral to an outpatient lymphedema specialist is beneficial if edema remains problematic at hospital discharge.

Finally, it is common for patients being treated by therapists in the acute care setting to have a **Foley catheter**. The Foley catheter is a flexible, balloon-tipped catheter placed directly into the bladder through the urethra (Figure 12-4). This catheter allows direct elimination of urine, protects the perineal region from urine leakage and skin breakdown, and allows for an accurate assessment of body fluid output. Fluid output is compared to fluid input (I & Os) to determine a patient's fluid balance. Fluid from the diet is the major source of fluid input while urine output is the largest proportion of fluid loss. As noted previously, UTIs are a large proportion of hospital-acquired infection and avoiding unnecessary urinary catheter use is the most important goal in prevention of CAUTI. The physical therapist may be an important member of the acute care team to help determine toileting and mobility safety allowing for catheter removal. Incontinence after catheter removal is common but should be of short duration.

Table 12-6

Genitourinary System Examination

Examination Technique	*Description of Technique*	*Examination Findings in Common Diseases/Disorders*
Common questions/history	• Abdominal pain: Note onset, duration, character (eg, sharp, dull, stabbing), location/radiation to other areas. Note anatomic location of pain (see Tables 11-18 and 11-19). • Urine characteristics: Color, amount, frequency, presence of blood, incontinence associated with activity, cough, sneeze (see Table 12-5) ¤ Urgency: Strong desire to urinate; often related to inflammation of bladder/prostate/urethra,; infection ¤ Frequency: Short duration between urination ¤ Nocturia: Voiding at night ¤ Dysuria: Burning or pain with urination, difficulty voiding (eg, pyelonephritis, cystitis, urethritis, vaginitis) ¤ Hematuria: Blood in urine (eg, UTI, renal disease, renal/bladder stones, GU cancer) ¤ Frothy urine: Proteinuria (eg, glomerulonephritis, nephrotic syndrome) • Fluid intake: How many glasses of water, caffeine • Characterization of pelvic pain: Onset, duration, location, character, severity, exacerbating or relieving factors • Vaginal or penile discharge: Amount, color, odor	• Pyelonephritis: Fever, chills, increased urgency and frequency, thoracic pain, cloudy urine • Cystitis: Frequent urination, urinary incontinence, hypogastric/pubic pain, cloudy/foul-smelling urine • Urethritis: Dysuria, urethral discharge, usually no complaints of frequency or urgency • Vaginitis (eg, candidiasis, trichomonisasis): Pain, soreness, itching of vagina, foul-smelling vaginal discharge, pain/discomfort with sexual intercourse • Kidney stone: Flank tenderness, radiating pain to groin, hematuria • Prostatitis: Perineal pain (region between scrotum and anus), dysuria, urethral discharge • Testicular cancer: Testicle swelling/hard mass or lump in testicle, gradual onset of pain • Inguinal hernia: Groin pain, scrotal swelling (increases with standing/decreases with lying down), palpable mass in scrotum or ingiunal canal

(continued)

Table 12-6 (continued)

GENITOURINARY SYSTEM EXAMINATION

Examination Technique	*Description of Technique*	*Examination Findings in Common Diseases/Disorders*
Inspection/observation	• Premenstrual complaints: Headaches, weight gain, edema, breast tenderness, mood changes • Menopausal complaints: Mood changes, hot flashes, post-menopausal bleeding • Observation of lower abdomen and/or genitalia: ¤ Rashes ¤ Lesions ¤ Masses ¤ Hernia • Examination for edema of the extremities (see Table 1-9). Consider review of clinical laboratory data (see Chapter 2 and Tables 2-2 through 2-11, 2-15): ¤ Serum creatinine ¤ Creatinine clearance ¤ BUN ¤ Electrolytes (sodium, potassium, chloride, calcium, magnesium) ¤ Arterial blood gas	• Genital herpes: Viral infection leading to superficial, small red vesicles ¤ Condyloma acuminatum (genital warts) ¤ Human papillomavirus (HPV) infection, flesh (white or reddish lesions) • Epididymitis: Inflammation of the epididymis, often associated with UTI, erythema and swelling of scrotum; pain relieved with scrotal elevation • Peripheral edema: Due to excessive loss of protein in urine (proteinuria) leading to a decrease in osmotic pressure within the vasculature (eg, nephrotic syndrome) or inability to excrete sodium and metabolic wastes (eg, renal failure) leading to excessive water retention • Liver disease: Due to portal hypertension or hypoalbuminemia (see Chapter 11)

Adapted from Fischbach FT, Dunning MB. *A Manual of Laboratory and Diagnostic Tests*. Philadelphia, PA: Lippincott Williams & Wilkins; 2004 and Seidel HM, Ball JW, Dains JE, Benedict GW. *Mosby's Guide to Physical Examination*. St. Louis, MO: Mosby, Inc; 2003.

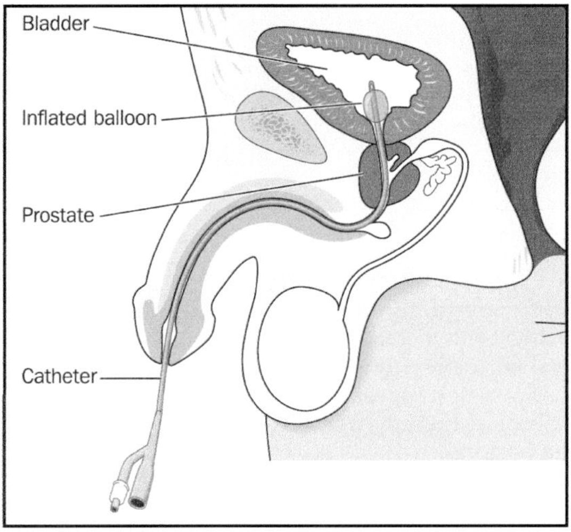

Figure 12-4. Anatomy of the male bladder and prostate showing the position of a balloon tipped catheter in the urethra and bladder. Note that the balloon is inflated. (Blamb/Shutterstock.com)

Case Study

Mr. Noresh is an 88-year-old (y/o) male who presented to emergency room with shortness of breath (SOB). He was found to have a UTI and started on an antibiotic, ceftriaxone. His wife stated that he vomited dark brown vomit the day before. While in the emergency room, he had coffee ground emesis again and the ECG revealed atrial flutter to the 140s. A nasogastric (NG) tube was placed to drain the stomach. He was transferred to the medical intensive care unit (MICU) due to hypotension, supraventricular tachycardia, and a presumed upper GI bleed. Mr. Noresh was last admitted 3 months ago for management of his atrial flutter. He has been on Coumadin (warfarin) since that time. International Normalization Ratio (INR) on admission was 6. A decision was made to withhold the Coumadin and not provide a reversal agent (ie, phytonadione [Vitamin K]).

Patient/Client History

General Demographics, Social History, and Living Environment

Mr. Noresh is married, and he is a retired mechanical engineer who lives in a ranch-style home with his wife of 66 years. There are 3 steps to enter the home with a railing on both sides. The master bathroom has a tub chair and a rail, which were installed 5 years ago after his wife's knee replacement.

General Health Status, Social/Health Habits, and Family History

Mr. Noresh denies current smoking and limited alcohol use (1 drink per day prior to dinner). He reports smoking "a long time ago" and reports stopping "cold turkey" more than 30 years ago. He reports being more sedentary recently and does not exercise regularly.

Medical/Surgical History

Mr. Noresh has a history of atrial flutter, diabetes, HTN, and CKD. Per patient, 3 to 4 years ago he had an episode of coffee ground emesis and underwent an esophagogastroduodenoscopy (EGD). He said they found strictures, no ulcer, varices, or arteriovenous malformations (AVMs). The patient denies non-steroidal anti-inflammatory drug (NSAID) or alcohol use.

Current Conditions

Mr. Noresh complains of (c/o) mild pubic burning sensation and SOB. He denies chest pain or palpitations. His admitting diagnoses are atrial flutter, upper gastrointestinal bleed (UGIB), and AKI with a creatinine of 1.54, which increased to 4, most likely due to decreased renal perfusion from the hypotension and supraventricular tachycardia (ie, prerenal syndrome). A repeat EGD reveals no active bleeding.

On day 2 of MICU admission, physical therapy was consulted. He states that he has been in bed since coming to the hospital.

Activities and Participation

Mr. Noresh was independent in functional activities, ADLs and instrumental activities of daily living (IADLs) prior to surgery. He states that he has not participated in any type of exercise program since playing spring and summer softball about 5 years ago. Mr. Noresh currently uses a cane when he is out doing errands because of right knee pain. He still drives, but limits this to daytime only due to failing vision. He states he did not need any assistance with walking, bathing, or climbing his 3 steps to get into the house. He states he can easily walk 3 or more blocks if needed.

Medications

Mr. Noresh is currently prescribed fluids for blood pressure support, Coumadin (restarted today) for atrial flutter and deep vein thrombosis prophylaxis, proton pump inhibitors related to the GI bleed and diltiazem (a calcium channel blocker) to slow the ventricular rate with the atrial flutter. He remains NPO (nils per os; nothing by mouth) allowing GI rest and healing of the stomach.

Other Clinical Tests

Abnormal laboratory findings: CBC revealed hemoglobin of 8.2 g/dL, WBCs of >23,000/mm^3, electrolytes revealed potassium of 7.3 mEq/L and the serum creatinine was 4 mg/dL. Laboratory findings are suggestive of infection, anemia, hyperkalemia, and renal insufficiency. The therapist should monitor the ECG secondary to electrolyte abnormalities and history of atrial flutter. A 24-hour urine collection is currently underway. Chest x-ray shows NG tube along with bilateral small pleural effusions with patchy pulmonary opacities, and an enlarged cardiac silhouette. Transthoracic echocardiogram (TTE) revealed an ejection fraction of 50% with ventricular dilation consistent with a diagnosis of heart failure with preserved ejection fraction (HFpEF). His present temperature is 36.5° C.

Systems Review

Cardiovascular and Pulmonary

Resting heart rate (HR) 112 beats per minute (bpm), pulse irregular, respiratory rate (RR) 20 breaths/minute and shallow using accessory muscles, BP 130/76 mm Hg, oxygen saturation (SpO_2) 91% on 3 liters nasal cannula oxygen and pain was 2/10 in his lower abdomen area. Mild edema was noted around both ankles (+2).

Integumentary

He has IV fluids, Foley catheter, nasal cannula, and an arterial line. He appears thin and presents with +2 edema of bilateral lower extremities (BLEs). His skin appears dry with notable thickened bilateral toenails and calluses on both heels. There was bilateral hair loss below his knees.

Musculoskeletal

Mr. Noresh's ROM was within functional limits (WFL), except for bilateral ankles to neutral dorsiflexion/plantar flexion and minimal inversion/eversion. He could move bilateral upper extremities (BUEs) and BLEs to command against gravity while lying in bed

Neuromuscular

Mr. Noresh had diminished sensation in BLEs. He complained of numbness and cold in his feet.

Communication, Affect, Cognition, Language, and Learning Style

English is his primary language. He is alert, awake, and oriented x 4.

Tests and Measures

Aerobic Capacity and Endurance

Following Manual Muscle Test (MMT), ROM, bed mobility, and transfer to the bed side chair, his vital sign response was HR 112 to 144 bpm and the rhythm remained atrial flutter, RR 20 to 26 breaths/minute, BP 130/76 to 110/82 mm Hg, SpO_2 increased from 91% to 95% and pain did not change. He did not report any dizziness with the drop in blood pressure. Vital signs (VS) returned to baseline after several minutes of out of bed (OOB) sitting in chair with feet elevated. Mr. Noresh appears deconditioned as demonstrated by the cardiovascular and pulmonary response to minimal activity; however, this could also be related to the UGIB with anemia and persistent atrial flutter.

Assistive and Adaptive Devices

Mr. Noresh transferred to the chair with moderate assistance of 1 using the bed rail and not his cane (Functional Status Score for the Intensive Care Unit [FSS-ICU] 3).

Balance, Gait, and Mobility (Including Locomotion)

Sitting unsupported at the edge of bed (EOB) balance was poor even with feet flat on the floor requiring minimal assistance to prevent loss of balance. The Function in Sitting Test (FIST) score was 18 out of 56. A stand pivot transfer to chair required moderate assist of 1 (FSS-ICU 3). Dynamic/standing balance and gait were not tested (FSS-ICU 0) due to fatigue and VS response to transfer to chair. The Activity Measure for Post Acute Care (AM-PAC) basic mobility score was 11/24.

Circulation (Arterial, Venous, Lymphatic) and Ventilation/Respiration

As noted previously, following strength testing and mobilization, his VS response was significant for an abnormal heart rhythm (atrial flutter) with an elevated HR (ventricular response range 112-144) combined with a 20 mm Hg decrease in systolic BP (systolic BP 130-110 mm Hg). The rapid ventricular rate in atrial flutter may decrease the cardiac output and may lead to symptoms such as palpitations, fatigue, dizziness, and SOB.

Mr. Noresh demonstrated improvement in the SpO_2 reading with mobilization. His breath sounds were crackles bilateral bases. His cough was weak, wet sounding, and productive of white to yellow secretions. He is at risk for pulmonary complications due to prolonged bedrest, decreased cough, fluid restriction, level of fatigue from persistent atrial flutter and pleural effusions with patchy opacities. His SpO_2 improved with OOB mobility, possibly due to improved ventilation sitting upright.

Mental Function

Mr. Noresh is awake, alert, and oriented x 4. He follows commands easily. There is no history of fluctuating mental status.

Muscle Performance

His strength was BUE 4/5 and BLE 4/5 with MMT. This is a Medical Research Council strength score of 48.

Pain

Mr. Noresh rated his pain at 2/10 in the lower abdomen area. The nurse informed that pain did not change during session.

Diagnosis

Mr. Noresh presents with limited cardiovascular and pulmonary reserve, muscle weakness and impaired functional mobility related to his GI bleed, persistent atrial flutter, new onset AKI superimposed on CKD, and bed rest.

Prognosis

Geriatric patients with multisystem involvement and prolonged ICU stay can respond to intervention to improve functional outcomes. The physical therapist recommended daily therapy to meet the goals of independence with bed mobility and transfers, improve airway clearance, muscle strength, and frequent transfers OOB as well as to progress to gait training. Discharge from the hospital to a post–acute care facility is expected

Intervention

Mr. Noresh participated in physical therapy 5 times/week to progress gait, transfers, airway clearance (ie, incentive spirometry, breathing exercises), therapeutic exercise to enhance extremity ROM and strength, and education regarding pain management, postoperative pulmonary complications, and ambulation safety. The patient education also supported the teachings of the diabetes and renal team.

ICF Clinical Reasoning Tool Case Study Summary								
Health Condition								
HPI: UGIB, AKI, atrial flutter, UTI, anemia, diabetes, bilateral small pleural effusions, mild pulmonary edema and BLL patchy pulmonary opacities; new diagnosis of HFpEF 60% ejection fraction PMHx: Atrial flutter, diabetes, HTN, CKD								
Precautions/Contraindications								
Frail looking older gentleman, Risk for falls due to deconditioning and hypotension/tachycardia; Possible ongoing infection with elevated WBC and abnormal CXR; anemia; universal precautions								
Body Structure and Function			*Activity/Task Limitations*			*Participation*		
Impairment/ Problem	*Tests and Measures*	*Intervention*	*Activity*	*Tests and Measures*	*Intervention*	*Participation*	*Tests and Measures*	*Intervention*
• Abnormal breath sounds • Decreased strength • Decreased endurance • Pain • Poor nutritional status	• Chest assessment • ROM/MMT • Pain/numeric scale • BMI	• Breathing exercises: huffing, IS • Bedside ROM as warm up • Progressive UE/LE resistance exercises • Education on fall risk • Consult diabetes and renal registered dietician	• ADLs • Bed mobility • Transfers • Gait • Balance	• FSS-ICU • AM-PAC "6 Clicks" • RPE • Berg Balance or Functional Reach Test when able	• Progressive functional retraining • Balance exercises in sitting and standing	• Unable to live independently or care for wife • Unable to drive and shop for groceries	• DQoL • RDQoL	• Continue physical therapy services • Consult social worker • Family meeting to discuss discharge plans

(continued)

ICF Clinical Reasoning Tool Case Study Summary (continued)

Personal Factors	*Other Considerations*	*Environmental Factors*
• Age: 88 y/o male • AAO x 4 • Primary language: English • Married and lives with wife who is s/p 2 myocardial infarctions in past 2 years • Uses cane for ambulation • Drives in daytime only • Sleeps only 5 hours at a time		Home: • Ranch style, 3 steps to enter, handrail • Tub seat and rail in bathroom x 5 years Hospital: • 6 days in ICU, arterial line, NC, urinary catheter, IV line; 4 days on step down floor NC, IV line

AAO = alert, awake, and oriented; BLL = bilateral lower lobes; BMI = body mass index; CXR = chest roentgenogram; DQoL = Diabetes Quality of Life Questionnaire; HPI = history of present illness; NC = nasal cannula; PMHx = past medical history; RDQoL = Renal-Dependent Quality of Life Questionnaire; RPE = rate of perceived exertion; s/p = status post; UE = upper extremity.

Adapted from American Physical Therapy Association. *Guide to Physical Therapist Practice*. 3rd ed. http://www.apta.org/Guide/. Updated October 21, 2015. Accessed October 5, 2018 and *Towards a Common Language for Functioning, Disability and Health*. World Health Organization. www.who.int/classifications/icf/icfbeginnersguide.pdf. Published 2002. Accessed April 29, 2019.

The physical therapist recommended referrals to occupational therapy, clinical dietician, and social work for ADL retraining, nutrition assessment, evaluation for depression-like symptoms, and discharge planning.

Outcomes

Ten days after admission Mr. Noresh had all lines removed, his laboratory values returned to baseline and his atrial flutter was controlled with a resting HR of 88. He was voiding regularly, eating small meals, and reported pain was 0/10. His strength had improved to 4+ to 5/5 throughout. Bed mobility, including supine-to-sit transfers, required supervision of 1 when using bed rail (FSS-ICU 5). Transfer to standing and to the chair required minimal assistance of 1 (FSS-ICU 4), and he could now ambulate 45 feet x 3 with rolling walker and minimal assistance (FSS-ICU 2). The HR, BP, RR, and SpO_2 responses were appropriate. The AM-PAC score increased from 11 to 17/24. The FIST score had improved from 18 to 29/56. Breath sounds were clearing on the right, but mild crackles were still auscultated over the left base. Mr. Noresh was recommended for acute rehabilitation.

Chapter Review Questions

1. What are the primary components of the GU systems?
   a. Liver, bladder, prostate, and pelvic floor muscles
   b. Kidneys, ureter, bladder, and urethra
   c. Pancreas, stomach, bladder, and prostate
   d. Adrenal gland, prostate, genitals, and urea
2. What is the primary waste product of protein metabolism?
   a. Ketones
   b. Erythropoietin
   c. Calcitriol
   d. Urea
3. Which of the following are clinical manifestations of renal failure?
   a. Hypokalemia, hypotension, pericardial tamponade
   b. Anemia, amenorrhea, hypophosphatemia
   c. Hyperkalemia, anemia, metabolic acidosis
   d. Pleural effusions, pruritus, metabolic alkalosis
4. Which of the following is a precaution when mobilizing a patient following hemodialysis?
   a. Monitor hemodynamic status closely during functional evaluation
   b. Place blood pressure cuff on ipsilateral extremity of arteriovenous fistula
   c. Expect dehydration, orthostatic hypertension, and complaints of fatigue with examination
   d. Modify plan of care related to physician order for bed rest

5. Which of the following are therapeutic interventions for a neurogenic bladder?
   a. Biofeedback and core exercises
   b. Electrical stimulation and biofeedback
   c. Timed voiding and core exercises
   d. Stress reduction and pelvic floor exercises

Answers: 1b, 2d, 3c, 4a, 5b

REFERENCES

1. Moore KL, Agur AM, Dalley AF. *Clinically Oriented Anatomy.* 7th ed. Philadelphia, PA: Lippincott Williams & Wilkins; 2013.
2. Merahn S. *PDxMD—Renal and Genitourinary Disorders.* Philadelphia, PA: Elsevier; 2003.
3. Weiss R, Nicholas G Jr, O'Reilly PH. *Comprehensive Urology.* London, United Kingedom: Mosby; 2001.
4. The National Institute of Diabetes and Digestive and Kidney Diseases. www.niddk.nih.gov. Accessed September 2014.
5. Guyton AC, Hall JE. *Textbook of Medical Physiology.* Philadelphia, PA: WB Saunders; 2000.
6. Rhoades RA, Tanner GA. *Medical Physiology.* Baltimore, MD: Lippincott Williams & Wilkins; 1995.
7. Koeppen BM, Stanton BA. *Renal Physiology.* St. Louis, MO: Mosby; 2001.
8. Huether SE, McCance KL. *Understanding Pathophysiology.* 5th ed. St. Louis, MO: Elsevier-Mosby; 2011.
9. Spargo BH, Haas M. The kidney. In: Rubin E, Farber JL, eds. *Essential Pathology.* 3rd Ed. Philadelphia, PA: Lippincott Williams & Wilkins, 2001.
10. Teichman JMH. *20 Common Problems in Urology.* New York, NY: McGraw-Hill; 2001.
11. Jones-Kalota SM, Greene LF, Parsons SL. Evaluation of the urologic patient. In: Stein BS, Caldamone AA, Smith JA, eds. *Clinical Urologic Practice.* New York, NY: WW Norton; 1995.
12. Tierney LM, McPhee SJ, Papadakis MA. *Current Medical Diagnosis and Treatment.* Norwalk, CT: Appleton & Lange; 1994
13. Wein AJ, Kavoussi LR, Partin AW, Peters CA. *Campbell-Walsh Urology.* 11th ed. Philadelphia, PA: Elsevier; 2016.
14. Nolan CR, Anderson RJ. Hospital-acquired acute renal failure. *J Am Soc Nephrol.* 1998;9:710-718.
15. Dimick JB, Pronovost PJ, Cowan JA, Lipsett PA. Complications and costs after high-risk surgery: where should we focus quality improvement initiatives? *J Am Coll Surg.* 2003;196:671-678.
16. Brenner BM. *Brenner & Rector's: The Kidney.* 7th ed. Philadelphia, PA: WB Saunders; 2004.
17. Agrawal M, Swartz R. Acute renal failure. *Am Fam Phys.* 2000;61:2077-2088.
18. National Kidney Foundation. Guidelines and commentaries. www.kidney.org/professionals/guidelines/guidelines_commentaries. Accessed July 17, 2019.
19. Mallick NP, Gokal R. Hemodialysis. *Lancet.* 1999;353:737-742.
20. Murphy GJ, White SA, Nicholson ML. Vascular access for hemodialysis. *Br J Surg.* 2000;87:1300-1315.
21. Work J. Hemodialysis catheters and ports. *Semin Nephrol.* 2002;22:211-220.
22. Gokal R, Mallick NP. Peritoneal dialysis. *Lancet.* 1999;353:823-828.
23. Dirkes SM. Continuous renal replacement therapy. dialytic therapy for acute renal failure in intensive care. *Nephrol Nurs J.* 2000;27:581-590.
24. Patton ME. Continuous renal replacement therapy: slow but steady. *Nursing.* 2003;33:48-50.
25. Brownback CA, Fletcher P, Pierce LN, Klaus S. Early mobility activities during continuous renal replacement therapy. *Am J Crit Care.* 2014;23(4):348-51. doi: 10.4037/ajcc2014889
26. Wang YT, Haines TP, Ritchie P, et al. Early mobilization on continuous renal replacement therapy is safe and may improve filter life. *Crit Care.* 2014;18(4):R161. doi: 10.1186/cc14001
27. Kreiger JN. Urinary tract infections in women: causes, consequences, and clinical management. In: Stein BS, Caldamone AA, Smith JA, eds. *Clinical Urologic Practice.* New York, NY: WW Norton; 1995.

28. Gould CV, Umscheid CA, Agarwal RK, Kuntz G, Pegues DA; the Healthcare Infection Control Practices Advisory Committee (HICPAC). *Guideline for Prevention of Catheter-associated Urinary Tract Infections, 2009. Centers for Disease Control.* https://www.cdc.gov/infectioncontrol/pdf/guidelines/cauti-guidelines.pdf. Updated February 15, 2017. Accessed February 28, 2019.
29. Preminger GM. Nephrolithiasis: pathogenesis, diagnosis, and medical therapy. In: Stein BS, Caldamone AA, Smith JA, eds. *Clinical Urologic Practice.* New York, NY: WW Norton; 1995.
30. MD Consult: clinical information for physicians. www.mdconsult.com. Accessed April 2, 2014.
31. Vallerand AH, Sanoski CA, Deglin JH, eds. *Davis's Drug Guide for Nurses.* 15th ed. Philadelphia, PA: FA Davis; 2017.
32. Painter P, Messer-Rehak D, Hanson P, et al. Exercise capacity in hemodialysis, CAPD, and renal transplant patients. *Nephron.* 1986;42(1):47-51.
33. Sagiv M, Rudoy J, Rotstein A, Fisher N, Ben-Ari J. Exercise tolerance of end-stage renal disease patients. *Nephron.* 1991;57(4):424-427.

Bibliography

American Physical Therapy Association. *Guide to Physical Therapist Practice.* 3rd ed. http://www.apta.org/Guide/. Updated October 21, 2015. Accessed October 5, 2018.

Craig CR, Stitzel RE. *Modern Pharmacology with Clinical Applications.* New York, NY: Little, Brown, and Co; 1997.

Deglin JH, Vallerand AH. *Davis's Drug Guide for Nurses.* 8th ed. Philadelphia, PA: FA Davis; 2003.

Karch AM. *Lippincott's Nursing Drug Guide.* Springhouse, PA: Lippincott Williams & Wilkins; 2004.

Ritter JM, Lewis LD, Mant TG. *Textbook of Clinical Pharmacology.* London, United Kingdom: Edward Arnold Co; 1995.

Appendix

Pharmacological Information: Genitourinary Diseases and Disorders Pharmacology

Diuretics

Action

Diuretics promote renal excretion of water by altering the secretion or reabsorption of electrolytes (sodium, potassium, chloride) within the loop of Henle or distal tubule of the nephron. Diuretics are commonly prescribed for HTN, hypervolemia as seen in heart failure, as well as pulmonary edema and effusions.

Side Effects

CNS: Dizziness, headache
CV: Hypotension (hypovolemia)
GI: Dry mouth, constipation, dyspepsia
Miscellaneous: Electrolyte abnormalities, including hyper-/hypokalemia, hyponatremia, hypochloremia, hypomagnesemia; metabolic alkalosis; muscle cramping

Common Medications

Loop diuretics: Bumex (bumetanide), Lasix (furosemide), Demadex (toresemide)
Osmotic diuretics: Mannitol
Potassium-sparing diuretics: Midamor (amiloride), Aldactone (spironolactone)
Thiazide diuretics: Hydrochlorothiazide

Electrolyte/pH/Mineral Modifiers and Replacement Solutions

Sodium Bicarbonate

Action

Alkalinizing agents are used to manage metabolic acidosis, neutralize gastric acid, and aid in the removal of certain drugs (eg, phenobarbital, aspirin). These agents release bicarbonate ions that buffer excess hydrogen ions raising the serum pH.

Side Effects

CV: Edema
GI: Flatulence, gastric distension
Miscellaneous: Metabolic alkalosis, hypernatremia, hypokalemia, hypocalcemia

Common Medications

Sodium bicarbonate (baking soda, soda mint); Bicitra, Oracit (sodium citrate)

Sodium Chloride

Action

Sodium chloride is primarily indicated for hydration and to supplement sodium in deficiency states. Normal saline (0.9%) is isotonic and primarily used for fluid replacement to expand extracellular fluid volume. Half normal saline (0.45%) is a hypotonic solution and may be used in hyperosmolar states (eg, diabetes). Hypertonic saline (3%, 5%) is used for rapid replacement of sodium and removal of excess extravascular fluid volume (eg, cerebral edema). Hypertonic saline can be used increase intravascular blood volume (eg, shock)

Side Effects
CV: Congestive heart failure (CHF), pulmonary edema
Miscellaneous: Hypernatremia, hypervolemia, hypokalemia, irritation at IV site

Calcium Salts

Action
Calcium salts are used to treat hypocalcemia and therapy for osteoporosis and peptic ulcer disease.

Side Effects
CNS: Tingling
CV: Cardiac arrest, dysrhythmias
GI: Constipation, nausea, vomiting, calculi (stones)

Common Medications
Calphron, PhosLo (calcium acetate); Alka-mints, Amitone, Calcitel, Caltrate, Maalox, Tums (calcium carbonate); Citrical (calcium citrate); Kalcinate (calcium gluconate)

Magnesium Salts

Action
Magnesium salts are used for the treatment of hypomagnesemia and may be used as a laxative or antacid.

Side Effects
CV: Bradycardia, hypotension
GI: Diarrhea
Misc: Flushing

Common Medications
Slo-Mag (magnesium chloride), magnesium citrate, magnesium gluconate, Phillips Milk of Magnesia (magnesium hydroxide), magnesium oxide, magnesium sulfate

Potassium and Sodium Phosphates and Potassium Supplements

Action
Potassium and sodium phosphates are indicated in states of phosphate depletion, to prevent urinary calculi, and as adjunctive therapy for UTIs. Potassium supplements are indicated in hypokalemia and in the treatment of dysrhythmias due to digoxin toxicity.

Side Effects
CNS: Confusion, weakness, flaccid paralysis
CV: Dysrhythmias, cardiac arrest
GI: Diarrhea, abdominal discomfort
Miscellaneous: Hypocalcemia, hyperkalemia

Common Medications
Neutra-Phos, K-Phos, K-Lyte, Klorvess, Kaylixir, Kolyum

Ringers and Lactated Ringers

Action

These isotonic solutions closely resemble the electrolyte composition of normal blood serum and are used to replace potassium, sodium, chloride, and calcium. These solutions do not provide calories or free water.

Dextrose and Saline Solutions

Action

These solutions are composed of varying tonicities (isotonic, hypotonic, and hypertonic). Isotonic solutions increase blood volume (eg, blood loss, dehydration). Hypertonic solutions promote expansion of blood volume by movement of intracellular fluid volume into the vasculature. Hypertonic solutions are most often used in the ICU (eg, shock, resuscitation, cerebral edema). Hypotonic solutions promote fluid movement into cells and tissues (eg, diabetic ketoacidosis). Dextrose solutions provide calories for nutrition, but do not correct electrolyte disturbances.

Common Medications

Hypotonic solutions: 1/2 NS – 0.45% NaCl

Isotonic solutions: 0.9% NS; D5W – 5% Dextrose in water; D5 1/4 NS – 5% Dextrose and 0.2 NaCl

Hypertonic solution: 3% NS; D10W – 10% Dextrose in water; D5 1/2 NS – 5% Dextrose and 0.45 NaCl; D5LR – 5% Dextrose in Lactated Ringers; Dextran, TPN

Other Medications

Other medications often prescribed include:

Anti-hypertensives (see Chapter 6: Angiotensin converting enzyme (ACE) inhibitors, Angiotensin II receptor blockers (ARBs), beta blockers)

Insulin (see Chapter 10)

Statins (See Chapter 6)

Chapter 13

Oncological Diseases and Disorders

Lora Packel, PT, PhD

Cancer rehabilitation is an emerging field that can address issues related to cancer and cancer treatment–related side effects throughout the continuum of care. Physical therapists can and should contribute to the prevention of cancer, rehabilitation during cancer treatment, restoration of function after treatment, long-term health promotion of the cancer survivor and amelioration of symptoms in those at the end of their life.[1] Rehabilitation specialists, notably physical therapists and physical therapist assistants, are uniquely qualified to address the musculoskeletal, neurological, integumentary, and cardiopulmonary ramifications of cancer treatment and empower people to return to an active lifestyle. This chapter will focus on the acute management of the person with cancer, as well as provide therapists with an understanding of issues that may arise after discharge from the acute setting. Physical therapists should have an understanding of the trajectory of the patient's disease so that they can intervene to stave off or reduce long-term effects of cancer treatments.

Anatomy and Physiology: An Overview of the Biology of Cancer

Cancer occurs when there is damage to a cell's DNA that causes it to divide in an uncontrolled manner, escaping the body's normal immunosurveillance.[2] Cancer may occur when cells are unresponsive to the typical signals for apoptosis, preprogrammed cell death. Cancerous cells may also become insensitive to suppressor genes or begin to make their own signals that perpetuate growth of the abnormal cell. These changes in combination with a supportive tumor environment are key factors in promoting cancer cells to divide, grow, and metastasize.[2]

Cancer cells have unique characteristics that differentiate them from healthy cells. Normal cells have a defined life span, **senescence**, with a balance between the number of new cells formed and those that die. Cancer cells, however, lack this preprogrammed life span and can continuously divide with adequate nutritional

Malone DJ, Bishop KL, eds. *Acute Care Physical Therapy: A Clinician's Guide, Second Edition* (pp 539-587).

Table 13-1 TNM Staging System	
T = Tumor Size	T0 = No evidence of primary tumor T1–T4 = Increasing size of tumor
N = Regional Lymph Nodes	N0 = No lymph node involvement N1–N3 = Increasing involvement of regional lymph nodes
M = Presence of Distant Metastases	M0 = No distant metastasis M1 = Distant metastasis
Adapted from Groenwald S, Frogge MH, Goodman M, Yarbro CH. *Cancer Nursing: Principles and Practice*. 4th ed. Sudbury, MA: Jones and Bartlett; 1997 and National Cancer Institute. Cancer staging. https://www.cancer.gov/about-cancer/diagnosis-staging/staging. Published March 9, 2015. Accessed July 15, 2019.	

support. Cancer cells also lack **contact inhibition**, or the signal to stop dividing when there is contact with an adjacent cell. This disrupts the orderly architecture of normal tissue, resulting in a mass of unorganized cells. Finally, cancer cells can divide without being anchored to a surface, which plays a role in metastasis.[3]

Cells with a mutation in their DNA can be categorized as benign or malignant. **Benign** refers to a mass of unorganized tissues, usually surrounded by a capsule, that grow slowly and will not spread or metastasize. Benign tumors are not cancerous, but they can cause symptoms by pressing on or obstructing surrounding tissues. **Malignant tumors** refer to cancers that have the potential to spread outside of their original location, **metastasis**. The exact mechanism of metastatic spread continues to evade researchers. In the present theoretical framework, metastasis requires the formation of new blood vessels, **angiogenesis**, bringing needed nutrition for cell growth. Next, the cancer cells must elude the normal immune response, which seeks out mutations and destroys cells. Finally, the cells extend into surrounding tissues and travel in the vascular system or the lymphatic system to a distant site that is capable of supporting the cancer's growth.[4]

Staging Systems

There are a variety of clinical staging systems used to provide health care professionals with a consistent language to characterize the extent of the cancer. Staging systems include the following information: site of primary tumor, cell type, size of tumor, regional lymph node involvement, metastasis, and tumor grade.[5] Staging systems help the medical team determine the best treatment and give an indication of prognosis.[5] The most widely used system is the TNM system: T indicates tumor size, N describes the nodal involvement, and M denotes the presence of metastases (Table 13-1). Another commonly used system stages cancers from 0 to IV, with 0 indicating a precancerous lesion and IV indicating metastatic disease (Table 13-2). There are four main types of staging. *Clinical staging* refers to how much cancer there is based on the physical exam, basic imaging, and biopsies. *Pathological staging* includes the previous information along with the surgical pathology findings. *Post-therapy staging* evaluates how much cancer is left after initial treatments, and *re-staging* is used when a cancer recurs.

Table 13-2

CANCER STAGING SYSTEM

Stage	*Description*
0	Carcinoma in situ (tumor that has not spread)
I, II, III	Higher stage indicates larger tumors that have spread beyond the initial organ to local lymph nodes and/or tissues.
IV	Tumor has spread to distant organs.

Adapted from Groenwald S, Frogge MH, Goodman M, Yarbro CH. *Cancer Nursing: Principles and Practice*. 4th ed. Sudbury, MA: Jones and Bartlett; 1997 and National Cancer Institute. Cancer staging. https://www.cancer.gov/about-cancer/diagnosis-staging/staging. Published March 9, 2015. Accessed July 15, 2019.

Table 13-3

EASTERN COOPERATIVE ONCOLOGY GROUP PERFORMANCE SCALE

Grade	*Performance Status*
0	Fully active, able to carry on all pre-disease performance without restriction
1	Restricted in physically strenuous activity but ambulatory and able to carry out work of a light or sedentary nature (eg, light house work, office work)
2	Ambulatory and capable of all self-care but unable to carry out any work activities; up and about more than 50% of waking hours
3	Capable of only limited self-care, confined to bed or chair more than 50% of waking hours
4	Completely disabled; cannot carry on any self-care; totally confined to bed or chair
5	Dead

Adapted from Oken M, Creech R, Tormey D, et al. Toxicity and response criteria of the Eastern Cooperative Oncology Group. *Am J Clin Oncol*. 1982;5:649-655.

PERFORMANCE SCALES

Oncologists utilize performance scales to describe the functional capacity of their patients. These scales are used as part of the inclusion/exclusion criteria for clinical trials and other treatment regimens to help determine which regimens may be too intensive for a debilitated patient. Two main systems are utilized: Eastern Cooperative Oncology Group Performance Scale (Table 13-3) and the Karnofsky Performance Scale. These scales should be included in the physical therapy examination to communicate functional status to the oncologist.[6]

Table 13-4 CONSIDERATIONS FOR TREATMENT PLANNING	
Disease Characteristics	• Type of cancer • Stage • Location • Size • Metastasis present or likely • Tumor is indolent or aggressive • Responsive to hormones
General Physical Health of Patient	• Can the patient tolerate the treatment plan? • Present performance status
Quality of Life	• Patient's present quality of life (QoL) • Potential QoL with treatment
Emotional Health	• Coping skills • Social support
Financial Health	• What financial constraints impact the treatment plan? • How will treatment affect the person's ability to work?

HEALTH CONDITIONS: SPECIFIC CANCERS, CANCER TREATMENTS, AND PHYSICAL THERAPIST MANAGEMENT

Oncologists use a variety of tests to diagnose cancer. These tests may include biopsy, biochemical markers, genetic testing, imaging, and physical examination. Once a definitive diagnosis is determined, the oncologist and patient must consider factors that influence the treatment plan (Table 13-4).

The goals for cancer treatment include cure, prevention of recurrence or metastasis, to control the cancer as long as possible, or palliation of symptoms. These goals may be achieved through surgery, radiation, chemotherapy, biological therapy, targeted therapy, or hormonal therapy.

Surgery

Surgery is the most common treatment for cancer and may be followed or preceded by other treatments depending on type and stage. Goals of surgery include:

- Debulking a tumor
- Diagnosing a tumor (ie, **biopsy**)
- Removing precancerous lesions
- Resecting a tumor
- Correction of life-threatening conditions caused by cancer
- Palliation
- Cure

The rehabilitation implications after surgery depend on the particular cancer surgery, some of which will be discussed in the following sections. Therapists need to consider what structures have been removed or altered and their effect on posture, muscle strength, balance, alignment, tissue pliability, and lymphatic flow. Muscles, bones, and nerves may be resected as part of the cancer surgery or they may be damaged as a result of the surgical approach. Therapists need to assess wound healing and determine how and when to increase load to the tissue based on the stages of tissue healing.

Common rehabilitation interventions for the postsurgical patients include early mobilization, pulmonary hygiene, and training in activities of daily living (ADLs). Early mobilization assists in the prevention of complications such as pneumonia, ileus, deep vein thrombosis (DVT), skin breakdown, and the loss of lean body mass. Pulmonary hygiene in the form of splinted coughing, deep breathing exercises, and postural education play an important role in preventing postoperative pulmonary complications. Finally, gait training and ADL training may be appropriate if surgery included an amputation, if there is a weightbearing restriction, if pain is limiting functional mobility, or if fatigue is impeding mobility. Education regarding the importance of physical activity for health promotion should also be included in acute care physical therapy sessions. There are many cancers for which physical activity is protective and may reduce cancer-related and overall mortality (eg, breast, colorectal, prostate).

Radiation Therapy

Another modality used in cancer treatment is radiation. Radiation is a **nonselective, localized treatment** that destroys cells by damaging DNA, impairing cell replication, or disrupting the milieu in which these cells thrive.[3,7] Radiation beams "excite" the tumor cells, damaging DNA. The goal of radiation is to maximize the effect on tumor cells, while minimizing the impact on healthy tissue. Healthy cells divide more slowly than cancerous ones and are more adept at repairing damage caused by radiation, thereby increasing cancer cell death while reducing damage to healthy cells.[7] The 2 primary methods to deliver radiation include external beam therapy and internal radiation (**brachytherapy**). In brachytherapy, radiation is delivered in seeds that are implanted into the tumor site. This is most often used in prostate and gynecological cancers. Radiation is fractionated, meaning smaller doses of radiation are given to reduce the impact on healthy tissues. There have been many advances in radiation therapy that enable the physician to more accurately deliver radiation to the tumor itself while protecting surrounding healthy tissue, such as intensity-modulated radiation therapy, image-guided radiation, and stereotactic conformal 3-dimensional (3D) therapy. The severity of side effects from radiation depend on dosing and the area being irradiated.

Radiation can be given as **adjuvant therapy** (after primary surgical treatment), or as **neoadjuvant therapy** (before cancer surgery). Radiation is most effective on cells that are rapidly dividing, such as cancer cells. However, radiation also impacts other cells that normally have a high turnover rate, such as cells in the gastrointestinal (GI) tract, hair follicles, and skin. Goals for radiation include:

- Cure
- Control of cancer
- Decrease tumor size
- Palliation
- Prevention of fracture

Radiation side effects can affect multiple tissue types and can be acute, early delayed (up to 3 months after treatment), or late delayed (more than 3 months after radiation) (Table 13-5).[8] Slowly proliferating cells may show radiation effects weeks,

Table 13-5

Common Side Effects of Radiation Therapy

- Immunosuppression:
  - Radiation to long bones, ilium, sternum
- Skin changes:
  - Fragile skin
  - Erythematous skin
  - Tissue fibrosis (acute or chronic), myofascial adhesions
- GI changes:
  - Vomiting/diarrhea, which can result in impaired nutrition, protein deficiency, and muscle catabolism
- Fatigue[8]:
  - Cumulative over the course of radiation therapy
  - May begin to resolve when radiation is complete or last 6 months to 1 year post-radiation.
  - Some people will experience long-term cancer-related fatigue.
- Avascular necrosis (AVN):
  - Loss of blood supply to an area resulting in necrosis of tissue
  - The most common area is the hip, potentially resulting in femoral head collapse and fracture.
  - Symptoms include pain with weightbearing, ache in the groin and anterior thigh, minimal relief with rest.
- Radiation myelitis:
  - Radiation may damage small blood vessels in the spinal column resulting in loss of blood flow, necrosis, and demyelination.
  - Symptoms include sensory dysfunction and motor weakness.
  - Time of onset is typically 4 to 12 months after the completion of radiation.
- Lymphedema:
  - Radiation over lymphatic beds increases the risk of developing lymphedema for many types of cancers.

months, or years after radiation treatment has ended. Tissues that may have a delayed radiation effect include skin, fascia, heart, and lungs.

An example of a late effect is radiation-induced fibrosis, which is characterized by a progressive change in tissues with a decrease in elasticity and atrophy.[9]

Preventative and restorative stretching should be prescribed to patients receiving radiation therapy. Radiation changes in the short and long term can affect range of motion (ROM), biomechanical alignment, lymphatic flow, and nerve integrity. The potential to develop fascial tightness after radiation needs to be considered. Exercises should continue for up to 6 months after the course of radiation is completed. One must also consider the risk for lymphedema if lymphatic beds are included in the radiation field. In women with breast cancer, axillary lymph node dissection and radiation therapy are 2 key risk factors for the development of lymphedema.[9]

Table 13-6 Common Side Effects of Chemotherapy
• Immunosuppression: Decrease in function of the components of the immune system. Patients may develop anemia or thrombocytopenia. In addition, there is a decrease in the white blood cell [WBC] count resulting in a diminished ability to resist infections. • Organ damage (eg, heart failure, liver toxicity, renal damage) • Nausea and vomiting • Alopecia (hair loss) • Diarrhea • Mucositis or mouth sores • Sterility • Peripheral neuropathy • Motor symptoms: ¤ Sense of heaviness in legs ¤ Tripping due to motor weakness of anterior tibialis ¤ Difficulty holding or manipulating objects ¤ Shaky handwriting • Sensory symptoms: ¤ Sensation of pins and needles ¤ Cold extremities ¤ Burning sensation ¤ Sharp, electrical, shooting pain • Autonomic symptoms: ¤ Orthostasis ¤ Feeling flush ¤ Tachycardia

Chemotherapy

Chemotherapy is a **systemic treatment** that does not distinguish between healthy and diseased tissue (ie, **nonselective**). Goals for chemotherapy include the following:

- Cure
- Control the cancer if it is not curable
- Shrink the tumor for palliation and to enable surgical resection

Chemotherapy is administered using a combination of drugs. Combination therapy helps to decrease toxic side effects, lowers the chances of drug resistance, and increases anti-neoplastic effectiveness. Similar to radiation therapy, chemotherapy has a higher kill rate for rapidly dividing cells. Thus, the side effects of chemotherapy are a result of the destruction of cells with rapid turnover, such as those cells found in the bone marrow, GI tract, reproductive tract, and hair follicles, as noted in Table 13-6.[3] Chemotherapy is given in cycles with rest breaks in between to allow healthy cells to recovery.

Certain chemotherapy agents may also affect the musculoskeletal system and the central nervous system (CNS) as listed in Table 13-7. For example, peripheral neuropathy is a common side-effect of chemotherapeutic agents including the taxanes and platinum compounds. **Peripheral neuropathy** refers to damage to the peripheral nerves resulting in myriad symptoms, such as sensory and motor changes, pain, and

Table 13-7

Chemotherapeutic Agents and Common Side Effects

Chemotherapeutic Agents	*Common Side Effects*
Cisplatin (eg, testicular, prostate, ovarian, uterine, head and neck, lung)	Ototoxicity, hypokalemia, hypomagnesemia, peripheral neuropathy
Ifosfamide (eg, ovarian, breast, testicular, lymphoma, lung)	Myelosuppression, lethargy, cerebellar toxicity
Cytarabine (eg, leukemia, lymphoma)	Cerebellar toxicity
Methotrexate (eg, breast, uterine, leukemia, head and neck, cervical)	Myelosuppression, pulmonary fibrosis, transverse myelitis, osteoporosis, cerebellar dysfunction
Doxorubicin (eg, breast, gastric, liver, bladder, prostate, sarcoma, lymphoma, multiple myeloma, leukemia)	Myelosuppression, cardiomyopathy
Vincristine (eg, lymphoma, breast, lung, leukemia)	Paraesthesia, ataxia, foot drop, cranial nerve palsies, loss of deep tendon reflexes
Tamoxifen (eg, breast)	Hot flashes, uterine bleeding, fluid retention
B-interferon (eg, leukemia, renal, melanoma, leukemia)	Myalgia, hypotension
Taxol (paclitaxel; eg, breast, ovarian, lung, bladder, prostate, melanoma, esophageal)	Myelosuppression, peripheral neuropathy

autonomic dysfunction. Motor impairment from chemotherapy has been associated with a higher risk of falls in cancer survivors.[10,11]

Symptoms of chemotherapy-induced peripheral neuropathy (CIPN) can occur during chemotherapy infusion or in the days or weeks afterward. Some patients will develop coasting, or CIPN that appears after chemotherapy has ended. Most people will have resolution of their neuropathy within 6 to 12 months after the completion of the chemotherapy regimen; however, some may have long-term symptoms.[12,13] Physical therapists should screen for CIPN prior to the initiation of chemotherapy and periodically during and after treatment. The Total Neuropathy Score clinical version or the Rasch-built Overall Disability Scale have evidence to support their reliability and validity as well as clinical sensitivity.[14-16] Oncologists typically utilize the NCI's Common Terminology Criteria for Adverse Events, which grades CIPN from loss of deep tendon reflexes or paresthesias that don't interfere with function (1) to permanent sensory loss that interferes with function (5).[17]

Treatment interventions for peripheral neuropathy may include medications such as serotonin-norepinephrine reuptake inhibitors.[14,18] In addition to medical therapy, physical and occupational therapy can be utilized for preventative and restorative therapy, including ADL training, bracing, strengthening, gait training, and balance training.[19]

Patients undergoing chemotherapy should be provided with education regarding the potential musculoskeletal side effects of their drug regimen. In addition, patients should be provided with an aerobic program to prevent loss of endurance and to mediate cancer-related fatigue. The intensity of the program should be individualized, taking into consideration age, stage of disease, and chemotherapy regimen. In addition, adjustments should be made for changes in blood counts, such as anemia and thrombocytopenia. Refer to the section on Exercise for the Person With Cancer and Chapter 2 (see Tables 2-12 and 2-13) for a more detailed discussion.

Targeted Therapies

Targeted therapies are directed at specific protein targets involved with the growth or spread of cancer. Targeted therapies prevent continued cell growth, whereas chemotherapy kills the cells. Targeted therapies are more specific than chemotherapy.[20] An example of a targeted therapy is used in leukemia where some people have a fusion of 2 proteins in their leukemic cells. Gleevec (imatinib), an oral agent, specifically targets this fusion, leaving healthy cells intact.

Other types of targeted therapies include hormonal treatment, anti-angiogenesis agents, signal transduction inhibitors, and immunotherapies. Hormonal treatments are given to people whose cancer grows when exposed to a particular hormone (eg, prostate and breast cancers). Hormonal therapies act to block a hormone from causing the tumor to grow. Anti-angiogenesis agents work to block the growth of blood vessels, which cancer cells need to grow and spread. These agents affect vascular endothelial growth factor (VEGF), which normally assists with the formation of new blood vessels. Immunotherapies may also be used by triggering the patient's own immune system to fight the cancer.[21] A recent advance in immunotherapy is CAR T-cell therapy. In CAR (chimeric antigen receptor) T-cell therapy, T cells are collected from the patient and altered to identify and attach to an antigen specific to the patient's cancer. CAR T is presently being used in refractory non-Hodgkins lymphoma and refractory acute lymphoblastic leukemia in children.

Bone Marrow Transplantation

Bone marrow transplantation (BMT) is a modality used to treat leukemia, myelodysplastic syndrome, lymphoma, and aplastic anemia. Transplants are being tested in clinical trials for ovarian, multiple myeloma, and colon cancers. There are 2 main types: autologous and allogeneic BMT. The mortality and morbidity associated with allogeneic transplants is higher than autologous due to prolonged immunosuppression, side effects of high dose chemotherapy, and graft-vs-host disease (GVHD).

In autogeneic transplants, the patient's own stem cells or marrow are used. Patients then undergo chemotherapy and/or total body irradiation followed by re-infusion of their own stem cells. Stem cells are pluripotent cells that have the ability to mature into any of the cells in the blood cell line, including monocytes, neutrophils, erythrocyte, and platelets. While awaiting recovery of their blood counts, patients are provided with intensive medical support as they experience the side effects of chemotherapy, including neutropenia, thrombocytopenia, anemia, electrolyte abnormalities, and nausea/vomiting.

In allogeneic transplants, the patient is rescued with cells from a human leukocyte antigen (HLA) matched relative or from a donor registry (matched unrelated donor [MUD]). Other types of allogeneic transplants include haploidentical or half-matched donors such as parents, transplants using umbilical cord blood, or reduced-intensity conditioning transplantation. The selection of the donor is one of the most critical components of the transplant. If the donor and recipient have a high degree of HLA compatibility there is a lower probability of developing GVHD, a condition associated with high morbidity and mortality. GVHD can occur either in the acute (first 100 days) or chronic phase (> 100 days) of allogeneic BMT. GVHD occurs when the donor's cells (graft) recognize the patient's body (host) as foreign and mount an immunological attack. This process is mediated by the donor T lymphocytes and is more likely to occur when there are HLA mismatches. Controlled GVHD may be beneficial to the leukemic patient, as the immunological attack may cause a graft vs leukemia affect, essentially helping to increase the kill rate of leukemic cells.[1] However, uncontrolled GVHD is associated with high morbidity and mortality.[1] GVHD typically attacks 3 body systems: skin, liver, and gut. GVHD skin appears as a rash in the acute phase progressing to soft tissue fibrosis in the chronic phase. Physical therapy can play an important role in providing a flexibility program to prevent and treat the loss of ROM with changes in the distensibility of soft tissue. In chronic GVHD involving skin, soft tissue mobilization may also help to restore ROM and flexibility. GVHD of the liver causes right upper quadrant pain and hepatic dysfunction with resultant confusion, encephalopathy, and jaundice. Finally, GVHD of the gut often results in sloughing of the intestinal lining leading to poor absorption of nutrients, vomiting, diarrhea, and loss of lean body mass. The treatment for GVHD involves increasing dosage of immunosuppressive drugs, such as corticosteroids, to diminish the immunological attack on the host. High-dose corticosteroids increase the likelihood of myopathy and osteopenia, both of which respond to physical therapy interventions. Steroid myopathy often presents with proximal hip weakness, manifesting in a difficulty with transfers and stairs. This may often go unnoticed, as walking is only impaired in later stages. A second manifestation of steroid myopathy is shoulder girdle weakness. Treatment for steroid myopathy should include weightbearing exercises and strengthening exercises emphasizing the patient's core and proximal muscle groups.

Exercise is important during and after BMT to minimize loss of lean body mass, endurance, and to maintain or improve quality of life.[22] Most BMT units place the patient in a single room for isolation during allogeneic transplants. Being confined to a room for 4 to 6 weeks places the patient at risk for loss of endurance, imbalance, and postural hypotension (see Chapter 4 and Table 4-1). In addition, chemotherapy, steroid regimens, malnutrition, and limited mobility due to illness can all contribute to progressive deconditioning. Instruction and demonstration of a daily exercise routine that includes both aerobic and strengthening components is essential. Moderate intensity aerobic exercise, such as stationary cycling, should be tailored to the patient's individual fitness levels and frequently modified to account for changes in his or her blood counts and overall medical condition.[23-26] Patients should also be provided with a home exercise program to restore strength and endurance.

The following sections will briefly describe some cancer types with the salient implications for the acute care physical therapist.

Breast Cancer

Aside from skin cancer, breast cancer is the most common type of cancer in American women.[27] Risk factors for breast cancer include years of menstruation, physical inactivity, elevated body mass index (BMI), alcohol consumption, smoking, high breast tissue density, use of long-term hormone replacement therapy, previous chest radiation previous chest radiation, and genetic predisposition.[28]

Staging is determined through multiple tests, including mammogram, breast ultrasound, fine needles aspiration, skeletal survey, lymph node dissection, or sentinel lymph node biopsy.

The primary treatment for breast cancer is surgery utilizing one of the following surgical approaches: lumpectomy, skin sparing mastectomy, or modified radical mastectomy.

- **Breast conserving surgery: Lumpectomy** or **partial mastectomy** is the removal of a suspicious breast lump and a small area of surrounding healthy tissue (clean margin). Lumpectomy is indicated for small tumors and is often followed by radiation. Breast conserving therapy with radiation is equivalent to mastectomy for small tumors, so the choice of approach is up to the patient and health care team.

- **Mastectomy** is the removal of breast tissue. Mastectomy is performed if the tumor is larger, there are multiple tumors, or the person chooses not to undergo radiation therapy. Types of mastectomy are:
  - **Simple mastectomy**: Removal of the entire breast, skin, and nipple
  - **Skin-sparing mastectomy** and **nipple-sparing mastectomy**: Tumor and breast tissue removed but the skin is kept intact for better cosmesis during immediate breast reconstruction. In skin sparing mastectomy the nipple is removed, however it is kept intact with a nipple sparing mastectomy.
  - **Modified radical mastectomy** (MRM): Removal of the entire breast, skin, nipple, and lining over the pectoralis muscles, with axillary node dissection or sentinel lymph node biopsy
- **Axillary staging** refers to an evaluation of the axillary lymph nodes to inform staging and treatment options. Two types of axillary staging are available: axillary lymph node dissection and sentinel lymph node biopsy.[27]
  - **Axillary lymph node dissection** (ALND): ALND used to be the standard of care to determine if the cancer has spread to the axillary region. If the cancer has spread to the axillary lymph nodes, it is likely that the cancer has spread beyond the breast. ALND is utilized when the sentinel lymph nodes are positive and involves removal of 10 to 30 of the level I and II lymph nodes. Level I nodes are located below the axillary vein and below the lower edge of the pectoralis minor muscle; level II nodes are located under the pectoralis minor, and level III is above the pectoralis.[29]
  - **Sentinel lymph node biopsy** (SLNB): To avoid the morbidity associated with extensive ALNDs, SLNBs are performed for those with small localized tumors. A radioisotope is injected around the tumor and is traced to the first lymph node or nodes, called the **sentinel nodes**. The sentinel nodes are colored by the radioisotope for easy identification and removed for further evaluation. If the sentinel nodes are negative for cancer cells, no further axillary dissection is warranted. If the biopsy is positive for cancer cells, the patient must return for a full axillary dissection to accurately stage the disease.

Common impairments after breast surgery and lymph node dissection include pain, poor ROM, paresthesias in the distribution of the intercostobrachial nerve, and swelling. Upper quarter dysfunction (UQD) has been reported in over 50% of patients who have undergone breast cancer surgery.[30] Patients undergoing surgery should be instructed in a progressive shoulder ROM program that addresses shoulder flexion, rotation, and abduction. Patients should also receive postural training to prevent shortening of the pectoralis musculature from a splinted or protected position of forward shoulders as well as strengthening of the scapular retractors and spine stabilizers. Two studies of patients 2.5 to 7 years after ALND or SLNB, found greater impairments in grip strength, increased pain, and higher rates of lymphedema in those who underwent a full axillary dissection.[31,32] This suggests that patients with a full ALND be monitored more closely with early physical therapy intervention. Shoulder dysfunction can also develop over time, indicating that survivors may benefit from a prospective surveillance system after primary treatment has ended.[33]

Exercises after breast cancer surgery should begin after removal of the drains, around postoperative days 7 to 10. Studies have reported decreased incidence of seroma formations when exercises are delayed after drain removal, without a significant impact on long-term shoulder function.[34,35] Demonstration of exercises should begin preoperatively if possible. If the patient will undergo radiation therapy after wound healing, it is imperative to restore shoulder flexion and external rotation so that he or she can be positioned optimally for radiation. Less common, but significant, issues in the acute setting are cellulitis, flap necrosis, and brachial plexopathy from surgical positioning. Therapists should adequately screen for these issues and contact the medical team if discovered for early intervention with medications, surgery, and continued rehabilitation.[31]

Edema in the breast, axilla, chest wall, and arm commonly occurs immediately after breast surgery. This postsurgical swelling will reduce over the next few weeks of recovery and does not usually indicate lymphedema. If arm swelling persists, the medical team should be consulted to determine the cause of edema, which could include postoperative infection, DVT, congestive heart failure (CHF), renal dysfunction, or disease recurrence. Risk factors for lymphedema include postoperative infection, elevated BMI, and ALND.[31]

Breast reconstruction is aimed at recreating a breast mound that is similar to the remaining breast. Reconstruction can be immediate (at the same time as mastectomy), or delayed.[36] Immediate reconstruction offers some women solace as they wake up from their Breast cancer surgery with a breast mound. Moreover, women have one surgery that attends to eradicating the tumor and recreating a breast. However, some women do not want to make a rushed decision about reconstruction and therefore opt to delay until curative treatment is completed. Other disadvantages of immediate reconstruction include longer operative time and possible delay of other cancer treatments if complications arise.[36] Delayed reconstruction occurs after the completion of cancer treatments, giving more time for consideration of surgical options. One disadvantage of the delayed approach is the changes in breast tissue and skin after radiation, which may impact surgical approach and cosmesis.[31] Presently, there is no clear evidence-based conclusion about the effectiveness of immediate vs delayed reconstruction.

There are many options for breast reconstruction including **implants**, **deep inferior epigastric perforator** (DIEP) **flaps**, and **transverse rectus abdominus myocutaneous** (TRAM) **flaps**. Any type of reconstruction that changes the length-tension relationships of muscle and the pliability of soft tissue and skin has the potential for short- or long-term musculoskeletal complications.

In skin sparing mastectomies, women can opt for a tissue expander and implant. The expander is placed under the pectoralis musculature and has a tube that is tunneled to the axilla. Over the course of weeks to months, saline is inserted into the tube, gradually filling the expander. When the final size is reached, the expander is removed and replaced with an implant.[37] Implants last approximately 10 to 15 years before needing replacement. Complications include pectoralis spasms, altered posture, capsular contracture around the implant, and infection. Capsular contracture around the implant oftentimes occurs outside of the acute care setting. Women will notice an altered position of the implant, or hardened skin.

Women who opt for breast implants should be taught postural exercises prior to this procedure. Depending on the size of the implant and the presence of pectoralis spasm, women may adopt a posture of rounded shoulders causing pectoralis tightness and weakness of scapular musculature. Gentle exercises may be employed early to avoid postural changes. A rigorous stretching program is not indicated until the final implant is in place. One should always monitor for areas of erythema, swelling, or necrosis triggering an immediate referral to the plastic surgeon.

The TRAM flap can be **pedicled** or a **free flap**. In a TRAM, the abdominal skin, fat, and some of the rectus abdominus muscle is used to recreate a breast mound. The epigastric artery and vein are kept intact and serve as the pedicle. In a free flap, the tissue and muscle are completely removed from the abdominal region and then reconnected to the blood supply in the axilla.[37] Surgeons may opt to use either the ipsilateral or contralateral rectus depending on the patency of the blood supply. If the contralateral rectus is used, patients will notice a medial bulge early in their recovery.

This bulge is the rectus muscle, which will atrophy over time due to denervation. Finally, mesh is placed at the donor site to prevent herniation of abdominal contents. In a DIEP flap, the rectus is spared and only the abdominal fat and tissue is used to recreate the breast mound. The epigastric artery is then connected to the mammary artery. Approximately 6 months after surgery, women can opt to have a nipple tattooed on or use a prosthetic nipple.

The acute care management of the TRAM reconstruction revolves around maintaining a healthy donor and recipient site. Mobility and lifting are limited by the physician to ensure this goal. Postoperatively, patients are instructed to remain in a flexed posture and limit lifting until the surgeon is comfortable with the health of the flap. This period may last from 3 weeks to a few months depending on tissue healing. The acute care role of the rehabilitation specialist includes teaching proper body mechanics within the limitations prescribed, transfer and bed mobility techniques, and lymphedema precautions. Importantly, patients should be educated regarding symptoms that may warrant a physical therapy consultation after the flap has healed. Patients who develop musculoskeletal complications may begin therapy after 6 to 8 weeks depending on flap viability. Common musculoskeletal and lymphatic consequences include breast and trunk lymphedema, adhesive capsulitis of the shoulder, poor posture, and low back pain. Appropriate therapy interventions may include a back stability program, shoulder ROM, strengthening, myofascial techniques for flexibility deficits, joint mobilization, body mechanics training, and complete decongestive therapy (see Lymphedema).[31,37]

In addition to surgery, radiation, and chemotherapy, some women will also undergo endocrine therapy if their tumors are sensitive to estrogen or progesterone.[37] Prior to menopause, the ovaries are the primary source of estrogen and after menopause estrogen is produced by adipose tissue. In some breast cancer, estrogen and/or progesterone stimulate the cancer cells to grow (estrogen receptor positive [ER +] tumors; progesterone receptor positive [PR+] tumors).[38] Women with ER or PR sensitivity will be eligible to take hormonal therapy, which attempts to block these hormones from binding to the breast tissue. One class of medications used is **selective estrogen receptor modulators** (SERMs). SERMS block estrogen in the breast tissue, but also act as a weak source of estrogen outside of the breast. The systemic effect of SERMs increases the risk of DVT, endometrial cancer, stroke, and, possibly, heart disease; however the benefits in reduced recurrence rates and reduced mortality outweigh these risks.[39] Therapists should be aware of these side effects and encourage aerobic exercise to possibly mediate the effects on clotting and cardiovascular disease. Therapists should also encourage women to have yearly visits with their primary care physician and oncologist to monitor for side effects. In post-menopausal women, **aromatase inhibitors** may be employed to stop adipose tissue from releasing estrogen into the blood stream. aromatase inhibitors can cause myalgias and arthralgias that are so significant that physicians may need to switch to a different aromatase inhibitor or terminate hormonal therapy. A risk factor for myalgia and arthralgia may include low Vitamin D levels.[39] Aromatase inhibitors also contribute to osteopenia, so patients should be encouraged to participate in weightbearing activities and strength training. There have been limited studies evaluating the impact of physical therapy interventions on hormonal therapy induced musculoskeletal symptoms.

Aerobic exercise is well tolerated and should be promoted during chemotherapy and radiation therapy.[1] Moderate intensity exercise can stem common decrements in fitness observed during treatment. Supervised exercise programs during chemotherapy have demonstrated no adverse events and positive findings in terms of fitness, endocrine symptoms, pain, and fatigue.[40]

Women with breast cancer should be followed prospectively beginning preoperatively and continuing after cancer treatment has ended.[40] Physical therapists should consider objective measurements in ROM, strength, sensation, posture, arm circumference, functional tasks, and quality of life. As many changes occur after the acute care stay, it is imperative to educate patients to follow up with their physicians regarding the function of their arms and seek out physical therapy as soon as any issues arise. Women should be encouraged to be as active as possible, as physical activity has been shown to improve quality of life and fitness, as well as improve overall mortality rates in women with breast cancer (Figure 13-1).[41]

Head and Neck Cancer

Head and neck cancers include cancer of the nasal cavity, nasopharynx, oral cavity, hypopharynx, salivary glands, and larynx. Treatment for head and neck cancer (HNCA) may include radiation, chemotherapy, and surgery. These treatments can cause significant dysfunction in mobility, speech, eating, and swallowing.[42] Additionally, surgeries can be quite disfiguring, causing emotional and interpersonal distress.

Physical therapists should screen those with HNCA early and throughout treatment due to their elevated risks for issues such as radiation-induced tissue fibrosis, cancer-related fatigue, deconditioning, lymphedema, and significant cervical and shoulder dysfunction. As the patient is undergoing or recovering from surgery or radiation, he or she is at risk for loss of lean muscle mass due to changes in nutritional intake. Patients are often on modified diets as they go through radiation due to nausea, mucositis, and xerostomia (dry mouth) and may experience smell sensitivity. Temporary or permanent access for enteral nutrition may be provided if their treatment has interfered with any part of their GI tract. Patients may also have temporary tracheostomies for airway protection and should be given a prophylactic pulmonary hygiene program including early mobility, deep breathing exercises, and cough instruction.

There are a variety of surgical approaches for HNCA depending on the location and size of the tumor.

- **Radical neck dissection** (RND): Removal of all 5 levels of lymph nodes, sacrifice of spinal accessory nerve (SAN), internal jugular vein, sternocleidomastoid (SCM), platysma, and omohyoid musculature. RND is used for large metastatic tumors and large palpable nodes (Figure 13-2).
- **Modified radical neck dissection** (MRND): Removal of lymph nodes levels I through V, with removal of one or more of the following:
  - SAN
  - Internal jugular vein
  - SCM
- **Selective neck dissection** (SND): Removal of the mass and any lymph nodes at highest risk of containing metastasis. Other structures removed are dependent upon the location of the tumor and its propensity to metastasize.
  - For **MRND and SND**, therapists should examine the operative record to determine which structures were removed as they vary surgery to surgery.

Acute care rehabilitation of the person after neck dissection should include a thorough examination of cervical ROM, posture, shoulder function, scapular kinematics, coughing techniques, mouth opening, and lymphedema education.[43,44] Therapy should proceed cautiously to allow for proper wound healing, with significant caution if the carotid artery is at risk for dissection. Some physicians will limit shoulder flexion to 90 degrees when drains are present to avoid seroma formation. Conservative cervical ROM can begin in the postoperative period unless limited by plastic surgery interventions such as flaps. Patients will often posture with forward

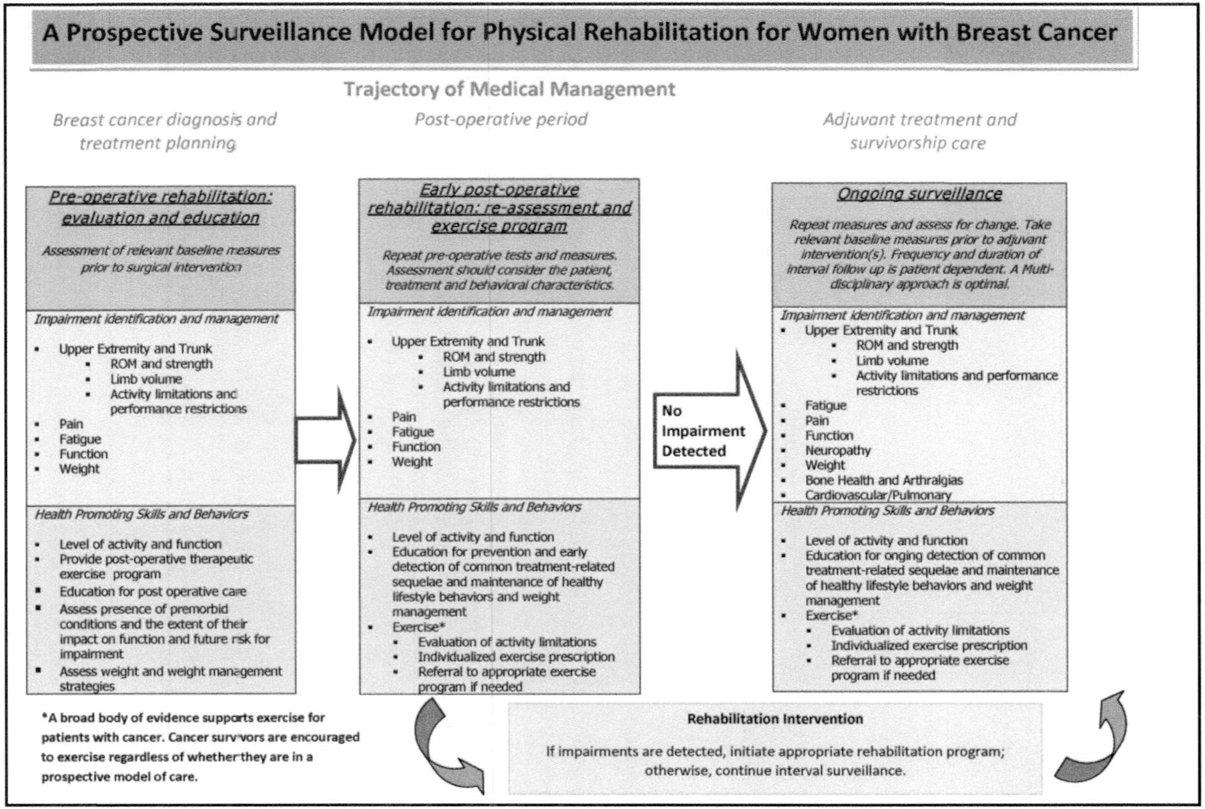

Figure 13-1. A prospective surveillance model for physical rehabilitation for women with breast cancer. (Reprinted with permission from Stout NL. Binkley JM, Schmitz KH, et al. A prospective surveillance model for rehabilitation for women with breast cancer. *Cancer.* 2012;15[18]:2191-2200.)

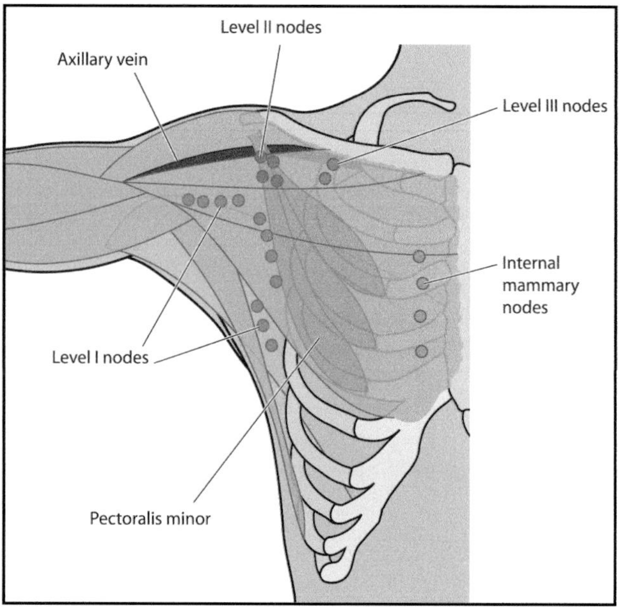

Figure 13-2. Diagram of axillary and internal mammary lymph nodes. Level I lymph nodes are inferior to the lower edge of pectorallis minor; level II lymph nodes are under or deep to the pectorallis minor; level III lymph nodes are subclavicular; and level IV lymph nodes are supraclavicular. (Blamb/Shutterstock.com)

head, rounded shoulders, and neck rotation due to pain, tracheostomy, and fear of damaging the surgical site. Posturing in this manner will exacerbate any shoulder dysfunction and decrease the ability to clear secretions. Postural exercises should include pectoralis stretching and strengthening of the trapezius and rhomboids. Neck dissection surgeries alter the venous and lymphatic drainage system of the head, neck, and face. Patient education regarding lymphedema needs to be stressed.

Many patients will undergo outpatient radiation therapy to the head and neck, which can contribute to ROM deficits in the cervical region, shoulder complex, and pterygoid muscles. Education regarding trismus, jaw muscle spasms, and the role of physical therapy for temporomandibular joint (TMJ) issues is needed, along with prophylactic stretching and ROM exercises.

Spinal Accessory Nerve

During neck dissection, the **spinal accessory nerve** (SAN) may be sacrificed or damaged from a traction injury due to the small surgical area of the posterior cervical triangle.[45-47] Even those without overt damage to the SAN often face weakness in the trapezius.[48] The SAN innervates the trapezius, which is an essential element for scapulohumeral rhythm and overhead motion. Statically, the trapezius holds the scapula on the thoracic cage. Dynamically, the trapezius contributes to medial stabilization and upward rotation of the scapula, allowing for full ROM of the humerus for overhead activities. If the SAN was removed or injured during surgery, the patient may demonstrate abnormal scapulohumeral rhythm and the following musculoskeletal abnormalities[47,49]:

- Atrophy of trapezius (chronic denervation)
- Limited shoulder flexion and abduction to 90 degrees or less
- Pain with shoulder flexion and abduction
- Scapular winging and upward rotation

- Scapular protraction and depression
- Subluxation of the humeral head

Altered static and dynamic biomechanics may cause other scapular muscles, such as the levator scapula, serratus anterior, and rhomboids, to become strained and may also contribute to capsular tightness and chronic pain.[49] Therapy of the patient with SAN impairment should focus on early identification of nerve palsy through testing of the trapezius and educating the patient on supporting the arm during sitting and standing activities.[45] Outpatient physical therapy referrals should be made to continue with positioning recommendations, training of the rhomboids and serratus to help compensate for loss of trapezius function, and to normalize scapulohumeral rhythm and overhead motions. Progressive resistance exercises, electrical stimulation, and postural education are important interventions to initiate in the outpatient setting, as long as there is adequate wound healing. This is even more essential if the patient is to undergo radiation therapy, which may contribute to loss of range and function.

Head and Neck Reconstruction

Patients who have large tumors or need resection of the mandible are potential candidates for osseocutaneous or myocutaneous reconstruction. The 3 most common techniques are **pectoralis flap**, **fibular flap**, and **radial forearm flap**. Pectoralis musculature is used when there is a need for muscle bulk due to a large resection. The motion of the pectoralis can be partially compensated for by the latissimus dorsi and subscapularis. However, if the patient has SAN damage, he or she has lost both posterior and anterior stabilization of the shoulder. Rehabilitation should focus on postural training and cervical ROM. Once wound healing is achieved, exercises should include scapular retraction and latissimus strengthening for posterior stability.

A fibular osseocutaneous flap can be used to reconstruct the mandible. Up to 10 cm of bone is resected, with preservation of the peroneal nerve.[1] The distal end of the fibula remains intact to allow for ankle stabilization. The long-term functional sequela of a fibular flap is unknown as the fibula serves mostly as a site for muscle attachment and is not a weightbearing bone. In the acute setting, patients are often non-weightbearing for 4 to 7 days. Evaluation of vascular integrity and peroneal nerve function are critical. Therapists should focus on normalizing gait, improving functional mobility, and preventing pulmonary complications through ambulation and deep breathing. One should provide verbal feedback to avoid compensatory gait deviations that will increase the energy requirements of walking and potentially lead to long-term postural pain. The surgical team usually evaluates TMJ function after initial healing has taken place and patients may be referred to outpatient physical therapy for treatment.

A radial forearm flap can be used to replace skin lost on the face or in the reconstruction of the oral pharynx. The patient should avoid weightbearing through the donor site during transfers and ADLs. ROM to the wrist, elbow, and shoulder should be taught as well as proper posture. ROM of the shoulder might be limited by the medical team to 90 degrees until drains are removed to avoid seroma formation.

Newer surgeries include different free flaps, such as the latissimus dorsi flap or the anteriolateral thigh flap. As newer techniques arise, therapists must consider the potential deficits that can occur from operative positioning and from disruption of both the donor and recipient sites.

Liquid Tumors: Leukemia, Lymphoma, and Multiple Myeloma

Leukemia is a hematological disorder that affects leukocytes, including neutrophils, basophils, eosinophils, lymphocytes, and monocytes. Leukemia results in proliferation of abnormal, malfunctioning cells that crowd out normal cell lines in the marrow, causing symptoms from failure of multiple cell lines.

Leukemia is classified according to the cell line that is affected (myeloid or lymphoid) and the stage at which cellular development became abnormal. Acute leukemias are characterized by dysfunction of immature, undifferentiated cells whereas chronic leukemia is characterized by dysfunction of mature, more differentiated cells. The onset of chronic leukemia is more gradual than acute leukemia, and the clinical course is often longer. There are many different subtypes within these categories, so treatment is dependent upon the patient's particular cellular characteristics. Leukemias are treated with one or more of the following: combination chemotherapy, targeted therapy, monoclonal antibodies, or stem cell transplant. Chemotherapy is given in 3 phases:

1. **Induction**: Initial cycle of chemotherapy used to induce remission. The chemotherapy causes bone marrow hypoplasia, allowing normal cells to grow and replenish the marrow.
2. **Consolidation**: A second round of chemotherapy aimed to prevent recurrence from resistant or microscopic residual disease
3. **Intensification**: A third round of chemotherapy often given for patients at high risk for recurrence

Many chemotherapy agents do not cross the blood-brain barrier and therefore require placement of an Ommaya shunt or lumbar puncture for direct delivery of chemotherapy when leukemic cells have infiltrated the central nervous system.[50]

Some people with acute lymphocytic or myelogeous leukemia will be eligible for tyrosine kinase inhibitors, which are a form of targeted therapy that target a specific protein on leukemic cells. Common side effects include fatigue, swelling of the eyes and hands, and myalgias.

Lymphoma is also a hematological disorder that arises from the lymphoreticular system, which is primarily responsible for the growth and development of B and T lymphocytes. The humoral response to a foreign antigen involves the B cell, which secretes antigen specific antibodies. T cells are a part of cell mediated immunity that develops specifically against a particular antigen (see Chapter 5).

There are 2 main categories of lymphomas: **Hodgkin's lymphoma** (Hodgkin's disease) and **Non-Hodgkin's lymphoma** (NHL). The Reed-Sternberg cell, a large multi-nucleated cell, characterizes Hodgkin's disease and is present in all 4 sub-types of Hodgkin's disease. Treatment for Hodgkin's disease includes radiation and/or chemotherapy, depending on stage, or stem cell transplant for resistant disease (Table 13-8). Due to advances in detection and treatment, Hodgkin's disease has a cure rate in the high 90s%.[28]

NHLs are a heterogeneous group of cancers that can range from slow-growing indolent tumors to rapidly growing tumors. NHL can affect either B or T cells and can appear in any organ of the body. Treatment may include radiation, chemotherapy, or bone marrow transplant.

The treatments for leukemia and lymphoma can be quite debilitating. The chemotherapy regimens often result in an immunosuppression that places the patient at a high risk for infection. Weakness, impaired aerobic capacity, fatigue, and peripheral neuropathies are all common side effects. Patients undergoing myeloablative chemotherapy can benefit from an aerobic and strength training program to minimize

Table 13-8

STAGES OF HODGKIN'S DISEASE

Stage	*Description*
I	One area of lymph node involvement
II	Two or more areas of lymph node involvement above the diaphragm
III	Two or more areas of lymph node involvement both above and below the diaphragm
IV	Widespread disease

decrements in aerobic capacity and strength.[51-53] Moreover, those who participate in an exercise program may have less fatigue and less nausea.[54] Home exercise prescription should include a progressive aerobic and strength training program to regain strength and endurance and to help mediate fatigue. Therapists should also prescribe programs for chemotherapy side effects, such as peripheral neuropathy, as needed. At the time of this writing, a newer treatment intervention is available for refractory disease called *CAR T-cell therapy*. Side effects can include a cytokine release syndrome with severe muscle and joint pain, cardiovascular instability, and neurologic events that require physical therapy intervention. Please refer to the sections on chemotherapy, radiation, and exercise intervention for more details.

MULTIPLE MYELOMA

Multiple myeloma is a disease of the plasma cell (See Chapter 5, Humoral Immunity). When B cells interact with a pathogen, they become plasma cells that produce antibodies. In multiple myeloma, plasma cells grow out of control and crowd out other cell lines resulting in anemia, thrombocytopenia, and an increased risk of infections.[55] If untreated, survival is approximately 7 months; however, with treatment, survival may be extended to 2 to 3 years.[3] Average age of onset is 65 years of age, and this disease is more common among Black people and in males.[3] Treatment options for multiple myeloma include chemotherapy, radiation, interferon, bisphosphosphonates, plasmapheresis, or BMT.

Multiple myeloma has a significant effect on skeletal stability. An antibody produced by the abnormal plasma cells disrupts the normal balance of osteoclastic and osteoblastic activity resulting in breakdown of bone. Growth factors stimulate the multiple myeloma cells to grow, creating a cycle that enables multiple myeloma to flourish.[56] As the disease progresses, lytic lesions appear in the bony skeleton, diminishing the structural integrity of bone increasing fracture risk, spinal cord compression, and hypercalcemia. Thorough patient history should be taken with an emphasis on radiological evidence of skeletal disease, pain, and functional mobility. Many physicians utilize the Mirel scoring system to determine bone stability (Table 13-9).[57,58] The Mirel system has low to moderate specificity and, therefore, may overestimate risk.[59] Exercise intervention should include weightbearing exercises to improve bone density if the skeleton is stable. Therapy should also include education regarding the signs and symptoms of cord compression and pathologic fracture as noted later in Tables 13-15 and 13-16. Patients will likely be placed on IV bisphosphonates, which interfere with osteoclast activity, preventing further decline in bone density. A rare side effect of bisphosphonate therapy is osteonecrosis of the jaw, so therapists should

Table 13-9 MIRELS' SCORING SYSTEM FOR PATHOLOGIC FRACTURE RISK			
	1 Point	*2 Points*	*3 Points*
Site	Upper extremity	Lower extremity	Peritrochanter
Pain	Mild	Moderate	Activity related
Lesion Type	Blastic	Mixed	Lytic
Size	<1/3 cortical diameter	1/3 to 2/3 cortical diameter	>2/3 cortical diameter
<7=radiation therapy; >8=prophylactic surgical fixation			
Adapted from Jawad MU, Scully SP. In brief: classifications in brief: Mirels' classification: metastatic disease in long bones and impending pathologic fracture. *Clin Orthop Relat Res*. 2010;468(10):2825-2827. doi: 10.1007/s11999-010-1326-4			

screen for temporomandibular disorders.[57] Other directed therapies are also being used to target proteins known to impact bone reabsorption.

If bone disease is present, patients may benefit from surgical intervention, bracing, functional mobility and ADL training, and education in pain management. Vertebroplasty or kyphoplasty may be indicated; however, some studies show that these procedures may increase the risk of subsequent fractures.[57] Finally, postural training may be beneficial if there is vertebral collapse from lytic disease of the spine. Compression fractures may cause increased thoracic kyphosis due to loss of vertebral height. Kyphotic posture may contribute to pain, poor ventilation, and weakness of the shoulder musculature. There are a few small studies that indicate strength training may be beneficial, if first screened carefully for fracture risk.[60] Refer to section on skeletal related events for additional information.

GYNECOLOGICAL CANCERS

Gynecological cancers include cervical, ovarian, endometrial, vulvar, and vaginal. Treatment may include surgery such as:

- **Hysterectomy**: Removal of the uterus and cervix
- **Bilateral salpingo-oophorectomy** (BSO): Removal of both ovaries and fallopian tubes
- **Pelvic and para-aortic lymph node dissection**: Removal of lymph nodes in the pelvic region to assist with staging of cancer; contributes to the development of lymphedema in some women.

Surgery is often followed by radiation therapy, chemotherapy, and, possibly, hormonal therapy, including leutenizing hormone–releasing hormone agonists, tamoxifen, or aromatase inhibitors, which are used to reduce circulating estrogen, which can cause ovarian cancers to grow and metastasize. Some of these agents increase the risk for blood clots and osteopenia, so therapists should screen carefully and institute strength training and weightbearing exercises. Aromatase inhibitors may also cause myalgias and arthralgias (see section on Breast Cancer). For women undergoing chemotherapy, a home walking program may improve physical functioning and quality of life.[61]

Side effects of gynecological cancer treatment include peripheral neuropathy, pelvic pain, urinary incontinence, lymphedema, sexual dysfunction, and menopausal symptoms. Radiation to the pelvic region may result in fibrosis of the muscles and connective tissues in the radiation field and increase the risk for lymphedema. These soft tissue changes can occur both acutely and chronically and lead to decreased flexibility, ROM, and adhesions to nerve fibers. Exercises should focus on the flexibility of hip and abdominal musculature, scar adhesions, and nerve gliding techniques.

Pelvic pain syndromes, defined as pain in the buttocks, groin, pelvis, upper thighs, or lower abdomen that lasts for more than 3 months after completion of cancer treatments, are common. Characteristics of pelvic pain include constant or intermittent pain described as an ache, burn, or "shock-like." Pain may be exacerbated by urination or bowel movements, sexual intercourse, or with extended periods of sitting.

Dyspareunia, or pain with sexual intercourse, may also occur after treatment. Removal or damage to the ovaries decreases circulating estrogen, which can cause dryness and thinning of the vaginal mucosa. Patients may benefit from referral to rehabilitation specialists in women's health for vaginal dilators, lubricants, and pelvic floor reeducation.

Another side effect of treatment for gynecological cancers is urinary incontinence. Local reflex arcs, as well as higher centers in the brain, control the act of urination. When the bladder is stretched, a signal is sent to the sacral portion of the spinal cord that then triggers the bladder to allow for contraction of the detruser muscle and concomitant relaxation of the external sphincter. Additionally, a signal is sent to the brain that controls the coordination of bladder emptying and allows for volitional control over the external sphincter.[63] Dysfunction in any one of these areas caused by surgery, radiation, or direct invasion by tumor may affect volitional urination[63]:

- **Stress incontinence**: Incomplete closing of the sphincter due to weakness resulting in incontinence. The primary symptom is leakage during high-impact exercises, laughing, lifting, coughing, sneezing, and running. Leakage usually ends when the activity stops. Stress incontinence can result from surgery, occur during surgery due to a neurological insult, or from stretching of the pelvic musculature. In addition, poor closing of the sphincter can result from treatment-induced thinning of the urethra.
- **Overflow incontinence**: Occurs when urine is blocked from leaving the bladder, limiting effective emptying. A tumor or scar tissue can cause this, or urinary incontinence can result from nerve damage decreasing the body's ability to sense bladder volume.
- **Urge incontinence**: Occurs when the detrusor muscle contracts inappropriately during filling of the bladder. Patients need to urinate frequently and have leakage due to inability to voluntarily stop the urine flow.

Evaluation of the person with incontinence should include the following:

- Frequency of urination
- Amount of fluids (eg, water, caffeine, alcohol)
- Frequency of night urination
- Pain or odor with urination
- Ability to stop urine stream
- Describe activity that increases leakage
- Use of validated outcome measures such as:
  - Urogenital Distress Inventory[63]
  - Incontinence Impact Questionnaire [64]
  - Geriatric Self Efficacy Scale for Urinary Incontinence[65]

A pelvic floor rehabilitation program should begin postoperatively and continue in the outpatient setting. Urinary incontinence is quite common after treatment for gynecological cancer and can significantly impact quality of life.[66] A comprehensive pelvic floor rehabilitation should include some or all of the following:

Table 13-10 **Kegel Exercises**
1. Contract the pelvic floor muscles during urination and attempt to slow or stop the flow of urine. 2. Hold this contraction for 5 seconds, then release. 3. Rest 10 to 15 seconds between trials. 4. Perform 15 contractions, 3 to 4 times per day. 5. Alternate this with trials of a quick hold and release. 6. Once the patient understands her anatomy and can perform the exercises, avoid practicing during urination.

- Kegel exercises (stress and urge incontinence) (Table 13-10)
- Biofeedback
- Medications if needed (eg, alpha-adrenergic drugs, tricyclics)
- Weighted vaginal cones
- Pelvic floor electrical stimulation
- Change in dietary habits and fluid intake

Lung Cancer

Peak incidence of lung cancer for males is between 50 to 60 years of age with poor 5-year survival. Smoking is associated with 90% of cases of lung cancer.[67] Smoking causes chronic irritation to bronchial ciliated epithelial cells. Epithelial cells can regenerate in response to irritation; however, with chronic smoking, they eventually become less differentiated, resulting in cancer.

Lung cancer is categorized into **small cell** and **non–small cell cancer** (NSCLCA). Small cell lung cancer has a high growth rate and a worse prognosis than NSCLCA. The presenting symptoms are often cough, hemoptysis, dyspnea, and wheezing. Patients may also present with shoulder pain, weakness, or nerve symptoms if there is invasion of the brachial plexus. Treatment for lung cancer may include surgical resection, chemotherapy, and radiation. Lung cancer is minimally responsive to the present chemotherapy regimens and, therefore, has poor survival.

Physical therapy interventions should focus on posture, breathing facilitation techniques inclusive of inspiratory muscle training, and conditioning, and conditioning of the cardiovascular and musculoskeletal system. As lung cancer tends to spread to bone and brain, treatment of patients with metastatic disease may focus on gait training, pain control, and cognitive rehabilitation. Patients who undergo surgical resection for lung cancer often develop an acute pain syndrome and altered biomechanics that can lead to diminished vital capacity. Posterolateral thoracotomy approaches can result in atrophy of the latissimus dorsi muscle and the lower serratus, impacting shoulder function. These musculoskeletal issues are diminished in muscle sparing techniques and video-assisted thoracotomy; however, patient positioning during surgery, mobilization, or fracture of the ribs, and placement of drainage tubes can all impact the musculoskeletal system.[68-70] Some patients will develop post-thoracotomy pain syndrome, which is thought to occur from injury to the intercostal neurovascular bundle during surgery, or from placement of chest tubes.[69] A preoperative timed stair climbing test may be used to predict morbidity; specifically, time to climb steps, change in pulse rate, and desaturation are used to determine risk of postoperative complications.[71] Moreover, prehabilitation may improve postoperative outcomes. After surgery and during chemotherapy, patients should initiate a low to moderate intensity exercise program that addresses both the aerobic and anaerobic systems. Exercise has been shown to reduce cancer-related fatigue and increase fitness, even amongst patients with advanced disease.[72-74]

Colorectal Cancer

Colorectal cancers (CRC) are the third most common types of cancer in the United States that impact both genders.[75] The highest incidence occurs among those older than 50.[76] The natural progression of CRC begins with benign polyps and then advances to form cancerous lesions. Poor prognostic indicators include malignant cells that perforate the bowel, and venous or lymph node invasion.

Rectal cancer is rare, with the incidence higher among females. The etiology is unclear, although associations have been made with HIV, immunosuppression, prior radiation, cigarette smoking, and human papiloma virus (HPV). The most frequent symptom is spontaneous bleeding and complaints of pressure or pain with defecation.[76]

Treatments for CRC include surgery, radiation, chemotherapy, and targeted therapy. Surgery is the primary treatment with adjuvant chemotherapy or radiation for metastatic disease. Surgery may be open or laparoscopic, and may remove all or some of the colon and surrounding lymph nodes (colectomy, hemi-colectomy). Those with rectal cancer may undergo neoadjuvant chemoradiation followed by surgery, which reduces recurrence rates. Surgery may include a local transanal resection, lower anterior resection, proctectomy with coloanal anastomosis, abdominal perineal resection, or pelvic exenteration (the surgical removal of all organs from a person's pelvic cavity, including the urinary bladder, urethra, rectum, and anus).[76] Surgery may result in a permanent or temporary colostomy. Side effects may include sexual dysfunction due to injury of the sympathetic and parasympathetic nerves that are essential for erectile function. Women may experience a decrease in the size of the vagina if repair is needed after tumor excision. Common side effects of radiation and chemotherapy are bowel dysfunction (eg, diarrhea, leaking, bleeding), fatigue, chemotherapy-induced peripheral neuropathy, or hand-foot syndrome.[77] Kegel exercises and biofeedback can assist with return of bowel continence.[78,79]

Physical therapists may be asked to perform and interpret preoperative functional aerobic testing, such as the Shuttle Walk Test or 6 Minute Walk Test (6MWT), as distance walked is associated with the risk of postoperative complications.[80,81] Postoperatively, it is recommended that patients undergo an early mobilization program as part of an Enhanced Recovery After Surgery (ERAS) protocol. There is evidence that early mobilization contributes to a shorter length of stay and quicker onset to flatus for patients who undergo open or laparoscopic colon surgery.[82-84] After discharge from the hospital, there is strong evidence that physical activity programs increase fitness, reduce symptoms, improve quality of life, and reduce the risk of recurrence, so patients should be counseled on increasing activity.[85]

Prostate Cancer

Prostate cancer is the most common cancer in men. Men with prostate cancer often die from other causes, commonly cardiovascular disease.[86] There is a subset of prostate cancer that is more aggressive, and those with metastatic disease have a median survival of 2 to 3 years. Prostate cancer can metastasize to the bladder, peritoneum, lungs, liver, and kidney. Most commonly, prostate cancer metastasizes to the pelvis or axial skeleton.[3,87]

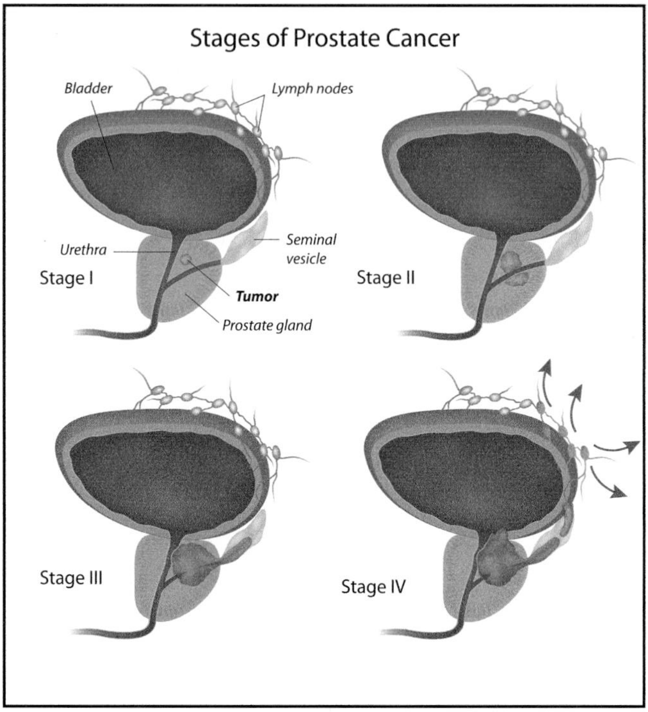

Figure 13-3. Stages of prostate cancer. Note the anatomical proximity of the prostate to the urinary tract with the urethra traveling through the prostate. (Alila Medical Media/Shutterstock.com)

Treatment for prostate cancer may include active surveillance, surgery, radiation, chemotherapy, brachytherapy, cryotherapy, vaccines, or hormone therapy. Active surveillance is for those with slow-growing tumors that have a low risk of metastasis. Primary surgical intervention can include a **radical retroperitoneal prostatectomy** through an abdominal incision, laparoscopic approach, or robotic surgery. In these surgeries, the prostate is removed and attempts are made to preserve the neurovascular bundle responsible for erections. The seminal vesicles and lymph nodes may also be removed. Surgery often includes excision of the bladder neck or internal sphincter, and part of the urethra; the bladder is then reattached to the remaining urethra. When part of the urethra is removed, the normal pressure of the system is changed, affecting continence.[88] Urinary incontinence is thought to occur due to damage to the sphincter or over activity of the detrusor muscle.[89] All men experience urinary incontinence in the short term and 14% to 28% experience urinary incontinence up to 5 years post-prostatectomy[90] (Figure 13-3). Patients are often responsive to biofeedback and biobehavioral techniques. See the section on Gynecological cancers for more information on urinary incontinence.

Side effects of surgery and radiation may also include temporary changes in bowel function, fascial tightness in the abdominal and pelvic region, sexual dysfunction, impotence, and lymphedema. If erectile function is to return, it often takes months to 2 years.[91]

Androgen deprivation therapy (ADT) is considered for patients whose cancer is likely to metastasize or has already spread. The aim of ADT is to reduce circulating androgens that stimulate the cancer to grow. Patients may undergo an orchiectomy or be prescribed hormonal blockers to slow tumor growth.[87] Hormone therapies can have significant side effects (Table 13-11). Bone mineral density may decrease in the

Table 13-11

Side Effects of Androgen Deprivation Therapy

• Fatigue • Hot flashes • Anemia • Sexual dysfunction • Penile and testicular atrophy • Increased fat mass • Insulin resistance	• Increased triglycerides, total cholesterol, high-density lipoprotein • Osteopenia and osteoporosis • Increased risk for fractures • Sarcopenia • Myalgias • Arthralgias

Adapted from Grossman, M, Cheung, A., Zajac, J. Androgens and prostate cancer; pathogenesis and deprivation therapy. *Best Pract Res Clin Endocrinol Metab*. 2013;27:603-616.

first year of ADT and may be underestimated by dual-energy x-ray absorptiometry (DEXA) scanning. Men may also lose 3% of their lean body mass in the first year of ADT, with continued loss seen if ADT is given continuously years following diagnosis.[87] Significant arthralgias and myalgias may impact physical activity levels, with severe issues causing a decrease in or discontinuation of the hormone therapy.

Acute therapy interventions may include mobility training, splinted coughing, and education regarding erectile dysfunction and urinary incontinence. Urinary incontinence training may begin pre- or postoperatively, although the efficacy of these interventions remains uncertain due to inadequate randomized clinical trials.[92,93] Weightbearing and strength training interventions may be important to stem the loss of muscle and bone density[94] (see section on skeletal-related events for therapy implications).

Testicular Cancer

The incidence of testicular cancer has been rising over the past few decades. Average age of onset is 33, although a small percentage are diagnosed in their teen and young adult years.[95] Risk factors include an undescended testicle, family history, HIV status, and White race (ACS, risk factors for testicular cancer). Most testicular cancers arise from germ tissue and demonstrate a rapid growth pattern. The metastatic pattern includes spread to lungs, liver, brain, and bone.[96]

Treatment for testicular cancer includes orchiectomy, retroperitoneal lymphadenectomy, radiation, chemotherapy, or stem cell transplant. Surgery may impact ejaculation, but nerve sparing approaches help to preserve sexual function. If ejaculation is impacted or if both testicles are removed, infertility may result. Moreover, loss of testosterone will contribute to osteopenia, muscle atrophy, hot flashes, and fatigue.[95] Chemotherapy is used for metastatic disease and has a high response rate; however, the commonly used regimens may cause peripheral neuropathy, lung impairment, and cold intolerance. Furthermore, testicular cancer survivors are at an elevated risk of cardiovascular disease, secondary cancers, and cancer-related fatigue.[97]

Considerations for the acute care therapist are similar to those mentioned under the section on prostate cancer. Refer to sections on metastasis, exercise, lymphedema, and neuropathy. Home programs should include aerobic and strength training to ameliorate the changes in muscle mass, bone density, and cardiovascular risk that accompany cancer treatment.[97]

Table 13-12 EXAMINATION OF CANCER-RELATED PAIN	
Temporal	Is the pain acute (onset days to weeks)? Is the pain chronic (>1 to 3 months)? Is it breakthrough pain or pain that significantly increases above and beyond your normal pain?
Intensity	On a scale of 0 to 10, with 0 indicating no pain and 10 maximal pain, what is your pain right now? Over the last 24 hours what has been the worst pain? Best pain?
Topography	Pain location (utilize description and body diagram)
Quality	Patient description of the pain without prompting; deep or superficial, localized or diffuse, burning/throbbing, shock-like, ache
Pain Goal Example	We would like for you to have no pain and we will work toward that. However, what is the level of pain, on a 0 to 10 scale, we can strive for that would provide you with good comfort and pain relief and also allow you to function well and carry out your daily activities?

CANCER PAIN

Pain is defined by the International Association for the Study of Pain[98] as "an unpleasant, multidimensional, sensory and emotional experience associated with actual or potential tissue damage." Chronic cancer pain affects up to 50% of patients diagnosed with cancer and up to 70% of those with advanced cancer.[99] Cancer pain should be managed by a multidisciplinary team that includes physical therapists and should be reassessed at every, or nearly every, interaction utilizing validated scales.

The physical therapy examination of cancer-related pain should begin with a thorough evaluation of the characteristics of pain and the patient's goal for pain relief (Table 13-12). Cancer pain can be musculoskeletal or neurologic in origin and may be a result of bone destruction, compression of nerves, collapse of vertebra, nerve inflammation, or altered biomechanics (Table 13-13). Cancer-related pain is often treated with a variety of medications, such as tricyclic antidepressants, anticonvulsants, corticosteroids, and baclofen. These medications can be effective; however, fine-tuning the dose can be an arduous process. There may be periods of oversedation or acute immobilizing pain as medications are titrated to their peak effective dose. During this process, the patient's ability to participate in therapy will vacillate. Patients and families should be taught safety awareness and fall prevention strategies as medications are adjusted.

Medications and rehabilitation strategies can be effective in the management of cancer-related pain.

- **Transcutaneous electrical nerve stimulation** (TENS): Uses low voltage electrical pulses transdermally to help reduce pain, as well as nausea.[25] High-frequency and low-intensity has been shown to be most effective for pain relief. TENS may be effective through blocking the afferent sensory information from higher sensors in the brain (Melzak-Wall Gate Theory). TENS may also be effective by causing local vasodilatation, possibly decreasing local ischemia. Finally, TENS may be effective by stimulating sensory nerves to signal the endogenous opiate

Table 13-13

CANCER-RELATED PAIN

Type of Pain	*Patient Descriptors*	*Possible Etiology*	*Exam Findings*
Neuropathic	• Tingling • Shock-like • Burning • Numbness • Temperature sensitivity	• Nerve irritation from tumor • Nerve irritation from surgery, radiation, chemotherapy • Vertebral collapse	• Motor weakness • Altered sensation • + neural tension tests • Pain along myotome or dermatome • Numbness/tingling distal to proximal
Skeletal	• Sharp • Escalating back pain • Pain in supine • Pain with ambulation • Pain in groin with weightbearing	• Altered bone stability from metastatic disease • Irritation of the periosteum from tumor • Spinal cord compression • Avascular necrosis	• Pain with weightbearing • Pain with joint compression • Pain that radiates to groin or anterior medial thigh with weightbearing • Pain with coughing
Joint	• Pain with function • Ache	• Tumor encroaching joint space • Arthralgia associated with chemotherapy, androgen deprivation, aromatase inhibitors	• Ache in non-weightbearing • Pain with passive and active ROM
Visceral	• Ache • Cramping • Stabbing • Poorly localized	• Tumor compressing viscera • Ischemia caused by tumor	• Pain not associated with movement • Difficult to reproduce with palpation or movement

Adapted from Cormie P, Newton RU, Spry N, Joseph D, Taaffe DR. Galvao DA. Safety and efficacy of resistance exercise in prostate cancer patients with bone metastases. *Prostate Cancer Prostatic Dis.* 2013;16:328-335.

release that decrease pain perception. TENS is indicated for postoperative incision, phantom limb, visceral, and bone pain. A 2012 Cochrane Review, which included 3 randomized controlled trials, was inconclusive regarding the effectiveness of TENS.[100,101]

- **Massage**: Assists with decreasing muscle spasms that occur from poor positioning or a change in muscle biomechanics. Anecdotal studies report that massage increases the overall quality of life of those with cancer.[101] There is some evidence that massage may help the emotional state of people with breast cancer.[102] Contraindications for massage include acutely irradiated skin, skin breakdown, massage directly over tumor, infection, thrombocytopenia, and coagulopathy.

- **Bracing**: Can be used to correct deformities caused by the tumor itself, surgery, or from nerve injury. Bracing can also position a joint for maximum comfort or to stabilize the spine.
- **Assistive devices**: Allow one to decrease weightbearing over painful or unstable bones.
- **Superficial heat**: Causes local changes in the skin, fascia, and muscle that may affect the sensation of pain. Local heat can increase oxygen and blood supply through vasodilatation to ease local ischemia or to aid in removal of waste products. Heat may also be used to relax muscle spasms, increase flexibility of soft tissue, or aid in relaxation. Heat is contraindicated directly over a tumor site, in the presence of DVT, and in a patient with poor or absent sensation.[103]
- **Cryotherapy**: Decreases muscle spindle sensitivity and, therefore, can assist in decreasing muscle spasm. Cryotherapy can also be used to decrease inflammation and may assist in dulling nerve pain by slowing the conduction velocity of nerves, thus delaying the transmission of pain impulses. Cryotherapy should not be used over insensate tissue, acutely irradiated tissue, or directly over a tumor site.[103]
- **Acupuncture**: May improve cancer-related pain and chemotherapy induced nausea.[104] It may also be beneficial for those who suffer from xerostomia, dry mouth, after head and neck irradiation. Caution should be taken in those with bleeding disorders, acutely irradiated tissue, insensate tissue, or at risk for infection.
- **Exercise**: Assists in pain that result from immobility, joint stiffness, or swelling. Exercise can also address postural changes that occur with pain, surgery, and fatigue.[105]
- **Relaxation and distraction**: May be used to divert attention away from pain. Focused deep breathing, imagery, and progressive relaxation techniques can be effective.[103]

Therapists should consider relative contraindications to the use of modalities in the person with a present or recent history of cancer. Modalities should not be used over areas of decreased sensation to touch or temperature or open skin, over reproductive organs, breast implants, or the spine, or directly over the tumor site. Other precautions used in the general population should be employed, including avoidance of traction over areas of instability or with positive vascular tests, over epiphyseal plates, or over implanted devices. Once the patient has reached approximately 5 years cancer free and with a low likelihood of recurrence, therapists can utilize precautions outlined for the general population.[87] Modalities may be employed distant from the cancer site with caution as there is no evidence regarding safety.

Skeletal-Related Events

Intractable pain, fracture, hypercalcemia, and spinal cord compression are skeletal-related events (SREs).[106] Bone metastasis is more common in breast, lung, thyroid, renal, and prostate cancers. SREs are associated with significant morbidity and mortality. The primary site for metastasis is the axial skeleton, followed by the appendicular skeleton (Table 13-14). There are 2 types of lesions that can potentially affect bone stability: lytic and blastic. **Lytic** lesions involve an increase in osteoclastic

Table 13-14

Location of Metastatic Bone Disease

Vertebrae	69%
Pelvis	40%
Femur	25%
Ribs	25%
Humerus	20%

Table 13-15

Pain Characteristics That May Indicate Fracture or Impending Fracture

- Pain with:
  - Weightbearing
  - Hip scour
  - Hip external rotation and abduction
  - Deep inspiration
- Pain in the groin
- Pain in a band around the chest wall
- Increased pain with:
  - Supine
  - Valsalva

activity, resulting in bone destruction and an increased risk for pathologic fracture. **Blastic** lesions involve an increase in bone formation, which can disrupt force distribution, thereby increasing the risk for instability and fracture.[107]

In the tumor microenvironment, cytokines are released that disrupt bone remodeling equilibrium leading to a microenvironment that promotes bone destruction and tumor growth. Pharmaceuticals are being developed to halt or slow the disruption of bone remodeling.[106,108]

The first sign of metastatic disease to bone is often subjective complaints of pain. Pain can originate from microfractures, stimulation of C fibers in the periosteum from tumor compression, reactive muscle spasm, or nerve root infiltration.[107] Pain can also occur from decreased blood flow causing bone necrosis. The diagnosis of anSRE includes subjective complaints, physical exam, and use of various forms of imaging, including x-ray, bone scan, magnetic resonance imaging (MRI), and computed tomography (CT) scan. There are systems to help determine bone stability and risk of pathologic fracture; however, the systems are imperfect (see section on multiple myeloma). Rehabilitation specialist should be aware of cancers that have a tendency to spread to bone, as well as signs and symptoms of impending fracture (Table 13-15).

When a person is diagnosed with bone involvement, multidisciplinary input is critical in determining appropriate treatment. The team, through subjective and objective assessments, needs to answer several essential questions to determine optimal treatment. The first question that the team needs to address is "What is the likelihood of fracture?" The medical team will use their physical examination in conjunction with imaging to determine the likelihood of pathologic fracture. Second, "What is the patient's expected life span?" If the patient has more than 3 months to live, surgery may be considered. If the patient's expected lifespan is short or the patient is not a surgical candidate, radiation and/or limited mobility with bracing may be considered. In addition to the potential to fracture and expected lifespan, the team needs to consider the patient's present and future quality of life. "What is the likelihood

Table 13-16

Signs and Symptoms of Spinal Cord Compression

• Pain that increases when lying supine	• Sensory deficits
• Pain with valsalva	• Bowel/bladder dysfunction
• Escalating back pain	• Hyperreactive reflexes
• Motor weakness	

that surgery will decrease pain and increase mobility? What is the patient's goal for pain relief? Can surgery help to attain this level of pain relief?" Finally, "What is the patient's rehabilitation potential?" Rehabilitation specialists play an important role in determining the patient's present functional mobility and potential for rehabilitation after treatment intervention. A thorough examination of strength, coordination, cognition, and social support will help guide the decision for treatment.

Interventions for metastatic bone disease include bisphosphonates for prevention or slowing of metastasis. Other interventions may include surgery, radiation therapy, pain management, and physical therapy. Goals for surgery include excision of tumor, cure, stabilization of bone, prevention of sequela from bed rest, and palliation. The method of fixation depends on the location of the fracture and extent of disease. Surgical fixation in oncology patients will usually include a larger area of bone, as the area surrounding the primary lesion is usually unhealthy tissue. If the bone lesion is stable or if the person is not a surgical candidate, radiation therapy is often used (see Table 13-9). Radiation to the bone causes degeneration and necrosis of tumor cells followed by bone regrowth. Chondrogenesis is initially inhibited, and there are a few reports of acute post-radiation fracture. Side effects of radiation to the bone include fatigue, skin erythema and hypersensitivity, impaired wound healing, avascular necrosis, and soft tissue fibrosis. Finally, there can be bone marrow suppression if the radiation field includes long bones or iliac wings.

Potential therapeutic physical therapy interventions include use of assistive devices to unload the joint, gait training, modalities for pain management, and strengthening. Resistance training prescription needs to be altered to manage the forces placed across potentially weakened bone to reduce the risk of fracture. Little evidence is available on the use of strength training in people with bone metastases.

Metastatic spinal cord compression (MSCC) occurs when disease spreads to the vertebra and impinges on the spinal column. This can occur by direct invasion into the vertebra and spinal canal, by disruption of the vascular supply to the cord, or when a tumor causes vertebral collapse with bony protrusion into the canal. MSCC can lead to demyelination, arterial compromise, and vasogenic edema, all of which affect the transmission of motor and sensory signals.[109] Symptoms of MSCC are presented in Table 13-16.

Physical therapists play a critical role in the early identification and treatment of the person with MSCC. The most optimal functional outcomes occur when treatment begins prior to neurological deficits or early in their course.[110] The neurological deficits at the time of diagnosis are the main determinant of ambulatory function after treatment.[109,111] Thus, MSCC is considered an oncologic emergency and therapists must refer to physicians immediately to optimize patient outcomes.[110]

Treatment is dependent upon evaluation of the stability of the spine and patient's lifespan prognosis. Some facilities may use the Spinal Instability Neoplastic Score, which takes predictive factors to determine stability and appropriate treatment interventions. Predictive factors for instability in this model are location of tumor, amount of pain, blastic or lytic characteristics, spinal alignment, extent of vertebral collapse and involvement of the posterior lateral complex.[112]

If surgery is not indicated, physicians may use radiation with corticosteroids. Physical therapy should focus on gait training, strengthening, ADL training, transfer training, and a bowel/bladder program. Bracing may be an asset to assist with limiting torsion and decreasing pain with mobility, although the impact on quality of life should be considered.[110] There is limited evidence to guide therapists on the timing of mobilization. Poor survival prognosis is associated with poor ambulatory status at the time of MSCC, shorter length of time between cancer diagnosis, development of MSCC, and number of extraspinal organs involved.[113]

Lymphedema

Lymphedema occurs when there is a disruption of the lymphatic system resulting in abnormal accumulation of protein rich lymph fluid.[114] Lymphedema occurs when the lymphatic load is normal, but transport capacity in not adequate, or when the lymphatic load is high and the transport capacity is inadequate. Risk factors for lymphedema include lymph node dissection, radiation over lymphatic beds, infections, tumor obstruction of lymph vessels, and possibly BMI.

The lymphatic system parallels the venous system and functions to maintain fluid balance, fight infections, and remove cellular debris and waste products. Up to 2 liters of fluid normally moves within the lymphatics. There are 3 main components to the lymphatic system: the pre-collectors, collecting lymphatics, and lymphatic ducts, which collect fluid and transport it back to the heart (Table 13-17).

In the acute care setting, therapists should discuss prevention techniques and overt signs of lymphedema. Anyone who receives cancer treatment that has the potential to damage the lymphatic system needs to adopt lifetime strategies to prevent the onset of lymphedema (Table 13-18).[115]

The present standard for treatment of lymphedema is **complete decongestive therapy** (CDT).[114] The first phase of CDT includes skin care, manual lymph drainage, bandaging, exercise, and a compression garment to maintain the volume of the limb. The second phase, or maintenance phase, consists of wearing a compression garment during the day and bandaging at night. Skin care and exercise are continued and progressed as appropriate. A lymphedema specialist who has extensively studied the anatomy and physiology of the lymphatic system, as well as the techniques of lymphatic massage, should administer CDT. The National Lymphedema Network (NLN) and the Lymphology Association of North America (LANA) provide guidelines for the education and practice of lymphedema management.

Fatigue and Deconditioning

Fatigue affects nearly every person who undergoes treatment for cancer.[116] **Cancer-related fatigue** (CRF) is a "distressing, persistent subjective sense of physical, emotional, and/or cognitive tiredness or exhaustion related to cancer or cancer treatment that is not proportional to recent activity and interferes with usual functioning."[116] Fatigue often occurs in symptom clusters, so patients should be screened for other issues, such as pain, nausea, depression, and insomnia.

The etiology of CRF is unclear. Potential contributors include the cancer treatment, the cancer itself, anemia, progression of disease, poor nutrition/cancer cachexia, infection, sleep disturbance, medications, electrolyte imbalance, depression, pain, decreased activity, and thyroid dysfunction.[117,118] Recent theories include disruption of the hypothalamic pituitary axis, dysregulation of cytokines, disruption of the circadian rhythm, and muscle catabolism.[119] In each of these theories, there is a disruption in the normal homeostasis of the systems that regulate sleep, cortisol levels, appetite, and energy.

Table 13-17

COMPONENTS OF THE LYMPHATIC SYSTEM

Pre-Collectors	*Collecting Lymphatics*	*Lymphatic Ducts and Trunks*
Location: Epidermis	**Location**: Dermis	**Location**: Central location in thorax
Defining Characteristics • One cell wall thick with overlapping cells with gaps to enable fluid to enter • Connected to tissues by filaments that pull cell junctions open with increases in tissue pressure • Responds to external pressure: Massage, muscle pump, breathing, gravity	**Defining Characteristics** • Contains valves for one-way flow • Contains smooth muscle to help fluid move through system	**Defining Characteristics** • Larger vessels that move lymphatic fluid into subclavian veins

Table 13-18

COMMON LYMPHEDEMA PRECAUTIONS

Lymphedema Prevention

- Maintain a healthy weight
- Prevent any trauma to the area that was affected by lymph node removal or damage (eg, arm, breast, and trunk for axillary dissection)
- No blood pressure on the affected arm
- No intravenous on the affected arm
- Keep skin and nails clean, avoid cutting cuticles
- Avoid cuts, scrapes, and burns
- Avoid tight-fitting clothes/jewelry

Signs of Lymphedema

- Heaviness in the limb where lymph nodes were removed or damaged
- Clothing or jewelry feeling tight
- Swelling
- Numbness or tingling
- Redness/warmth in limb where lymph nodes were removed or damaged

CRF often begins in the second or third week of radiation therapy and peaks approximately halfway through the total number of radiation sessions. Fatigue begins to abate after cessation of radiation.[118,120,121] During chemotherapy, CRF peaks about 1 week after infusion and slowly improves. However, the cycle of CRF repeats itself with the next infusion and may not return to baseline levels after chemotherapy has ended.[118,120,121] Upwards of 50% of long-term cancer survivors report that they still struggle with CRF and it diminishes their quality of life.[122,123]

CRF is pervasive and impacts quality of life and, therefore, should be screened for regularly throughout the continuum of disease. Medical causes of fatigue should be ruled out prior to the initiation of other treatment modalities. Physicians will determine if there are medical causes of CRF that can be treated, such as anemia, thyroid dysfunction, heart disease, or mood disorders.[116] Adults should be asked to rate their fatigue over the last 7 days on a scale of 0 to 10, with 0 representing no fatigue and 10 representing the worst imaginable. The National Comprehensive Cancer Network's (NCCN) Clinical Practice Guidelines categorize cancer-related fatigue as mild (0 to 3), moderate (4 to 6), or severe (7 or more), with suggested interventions for each level.[116]

The NCCN scale should be used for screening; however, if a more comprehensive evaluation of CRF is warranted, therapists should consider the use of a validated tool, such as the Functional Assessment of Cancer Therapy—Fatigue subscale.[124] Therapist should consider other outcomes measures to evaluate the effect of fatigue on function in addition to quality of life.

There is strong evidence to support exercise as an intervention for CRF. Moderate intensity exercise, with appropriate adjustments for changes in blood counts, bone disease, and comorbidities that impact exercise prescription, is recommended.[125-129] The exact dose of exercise that is most beneficial remains elusive; however, the general recommendation is that patients should maximize their activity. In the survivorship phase, people should aim for 150 minutes of moderate intensity exercise over the course of 1 week.[130] In addition to exercise, psychosocial interventions, such as relaxation and cognitive behavioral therapy techniques, have also shown to reduce CRF and should be used in combination with activity.

Exercise for the Person With Cancer and Survivorship

Survivorship begins with the cancer diagnosis and extends to the end of life.[131] The NCCN has identified key priorities of care in the survivorship phase[132]:

1. "Prevention of new and recurrent cancers and other late effects.
2. Surveillance for cancer spread, recurrence, or new cancers
3. Assessment of late psychosocial and physical effects
4. Intervention for consequences of cancer treatment
5. Coordination of care between primary care providers and specialists to ensure that all of the survivor's needs are met."

Exercise plays an important role in prevention and restoration of physical mobility and well-being across the trajectory of disease. It has been shown to elevate mood, decrease anxiety, and improve physical functioning and overall quality of life in people with cancer.[1,24,25,117,133-135] In certain cancer types (eg, breast, colorectal), physical activity can also reduce the risk of recurrence as well as lower the all-cause mortality rate.

It is of utmost importance that people with cancer reduce inactivity and strive toward reaching the recommended dose of 150 minutes of moderate intensity activity per week, 2 days of strength training, and flexibility training. For survivors who are older than 60 or who have balance issues, physical therapists should incorporate balance training into the exercise prescription. It is critical for therapists to begin the survivor's path to recovery in acute care, with an emphasis on slowly resuming and increasing physical activity once the patient is stabilized. According to the NCCN survivorship guidelines, there are 3 exercise risk levels that should be considered. Survivors with early stage cancer who have a history of exercise and no significant comorbidities may benefit from community programs for physical activity and are considered low risk. Those with more significant cancer burden, with peripheral neuropathy, lymphedema, bone involvement, anemia, thrombocytopenia, or other health issues should be referred to a physical therapist with training in cancer rehabilitation.[131] Therapists should refer to the NCCN guidelines for a full description of survivorship plans, including recommendations for aerobic exercise and strength training.

Physical therapists play a key role in risk reduction, functional recovery, and improving psychosocial well-being. Therapists should play an active role in the acute care setting, helping to improve patients function and set them on the road to being a lifetime exerciser. Rehabilitation services have a role throughout the trajectory of care, from prevention to end of life, and must actively seek to contribute to patient care through evidenced-based collaborative practice.

Case Study

Ms. Geraldine Connor, a 66-year-old woman who presents to outpatient physical therapy status-post (s/p) FOLFOX regimen for stage III colon cancer (FOLFOX is a combination of chemotherapy drugs: leucovorin calcium, fluorouracil, oxaliplatin). She underwent surgical resection of her tumor 6 months prior. Physical therapy is consulted for CIPN.

Patient/Client History

General Demographics, Social History, and Living Environment

Ms. Connor is married with 2 adult children ages 38 and 42. She lives in a 2-story rowhome with 10 steps to enter, railing on right, half bath on the first floor, and her bedroom on the second floor. She is a retired schoolteacher who actively volunteers at her local elementary school and at her church's food pantry.

General Health Status, Social/Health Habits, and Family History

Prior to her colorectal surgery and chemotherapy she was active in the community. She has a family history of colon cancer, and it was the cause of death of her mother after a lengthy illness.

Medical/Surgical History

Segmental colon resection, FOLFOX chemotherapy, osteoarthritis in her right knee

Current Condition

Ms. Connor's chief complaint is numbness and tingling in both legs and feeling "wobbly." She reports one near fall when navigating a parking lot at night. She has been hesitan to volunteer at the local school for fear of falling.

Activities and Participation

Patient was independently ambulating at home and in the community.

Medications

Elavil (amitriptyline)

Other Clinical Tests

Laboratory Values: WBCs are normal at 9000 cells/mL, hemoglobin is decreased at 9 g/dL, and platelets are normal at 178,000/µL.

Systems Review

Cardiovascular and Pulmonary

Resting vital signs (VS) demonstrate a heart rate (HR) of 88 beats per minute (BPM), blood pressure (BP) taken in the right arm 140/70 mm Hg and left arm 138/70 mm Hg (non-significant difference). The respiratory rate (RR) 16 breaths/minute and pulse quality of the radial artery is 2+ and regular. There is no edema noted in bilateral lower extremities (BLEs).

Integumentary

There is a port in left upper chest covered by gauze. The skin appears clean and intact. Otherwise, the integument is unremarkable.

Musculoskeletal

Gross movement of bilateral upper extremities (BUEs) and BLEs appears normal but a more thorough examination is indicated due to CIPN.

Neuromuscular

BUE and BLE reflexes are within normal limits (WNL). Light touch was decreased bilaterally in a stocking glove pattern below patella extending to toes.

Communication, Affect, Cognition, Language, and Learning Style

Alert and oriented, English is primary language, slightly hard of hearing. Ms. Connor follows multistep commands easily.

Tests and Measures

Aerobic Capacity and Endurance

A 6MWT was performed with the following results: total walk distance was 580 feet for an average speed of 1.1 miles per hour (mph). The VS range during the test was HR range: 88-130 bpm, BP range 140/70-158/70, rate of perceived exertion (RPE) range: 6-14/20 on the Borg Scale. The predicted walk distance was 1534 feet. Her walk distance of 580 feet was 38% of predicted for her age and gender.

Balance, Gait, and Mobility (Including Locomotion)

Gait analysis was performed revealing a slow gait speed with occasional decreased foot clearance during swing phase on the right. She also demonstrated a wide base of support and appeared to use her visual system to gaze at surface during ambulation. Sitting balance unsupported was unremarkable with no loss of balance noted. In standing, it was noted that Ms. Connor had a narrow base of support and she would lose her balance posteriorly with moderate perturbation force. Timed Up and Go (TUG) Test was performed with a result of 17 seconds. Fullerton Advanced Balance Scale was 24/40.

Muscle Performance

BUE and BLE muscle testing revealed 4+/5 throughout, except bilateral dorsiflexion, which was 4/5. There were no deficits in ROM.

Pain and Sensory Integrity

Patient reported numbness in her BLEs 4/10 below knees. She reported the worst discomfort is 5/10 in the evenings and noted difficulty sleeping due to discomfort of bed sheets on her legs.

Neuropathy Specific Outcome Measures

Functional Assessment of Cancer Therapy/Gynecologic Oncology Group–Neurotoxicity—32/44 (higher score indicates better quality of life). Modified Total Neuropathy Score (mTNS) was 23/28 (higher score indicates worse neuropathy).

Diagnosis

Ms. Connor presents with CIPN s/p FOLFOX regimen for stage II colon cancer. Impairments include dysesthesia and allodynia, decreased sensation bilaterally below knees, and strength decrements in lower extremities. These impairments have resulted in activity limitations in the area of gait distance and an elevated TUG time compared to age-matched norms. Balance measures indicate an elevated risk for falls and limit her participation in community volunteer activities. The patient would benefit from continued physical therapy for gait training with the least restrictive assistive device. Recommend outpatient physical therapy upon discharge and prescription of assistive device for stability.

Prognosis

CIPN often improves over the course of 6 months to 1 year, with some patients experiencing long-term functional impairments. Patient has a good prognosis to return to community activities with outpatient therapy that focuses on gait and balance training.

Intervention

The plan of care will focus on balance and include challenges to the visual, somatosensory, and vestibular systems. Strength training with a focus on muscular endurance for standing activities will be included, as well as gait training with the least restrictive assistive device. Patient will be educated on skin integrity checks of her feet.

Outcomes

The patient received a total of 12 sessions. TUG decreased from 18 seconds to 12 seconds and the 6MWT improved to 1304 feet, which is 85% of the predicted value for age-matched controls. Fullerton Advanced Balance Scale increased to 34/40, below

ICF Clinical Reasoning Tool Case Study Summary

Health Condition								
HPI: CIPN PMHx: Colon cancer treated by chemotherapy (FOLFOX regimen) and colon resection (colectomy); osteoarthritis (primarily right knee)								
Precautions/Contraindications								
Fall precautions; abnormal lab values including leukopenia and anemia; standard precautions related to infection control								
Body Structure and Function			*Activity/Task Limitations*			*Participation*		
Impairment/ Problem	*Tests and Measures*	*Intervention*	*Activity*	*Tests and Measures*	*Intervention*	*Participation*	*Tests and Measures*	*Intervention*
• Decreased BUE/BLE strength • Decreased endurance • Impaired sensation (stocking glove pattern) • Impaired balance • Hard of hearing • Pain (allodynia) • Abnormal lab values	• ROM/MMT • 6MWT • Integumentary examination • Sensation testing including FACT/ GOG-Ntx • Pain/numeric scale • Lab values	• Progressive resistance exercises and balance tasks	• ADLs • Transfers • Gait	• TUG • 6MWT • RPE	• Progressive resistance exercises • Progressive aerobic exercise	• Unable to return to volunteer work	• MMSE • FACT/ GOG-Ntx	• Continue physical therapy services

(continued)

ICF Clinical Reasoning Tool Case Study Summary (continued)

Personal Factors	*Other Considerations*	*Environmental Factors*
• Age: 66 y/o female • A x O • Primary language: English • Married with 2 grown children (38 and 42) • Retired school teacher • Active in community: Volunteer at elementary school and food pantry		Home: • 2 story row house • 10 steps to enter; half bath on 1st floor, full bathroom and bedroom on 2nd floor Hospital: • Port in left upper chest for chemotherapy infusion

A x O = awake and oriented; FACT/GOG-Ntx = Functional Assessment of Cancer Therapy/Gynecologic Oncology Group-Neurotoxicity; HPI = history of present illness; MMSE = Mini-Mental State Examination; MMT = Manual Muscle Test; MWT = Minute Walk Test; PMHx = past medical history; y/o = year old.

Adapted from American Physical Therapy Association. *Guide to Physical Therapist Practice*. 3rd ed. http://www.apta.org/Guide/. Updated October 21, 2015. Accessed October 5, 2018 and *Towards a Common Language for Functioning, Disability and Health*. World Health Organization. www.who.int/classifications/icf/icfbeginnersguide.pdf. Published 2002. Accessed April 29, 2019.

the threshold for falls and mTNS decreased to 15/28. Ms. Connor was able to leave the floor and could ambulate in the community without an assistive device, although gait speed remained slow at approximately 2.5 mph. She was referred to outpatient physical therapy.

Chapter Review Questions

1. What is the most common clinical sign of bone metastasis?
    a. Ache or sharp pain
    b. Redness and swelling
    c. Muscle atrophy
    d. Bruising and petechiae
2. Which of the following is the key influence in determining a patient's medical treatment for cancer?
    a. Type and stage of cancer
    b. Patient's past quality of life
    c. Financial potential
    d. Previous surgery
3. Three side effects of radiation treatment for cancer are:
    a. Avascular necrosis, acne, shingles
    b. Immunosuppression, radiation myelitis, fatigue
    c. Upper GI bleeding, muscle catabolism, weight gain
    d. Tissue fibrosis, myofascial adhesions, enhanced sleep
4. Which of the following are 2 neurologic side effects related to chemotherapy?
    a. Hearing loss and hyperkalemia
    b. Balance disorders and HTN
    c. Peripheral neuropathy and myalgia
    d. Lethargy and bronchiolitis obliterans
5. What are signs and symptoms of possible spinal cord compression?
    a. Pain with hip scour
    b. Decreased pain with valsalva
    c. Pain that decreases with lying down
    d. Escalating back pain

Answers: 1a, 2a, 3b, 4c, 5d

References

1. Courneya K, Friedenreich C. Physical exercise and quality of life following cancer diagnosis: a literature review. *Ann Behav Med.* 1999; 21(2):171-179.
2. Goubran H, Kotb R, Stakiw J, Emara M, Burnouf T. Regulation of tumor growth and metastasis: The role of tumor microenvironment. *Cancer Growth Metastasis.* 2014;7: 9-18.
3. Abeloff M. *Clinical Oncology.* 2nd ed. Orlando, FL: Churchill Livingstone; 2000.
4. Talmadge JE, Fidler IJ. AACR Centennial Series: The biology of cancer metastasis: historical perspective. *Cancer Research.* 2010;70:5649-5669.
5. National Cancer Institute. *Cancer staging fact sheet.* www.cancer.gov/cancertopics/factsheet/Detection/staging. Published March 9, 2015. Accessed March 1, 2019.
6. National Cancer Institute. ECOG performance status. https://training.seer.cancer.gov/followup/procedures/dataset/ecog.html. Accessed July 15, 2019.
7. Baskar R, Lee KA, Yeo R, Yeoh KW. Cancer and radiation therapy: current advances and future directions. *Int J Med Sci.* 2012;9(3):193-199. doi: 10.7150/ijms.3635.
8. Janaki MG, Kadam AR, Mukesh S, Nirmala S, Ponni A, Ramesh BS, Rajeev AG. Magnitude of fatigue in cancer patients receiving radiotherapy and its short term effect on quality of life. *J Cancer Res Ther.* 2010;6(1):22-26.
9. Stubblefield M. Radiation fibrosis syndrome: Neuromuscular and musculoskeletal complications in cancer survivors. *PMR.* 2011;3(104):1041-1054.
10. Monleon S, Murta-Nascimento C, Bascuas I, Macia F, Duarte E, Belmonte R. Lymphedema predictor factors after breast cancer surgery: a survival analysis. *Lymphat Res Biol.* 2015;13(4):268-274.
11. Gewandter JS, Fan L, Magnuson A, et al. Falls and functional impairments in cancer survivors with chemotherapy-induced peripheral neuropathy (CIPN): a University of Rochester CCOP study. *Support Care Cancer.* 2013;21(7):2059-2066.
12. Tofthagen C, Overcash J, Kip K. Falls in persons with chemotherapy-induced peripheral neuropathy. *Support Care Cancer.* 2012;20(3):583-589.
13. Quasthoff S, Hartung HP. Chemotherapy-induced peripheral neuropathy. *J Neurol.* 2002;249:9-17.
14. Argyriou AA, Kyritsis AP, Makatsoris T, Kalofonos HP. Chemotherapy-induced peripheral neuropathy in adults: a comprehensive update of the literature. *Cancer Manag Res.* 2014;19(6):135-147.
15. Cavaletti G, Frigeni B, Lanzani F, et al. The total neuropathy score as an assessment tool for grading the course of chemotherapy-induced peripheral neurotoxicity: comparison with the National Cancer Institute-Common Toxicity Scale. *J Peripher Nerv Syst.* 2007;12(3):210-215.
16. Cavaletti G, Alberti P, Frigeni B, Piatti M, Susani E. Chemotherapy-induced neuropathy. *Curr Treat Options Neurol.* 2011;13:180-190.
17. Binda D, Vanhoutte EK, Cavaletti G, et al. Rasch-built overall disability scale for patients with chemotherapy-induced peripheral neuropathy (CIPN-R-ODS). *Eur J Cancer.* 2013;49(13):2910-2918.
18. National Cancer Institute. Common terminology criteria for adverse events, v.4. http://evs.nci.nih.gov/ftp1/CTCAE/About.html. Accessed July 3, 2014.
19. Hershman DL, Lacchetti C, Dworkin RH, et al. Prevention and management of chemotherapy-induced peripheral neuropathy in survivors of adult cancers: American Society of Clinical Oncology clinical practice guideline. *J Clin Oncol.* 2014;32(18):1941-1967.
20. Pachman DR, Watson JC, Lustberg MB, et al. Management options for established chemotherapy-induced peripheral neuropathy. *Support Care Cancer.* 2014;22(8):2281-2295. doi: 10.1007/s00520-014-2289-x
21. National Cancer Institute. Fact sheet on targeted cancer therapies. www.cancer.gov/cancertopics/factsheet/Therapy/targeted. Updated February 6, 2019. Accessed March 1, 2019.
22. Chang S, Traynor A, Burt RK. Update on stem cell transplantation. *Resident & Staff Physician.* 2001;47(2):44-54.
23. Hung YC, Bauer J, Horsley P, Waterhouse M, Bashford J, Isenring E. Changes in nutritional status, body composition, quality of life, and physical activity levels of cancer patients undergoing autologous peripheral blood stem cell transplantation. *Support Care Cancer.* 2013;21(6):1579-1586
24. Dimeo F, Stieglitz RD, Novelli-Fischer U, et al. Effects of physical activity on the fatigue and psychologic status of cancer patients during chemotherapy. *Cancer.* 1999;85(10):2273-2277.

25. Dimeo F, Fetscher S, Lange W, et al. Effects of aerobic exercise on the physical performance and incidence of treatment-related complications after high-dose chemotherapy. *Blood.* 1997;90(9):3390-3394.
26. Baumann FT, Kraut L, Schule K, Bloch W, Fauser AA. A controlled randomized study examining the effects of exercise therapy on patients undergoing haematopoietic stem cell transplantation. *Bone Marrow Transplant.* 2010;45(2):355-362.
27. Wiskemann J, Huber G. Physical exercise as adjuvant therapy for patients undergoing hematopoietic stem cell transplantation. *Bone Marrow Transplant.* 2008;41(4):321-329.
28. American Cancer Society. 2014 cancer facts and figures. http://www.cancer.org/acs/groups/content/@research/documents/webcontent/acspc-042151.pdf. Accessed May 10, 2019.
29. Karam A. Update on breast cancer surgery approaches. *Curr Opin Obstet Gynecol.* 2013;25:74-80.
30. American Cancer Society. How is breast cancer treated? http://www.cancer.org/cancer/breastcancer/overviewguide/breast-cancer-overview-treating-surgery. Accessed May 10, 2019.
31. McNeely ML, Binkley JM, Pusic AL, Campbell KL, Gabram S, Soballe PW. A prospective model of care for breast cancer rehabilitation: postoperative and postreconstructive issues. *Cancer.* 2012;118(8s):2226-2236.
32. Sagen A, Kaaresen R, Sandvik L, Thune I, Risberg MA. Upper limb physical function and adverse effects after breast cancer surgery: a prospective 2.5-year follow-up study and preoperative measures. *Arch Phys Med Rehabil.* 2014;95(5):875-881.
33. Kootstra JJ, Dijkstra PU, Rietman H, et al. A longitudinal study of shoulder and arm morbidity in breast cancer survivors 7 years after sentinel lymph node biopsy or axillary lymph node dissection. *Breast Cancer Res Treat.* 2013;139(1):125-134.
34. Shamley D, Lascurain-Aguirrevena I, Oskrochi R, Srinaganathan R. Shoulder morbidity after treatment for breast cancer is bilateral and greater after mastectomy. *Acta Oncologica.* 2012;51:1045-1053.
35. Schultz I, Barholm M, Grondal S. Delayed shoulder exercises in reducing seroma frequency after modified radical mastectomy: a prospective randomized study. *Ann Surg Oncol.* 1997;4(4):293-297.
36. Harris S, Hugi MR, Olivotto IA, et al. Upper extremity rehabilitation in women with breast cancer after axillary dissection: clinical practice guidelines. *Crit Review Phys Rehabil Med.* 2001;13(2,3):91-103.
37. Harmer V. Reconstruction for breast cancer in a nutshell. *Br J Nurs.* 2012;21(15):904-909.
38. Carlson N, King J. Overview of breast cancer treatment and reconstruction for primary care providers. *J Midwifery Womens Health.* 2012;57:558-568.
39. American Cancer Society. Hormone therapy for breast cancer. http://www.cancer.org/cancer/breastcancer/detailedguide/breast-cancer-treating-hormone-therapy. Accessed on May 10, 2019.
40. Courneya K, McKenzie D, Mackey J, et al. Effects of exercise dose and type during breast cancer chemotherapy: Multicenter randomized trial. *J Natl Cancer Inst.* 2013;105:1821-1832.
41. Stout NL, Binkley JM, Schmitz KH, et al. A prospective surveillance model for rehabilitation for women with breast cancer. *Cancer.* 2012;15(118):2191-2200.
42. Zhong S, Jiang T, Ma T, et al. Association between physical activity and mortality in breast cancer: a meta-analysis of cohort studies. *Eur J Epidemiol.* 2014;29(6):391-404.
43. Campbell B, Marbella A, Layde PM. Quality of life and recurrence concern in survivors of head and neck cancer. *Laryngoscope.* 2000;110:895-906.
44. Cheville A, Packel L. Rehabilitation of the person s/p neck dissection. *Acute Care Perspectives—J Am Phys Ther Assoc.* 2001;10:37-39.
45. Guru K, Manoor U, Supe, S. A comprehensive review of head and neck cancer rehabilitation: Physical therapy perspectives. *Indian J Palliat Care.* 2012;18(2):87-97.
46. Cheng PT, Hao SP, Lin YH, Yeh AR. Objective comparison of shoulder dysfunction after three neck dissection techniques. *Ann Otol Rhinol Laryngol.* 2000;109:761-766.
47. Brown H, Burns S, Kaiser CW. The spinal accessory nerve plexus, the trapezius muscle and shoulder stabilization after radical neck cancer surgery. *Ann Surg.* 1988;208:654-661
48. Thawley SE, Panje WR, Batsakis JG, Lindberg RD. *Comprehensive Management of Head and Neck Tumors. Vol 1 and 2.* 2nd ed. Philadelphia, PA: WB Saunders; 1999.
49. McGarvey AC, Osmotherly PG, Hoffman GR, Chiarelli PE. Scapular muscle exercises following neck dissection surgery for head and neck cancer: a comparative electromyographic study. *Phys Ther.* 2013;93(6):786-797.

50. Minami A, Kasashima T, Iwasaki N, et al. Vascularised fibular grafts. An experience of 102 patients. *J Bone Joint Surg Br.* 2000;82(7):1022-1025.
51. American Cancer Society. How is ALL treated—detailed guide. www.cancer.org/cancer/leukemia-acutelymphocyticallinadults/detailedguide/leukemia-acute-lymphocytic-treating-chemotherapy. Accessed May 10, 2019.
52. Dimeo F, Schwartz S, Fietz T, Wanjura T, Boning D, Thiel E. Effects of endurance training on the physical performance of patients with hematological malignancies during chemotherapy. *Supportive Care Cancer.* 2003;11(10):623-628.
53. Braam KI, van der Torre P, Takken T, Veening MA, van Dulmen-den Broeder E, Kaspers GJ. Physical exercise training interventions for children and young adults during and after treatment for childhood cancer. *Cochrane Database Syst Rev.* 2013;30(4). doi: 10.1002/14651858.CD008796.pub2
54. Paul KL. Rehabilitation and exercise considerations in hematologic malignancies. *Am J Phys Med Rehabil.* 2011;90(5 suppl 1):S88-94. doi: 10.1097/PHM.0b013e31820be055
55. Oechsle K, Aslan Z, Suesse Y, Jensen W, Bokemeyer C, de Wit M. Multimodal exercise training durin gmyeloablative chemotherapy: a prospective randomized pilot trial. *Support Care Cancer.* 2014;22(1):63-69.
56. American Cancer Society. Multiple myeloma. http://www.cancer.org/cancer/multiplemyeloma/detailedguide/multiple-myeloma-what-is-multiple-myeloma. Accessed May 10, 2019.
57. Terpos E, Berenson J, Raje N, Roodman G. Management of bone disease in multiple myeloma. *Exp Rev in Hematology.* 2014;7(1):113-125.
58. Mirels H. Metastatic disease in long bones. A proposed scoring system for diagnosing impending pathologic fractures. *Clin Orthop Relat Res.* 1989;(249):256-264.
59. Campos M, Urrutia J, Zamora T, et al. The Spine Instability Neoplastic Score: an independent reliability and reproducibility analysis. *Spine J.* 2014;14(8):1466-1469. doi: 10.1016/j.spinee.2013.08.044
60. Kronisch C, Balagué F, Dudler J. Fear of impending fractures: when to refer? A case-based review. *Clin Rheumatol.* 2015;34(7):1303-1309.
61. Groeneveldt L, Mein G, Garrod R, et al. A mixed exercise training programme is feasible and safe and may improve quality of life and muscle strength in multiple myeloma survivors. *BMC Cancer.* 2013;13:31. doi: 10.1186/1471-2407-13-31
62. Newton MJ, Hayes SC, Janda M, et al. Safety, feasibility and effects of an individualised walking intervention for women undergoing chemotherapy for ovarian cancer: a pilot study. *BMC Cancer.* 2011;11:389. doi: 10.1186/1471-2407-11-389
63. Curtis LA, Dolan TS, Cespedes RD. Acute urinary retention and urinary incontinence. *Emerg Med Clin North Am.* 2001;19(3):591-619.
64. Hagen S, Hanley J, Capewell A. Test-retest reliability, validity, and sensitivity to change of the Urogenital Distress Inventory and the Incontinence Impact Questionnaire. *Neurourol Urodyn.* 2002;21(6):534-539.
65. Wang YC, Hart DL, Deutscher D, Yen SC, Mioduski JE. Psychometric properties and practicability of the self-report urinary incontinence questionnaire in patients with pelvic-floor dysfunction seeking outpatient rehabilitation. *Phys Ther.* 2013;93(8):1116-1129. doi: 10.2522/ptj.20120134
66. Tannenbaum C, Brouillette J, Michaud J, et al. Responsiveness and clinical utility of the geriatric self-efficacy index for urinary incontinence. *J Am Geriatr Soc.* 2009;57(3):470-475.
67. Yang EJ, Lim JY, Rah UW, Kim YB. Effect of a pelvic floor muscle training program on gynecologic cancer survivors with pelvic floor dysfunction: a randomized controlled trial. *Gynecol Oncol.* 2012;125:705-711.
68. Alberg AJ, Samet JM. Epidemiology of lung cancer. *Chest.* 2003;123(1 suppl):21S-49S.
69. Hopkins KG, Rosenzweig M. Post-thoracotomy pain syndrome: Assessment and intervention. *Clin J Oncol Nurs.* 2012;16(4):365-370.
70. Elshiekh MA, Lo TT, Shipolini AR, McCormack DJ. Does muscle-sparing thoracotomy as opposed to posterolateral thoracotomy result in better recovery? *Interact Cardiovasc Thorac Surg.* 2013;16(1):60-67. doi: 10.1093/icvts/ivs295
71. Nosotti M, Baisi A, Mendogni P, Palleschi A, Tosi D, Rosso L. Muscle sparing versus posterolateral thoracotomy for pulmonary lobectomy: randomised controlled trial. *Interact Cardiovasc Thorac Surg.* 2010;11(4):415-419. doi: 10.1510/icvts.2010.238840
72. Rodriguez-Larrad A, Lascurain-Aguirrebena I, Abecia-Inchaurregui LC, Seco J. Perioperative physiotherapy in patients undergoing lung cancer resection. *Interact Cardiovasc Thorac Surg.* 2014; 19(2):269-281. doi: 10.1093/icvts/ivu126

73. Hoffman AJ, Brintnall RA, von Eye A, et al. Home-based exercise: promising rehabilitation for symptom relief, improved functional status and quality of life for post-surgical lung cancer patients. *J Thorac Dis.* 2014;6(6):632-640. doi: 10.3978/j.issn.2072-1439.2014.06.08
74. Kuehr L, Wiskemann J, Abel U, Ulrich CM, Hummler S, Thomas M. Exercise in patients with non-small cell lung cancer. *Med Sci Sports Exerc.* 2014;46(4):656-663.
75. Chang NW, Lin KC, Lee SC, Chan JY, Lee YH, Wang KY. Effects of an early postoperative walking exercise programme on health status in lung cancer patients recovering from lung lobectomy. *J Clin Nurs.* 2014; 23(23-24):3391-3402. doi: 10.1111/jocn.12584
76. American Cancer Society. What are the key statistics for colo-rectal cancer? http://www.cancer.org/cancer/colonandrectumcancer/detailedguide/colorectal-cancer-key-statistics. Accessed May 10, 2019.
77. American Cancer Society. Surgery for colo-rectal cancer. http://www.cancer.org/cancer/colonandrectumcancer/detailedguide/colorectal-cancer-treating-colon-surgery. Accessed May 10, 2019..
78. American Cancer Society. Chemotherapy for colo-rectal cancer. http://www.cancer.org/cancer/colonandrectumcancer/detailedguide/colorectal-cancer-treating-chemotherapy. Accessed May 10, 2019..
79. Liu CH, Chen CH, Lee JC. Rehabilitation exercise on the quality of life in anal sphincter-preserving surgery. *Hepatogastroenterology.* 2011;58(110-111):1461-1465.
80. Bartlett L, Sloots K, Nowak M, Ho YH. Biofeedback therapy for symptoms of bowel dysfunction following surgery for colorectal cancer. *Tech Coloproctol.* 2011;15(3):319-326.
81. Lee L, Schwartzman F, Carli GS, et al. The association of the distance walked in 6 min with pre-operative peak oxygen consumption and complications 1 month after colorectal resection. *Anaesthesia.* 2013;68:811-816.
82. Nutt CL, Russell JC. Use of the pre-operative shuttle walk test to predict morbidity and mortality after elective major colorectal surgery. *Anaesthesia.* 2012;67:839-849.
83. Ahn K, Hur H, Kim D, et al. The effects of inpatient exercise therapy on the length of hospital stay in stages I-III colon cancer patients: randomized controlled trial. *Int J Colorectal Dis.* 2013;28:643-651.
84. Kim DW, Kang SB, Lee SY, Oh HK, In MH. Early rehabilitation programs after laparoscopic colorectal surgery: Evidence and criticism. *World J Gastroenterol.* 2013;19(46):8543-8551.
85. Gustafsson UO, Scott MJ, Schwenk W, et al. Guidelines for perioperative care in elective colonic surgery: Enhanced Recovery After Surgery (ERAS) Society recommendations. *Clin Nutr.* 2012;31(6):783-800.
86. Cramer H, Lauche R, Klose P, Dobos G, Langhorst J. A systematic review and meta-analysis of exercise interventions for colorectal cancer patients. *Eur J Cancer Care (Engl).* 2014;23:3-14.
87. Grossman, M, Cheung, A., Zajac, J. Androgens and prostate cancer; pathogenesis and deprivation therapy. *Best Pract Res Clin Endocrinol Metab.* 2013;27:603-616.
88. Groenwald S, Frogge MH, Goodman M, Yarbro CH. *Cancer Nursing: Principles and Practice.* 4th ed. Sudbury, MA: Jones and Bartlett; 1997.
89. Goodman CC, Fuller KS. *Pathology Implications for the Physical Therapist.* 3rd ed. St. Louis, MO: Saunders Elsevier; 2009.
90. Patel M, Yao J, Hirschhorn A, Mungovan S. Preoperative pelvic floor physiotherapy improves continence after radiacal retropubic prostatectomy. *Int J Urol.* 2013;20(10):986-992.
91. Penson DF. Treatment for post prostatectomy incontinence: is this as good as it gets? *JAMA.* 2011;305(2):197-198.
92. American Cancer Society. Surgery for prostate cancer. http://www.cancer.org/cancer/prostatecancer/detailedguide/prostate-cancer-treating-surgery. Accessed May 10, 2019.
93. Butoescu V, Tombal B. Practical guide to bone health in the spectrum of advanced prostate cancer. *Can J Urol.* 2014;21(suppl 1):84-92.
94. Campbell SE, Glazener CM, Hunter KF, Cody JD, Moore KN. Conservative management for postprostatectomy urinary incontinence. *Cochrane Database Syst Rev.* 2012;18:1. doi: 10.1002/14651858.CD001843.pub4
95. Cormie P, Newton RU, Spry N, Joseph D, Taaffe DR. Galvao DA. Safety and efficacy of resistance exercise in prostate cancer patients with bone metastases. *Prostate Cancer Prostatic Dis.* 2013;16:328-335.
96. Cancer treatment and care. Health Communities. www.oncologychannel.com/testicularcancer/riskfactors.shtml. Updated September 3, 2015. Accessed March 1, 2019.
97. American Cancer Society. Key statistics for testicular cancer. http://www.cancer.org/cancer/testicularcancer/detailedguide/testicular-cancer-key-statistics. Accessed July 25, 2014.

98. International Association for the Study of Pain. IASP terminology. https://www.iasp-pain.org/Education/Content.aspx?ItemNumber=1698#Pain. Updated December 14, 2017. Accessed July 15, 2019.
99. Abouassaly R, Fossa S, Giwercman A, et al. Sequelae of treatment in long-term survivors of testis cancer. *Eur Urol.* 2011;60:516-526.
100. Dalal S, Tanco KC, Bruera E. State of art of managing pain in patients with cancer. *Cancer J.* 2013;19(5):379-389. doi: 10.1097/PPO.0b013e3182a631c5
101. Hurlow A, Bennett MI, Robb KA, Johnson MI, Simpson KH, Oxberry SG. Transcutaneous electrical nerve stimulation (TENS) for cancer pain in adults. *Cochrane Database Syst Rev.* 2012;(3):CD006276. doi: 10.1002/14651858.CD006276.pub3
102. Bao Y, Kong X, Yang L, et al., Complementary and alternative medicine for cancer pain: an overview of systematic reviews. *Evid Based Complement Alternat Med.* 2014;2014:170396. doi:10.1155/2014/170396
103. Pan YQ, Yang KH, Want YL, Zhang LP, Liang HQ. Massage interventions and treatment-related side effects of breast cancer: a systematic review and meta-analysis. *Int J Clin Oncol.* 2014;19(5):829-841.
104. Hecox B, Mohrotoab TA, Weisberg J. *Physical Agents: A Comprehensive Text for Physical Therapists.* Norwalk, CT: Appleton & Lange; 1994.
105. Tas D, Uncu D, Sendur MA, Koca N, Zengin N. Acupuncture as a complementary treatment for cancer patients receiving chemotherapy. *Asian Pac J Cancer Prev.* 2014;15(7):3139-3144.
106. Portenoy RK. *Pain in Oncologic and AIDS Patients.* 2nd ed. Newtown, PA: Handbooks in Health Care; 1998.
107. Ell B, Kang Y. Snap shot: bone metastasis. *Cell.* 2012;151(3):690-691.
108. Papachristou DJ, Basdra EK, Papavassiliou AG. Bone metastases: molecular mechanisms and novel therapeutic interventions. *Med Res Rev.* 2012;32(3):611-636.
109. Kilbride L, Cox M, Kennedy CM, Lee SH, Grant R. Metastatic spinal cord compression: a review of practice and care. *J Clin Nurs.* 2010;19(13-14):1767-1783.
110. Coleman RE. Metastatic bone disease: clinical features, pathophysiology and treatment strategies. *Cancer Treatment Reviews.* 2001;27:165-176.
111. Helweg-Larsen S. Prognostic factors in metastatic spinal cord compression: a prospective study using multivariate analysis of variables influencing survival and gait function in 153 patients. *Int J Radiat Oncol Biol Phys.* 2000;46(5):1163-1169.
112. Lu C, Stomper PC, Drislane FW, et al. Suspected spinal cord compression in breast cancer patients: a multidisciplinary risk assessment. *Breast Cancer Research and Treatment.* 1998;51:121-131.
113. Fisher CG, DiPaola CP, Ryken TC, et al. A novel classification system for spinal instability in neoplastic disease: an evidence-based approach and expert consensus from the Spine Oncology Study Group. *Spine (Phila Pa 1976).* 2010;35(22): E1221-E1229.
114. Rades D, Weber A, Karstens JH, Schild SE, Bartscht T. Prognostic role of the number of involved extraspinal organs in patients with metastatic spinal cord compression. *Clin Neurol Neurosurg.* 2014;118:12-15.
115. Kelly DG. *A Primer on Lymphedema.* Upper Saddle River, NJ: Prentice Hall; 2002.
116. National Lymphedema Network. 18 Steps to Prevention. https://www.krh.org/data/content/Du3iPrK7_lymphedema.pdf. Published 2008. Accessed July 15, 2019.
117. National Comprehensive Cancer Network. Cancer-related fatigue practice guidelines v.2014. http://www.nccn.org/professionals/physician_gls/pdf/fatigue.pdf. Accessed August 4, 2014.
118. Marty M, Pecorelli S, eds. *Fatigue and Cancer.* New York, NY: Elsevier Science; 2001.
119. National Cancer Institute. Cancer Related Fatigue PDQ. https://www.cancer.gov/about-cancer/treatment/side-effects/fatigue/fatigue-hp-pdq. Updated June 29, 2017. Accessed July 15, 2019.
120. Wang XS. Pathophysiology of cancer-related fatigue. *Clin J Oncol Nurs.* 2008;12(5 suppl):11-20.
121. Lucia A, Earnest C, Perez M. Cancer-related fatigue: can exercise physiology assist oncologists? *Lancet Oncol.* 2003;4(10):616-625.
122. Manzullo E, Escalante C. Research into fatigue. *Hematol/Oncol Clin North Am.* 2002;16(3):619-628.
123. Narayanan V, Koshy C. Fatigue in cancer: a review of literature. *Indian J Palliat Care.* 2009;15(1):19-25.
124. Escalante CP, Manzullo EF. Cancer-related fatigue: the approach and treatment. *J Gen Intern Med.* 2009;24(suppl 2):S412-S416. doi: 10.1007/s11606-009-1056-z

125. National Cancer Institute. Cancer-related fatigue healthcare professional version. http://www.cancer.gov/cancertopics/pdq/supportivecare/fatigue/Health Professional/page4. Updated June 29, 2017. Accessed March 1, 2019.
126. Stubbe CE, Valero M. Complementary strategies for the management of radiation therapy side effects. *J Adv Pract Oncol.* 2013;4(4):219-231.
127. Tomlinson D, Diorio C, Beyene J, Sung L. Effect of exercise on cancer-related fatigue: a meta-analysis. *Am J Phys Med Rehabil.* 2014; 93(8):675-686.
128. Backman M, Wengström Y, Johansson B, et al. A randomized pilot study with daily walking during adjuvant chemotherapy for patients with breast and colorectal cancer. *Acta Oncol.* 2014;53(4):510-520.
129. Gardner JR, Livingston PM, Fraser SF. Effects of exercise on treatment-related adverse effects for patients with prostate cancer receiving androgen-deprivation therapy: a systematic review. *J Clin Oncol.* 2014 1;32(4):335-346.
130. Oechsle K, Aslan Z, Suesse Y, Jensen W, Bokemeyer C, de Wit M. Multimodal exercise training during myeloablative chemotherapy: a prospective randomized pilot trial. *Support Care Cancer.* 2014;22(1):63-69.
131. Schmitz KH, Courneya KS, Matthews C, et al; American College of Sports Medicine. American College of Sports Medicine roundtable on exercise guidelines for cancer survivors. *Med Sci Sports Exerc.* 2010;42(7):1409-1426.
132. Division of Cancer Control & Population Sciences. Definitions. National Cancer Institute. https://cancercontrol.cancer.gov/ocs/statistics/definitions.html. Accessed July 15, 2019.
133. National Comprehensive Care Network. Survivorship guidelines. http://www.nccn.org/professionals/physician_gls/pdf/survivorship.pdf. Accessed August 4, 2014.
134. Schwartz AL. Fatigue mediates the effects of exercise on quality of life. *Qual Life Res.* 1999;8:529-538.
135. Mock V, Dow KH, Meares CJ, et al. Effects of exercise on fatigue, physical functioning, and emotional distress during radiation therapy for breast cancer. *Oncol Nurs Forum.* 1997;24(6):991-1000.
136. American Cancer Society. Cancer glossary. http://www.cancer.org/cancer/cancerglossary/index. Accessed August 6, 2019.

Appendix A

Cancer Terminology

Benign tumor: "An abnormal growth that is not cancer and does not spread to other areas. May still cause problems or symptoms in the local area."[136]

Malignant tumor: "A mass of cancer cells that may invade nearby tissues or spread (metastasize) to distant areas of the body"[136]

Metastasis: "The spread of cancer cells to one or more areas elsewhere in the body through the lymph system or bloodstream"[136]

Recurrence: "A return of the cancer to the original site or at a distant site."

Apoptosis: "Pre-programmed or determined cell death."[136]

Carcinoma: "Cancer that occurs in the lining or epithelium of passages or organs"[136]

Adenocarcinoma: "Cancer that occurs in gland cells or cells that secrete substances"[136]

Sarcoma: "Cancers that originate in bone tissue, cartilage, fat, muscle, or other connective tissue"[136]

Adjuvant chemotherapy: "Chemotherapy given after cancer surgery to rid the body of any remaining cancer cells. Adjuvant chemotherapy can also be delivered after radiation therapy with the same aim of ridding the body of microscopic cancer cells."[136]

Neoadjuvant chemotherapy: "Chemotherapy that is delivered before the main type of cancer treatment, such as surgery. The goal is to shrink the tumor so that surgeons can more easily remove it."[136]

Appendix B

Pharmacological Information: Oncological Diseases and Disorders Pharmacology (Antineoplastics)

Daniel J. Malone PT, PhD, CCS and Lora Packel PT, PhD

Alkylating Agents

Action

Alkylating agents cause cross-linking of DNA strands, abnormal base pairing of DNA or DNA strand breaks. The abnormalities inhibit DNA replication and transcription preventing cell division. Cell-cycle nonspecific.

Side Effects

CV: Dysrhythmias, CHF
GI: Nausea and vomiting
GU: Cystisis, sterility
Miscellaneous: Myelosuppression (leukopenia, thrombocytopenia), alopecia
Pulmonary: Pulmonary fibrosis

Common Medications

Nitrogen mustard: Mustargen (mechlorethamine), Cytoxan (cyclophosphamide), chlorambucil, thiotepa, busulfan, Alkeran (melphalan)

Antimetabolites

Action

Antimetabolites are drugs that compete for binding sites on enzymes or mimic and replace natural substances in DNA and RNA. These agents alter cell metabolism and protein synthesis, resulting in altered cell growth and death. Antimetabolites affect cells during the S-phase of cell division.

Side Effects

CNS: Encephelopathy, cerebellum dysfunction (cytarabine)
GI: Diarrhea, nausea, vomiting
GU: Cystisis, sterility
Miscellaneous: Myelosuppression (leukopenia, thrombocytopenia), joint pain, mucositis, alopecia

Common Medications

5-FU (Fluorouracil), Hydrea (hydroxyurea), methotrexate, cytarabine, gemcitabine

Hormonal and Enzyme Therapy

Action

Hormones may be used as chemotherapeutic agents by binding to specific receptors on cancer cells and inhibiting cell growth. These agents may actively compete with endogenous hormones leading to receptor blockade (eg, tamoxifen) or augment the effects of a particular hormone (eg, octreotide)

Side Effects

CV: Thromboembolism/pulmonary embolism
GI: Nausea, vomiting
GU: Cystisis, sterility
Miscellaneous: Hot flashes, weight gain, loss of libido, impotence

Common Medications

Breast cancer: Nolvadex (tamoxifen), raloxifene
Prostate cancer: Eulexin (flutamide), Suprefact (buserelin), Lupron (leuprolide)
Pancreatic/metastatic cancer: Sandostatin (octreotide acetate)
Lymphoma: Corticosteroids (prednisone, prednisolone)

Anti-Tumor Antibiotics

Action

Anti-tumor antibiotics bind to DNA preventing DNA and RNA synthesis. Additionally, these agents may cause DNA uncoiling and strand breaks. Cell-cycle nonspecific.

Side Effects

CNS: Encephelopathy, cerebellum dysfunction (cytarabine)
CV: Cardiomyopathy (daunorubicin, doxorubicine),
GI: Diarrhea, nausea, vomiting
GU: Renal dysfunction, cystisis
Miscellaneous: Myelosuppression (leukopenia, thrombocytopenia), alopecia
Pulmonary: Pneumonitis/pulmonary toxicity (bleomycin)

Common Medications

Anthracyclines: Daunorubicin, idarubicin, mitoxantrone
Bleomycins: Bleomycin, mitomycin

Aromatase Inhibitors

Action

Aromatase inhibitors block the effects of estrogen on estrogen sensitive tumors.

Side Effects

CNS: Headache, dizziness
CV: Edema
GI: Nausea, vomiting, diarrhea, constipation, abdominal pain
Miscellaneous: Hot flashes, back/bone pain, weakness
Pulmonary: Bronchospasm, dyspnea

Common Medications

Anastrozole (Arimidex)

Plant Alkaloids/Antimicrotubules

Action

Plant alkaloids are substances derived from plants that impair the ability of a cell to divide. These agents interfere with cell structure and cell division by binding with tubulin, a necessary protein to form the mitotic spindle during cell division. Plant alkaloids are more effective during S and M phases of cell division.

Side Effects

CNS: Lethargy
CV: Hypotension, bradycardia
GI: Constipation, abdominal pain
Miscellaneous: Peripheral neuropathy (decreased tendon reflexes/paresthesias/weakness), myalgias, myelosuppression (neutropenia, leukopenia, thrombocytopenia), weakness
Pulmonary: Bronchospasm, dyspnea

Common Medications

Vinca alkaloids: Vincristine, vinblastine, vinorelbine
Epipodophyllotoxins: Etoposide
Taxanes: Taxol (paclitaxel), Taxotere (docetaxe)

Platinum Compounds

Action

Platinum compounds are believed to produce cross-linking of DNA base pairs similar to the alkylating agents, as well as binding to various cellular proteins. The result is impaired cell division, growth, and promotion of cell death.

Side Effects

CNS: Tremor
GI: Nausea, vomiting
GU: Renal toxicity
Miscellaneous: Peripheral neuropathy, myalgias, myelosuppression (leukopenia, thrombocytopenia), anemia, weakness

Common Medications

Platinol (cisplatin), Paraplatin (carboplatin)

Monoclonal Antibody Therapy

Action

Monoclonal antibodies are genetically engineered antibodies. An antigen of interest (eg, cancer cells) is infected into an animal (eg, mouse) triggering an immune reaction. The immune reaction generates lymphocytes producing specific antibodies against the antigen of interest.

Side Effects

CNS: Dizziness, depression, fatigue
CV: Cardiomyopathy (trastuzumab), HTN, hypotension, tachycardia
GI: Abdominal discomfort, anorexia, constipation, nausea, vomiting
Miscellaneous: Fevers, chills, back pain

Common Medications

Campath (alemtuzumab), Mylotarg (gemtuzumab ozogamacin), rituximab, trastuzumab

GU = genitourinary.

Chapter 14

TRANSPLANTATION

Kathy Lee Bishop, PT, DPT, CCS and Daniel J. Malone, PT, PhD, CCS

Organ transplantation as a feasible treatment for advanced disease is a fairly recent development and the primary hurdles that medical teams continue to confront are limited patient survival and limited organ availability.[1-7] The introduction of the immunosuppressive drug cyclosporine, a calcineurin inhibitor, combined with surgical advances have dramatically improved organ and patient survival.[8-10] The introduction of other immunosuppressive drugs, improved preservation of the harvested organs, advances in surgical techniques, and judicious patient selection have dramatically improved patient survival.[4,6,11,12] Survival is not the only important outcome, but the quality of that survival is important to the health care team and to the patient and family.[11] This highly technical and demanding specialty is now considered the standard of care for end-stage organ disease.

Therapists are likely to encounter the patient who has undergone organ transplantation regardless of practice setting. Patients may be followed at the transplant medical center during the perioperative and early postoperative periods, but hospital admission can occur at any hospital long term. As patients become more active and resume regular activities of daily living (ADLs), including physical exercise, they are susceptible to a variety of complications, including musculoskeletal injuries. Transplant recipients may be followed for physical therapy services in all clinical settings, including outpatient clinics. Improved understanding of transplant anatomy, physiology, precautions, risk factors, and impact on other body systems is key for appropriate care.

The primary goals of this chapter are to introduce thoracic and abdominal organ transplantation to the therapist working in the acute care setting. Intestinal transplantation is beyond the scope of this chapter and will not be covered due to the limited number of transplants each year.[13] The first sections present an overview of the common solid organ transplants and rehabilitation; recommended goals and precautions will be provided for transplant recipients. Subsequent sections will focus on common concerns in transplantation, a case study, and chapter review questions.

Malone DJ, Bishop KL, eds. *Acute Care Physical Therapy: A Clinician's Guide, Second Edition* (pp 589-637).

Overview of Candidate Selection

Who are the potential candidates for organ transplantation? Which patients would best benefit from the limited supply of organs in the United States is a challenging question.[14] Inclusion criteria as well as absolute and relative contraindications for performing the procedure exist, but there is variability among transplant centers (Table 14-1).[14-27] Typically, patients with end-stage, single organ disease who have exhausted remaining medical and surgical interventions with reversible non-transplant organ dysfunction are considered for transplant. In addition to the primary health condition, comorbidities, functional status, quality of life, psychosocial and financial considerations, and dependencies on drugs, alcohol, and nicotine are assessed. The cut off was often 65 years of age, but more recent studies have demonstrated that older candidates have similar outcomes to candidates under 65 at 1 and 3 years.[14] Wait list duration is an important factor, and patients are typically referred for transplantation when life expectancy is limited. For example, lung transplant patients are typically referred when life expectancy is 18 to 24 months. Determination of when to refer is a balancing act among life expectancy, disease progression, and surgical risk. To optimize candidate selection and donor-recipient match, patients undergo extensive testing, as noted in Table 14-2.[7,18-28] Additional information includes medication history and comorbidities. For example, prolonged exposure to corticosteroids impairs wound healing and increases risk for osteoporosis and pathologic fractures.[4,27,29-32] The negative impact from wound dehiscence, pain, and limited mobility can impair post-transplant outcomes and quality of life. The evaluation process continues to adapt as transplant experience advances. Characteristics of the donor also have a profound role in survival outcomes.[14,28,33,34] Donor age, height, cytomegalovirus (CMV) mismatch, and comorbidities like smoking and diabetes are just a few factors considered.[35,36] The transplant team deciding patient candidacy is usually multidisciplinary.[7] Team members include the primary physicians (eg, nephrologist, cardiologist, pulmonologist, hepatologist), nursing coordinators, transplant surgeons, dietitians, social workers, and respiratory, occupational, and physical therapists. Physical therapists evaluate activity limitations, participation restrictions, postural deficiencies, and identify fixed vs reversible musculoskeletal pathologies. The physical therapist will work with each team member to support the goals of the team. For example, if the patient is at risk prior to transplant for osteoporosis due to low bone mass with poor nutritional status and corticosteroid exposure, the therapist may prescribe progressive resistive training and weightbearing exercise. If the patient has lung disease and a productive cough, the therapist may prescribe and instruct the patient in a home airway clearance program. The rehabilitation program should be designed to optimize the patient's overall exercise tolerance to prepare for the rigors of surgery.

All patients following thoracic transplant and discharge from the acute care setting are recommended to undergo cardiopulmonary rehabilitation to optimize recovery of function and quality of life. This monitored time also provides ongoing surveillance of infection and rejection.

Table 14-1

LUNG TRANSPLANTATION

Inclusion Categories

Cystic Fibrosis	Chronic Obstructive Pulmonary Disease	Idiopathic Pulmonary Arterial Hypertensions	Idiopathic Pulmonary Fibrosis	Sarcoidosis
• FEV_1 <30% predicted or a rapid decline in FEV_1 • Hypercapnia • Pulmonary hypertension • Increasing oxygen requirements • Exacerbation of lung disease resulting in ICU admission • Recurrent or refractory pneumothorax • Recurrent hemoptysis not managed by embolization	• BODE index of 7 to 10 or at least 1 of the following: ¤ Hospitalization for exacerbation associated with acute hypercapnia ¤ Pulmonary hypertension and/or cor pulmonale despite oxygen therapy ¤ FEV_1 <20% ¤ DLCO of <20% ¤ Homogeneous distribution of emphysema	• NYHA class III or IV on maximal medical therapy • ≤350 m or declining 6MWT • Cardiac index of <2 L/min/m^2 • Failing therapy with intravenous epoprostenol, or equivalent • RAP >15 mm Hg	• Evidence of UIP via histology or radiography and any of the following: ¤ ≥10% decrement in FVC during 6 months of follow up ¤ DLCO <39% predicted ¤ ≤88% SpO_2 during 6MWT ¤ Honeycombing on HRCT ¤ Fibrosis score of >2	• NYHA class III or IV and any of the following: ¤ Pulmonary hypertension ¤ RAP >15 mm Hg ¤ Hypoxemia at rest

(continued)

Table 14-1 (continued)

LUNG TRANSPLANTATION

Exclusion Criteria

- Previous malignant neoplasm within 2 years
- Untreatable advanced dysfunction of another major organ system
- Hepatitis B with positive surface antigen
- Hepatitis C with biopsy-proven liver disease
- Inability to adhere to complex medical plan
- Financial instability
- Lack of psychosocial support
- Significant left/right ventricular dysfunction
- HIV positive
- Progressive neuromuscular disorder
- Advanced connective tissue diseases
- Active extrapulmonary infection
- Substance addiction within 6 months
- ≤600 feet on 6MWT
- Nonambulatory without any rehabilitation potential

Relative Contraindications for Cystic Fibrosis

- Previous thoracotomy/thoracic surgery
- Corticosteroid use >20 mg/day
- Pseudomonas cepacia infections
- Pleurodeses
- Preoperative evidence of multiresistant organisms
- *Burkholderia cepacia* complex

BODE = body mass index, airflow obstruction, dyspnea, exercise capacity; DLCO = diffusing capacity of carbon monoxide; FEV_1 = forced expiratory volume in 1 second; HRCT = high-resolution computed tomography; ICU = intensive care unit; NYHA = New York Heart Association; RAP = right atrial pressure; 6MWT = 6 Minute Walk Test; UIP = usual interstitial pneumonia.

Adapted from Kreideret al[14]; Braun and Merlo[15]; Lynch et al[16]; and Whitson and Hayes.[17]

Table 14-2

POTENTIAL PREOPERATIVE TESTING FOR TRANSPLANTATION

Lung	*Heart*	*Liver*	*Kidney*	*Pancreas*
• ABG • Cardiac catheterization • CT scan/MRI/ multigated acquisition or angiogram imaging • ETT • Oxygen saturation • Posture/functional tests • 6MWT • Sputum culture • Ventilation/perfusion scan	• Abdominal ultrasound • Cancer screening tests • Carotid artery studies • CT scan • ETT • Peripheral vascular studies • Right heart catheterization • 6MWT	• Cardiac catheterization • Detailed cardiovascular history • Dobutamine stress • Myocardial perfusion scintigraphy with gated single-photon emission computed tomography • 24-hour holter • Ultrasound	• CT scan • MRI • Ultrasound with doppler	• Screening for neuropathy • Eye and dental examination

(continued)

Table 14-2 (continued)

POTENTIAL PREOPERATIVE TESTING FOR TRANSPLANTATION

Common Pretransplant Screening
• Blood tests: Varicella zoster, hepatitis, toxoplasmosis, CMV, HIV, evaluate cardiovascular, endocrine, kidney, liver, and thyroid function • Other tests: Addiction screening and counseling, ABG, blood glucose/HbA1C, blood typing (cross-match testing), cardiovascular risk factor screening, chest radiograph, colonoscopy, dental evaluation, detailed laboratory panel, echocardiogram, ECG, financial evaluation, lower GI series, mammogram, nutritional screening, panel reactive antibody, pap smear, PPD, PSA (men >50), psychosocial evaluation, PFT, quality of life assessment, tissue typing, upper gastrointestinal series, urine analysis, viral testing

ABG = arterial blood gas; ECG = electrocardiogram; ETT = exercise tolerance test; MRI = magnetic resonance imaging; PFT = pulmonary function test; PPD = purified protein derivative; PSA = prostate-specific antigens.

Adapted from Versluis-Burlis and Downs[7]; Ghant and Jim[18]; Glicklich and Vohra[19]; Krowka et al[20]; Maddur et al[21]; Martinex-Palli and Cardenas[22]; Mayo Clinic[23]; Penn Medicine[25]; and National Kidney Foundation.[26]

Table 14-3

FACTORS USED TO CALCULATE LUNG ALLOCATION SCORE

Characteristics	*Post-Transplant Survival Predictive Factors*
• Age at offer • Bilirubin • BMI • Cardiac index • Central venous pressure at rest • Continuous mechanical ventilation • Diabetes • Diagnosis • FVC % predicted • Functional status • Oxygen required at rest (liters/minute) • PCO_2 • Pulmonary artery systolic pressure • 6MWD	• Age at transplant • Continuous mechanical ventilation • Diagnosis • FVC % predicted • NYHA functional status • PCWP (mean) >20 mm Hg • Serum creatinine (mg/dL)
Raw LAS = net transplant benefit (1 year survival with transplant - 1 year survival without transplant) minus medical urgency (1 year survival without transplant). Score is then normalized to a 0 to 100 scale.	

BMI = body mass index; FVC = forced vitalcapacity; PCO_2 = partial pressure of carbon dioxide; PCWP = pulmonary capillary wedge pressure; 6MWD = 6 Minute Walk Distance.

Adapted from Eberlein M, Garrity ER, Orens JB. Lung allocation in the United States. *Clin Chest Med.* 2011;32(2):213-222; Kotloff KM, Thabut G. Lung transplantation. *Am J Respir Crit Care Med.* 2011;184:159-171; and UNOS. Preparing your patients for changes to the lung allocation system. *Heart/Lung News.* https://unos.org/news/preparing-patients-changes-lung-allocation-system. Published January 19, 2014. Accessed July 18, 2019.

THORACIC ORGAN TRANSPLANTATION

Lung Transplantation

Lung transplantation includes single lung transplantation (SLT), double lung transplantation (DLT), sometimes called **bilateral single sequential**, and living-related donor procedures. One-year survival for pediatric thoracic transplants is approximately 87%.[37] Survival rates in adults are more diverse, with 1-year survival being 88% for lung and 65% for heart–lung.[13,37-42] Survival rates are worse overall for older male recipients compared to younger female recipients. Recipients with primary pulmonary hypertension, sarcoidosis, and idiopathic pulmonary fibrosis have higher mortality rates during the initial 3-month period following transplantation.[36,38]

Indications/Candidate Selection

The Lung Allocation Score (LAS) system was implemented in 2005. The goal of the LAS was to allow for a fairer distribution of donor lungs. Tables 14-3 and 14-4 list the diagnoses, characteristics, and scoring process. The LAS is only for candidates older than 12 years. These changes were necessary to help identify those patients most in need of transplant, avoid futile transplants, deemphasize wait time as a determining

Table 14-4

Diagnostic Groups for Lung Transplantation and Transplant Type

LAS Group A	*LAS Group B*	*LAS Group C*	*LAS Group D*
Obstructive Lung Disease	**Pulmonary Vascular Disease**	**Cystic Fibrosis or Immunodeficiency Disorders**	**Restrictive Lung Disease**
• A 1-Antitrypsin Deficiency (BLT, SLT) • Bronchiectasis (BLT, HLT) • COPD (BLT, SLT) • Emphysema (BLT, SLT) • Lymphangioleiomyomatosis (BLT, SLT) • Sarcoidosis (PAP <30 mm Hg) (BLT, SLT)	• Eisenmenger syndrome (BLT, HLT) • Primary pulmonary hypertension (BLT, SLT) • Pulmonary capillary hemangiomatosis (BLT, HLT, SLT) • Secondary pulmonary hypertension (BLT)	• Common variable immune deficiency (BLT, HLT) • Cystic fibrosis (BLT, HLT) • Hypogammaglobulinemia (BLT, HLT)	• ABCA 3 transporter hemangiomatosis (BLT, SLT) • Acute respiratory distress syndrome/pneumonia (BLT, SLT) • Bronchiolitis obliterans and organizing pneumonia (BLT, HLT) • Bronchoalveolar carcinoma (BLT, SLT) • Hypersensitivity pneumonitis (BLT, SLT) • IPF (BLT, SLT) • Idiopathic interstitial pneumonia (BLT, SLT) • Lung retransplant/graft failure (BLT, HLT, SLT) • Pulmonary lymphangiectasis (BLT, SLT) • Secondary pulmonary fibrosis (BLT, SLT) • Surfactant protein C mutation (BLT, SLT)

BLT = bilateral lung transplantation; COPD = chronic obstructive pulmonary diease; HLT = heart–lung transplantation.

Adapted from Kreider et al[14]; Eberlein et al[28]; Organ Procurement and Transplantation Network[34]; and UNOS.[144]

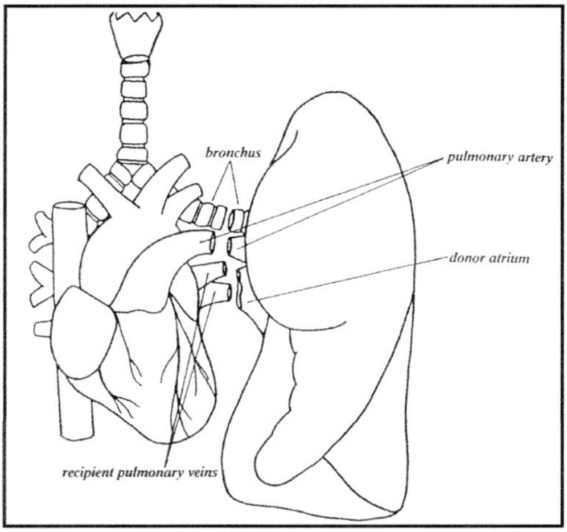

Figure 14-1. Lung transplant. Schematic illustrates the 3 anastomoses: (1) mainstem bronchus, (2) pulmonary artery, and (3) left atrium with pulmonary veins.

factor, and decrease wait list mortality. Since implementation of the LAS, waiting time for transplant has decreased from 2 to 3 years to less than 35 days and has substantially decreased wait list mortality.[40] This new process has essentially eliminated the need for living-donor lobar lung transplantation in the United States.[43] Survival is lowest for LAS of less than 50, recipients older then 65, and category B (see Table 14-4). Improved survival may be attributed to many factors, including choice of procedure (bilateral and single right lung transplant had a greater survival then left SLT), the LAS for candidate selection, limiting ischemia-reperfusion injury, timing of immune suppression, antiviral prophylaxis, and donor organ preservation.[13,40]

The type of surgery will depend on the disease process, organ availability, recipient matching, and age. Interestingly, there is an increasing percentage of patients who are in the intensive care unit (ICU) prior to the time of transplant.[44] Mechanical ventilation and extracorporeal membrane oxygenation (ECMO) are not absolute contraindications to transplantation, but mechanical ventilation duration, current infectious pathogens, and immobility may adversely affect outcomes.[42] Patients on ECMO represented 5.3% of lung transplant recipients in 2014.[44] Transplantation following ECMO is limited to certain centers and survival is lower compared to nonsupported patients.[45-48]

Operative Procedure

The SLT operation is usually performed through a posterolateral thoracotomy through the fourth and fifth intercostal spaces.[4,31,49] This approach helps to spare the serratus anterior and latissimus dorsi muscle groups.[31] An anterolateral thoracotomy with transverse sternotomy, or "clamshell," has been used in patients who have emphysema and are simultaneously having lung volume reduction on the opposite side.[49] The surgeon dissects the superior and inferior pulmonary veins, the pulmonary artery, and the main stem bronchus. The phrenic nerve and the hilum are exposed when the pericardium is opened, and the left atrium is accessed via an extended incision. Some cartilages of the recipient bronchus are removed and shortened to allow telescoping of the donor bronchus within the recipient's bronchus improving blood supply and healing.[49] The donor and recipient pulmonary arteries are anastomosed along with the left atrial cuff including the pulmonary veins to the recipient's left atrium as noted in Figure 14-1.[4]

The bilateral single sequential lung transplant has replaced the en bloc DLT in the United States. This procedure lessens bronchial anastomosis dehiscence and limits

Table 14-5

Risks for Complications and Prolonged Length of Stay in Intensive Care Unit Post-Transplantation

• Advanced age • APACHE II score • Cardiopulmonary bypass duration • Cardiovascular instability • ECMO at time of transplant • Graft dysfunction/gas-exchange impairment/carbon dioxide retention • Lower pretransplant FEV_1	• Infection (persistent purulent sections with donor or aspiration) • Infiltrates on donor chest roentgenogram • Longer ischemic time • Mechanical ventilation at time of transplant • Obesity • Pulmonary hypertensive disorders • Respiratory muscle weakness

APACHE = Acute Physiology and Chronic Health Evaluation.

Adapted from Toyada and Toyada[39]; Mason et al[42]; Weill et al[45]; Gottlieb et al[46]; Hoopes et al[47]; Chiumello et al[48]; de Perrot et al[49]; Algar et al[50]; Ferdinande et al[51]; and Burns and Iacono.[52]

complications associated with cardiopulmonary bypass.[7] The procedure is similar to the SLT except the incision is a median sternotomy or the anterolateral thoracotomy with transverse sternotomy (clamshell).[31]

Acute Care Management and Complications

Patients frequently require mechanical ventilation for 24 to 48 hours following transplantation, but rapid extubation is common. An early goal is to liberate the patient from mechanical ventilation, but potential difficulties with the weaning process and factors prolonging the ICU duration are outlined in Table 14-5.[39,42,45-52] Early mobilization and prophylaxis for deep vein thrombosis (DVT) are an important component of acute care management for any surgical patient. Universal precautions are the standard of care for all patients in a hospital setting but are fundamental to care of transplant recipients. Risk of infection and rejection are ever present. Signs and symptoms of possible lung rejection are outlined in Table 14-6.[7,40,41,53] Complications following lung transplantation can be divided into early and late categories as described in Table 14-7.[54-57] Primary causes of death and other complications can be found in Table 14-8. Rejection falls into both categories but can be further subdivided into acute and chronic conditions. Acute cellular rejection has been reported to occur in 36% of recipients in the first year.[40] Acute graft dysfunction, also called **primary graft failure**, has been shown to occur in 2.3% of the transplant population and is the leading cause of death in the perioperative period.[38,40] Chronic rejection is synonymous with bronchiolitis obliterans syndrome (BOS), and is the leading cause of late morbidity and mortality following lung transplantation and HLT.[38] BOS is characterized by fibrosis and scar formation in the smaller airways (see Chapter 7).[40] Upwards of 50% of lung transplant recipients will have BOS 5 years after surgery and 75% by 10 years.[40]

Airway anastomotic dehiscence is a complication that occurs early in the development of lung transplantation. Exposure to corticosteroids, inability to reconnect the bronchial circulation, end-to-end suturing, and immunosuppressive medications have been implicated in impaired wound healing. Various improvements in the surgical anastomosis along with modifications of the drug regimen have decreased ischemic and stenotic complications of the airway.[10,49,58]

Table 14-6

Signs and Symptoms of Lung Transplant Rejection

• Chest congestion	• Leukocytosis
• Coughing	• Lethargy
• Desaturation with activity/exercise	• Low-grade temperature
• Decrease in exercise tolerance	• Myalgias
• Feeling unwell	• New pain around lungs
• Fever and flu-like symptoms	• Palpitations
• General malaise	• Restrictive pattern on spirometry (↓ FVC, ↓ FEV_1)
• Increased SOB/DOE	

DOE = dyspnea on exertion; SOB = shortness of breath.

Adapted from Kotloff KM, Thabut G. Lung transplantation. *Am J Respir Crit Care Med.* 2011;184:159-171; Lung transplant. National Heart, Lung, and Blood Institute. https://www.nhlbi.nih.gov/health/health-topics/topics/lungtxp/risks. Accessed March 19, 2019; and Versluis-Burlis T, Downs AM. Thoracic organ transplantation: heart, lung, and heart-lung. In: Hillegass EA, Sadowsky HS, eds. *Essentials of Cardiopulmonary Physical Therapy.* 2nd ed. Philadelphia, PA: WB Saunders; 2001.

The immunosuppressed patient is at risk for opportunistic infections, but lung transplant and HLT recipients have the added challenge of environmental exposure with every breath. The most frequently encountered infection is bacterial pneumonia within 1 month of transplant. Risk factors include mechanical ventilation, aspiration, poor cough, impaired mucociliary clearance, and immunosuppression.[40] The most common viral pathogen is CMV, which may lead to as much as 1/3 of recipients at risk during the first year post-transplant. Patient education should include avoidance of unnecessary exposures, such as crowded locations, children or adults with active infections, and using a mask during times of poor air quality. Patients should be cautioned to avoid gardening and construction projects because of exposure to mold and fungi.

Physical Therapist Management of Lung Transplantation

Following transplantation, rehabilitation is initiated in the ICU. Goals during the acute care phase of rehabilitation focus on independence with mobility and ADLs, effective coughing and airway clearance, pain control, and patient education (Table 14-9). The normal cough reflex and lymphatic drainage are absent below the level of the bronchial anastomosis due to denervation. Deep breathing exercises and splinted incision coughing should be performed every waking hour to prevent atelectasis and pneumonia. Evaluation for orthostatic hypotension should be considered during early therapy sessions. The therapist needs to appreciate fluid status, effects of immobility, and side effects from pain medications on cardiovascular responsiveness to position changes.

The functional status at hospital discharge may be similar to admission due to the effects of surgery and hospitalization (eg, incision pain, sleep deficits, limited nutrition, anesthesia, limited mobility), immunosuppressive medications, prior deconditioning, and the native disease. Patients may frequently complain of dyspnea and fatigue on exertion. These complaints may not be due to pulmonary impairments but rather preoperative deconditioning. Potential exercise capacity changes following lung transplantation are outlined in Table 14-10.[11,49,59-70] Overall concerns and areas to monitor are outlined in the rehabilitation section for all solid organ transplantations.

Therapists must be aware of the signs and symptoms of infection and rejection (see Table 14-6).

Table 14-7
Categories of Lung Transplantation Complications by Onset

Onset	*Type of Complication*	
Perioperative	Primary graft dysfunction	
Early	**Acute Lung Allograft Dysfunction (ALAD)**	
	• Allograft related: ¤ Acute rejection (cellular/ humoral) ¤ ABPA ¤ AFOP/ARDS ¤ Anastomosis problem ¤ Infection ¤ Lymphocytic bronchitis/ bronchiolitis ¤ Pneumothorax ¤ Pulmonary embolus ¤ Other causes	• Nonallograft related: ¤ Donor-specific antibodies ¤ Pleural disease (pleuritis) ¤ Spirometry (poor technique or device malfunction)
Chronic >3 months	**Chronic Lung Allograft Dysfunction (CLAD) Non-Reversible**	
	Chronic decline in FEV_1 >20% and/or FVC >20% compared to baseline values	
	Restrictive: RAS FVC <80% baseline FVC at diagnosis >3 weeks	*Obstructive:* BOS FEV_1 <80% baseline FEV_1 >3 weeks
	Mean of best 2 postoperative measurements minimum of 3 weeks apart	
	Non-Chronic Rejection Causes of Pulmonary Function Test Decline	
	• Allograft-related ¤ Anastomotic stricture ¤ ARAD ¤ Disease reoccurrence ¤ Follicular bronchiolitis ¤ Infection/colonization ¤ Persistent acute rejection	• Extra-allograft ¤ Diaphragm dysfunction ¤ Environmental interface ¤ GERD ¤ Inherited risk factors ¤ Native lung (fibrosis, hyperinflation, infection) ¤ Neuromuscular ¤ Pleural disease ¤ Other causes

ABPA = allergic bronchopulmonary aspergillosis; AFOP = acute fibrinoid-organizing pneumonia; ARAD = azithromycin-responsive allograft dysfunction; ARDS = acute respiratory distress syndrome; GERD = gastroesophageal reflux disease; RAS = restrictive allograft syndrome.

Adapted from De Vlaminck et al[54]; Verleden et al[55]; Verleden et al[56]; and Vos et al.[57]

Therapists may be the first health care providers to recognize these markers because the therapist is mobilizing the patient and monitoring daily changes in activity levels. Deterioration of the patient's status should be reported to the transplant

Table 14-8

PRIMARY CAUSE OF DEATH AND COMPLICATIONS FOLLOWING LUNG TRANSPLANTATION

Early (<30 days)	*Late (>1 Year)*
• Graft failure • Infection, non-CMV • Cardiovascular • Technical • Acute rejection • Other causes	• Bronchiolitis • Infection, non-CMV • Graft failure • Malignancy, non-lymphoma • Cardiovascular • Lymphoma • Cytomegalovirus • Other causes

Adapted from Yusen RD, Edwards LB, Kucheryavaya AY, et al; International Society of Heart and Lung Transplantation. Registry of the International Society for Heart and Lung Transplantation: Thirty-Second Adult Lung and Heart-Lung Transplant Report-2015; focus theme: early graft failure. *J Heart Lung Transplant.* 2015;34:1264-1277.

Table 14-9

POTENTIAL REHABILITATION GOALS BEFORE AND FOLLOWING TRANSPLANTATION

Educate	*Optimize and Improve*
• Body mechanics during ADLs • Breathing efficiency during ADLs • Effective coughing/ splinting • Medications and side effects • Precautions, signs/symptoms of infection/rejection • Identification of infection and rejection • Stress management and relaxation techniques • Team roles • Use of scales for self-monitoring: Borg, pain during ADLs, IADLs, dyspnea, and return to normal activity • Use of home self-monitors (eg, spirometry, glucometer, daily weight)	• Airway clearance and breathing control • Cardiovascular pulmonary endurance and exercise capacity • Functional level to return to work • Independence with ADLs and IADLs • Overall function • Pain control • Posture and flexibility • ROM and strength

IADLs = independent activities of daily living; ROM = range of motion.

team. The signs and symptoms of infection and rejection are often subtle and early recognition is crucial. During periods of acute rejection, exercise can be performed cautiously. The progression of rehabilitation follows an early mobilization (see Chapter 4) and pulmonary rehabilitation philosophy (see Chapter 7). Activity/exercise intensity is performed to Modified Borg Scale ratings of 4 to 6 (0 to 10 scale) while monitoring for appropriate pulse oximetry and other vital sign responses.

Table 14-10

Long-Term Exercise Responses Following Lung, Heart, and Heart–Lung Transplantation

Lung
• Exercise capacity and pulmonary function below normal values • Limitations multifactorial but mostly thought to be peripheral (circulation/muscle) • VO_{2max} 40% to 60% • Predicted DLT VO_2 > SLT/HLT • ↓ in physiologic dead space (Vd/V_T) and alveolar-arterial oxygen gradient • ([A-a] PO_2) • Elevated RR, HR, and minute ventilation at rest • High respiratory exchange ratio • Early onset of lactic acidosis • Impaired oxidative capacity of peripheral muscles, lower type 1 fibers • %HRR improves • Decreased muscle mass • Reduced total leg strength • Decreased mitochondrial enzyme activity • Decreased calcium uptake and release
Heart
• Exercise capacity and pulmonary function below normal values • Limitations multifactorial but mostly thought to be peripheral (circulation/muscle) • VO_{2peak} 51% to 101% predicted • Lower maximum HR (~25% < controls) • 74% to 93% of age predicted HR_{max} • Lower anaerobic threshold maximum HR 20% to 25% less than controls • Lower maximum oxygen pulse • Exaggerated neuroendocrine response
Heart–Lung
• Exercise capacity and pulmonary function below normal values • Limitations multifactorial but mostly thought to be peripheral (circulation/muscle) • VO_{2max} 39% to 62% predicted • Blunted chronotropic/inotropic responses to exercise • Lower anaerobic threshold • Pulmonary function typically restrictive pattern
A-a = alveoli to arterial; HR = heart rate; HRR = heart rate reserve; RR = respiratory rate; Vd/V_T = ventilation deadspace over tidal volume; VO_2 = oxygen consumption.
Adapted from Braith and Edwards[11]; de Perrot et al[49]; De Jonge et al[59]; Reinsma et al[60]; Wickerson et al[61]; Nytroen and Gullestad[62]; Squires[63]; Wilhem[64]; Chaudry et al[65]; Langer et al[66]; Marconi and Marzorati[67]; Didsbury et al[68]; Armstrong et al[69]; and Fink et al.[70]

Patient education focuses on incentive spirometry, effective coughing, maintaining daily records of weight, temperature, overall perception of well-being, and spirometry. Patients are often provided hand-held spirometers (microspirometers) to measure daily changes in pulmonary function including the FEV_1 and FVC and the accurate performance and recording of this data should be reviewed daily.

Heart Transplantation

The 1-year survival rate for heart transplant is 90%, and is the highest among thoracic transplant recipients.[35,41,71] The number of transplants performed each year is approximately 4100.[35] This fairly flat number of heart transplants is due to limited donor organ availability, promoting advances in surgical techniques and medications and devices for patients with cardiac disease.[35] Advances include valve repair and coronary artery bypass grafting in higher risk populations, biventricular pacemakers, and mechanical circulatory assist devices (eg ventricular assist devices [VADs], ECMO).[6,59,72] Earlier and more aggressive intervention following cardiac events, such as angioplasty for unstable angina or a myocardial infarction, is becoming the standard of care.[3] Mechanical circulatory assist devices are not only serving as a bridge to transplant, but also as a destination option for patients with severe heart failure.[64,71] Survival rates with mechanical assist devices have begun to approach the level of heart transplant.[64,71] See Chapter 6 for more detail on VAD/ECMO. The United Network of Organ Sharing (UNOS) guidelines are used to set criteria for determining heart transplant recipient status (Table 14-11).

Indications/Candidate Selection

The primary indication for heart transplantation is end-stage cardiac disease or heart failure (Table 14-12).[3,4,6,31,52,71,73,74] Heart transplant is recommended for patients with maximal oxygen consumption (VO_{2max}) less than 14 mL/kg/min, recurrent symptomatic ventricular dysrhythmias refractory to all therapeutic modalities, and severe ischemia, which is not treatable with angioplasty or coronary bypass surgery.[6] Candidate evaluation is extensive as previously noted for lung transplantation.

Operative Procedure

Orthotopic heart transplantation (Figure 14-2), the primary form of cardiac transplant, refers to the removal of the recipient heart followed by replacement with the donor's heart in the same anatomic location. A median sternotomy is made, and the patient is placed on cardiopulmonary bypass. The donor atria are incised to allow anastomosis to the recipient atria. This biatrial method allows for short operative time by anastomosing the donor left and right atria to the recipient's heart at the midatrial level. This method has a higher incidence of mitral and tricuspid insufficiency. An alternative method is the bicaval technique involving individual anastomoses of the inferior and superior vena cava instead of the right atrial cuff. Additional modifications include an anastomosis of paired pulmonary veins to replace the left atrial cuff anastomosis.[3] This technique has proven effective with fewer electrophysiological complications requiring pacemaker support.[3,6]

Heterotopic heart transplantation is indicated in select cases and is referred to as the **piggyback technique**.[6,7] The donor and recipient hearts remains intact, and the right and left atria are anastomosed to allow the 4 atria to function as 2. The aorta and pulmonary arteries are adjoined. The 2 hearts function in parallel sharing the venous return and contributing to the cardiac output. The primary indications for this type of transplant are poor donor heart function, pulmonary hypertension, and mismatched size between donor and recipient. The advantage of the technique is to allow the recipient heart to assist during periods of rejection or impaired function. Disadvantages of this technique are dysrhythmias, angina related to the native heart, risk of pulmonary emboli, and long-term use of anticoagulation therapy.

Acute Care Management and Complications

Bleeding, persistent pulmonary hypertension, valve dysfunction, renal dysfunction, rejection, and infection are complications in the initial postoperative phase.[6,74] Bleeding risk is increased in those who have had multiple operations, anticoagulation

Table 14-11

United Network for Organ Sharing Guideline for Heart Transplant Recipient

UNOS Status 1A	*UNOS status 1B*	*UNOS Status 2*
• Continuous infusion of high-dose inotropes • Life expectancy <7 days without transplant • Mechanical circulatory support >30 days with device related complications • Mechanical ventilation • Patient requiring MCS with 1 or more of the following: ¤ ECMO ¤ IABP ¤ LVAD or RVAD <30 days ¤ TAH	• At least 1 of the following devices or ongoing therapies: ¤ Continuous infusion of intravenous inotropes ¤ LVAD or RVAD >30 days	• Any other patients who do not meet criteria for Status 1A or 1B

IABP = intra-aortic balloon pump; LVAD = left ventricular assist device; MCS = mechanical circulatory support; RVAD = right ventricular assist device; TAH = total artificial heart.

Adapted from Toyoda Y, Guy TS, Kashem A. Present status and future prospectives of heart transplantation. *Circ J*. 2013;77:1097-1110.

therapy, and prior liver or renal dysfunction. Perioperative kidney dysfunction may be related to fluid shifts during the surgery, impaired donor heart function, and use of nephrotoxic immunosuppressive medications.[6,74] Liberating the patient from mechanical ventilation and aggressive pulmonary hygiene is important until the patient begins out of bed (OOB) activity. Standard precautions apply for all patients, but in the transplant population, should be overzealously applied.

Rejection of the transplanted heart is a life-long challenge, and common signs and symptoms are presented in Table 14-13.[75] Hyperacute rejection is rare and occurs within hours after surgery.[6] Acute cellular rejection is more common and occurs within the first 30 days. Identification and treatment of rejection is the most important component of after care for heart transplant patients. Patients undergo frequent endomyocardial biopsies for histologic examination as the standard method to detect rejection. Routine biopsy of heart tissue is performed regardless of symptoms. The biopsy is graded on a scale of 0 to 3 with 0 being no rejection and 3 being severe diffuse infiltrate with tissue damage, with or without hemorrhage, vasculitis, or edema.[74] Patients may have to be admitted to the ICU if there is hemodynamic compromise from the acute rejection. Therapy will have to be adjusted until acute rejection has been medically stabilized.

Infection is also a persistent complication of immunosuppressive treatment. Bacterial infections are more common early while viral infections are one of the leading long-term causes of morbidity and mortality.[64,74]

The primary late complication of heart transplantation is graft coronary artery disease (CAD), also termed **cardiac allograft vasculopathy** (CAV) or **transplant coronary disease**.[3,6,64,74] CAV occurs in approximately 8% within the first year and up to 32% by the fifth year following heart transplant. Transplant vasculopathy is challenging because the stenotic lesion can be diffuse or focal and is often asymptomatic.[76] A correlation has been demonstrated with a higher degree of human leukocyte antigen

Table 14-12

Heart Transplantation, Inclusion/Exclusion Categories

Inclusion/Indications	*Exclusion/Contraindications*
• Recurrent refractory symptomatic ventricular arrhythmia • Maximal oxygen consumption <14 mL/kg/min • Severe ischemia limiting routine activity not responsive or amenable to revascularization • End-stage heart disease with optimal medical and surgical therapy with irreversible pulmonary hypertension • Heterotopic heart transplant • Refractory heart failure (inotropes or VAD) • Functional classes III or IV on optimal therapy and with prognosis <1 year survival <75% • 6MWT <300 m or V_E/V_{CO2} >35	• ABO incompatibility for cross matching recipient and donor • Active smoker • Age >70 years old • Cancer <5 years other than localized skin or stage 1 breast or prostate • HIV • Pulmonary hypertension (PVR >5 Wood units) • Severe liver failure, pulmonary disease, CVD, PVD • Severe psychiatric disease, poor compliance to treatment, and chemical dependence • Severe neurologic deficit
Relative Contraindications	
• Acute pulmonary thromboembolism • Active GI disease • Cachexia • Documented PVD or CVD • IDDM with end organ damage • Pulmonary dysfunction: <40% predicted FEV_1 and FVC	• Irreversible renal or hepatic dysfunction • Inability to make a strong commitment to transplantation • Morbid obesity >140% of IBW • No psychosocial support • Severe pulmonary hypertension

ABO = blood type designation; CVD = cerebrovascular disease; GI = gastrointestinal; IBW = ideal body weight; IDDM = insulin-dependent diabetes mellitus; PVD = peripheral vascular disease; PVR = peripheral vascular resistance; V_E/V_{CO2} = ventilatory equivalent for carbon dioxide.

Adapted from Miniati and Robbins[3]; Harringer and Haverich et al[4]; Radovancevic and Frazier[6]; Gilbert et al[31]; Toyoda et al[71]; Mangini et al[73]; Birati and Rame[74]; and International Society for Heart and Lung Transplantation.[145]

(HLA) mismatch and persistent inflammation.[74] Focal lesions have been treated with angioplasty, but traditional treatments for CAD, like bypass grafting, have limited success. Prevention, similar to typical atherosclerosis management, may play a role by influencing lipid deposition, diabetes, HTN, and reducing opportunistic infections.[3,6,74] Superior vena cava stenosis and tricuspid regurgitation have also been documented as late complications.[3,8]

Physical Therapist Management of Heart Transplantation

Hemodynamic stability, side effects of immunosuppressive medications, and incision pain are challenges to the physical therapist. The transplanted heart is denervated leading to an elevated resting HR, blunted HR and BP responses to a given activity, and the patient will require a prolonged time for the vital signs to return

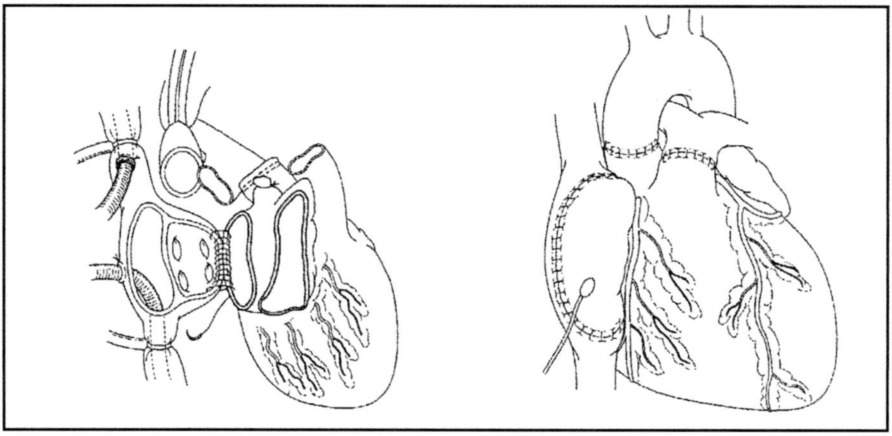

Figure 14-2. Orthotopic heart transplant. Schematic illustrates the biatrial method. Note epicardial pacemaker electrode in place. (Reprinted from Sadowsky HS. Cardiac transplantation: a review. *Phys Ther.* 1996;76:498-515. With permission from the American Physical Therapy Association.)

to baseline with the cessation of activity. Patients rely on venous return to augment end diastolic volume (see Chapter 6, Frank-Starling mechanism,) and circulating catecholamines to elevate HR and stroke volume to increase cardiac output and BP. These physiologic mechanisms take several minutes to activate necessitating the performance of warm-up and cool-down activities prior to activity and exercise. Rate of perceived exertion, HR/pulse rate, ECG, BP, oxygen saturation, RR and breathing pattern, and patient color are all helpful signs of subtle changes in the cardiovascular and pulmonary systems' ability to respond to activity. As noted previously, the progression of rehabilitation includes early mobilization (see Chapter 4) and patients who have undergone heart transplant should be participating in phase 1 cardiac rehabilitation (see Chapter 6). Tables 14-9 and 14-13 outline some of the more specific challenges as well as goals the physical therapist should be focused on for patients following heart transplantation.

Heart–Lung Transplantation

Indications/Candidate Selection

The number of HLTs continue to decline since the mid-1990s, possibly related to the successful use of lung transplantation for cystic fibrosis and primary pulmonary hypertension, as well as donor organ shortage.[31,77] Table 14-4 lists the diagnostic groups who have benefited from a HLT. Typically, the patient is listed on both the heart and lung allocation systems through UNOS.[77]

Operative Procedure

The HLT incision is a median sternotomy or bilateral transverse thoracotomy.[4,7,49] Right and left pneumonectomies are carefully performed to avoid damaging the vagal and phrenic nerves.[4] En bloc implantation involves dissection of the trachea near the carina, and anastomoses of the recipient's aorta, right atria, and trachea. Domino transplants, where one recipient receives a donor's heart and lungs and then that transplant recipient's heart is transplanted into another patient, are not performed frequently, but the domino procedure may be more advantageous compared to routine cadaveric donor transplantation.[77] Some specific benefits include improved HLA matching and tighter control of ischemia time during organ procurement. Also,

Table 14-13 Signs and Symptoms of Heart Transplantation Rejection	
• Decrease in exercise tolerance	• Myalgias
• Elevated resting BP	• Palpitations
• General malaise	• Reduction in urine production
• Hypotension with activity	• Soft heart sounds/S_3 gallop
• Increased SOB/DOE	• Ventricular dysrhythmias
• Lethargy	• Weight gain
• Low-grade temperature	

Adapted from Heart transplant. National Heart, Lung, and Blood Institute. https://www.nhlbi.nih.gov/health/health-topics/topics/ht/after. Accessed March 19, 2019.

the complications of the airway and vascular anastomoses in younger children is decreased with the domino procedure.

Acute Care Management and Complications

Management of the patient following HLT is similar to aspects of both postoperative lung and heart transplant care. The challenge for the patient and care team is the denervated heart and lungs. The therapist must remember the absence of cough reflex and autonomic nervous system input to the heart and lungs. Additionally, the continuous threats of infection and rejection necessitate careful observation for all potential signs and symptoms of untoward events.

Abdominal Organ Transplantation

Kidney Transplantation

More than 15,000 kidney transplants are performed every year and 1-year patient survival after transplant from a living related donor is greater than 96% and greater than 93% from a cadaver.[78,79] Transplantation clearly improves the quality and quantity of life compared with other modalities of renal replacement therapy, such as hemodialysis, especially for younger and diabetic patients.[80]

In the United States, many recovered kidneys are not used for transplant. To improve kidney distribution, a new kidney allocation system was introduced in 2014. The newer kidney allocation system, the Kidney Donor Risk Index (KDRI), uses 10 donor characteristics to determine the relative risk of post-transplant graft failure. The characteristics include donor age, weight, height, race/ethnicity, cause of death, history of HTN or diabetes, serum creatinine, hepatitis C status, and donation after cardiac death status. The KDRI of each kidney is then mapped into a Kidney Donor Profile Index (KDPI) from 1 (Best) to 100 (Worst).[80] Longer graft survival is related to a lower KDPI score. To better match donated kidneys that have a longer estimated survival, kidneys with a KDPI percentile of less than or equal to 20% are preferentially allocated to transplant candidates in the upper 20% for post-transplant survival. Candidates are given priority if the candidate is a pediatric patient, prior living donor, awaiting multiple organs, and zero-HLA mismatch kidneys or has calculated panel-reactive antibodies (PRA) of 98% and above (often related to prior blood transfusions, pregnancy, transplant; high PRA increases the risk of rejection).[79,80]

Indications/Candidate Selection

Candidates for kidney transplantation undergo an extensive evaluation to identify important medical and psychosocial factors that may lead to adverse outcomes as previously noted for thoracic organ transplantation. There is a diverse array of pathologies that destroy renal function as noted in Chapter 12, but the most common cause of end-stage renal disease (ESRD) is diabetes.[81] Table 14-14 provides a list of the most common renal disorders leading to transplant as well as exclusion criteria.[80,82] The patient with ESRD has several treatment options, including long-term dialysis, cadaveric kidney transplant, living kidney transplant, and for those with diabetes and renal failure, simultaneous kidney-pancreas transplantation. Cardiovascular disease is the most prevalent comorbid condition in patients with ESRD and traditional risk factors for atherosclerosis factor into the high incidence of cardiovascular disease in patients with ESRD, including HTN, dyslipidemia, and diabetes.[78-82]

Operative Procedure

The surgical approach is a curved incision in the patient's lower quadrant and proceeds through the external oblique to the peritoneum. The transplant site is usually the extra peritoneal space of the right or left lower abdominal quadrant and is often **heterotopic**, the native kidneys are left in place while the transplanted kidney is positioned in a different location. The surgical technique involves anastomoses of the renal artery and vein and ureter (Figure 14-3). The surgeon performs an end-to-side anastomosis of the donor renal artery to the recipient's external iliac, common iliac, or hypogastric artery. The renal vein is customarily anastomosed to the corresponding vein. The transplant ureter is either placed directly into the bladder wall or anastomosed to the recipient ureter.[83] Precise wound closure is important to prohibit hernia formation. Temporary suction drains are usually present during the perioperative period.[84] The technique for living donor kidney transplantation is similar to that described for cadaveric donor transplantation.[83] Minimally invasive robotic-assisted kidney transplantation is an option at certain transplant centers.[85] A form of this surgery has been done since 2002, but the first true robotic-assisted laparoscopic kidney transplant (RAKT) was done in 2010. This type of surgery has been shown to have better outcomes with morbidly obese patients compared to the traditional operative approach.

Acute Care Management and Complications

The incidence of postoperative complications has decreased, but acute rejection and infections remain a concern (Table 14-15).[79] The most common complication during the acute care period is allograft dysfunction that may progress to graft loss. Renal failure persisting after transplantation is called **delayed graft function** (DGF) and is associated with oliguria, diminished urine formation, or the need for dialysis after the operation. DGF is usually due to ATN or nephrotoxicity because of the immunosuppressive medications (especially cyclosporine or tacrolimus). A newer immunosuppressive medication, belatacept, has been shown to be superior to traditional calcineurin inhibitor medications (cyclosporine, tacrolimus) for rejection. DGF may occur in 20% to 30% of cadaveric transplants and is rare after living donor.[79,86] Other early but infrequent graft problems include accelerated acute or hyperacute rejection. Risk for serious infections persist over the life of the transplant. Common symptoms of rejection are presented in Table 14-16.[79,87]

The gold standard for early detection of acute rejection is a renal biopsy. Because the biopsy puts the new allograft at risk, noninvasive imaging is preferred.[88] The diagnosis of rejection is confirmed by ultrasonography to rule out urinary obstruction or anastomotic thrombus or leak followed by biopsy and histologic examination. Magnetic resonance imaging (MRI), positron emission tomography (PET), and single

Table 14-14

KIDNEY TRANSPLANTATION, INCLUSION/EXCLUSION CATEGORIES

Inclusion/Indications	*Exclusion/Contraindications*
• ESRD (serum creatinine >5 mg/dL; BUN >70 mg/dL) • Diabetes • Chronic glomerulonephritis • Polycystic kidney disease • Nephrosclerosis • Interstitial nephritis • Systemic lupus erythematosus • Congenital malformations • Kidney stone obstructions • Repeated urinary tract infections	• Reversible renal disease • Recent malignancy • Untreated active infection • Active substance abuse • Severe and/or uncontrolled psychiatric illness • Irreversible extrarenal disease limiting life span • Morbid obesity • Extrarenal complications • CAD with limitation of life span • Severe PVD • Primary amyloidosis with extrarenal disease • HIV with CD4 counts <200/μm or AIDS-defining illness • Advanced dementia • Advanced age • Active glomerulonephritis • Noncompliance

BUN = blood urea nitrogen; CD = cluster destination.

Adapted from Ghanta M, Jim B. Renal transplantation in advanced chronic kidney disease patients. *Med Clin N Am.* 2016;100:465-476 and Scheuber C. A review of organ transplantation: heart, lung, kidney, liver, and simultaneous liver-kidney. *Crit Care Nurse Q.* 2016;39(3):199-206. doi: 10.1097/CNQ.0000000000000115

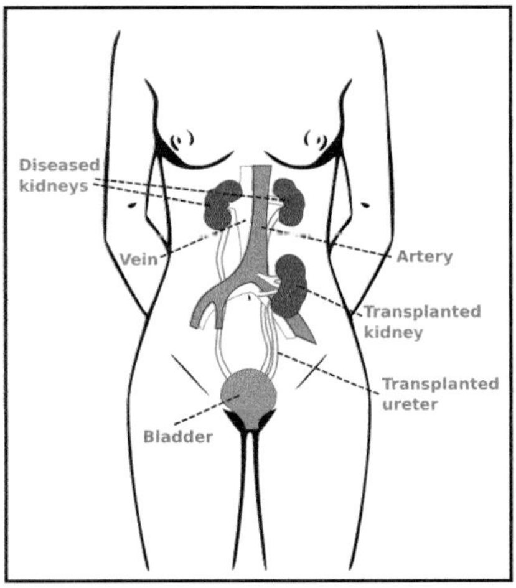

Figure 14-3. Kidney transplant. Schematic illustrates 3 anastomoses: (1) renal artery, (2) renal vein, and (3) ureter. Note how native kidneys are left in place. (Reprinted with permission via Creative Commons Attribution 3.0 Unported license. Wiremu Stadtwald Demchick.)

Table 14-15

COMPLICATIONS POST–KIDNEY TRANSPLANTATION

Early (<3 Months)	*First Year*	*Beyond First Year*
• Acute rejection • Urinary retention • Urine leak • Ureteral obstruction • Delayed graft function • Thrombotic microangiopathy • Acute tubular necrosis (ATN)	• Recurrent disease • BK virus (polyomavirus BK)	• Chronic allograft failure • Late allograft failure

Adapted from Chandran S, Vincenti F. Clinical aspects: focusing on key unique organ-specific issues of renal transplantation. *Cold Spring Harb Perspect Med.* 2014;4(2):a015644.

Table 14-16

SIGNS AND SYMPTOMS OF KIDNEY REJECTION

- Decreased renal function
- Increased serum creatinine/BUN
- Edema
- Decreased urine output
- HTN
- Weight gain
- Tenderness and swelling at graft site
- Fever
- Presence of sediment in urine

Adapted from Chandran S, Vincenti F. Clinical aspects: focusing on key unique organ-specific issues of renal transplantation. *Cold Spring Harb Perspect Med.* 2014;4(2):a015644 and Vincenti F, Rostaing L, Grinyo J, et al. Belatacept and long-term outcomes in kidney transplantation. *New Enlg J Med.* 2016;374:333-343.

photon emission computed tomography (SPECT) are also being used to detect acute rejection in renal allografts.[88]

The most frequent postoperative infections are those similar for all surgical patients and include infections of the urinary tract, indwelling catheters, vascular access and drains, and postoperative pneumonia. Bacterial infections are more common than fungal and viral infections in the early postoperative period. Opportunistic infections typically occur after the first month and are due to intensive immunosuppression.[79,81] Thirty to 60% of patients suffer some type of infection during the first transplant year and infection is linked to half of the deaths post-transplant.[81]

Physical Therapist Management of Kidney Transplantation

The acute care physical therapist needs to monitor laboratory values and determine potential signs and symptoms of infection or rejection. The physical therapist needs to consider that kidney transplant candidates are typically physically inactive with reduced exercise capacity and present with multisystem impairments (see Table 12-1).[89] The limited exercise capacity and poor physical functioning has been linked to low quality of life and high mortality in this population. The reason for the debility of patients with ESRD and dialysis is far from clear. The anemias of chronic renal disease, uremic myopathy, and resulting decreased muscle oxygen utilization, and disuse atrophy have a significant impact on physical function.[89,90] Immediately after transplant, these impairments and activity limitations persist, and therapeutic interventions are aimed to restore functional independence with an emphasis on transfers, gait training, and performance of ADLs. Airway clearance is recommended during the initial postoperative period because pulmonary complications are a leading cause of morbidity and prolonged hospitalization for all abdominal surgery patients. Once functional independence has been attained, the exercise prescription can address hobbies, fitness, and sports-related goals.

Exercise training after kidney transplant results in higher levels of measured and self-reported physical functioning. Patients who participate in an outlined exercise program demonstrated increased exercise adherence and participation long term.[91] Therefore, the initiation of a home exercise program early in the postoperative rehabilitation course is essential. Close monitoring of hemodynamic status and patient complaints is imperative due to the increased incidence of cardiovascular disease in this population. Brisk diuresis often accompanies successful graft function leading to potential dehydration. Alternatively, patients with DGF may exhibit fluid overload and electrolyte abnormalities.[83] For reasons not entirely clear, but generally attributed to intensive or persistent steroid administration, previously normoglycemic patients may develop diabetes during the post-transplant period.[83,84] An additional consideration is the fact that the colon is especially vulnerable to ischemia and perforation, and all patient complaints of abdominal pain or distress should be forwarded to the medical/surgical team.[83,84]

Liver Transplantation

Similar to all solid organ transplants, liver transplantation is now a well-established, definitive treatment for irreversible acute and chronic end-stage liver disease (ESLD).[92] In 2014 nearly 6800 liver transplants were performed in adults with nearly 15,000 candidates registered on the waiting list. Illness and death prohibited nearly 3000 patients on the waiting list from receiving a transplant.[92] The number of liver transplants has grown over the past 2 decades, and the list of indications for transplantation has been extended. Optimally, transplantation should improve both quality and quantity of life. Patient survival at 1 year is 85% and approximately 75% at 5 years.[33,93]

Indications/Candidate Selection

Similar to kidney and lung transplantation, a new process for liver transplant allocation was implemented in 2002 called the Model for End-Stage Liver Disease (MELD).[33] The MELD score defines how urgently a patient over the age of 12 needs a liver transplant within the next 3 months. The MELD score is a numerical scale ranging from 6 (less ill) to 40 (gravely ill). A MELD score greater than 35 is associated with a high mortality rate. The calculation is based on 3 routine lab tests: creatinine, prothrombin time, and bilirubin. There has been a reduction in waiting list mortality since adoption of this new system.[92,93] Patients awaiting living transplant may be in the ICU, often requiring vasopressor support, mechanical ventilation, and dialysis. Outcomes improve for these patients if they can recover prior to transplantation. Table 14-17 lists indications and exclusions for liver transplantation.[92-95]

Operative Procedure

Standard Surgical Procedure

Similar to other transplants, the donor organ is usually procured as part of multi-organ retrieval from a heart-beating, brain dead donor. **Orthotopic liver transplantation** is the removal of the native organ, a hepatectomy, while the donor organ is placed in the same anatomic location. The abdominal cavity is entered through a bilateral subcostal incision with a mid-line extension toward the xiphoid.[96] Coagulopathy is common in ESLD due to the combination of portal hypertension and

Table 14 -17

Liver Transplantation, Inclusion/Exclusion Categories

Inclusion/Indications	*Exclusion/Contraindications*
• Acute liver failure (eg, hepatitis A/B) • Chronic liver failure: Noncholestatic cirrhosis (eg, alcohol-induced cirrhosis) • Chronic liver failure: Cholestatic cirrhosis (eg, primary biliary cirrhosis, sclerosing cholangitis) • Chronic liver failure: Metabolic: (eg, cystic fibrosis, amyloidosis, Wilson's disease) • Chronic liver failure: Vascular (eg, Budd-Chiari syndrome) • Other indications (eg, hyperlipidemia, polycystic liver disease) • Malignant disease (eg, hepatoblastoma) • Benign liver tumors (eg, denomatosis)	• Active alcohol or drug abuse • Uncontrolled medical conditions, extrahepatic malignancy, systemic infections • Advanced cardiovascular or pulmonary disease *Relative Contraindications* • Psychosocial conditions • Advanced age • Severe hepatopulmonary or severe hepatorenal syndrome • Morbid obesity or malnutrition • HIV positive

Adapted from Kim et al[92]; Farkas et al[93]; Wan Song et al[94]; and Joshi and Agarwal.[95]

reduced production of clotting factors leading to defective clotting and fibrinolysis.[93] Prior upper abdominal surgery also complicates the surgical removal of the liver due to potential scar tissue and bleeding risk.

Segmental and Lobar Liver Procedure

The shortage of donor organs and the necessity to maximize the number of liver grafts is the most serious challenge to liver transplantation. Living-donor transplantation and surgical innovations, including the transplantation of "split livers" from cadaveric and living donors, have increased organ availability.[93] These procedures, termed **segmental** and **lobar liver transplant**, are possible owing to the unique segmental anatomy of the liver and its regenerative capacity. Current methods include the removal of the left lateral segment or the entire right or left lobe from a living donor with subsequent transplantation into the recipient. Similarly, a cadaveric liver can be split into 2 parts that can be transplanted into 2 size-matched recipients.

The postoperative treatment of the liver transplant patient is complicated by the physiologic derangements that accompany ESLD. Complications can be divided by time as well as hepatic and non-hepatic categories (Table 14-18).[92,97-100] The most serious hepatic complications are graft dysfunction and primary nonfunction (PNF). These complications range from minor abnormalities in liver functioning to overt graft failure, hemodynamic compromise, multiorgan failure, and death.

Massive fluid shifts, transient renal insufficiency resulting from the surgery, and premorbid liver dysfunction may leave the patient volume overloaded during the immediate postoperative period. Hypervolemia can impair cardiopulmonary function leading to heart failure and pulmonary edema. Pulmonary function may be further compromised due to right hemidiaphragmatic dysfunction and incision

Table 14-18

COMPLICATIONS POST–LIVER TRANSPLANTATION

Early	*Long-Term*	*Recurrent Disease*	*Non-Hepatic*
• Primary dysfunction • Graft rejection • Infections • Biliary complications • Surgical complications	• Recurrent viral hepatitis • Drug hepatotoxicity • Chronic renal failure • HTN • Diabetes • Dyslipidemia • Obesity • Bone or neurological complications • De novo tumors	• Hepatitis B • Hepatitis C • Hepatocellular carcinoma • Autoimmune disease from donor • Primary sclerosing cholangitis	• Anemia • Bleeding • Coagulopathy • Depression • Encephalopathy • Fluid overload • Heart failure • Pneumonia • Pulmonary vascular permeability • Renal insufficiency • Seizures • Thrombocytopenia

Adapted from Kim et al[92]; Moon and Lee[97]; Dansinger[98]; Barnes Jewish Hospital[99]; and Zieve.[100]

discomfort limiting ventilation and cough effectiveness. Acute rejection occurs in approximately 18% of patients while chronic rejection is rare.[97] The clinical signs of rejection are listed in Table 14-19.[98-100] The diagnosis of rejection is confirmed by liver biopsy. Common infectious complications include pneumonia, wound infections, intravenous line infections, and urinary tract infections.[92,97]

Physical Therapist Management of Liver Transplantation

Wait times have decreased for MELD scores 35 or higher, but higher risk patients have greater challenges with postoperative return to normal function.[33,92,101,102] The metabolic consequences of liver diseases increase the risk of patients presenting with malnutrition and anorexia, osteoporosis, insulin resistance, fluid imbalances, coagulopathy, variceal bleeding, and encephalopathy leading to pre-transplant physical inactivity (see Tables 11-5 and 11-16).[103-105] This inactivity is due to the disease as well as self-imposed bed rest with resultant muscle atrophy and limited strength and endurance.[106] Loss of muscle mass may impact both peripheral and respiratory muscles.[101] Chronic dyspnea and hypoxemia have been reported prior to liver transplantation.[101,105,107,108] Factors that lead to pulmonary dysfunction include pleural effusions, interstitial lung edema, and respiratory muscle wasting.[102,105,108] Studies have revealed there is a 40% to 60% lower maximal oxygen consumption in liver transplant recipients.[107]

The most common complaints post-transplant include weakness, fatigue, SOB)and bone/joint discomfort. The 6MWT and Borg Balance Scale (BBS) have been utilized to track improvements in functional capacity in the immediate postoperative days following liver transplant.[109] MELD scores have been shown to inversely correlate with the 6MWT distance as well as the maximal inspiratory pressure (a measure of inspiratory muscle strength) prior to transplant.[110] Patients should return to independent ADL and IADL functioning, and many will return to work and leisure pursuits and may even participate in the transplant Olympics. It is important to note, however, that recipients who engage in regular physical activity score higher on quality of life measures providing further credence to the initiation of home exercise programs.[111]

Table 14-19

COMMON SIGNS AND SYMPTOMS OF LIVER REJECTION

• Early symptoms:	• Late symptoms:
¤ Change in heart rate	¤ Abdominal swelling
¤ Decrease in urination	¤ Confusion
¤ Edema	¤ Dark urine
¤ Fever > 101°	¤ Discolored stools
¤ Flu-like symptoms	¤ Increased fatigue
¤ General malaise	¤ Yellowing of skin and eyes
¤ Leukocytosis	
¤ Pain in area of transplant	
¤ SOB	
¤ Weight changes	

Adapted from Dansinger M. Life after your transplant: signs of rejection. WebMD. http://www.webmd.com/a-to-z-guides/life-after-transplant-signs-rejection. Published 2017. Accessed March 20, 2019; Liver transplant: what to expect. Barnes Jewish Hospital. http://www.barnesjewish.org/Medical-Services/Transplant/Liver-Transplant/Liver-Transplant-Process/After-Liver-Transplant#Rejection. Accessed March 20, 2019; and Zieve D. Transplant rejection. *Medline Plus*. https://medlineplus.gov/ency/article/000815.htm. Published May 21, 2017. Accessed March 20, 2019.

Pancreas and Islet Transplantation

Hyperglycemia is the most important factor in the development and progression of the secondary complications of diabetes. Pancreas transplantation is unique among organ transplants because this is primarily a therapy that attempts to stabilize and prevent the devastating end organ complications associated with type 1 diabetes. As a treatment option for adults with insulin-dependent diabetes, pancreas transplantation has proven to be superior to intensive insulin therapy for control of secondary complications and for achieving normoglycemia.[112] Indications for pancreas transplant are extremely narrow due to the profound organ shortage in relationship to the prevalence of diabetes, the significant surgical risk, and the requirement of life-long immunosuppression. The number of pancreas transplants has decreased since 2004 with less than 1100 being performed in 2012.[113] Some of this decline may be attributed to improved insulin delivery systems, islet transplant, and concerns about solitary pancreas transplant outcomes. The survival rates are approximately 97% at 1 year and 92% at 3 years.[112,113]

Indications/Candidate Selection

There are essentially 3 types of pancreas transplant options available for type 1 diabetes candidates: simultaneous pancreas and kidney (SPK) transplantation, pancreas transplant after kidney (PAK) transplantation, and pancreas transplantation alone (PTA).[112] SPKs account for 70% of all pancreas transplants performed in the United States.[112] PTA makes up the smallest percentage of transplants and is indicated in only selected patients with type 1 diabetes and normal kidney function.[112] Additional considerations are similar to other solid organ transplants including freedom from substance abuse, psychiatric disease, malignancy, end organ damage, or disease including CAD and congestive heart failure (see Table 14-1, exclusion criteria).

Islet transplantation for patients with type 1 diabetes is no longer considered experimental with over 1000 patients receiving either an allograft or autograft since 2000.[114,115] There are presently 2 options for this type of transplantation: islet after kidney transplantation and islet transplantation alone. The islet transplantation involves isolating and purifying the islet cells from the pancreas of one or more deceased organ donors (allotransplant) or in select patients with type 2 diabetes, performing a pancreatectomy, followed by extraction and purification of the islets from the removed pancreas (autotransplant). The purified islet cells are then infused into the liver of the recipient via the portal vein. The goal is for the islet cells to produce insulin to normalize glycemic control with or without insulin injections and potentially reverse the secondary complications from the diabetes. However, this often takes time, may require several infusions and patients may not be free of exogenous insulin. Improved outcomes relate to identification of the benefit of single donor islet cells and improved immunosuppression protocols.[115]

Operative Procedure

Most pancreas transplants are cadaveric but living related donors who undergo a hemipancreatectomy may be used for transplant. The procedure is heterotopic with the native organ remaining in place. A midline abdominal incision is the usual surgical approach. Surgical technique for the transplant vary but some commonalties exist. The donor graft is explanted with a cuff of duodenum for future buttressing of the exocrine portion of the pancreas. The pancreatic graft's arterial supply is from the patient's right common or external iliac artery and venous outflow is to the portal, right common, or external iliac veins.[112] Exocrine drainage is primarily handled by anastomosis of the duodenal segment to the bladder or to the small intestine.

Acute Care Management and Complications

Complications after pancreas transplant are similar to other abdominal organ procedures including infection, rejection, metabolic abnormalities, anastomotic leaks and obstruction, and vascular thrombosis at the anastomotic sites. Rejection can occur within days or years after the transplant. Increase in pancreatic enzymes, especially lipase, is a more sensitive marker than amylase.[112] For patients who undergo the SPK transplant, renal function is used as a surrogate marker for pancreatic functioning. The serum creatinine is monitored and kidney biopsy results allow the diagnosis of rejection.

Solid organ pancreas transplant is associated with higher surgical complications, including hemorrhage, thrombosis, pancreatitis, and sepsis, resulting in reoperation.[114] Improvement has been made in venous thrombosis through careful monitoring of coagulation.[114]

Physical Therapist Management of Pancreas and Islet Transplantation

The physical therapy regimen post-transplant is similar to that for the kidney transplant patient with one notable difference: postoperative monitoring of laboratory values with special emphasis on blood glucose, electrolytes, and fluid status is vital. The normal pancreas secretes vast quantities of bicarbonate and water in addition to amylase, lipase, and proenzymes that are activated in the duodenum necessary for digestion. However, the transplanted pancreas with bladder attachment may lead to the urinary loss of large volumes of bicarbonate and water with subsequent metabolic acidosis, dehydration, orthostatic hypotension, and cardiac dysrhythmias secondary to electrolyte abnormalities.[112]

Successful pancreatic and islet transplant achieves normal blood glucose levels, euglycemia, and glycosylated hemoglobin (HbA1C) without the need for exogenous insulin. Normal glycemic control slows, and potentially reverses, diabetic nephropathy, motor and sensory neuropathy, and HTN, decreases the incidence of cardiac disease, and improves quality of life.[112-115]

Common Concerns Post–Solid Organ Transplantation

Transplantation and chronic illness are associated with significant psychosocial stressors as noted in Table 14-20.[7,116-122] The therapist should be aware of these potential complications and consult with appropriate mental health workers.

Infection, Rejection, and Immunosuppression

The allograft, or a transplanted organ, can be rejected acutely or after many years. Rejection is a host-vs-graft immune response that leads to graft dysfunction and tissue destruction. Allograft rejection is classified as hyperacute, acute, or chronic, and rejection is either a cell-mediated (innate immunity) or humoral (adaptive immunity) immune event.[84] **Natural** or **innate immunity** refers to the nonspecific immune events involving macrophages, neutrophils, natural killer cells, complement proteins, and various cytokines. **Adaptive immunity** involves recognition of specific antigens present on the cell membrane from the allograft and activation of specific T and B lymphocytes (see Chapter 5).[123-125]

Hyperacute and **accelerated rejection**, in which the graft becomes nonfunctional within hours or days, is due largely to ABO blood group or HLA incompatibility. HLAs are cell-surface proteins found on virtually all nucleated cells of the body and platelets, and the placement of an incompatible organ into a recipient with preformed antibodies against the donor antigen stimulates a vigorous immune response. The immune response results in rapid destruction of the graft's vascular endothelium, vessel thrombosis, and organ infarction. Hyperacute rejection is typically nonresponsive to immunosuppressive therapy and medical care is supportive. Sometimes accelerated rejection can be reversed by vigorous pharmacological therapy.[123-125]

Acute rejection of organ allografts is an adaptive immune response involving T cells mediated by CD8 T cells, CD4 T cells, or both. Acute rejection is usually treated by bolus intravenous steroid therapy, with or without temporary increases in the maintenance immunosuppression. Damaged areas of the allograft heal by fibrosis and the remainder of the graft continues to function.[123-125]

Minimizing the differences between the donor and recipient by verification of ABO compatibility and crossmatching decreases the likelihood of acute rejection. **Crossmatching** refers to testing the recipient's serum antibodies against donor white blood cells (WBCs; lymphocytes). Although HLA matching significantly improves the success rate of organ transplantation, it does not prevent all rejection reactions.

Chronic rejection describes the late process of graft destruction resulting in graft ischemia and fibrosis and is believed to be an antibody-mediated process involving T and B lymphocytes. Other potential factors include ischemia between the harvesting and implantation surgeries, the reduced mass of transplanted tissue (especially in the case of kidney and split liver transplants), denervation of the transplanted organ, hyperlipidemia and HTN associated with immunosuppressive drugs, immunosuppressive drugs themselves, and chronic viral injury.[123-125] Chronic rejection manifests differently in each organ. Chronic rejection in lung transplantation is termed **bronchiolitis obliterans syndrome** (BOS) and results in progressive narrowing of the bronchioles.[40] Chronic rejection in heart transplantation, CAV, is a diffuse myointimal hyperplasia, or accelerated atherosclerosiss, proceeding to fibrosis of the coronary arteries and eventual ischemic heart disease and heart failure.[73,74,125] Chronic rejection of a kidney is termed **transplant nephropathy/transplant glomerulopathy** or, recently, **interstitial fibrosis and tubular atrophy** (IF/TA), without evidence of any specific etiology. Transplant nephropathy is the leading cause of transplant

Table 14-20

POTENTIAL TRANSPLANTATION PSYCHOSOCIAL ISSUES

Pre-Transplant	*Post-Transplant*
• Lack of social support	• Life-long adherence to immunosuppressant medications
• Impaired physical functioning	• Life-long side effects of immunosuppressant medications
• Female gender	• Risk of long-term complications
• Active psychopathology	• Anxiety and depression
• Substance use disorders	• Delirium
• Cognitive dysfunction	• Social role functioning
• Managing chronic health care regimen	• Physical role functioning
• Patient adherence	• Emotional psychological functioning
• Wait time	• Occupational choice
• Generalized distress and fatigue	• Limitations on emotional stability
• Family history of personality disorders, poly-substance abuse, alcohol use	• Post-traumatic stress syndrome
• Negative emotions	• Modification in lifestyle
• Coping strategies	• Changes in body image
• Unmarried	• Return to work
• Lack of physical activity	• Donor guilt
• Obesity	• Stress
• Coping with disabling or life-threatening illness	• Change in life expectancy
• Delirium	• Change form sick to well role
• Finances	• Relapse of negative lifestyle behaviors
	• Finances

Adapted from Versluis-Burlis and Downs[7]; Wrightson et al[116]; Kuntz et al[117]; Rainer et al[118]; Coglianes et al[119]; Spaderna et al[120]; Maldonado et al[121]; and Grover and Sarkar.[122]

failure and results from interstitial fibrosis, renal tubular atrophy and thickening of the glomerulus. The patient's creatinine concentration will slowly increase, proteinuria will occur, and HTN worsens.[125-127] Chronic liver rejection is termed **ductopenic rejection/vanishing bile duct syndrome**, and is due to progressive hepatic tissue fibrosis, hepatic arteriolar thickening, and loss of bile ductules. Liver rejection presents as jaundice, loss of synthetic function, and portal hypertension and is associated with elevated bilirubin, elevated liver function tests (LFTs; see Chapter 2, Table 2-1) and cholestasis.[92,97,125,128]

Immunologic control and suppression are vital to the prevention of allograft rejection. Common immunosuppressive drugs include corticosteroids, azathioprine, mycophenolate mofetil, tacrolimus, cyclosporine, and rapamycin. Immunosuppression dosing is more intensive immediately post-transplant and then gradually diminishes during the first year as the recipient's immune system adapts and the allograft becomes less immunoreactive.[124,128] Although the graft becomes less immunoreactive and the dosing of immunosuppressive drugs decrease, patients rarely reach a point where these drugs can be discontinued. The patient's drug regimen is constantly modified, and as new products are introduced, clinical immunosuppression regimens are adjusted. Immunosuppressive drugs have many side effects, such as HTN, nephrotoxity, lymphocytic proliferative syndrome, neurotoxicity, impaired wound healing, osteoporosis, gingival hyperplasia, proximal muscle weakness, and weight gain.[116,124,128,129] Immunosuppression also leads to an increased risk of infectious complications, and opportunistic infections can lead to significant morbidity and mortality. Consistent observation of infection control precautions is vital with all physical therapy management of the transplant population (infection control/standard precautions are outlined in Chapter 5).

Patients can participate in physical therapy services during active episodes of infection and rejection if stable; however, modifications in the care plan, such as reduced exercise intensity and duration and closer vital sign monitoring, should be standard procedures. The physical therapist will need to add specific organ examination items, such as closer observation of laboratory values including electrolytes, blood glucose, and coagulation profiles for the kidney, liver, and pancreas transplant patient; ECG (heart rate and rhythm), blood pressure and perceived exertion for the heart transplant patient; and noting pulse oximetry, sputum production, airflow, and perceived exertion in the lung transplant patient.

Common Late Complications

HTN is a common postoperative complication in the transplant patient. The development of HTN is multifactorial and may include nephrotoxic effects of cyclosporine and prednisone, preexisting or progressive renal insufficiency, and weight gain.[124,130,131] **New onset diabetes after transplantation** (NODAT) is primarily medication-related and is associated with increased mortality and poorer graft survival.[129,130] Corticosteroids increase blood glucose levels by increasing gluconeogenesis and increase peripheral insulin resistance, while cyclosporine and tacrolimus inhibit insulin release and promote beta cell toxicity. **Osteoporosis** is common after solid organ transplantation, and the majority of bone loss occurs within the first 6 months post-transplant. The principal cause of bone demineralization is the direct inhibition of osteoblastic activity, increased calcium urinary excretion, impaired GI absorption of calcium, and sex hormone inhibition by steroids.[132,133] **Hyperlipidemia** and **hypertriglyceridemia** are common post-transplant and are also believed to be drug side effects.[124,128] Patients who have undergone transplant are at an increased risk of **malignancy**, especially lymphomas, skin cancer, and Kaposi's sarcoma.[124,128-130,134,135] Other potential late complications of transplantation include steroid-induced myopathy and skin alterations, aseptic necrosis of bone, gout, visual abnormalities associated with cataracts, heart failure, herpes zoster, and obesity.[84,124,128,136] Finally, neurotoxicity related to cyclosporine and tacrolimus has been noted and may be manifested as seizures, severe headaches, confusion, and stroke. as well as varying levels of delirium.[124,136]

The role of the physical therapist as it relates to the long-term consequences of transplantation is not well developed. Exercise programming has been demonstrated to limit many of the secondary effects of immunosuppression. Specifically, exercise training has been shown to reverse steroid-induced myopathy with improvements noted in strength, muscle cross-sectional area, and fat-free mass.[137,138] Strengthening and weightbearing exercise are standard recommendations for patients with osteoporosis.[139] Cardiorespiratory fitness and exercise training have demonstrated positive impacts on patients with diabetes, are an essential aspect of weight control, and have been associated with reduced incidences of cancer.[140,141] Finally, participation in exercise programs leads to enhanced quality of life after transplantation. Although improvements in exercise capacity are noted for each type of transplantation, recipients demonstrate consistent decrements in maximal exercise capacity compared to age-matched individuals (see Table 14-10). Deconditioning, abnormal mitochondrial functioning, and pulmonary deficits have been proposed to contribute to the reduction in exercise capacity following transplant.[48,59-63,91,101,110]

Summary

Physical therapy consultation and interventions for the patient who has undergone solid organ transplantation is common during the immediate postoperative period. However, patients frequently seek treatment at community and regional hospitals for multiple postoperative and general age-related complications. Transplantation is not a cure, but the patient inherits a variety of post-transplant complications, most notably the constant battle between infection and rejection. Exercise plays a large role in maintaining the quality of life for these patients, and it is important for therapists to understand many of the acute and long-term complications of transplantation as they prescribe safe and effective therapeutic interventions. The physical therapist and physical therapist assistant are important members of the transplant team. Physical therapy services play a pivotal role in the acute care setting to assist with pain management and observation for infection/rejection, promote pulmonary hygiene and early mobilization, and institute appropriately designed therapeutic programs to reduce activity limitations and return the patient to an independent lifestyle. Common goals for pre- and post-transplantation are summarized in Table 14-9.

Case Study

Mrs. Cantrell is a 55-year-old (y/o) female who received a left SLT. Mrs. Cantrell has a history of (h/o) end-stage COPD. Physical therapy was consulted for evaluation and treatment 1 day following the transplant.

Patient/Client History

General Demographics, Social History, and Living Environment

Mrs. Cantrell lives with her husband of 34 years in a 2-story, older home. She has 5 steps to enter from the outside, the bathroom and bedroom are on the second floor, and there is no handrail for either stairs. Mrs. Cantrell is a retired elementary school teacher. She has 3 daughters who live locally. Her middle daughter is expecting a child soon, the first grandchild for the family. Her husband is a truck driver and is on the road 6 days per week.

General Health Status, Social/Health Habits, and Family History

Mrs. Cantrell is diagnosed with COPD and was dependent on oxygen (O_2) and on chronic steroids prior to the surgery. She was a 3 packs/day smoker for more than 20 years but stopped 3 years ago. She has been on anti-anxiety medication off and on for 2 years and was cachectic in appearance prior to surgery.

Medical/Surgical History

Her hospital course following transplantation was complicated by failure to wean from mechanical ventilation, and she underwent a tracheotomy 1-week following transplantation. Mrs. Cantrell was transferred from the surgical ICU to the medical ICU for continued care 1 month following transplantation. The hospital course continued to be complicated by pseudomonas pneumonia, poorly controlled HTN, positive methicillin resistant *Staphylococcus aureus* (MRSA; on contact isolation) and candida in sputum, compression fractures, *Clostridium difficile* with associated severe diarrhea, new onset atrial flutter, and diabetes. She also had profound deconditioning and difficulty in weaning from mechanical ventilation.

Current Conditions

Mrs. Cantrell is unable to audibly verbalize her complaints but can mouth words. She appears uncomfortable and confirms feeling SOB and very anxious. She is on a mechanical ventilator with the following settings: synchronized intermittent mandatory ventilation (SIMV) 10, pressure support 15, fraction of inspired oxygen (F_IO_2; 40%), positive end expiratory pressure (PEEP) of 5 cm H_2O. She rates her pain on a scale of 0 to 10 as 7, a RPE while in bed at with her head elevated 30 degrees a 9 (on the modified Borg RPE scale [0 to 10]) by pointing to the scale. Her activity status is fully dependent for all ADLs, bed mobility, and transfers. Her OOB tolerance is less than 45 minutes with a Hoyer transfer.

Activities and Participation

Mrs. Cantrell did not use an assistive device prior to surgery and was independent with her ADLs but needed additional time to complete tasks due to her SOB. She did attend pulmonary rehabilitation in the outpatient physical therapy department as part of her pre-transplant program. She was able to walk on a treadmill for 17 minutes at 1.7 miles per hour on 3 L of O_2 with an SpO_2 of 91% and dyspnea score of 4 on the modified Borg scale.

Medications

Her medications upon transfer from the surgical ICU to the medical ICU were vancomycin, Bactrim (sulfamethoxazole/trimethoprim), nystatin, Atrovent (ipratropium bromide), Alupent (metaproterenol), cyclosporine, Imuran (azathioprine), Solu-Medrol (methylprednisolone), acyclovir, Imodium (loperamide), digoxin, Reglan (metoclopramide), Vasotec (enalapri), Carafate (sucralfate), Haldol (haloperidol), and Ativan (lorazepam).

Other Clinical Tests

Recent ABG revealed a compensated respiratory acidosis: pH 7.40/PCO_2 49/PO_2 80/HCO_3^-32. The complete blood count (CBC) and electrolyte panel revealed anemia with an Hb 8.2 g/dL and leukocytosis (WBC 22,000/uL). The electrolyte panel revealed hyponatremia (sodium 124 mEq/L) necessitating a free water restriction (ie, no ice chips). A lung perfusion scan shortly after the surgery showed 46% of blood flow to transplanted lung, but a recent perfusion scan showed a further decline in perfusion to 37%. A lung biopsy revealed acute lung allograft rejection. Mrs. Cantrell was treated with a course of high-dose steroids and anti-thymocyte globulin (ATGAM) that resulted in a 6% increase in perfusion.

SYSTEMS REVIEW

Cardiovascular and Pulmonary

Resting vital signs in supine with head of the bed raised 30 degrees are SpO_2 94% on F_IO_2 0.50 (50%) and mechanical ventilation settings of SIMV 10, pressure support (12, PEEP 5, RR 28 breaths/minute, BP 140/70 mm Hg, HR 110 beats per minute (bpm; sinus tachycardia).

Integumentary

Mrs. Cantrell appears cachectic, with multiple areas of ecchymosis on both forearms, muscle wasting of all 4 extremities, and her skin appears grayish, very dry, and scaly. She has a large thoracic incision on the left chest wall with multiple smaller incisions from chest tubes in the same chest region. She has a tracheostomy, which appears moist and clean. Kneehigh pneumatic compression stockings for BLEs are present. Mrs. Cantrell has an arterial line in her left radial artery and has a central venous line in the right subclavian vein.

Musculoskeletal

Mrs. Cantrell moves her bilateral upper extremities (BUEs) and bilateral lower extremities (BLEs) to command but appears to have difficulty with antigravity movements.

Neuromuscular

Mrs. Cantrell is oriented to place and year only. Sensation was intact and reflexes were diminished. She has profound motor weakness, but movement patterns appeared normal.

Communication, Affect, Cognition, Language, and Learning Style

Mrs. Cantrell presently communicates by mouthing words and pointing to sentences on a communication board. She is very expressive with her eye contact. She is alert and awake, and is challenged by multi-step commands at this time. Her Richmond Agitation and Sedation Scale (RASS) is 0 and she is Confusion Assessment Method for the ICU (CAM-ICU) negative.

TESTS AND MEASURES

Aerobic Capacity and Endurance

The vital sign (VS) response to ROM, manual muscle testing (MMT), and bed mobility was HR 110-132 bpm, BP 140/70-126/74 mm Hg, RR 28-40 breaths/minute and SpO_2 94% to 90%. Mrs. Cantrell required 4 minutes of rest for vital signs to return to baseline.

Assistive Technology

Recommended resting BLE splints to limit heel pressure and prevent contractures and a pressure relief mattress cushion for the bed and bedside chair.

Circulation (Arterial, Venous, Lymphatic) and Ventilation/Respiration

Mrs. Cantrell's pulses were rapid and thready, but regular. She has 1+ edema in BLEs at ankles and distal. As noted, HR was tachycardic at rest and increased significantly with bed mobility. BP was elevated at rest and decreased while sitting at the edge of the bed, indicating orthostasis.

As noted previously, Mrs. Cantrell has significant tachypnea with RR 28-40, desaturation to 90% by SpO_2 during mobilization. Her breath sounds were distant on the right, crackles at the bases, left > right. Cough was ineffective. Mrs. Cantrell complained of (c/o) severe SOB and extreme anxiety and she was transferred back to supine with head of bed elevated 30 degrees. VS returned to baseline in 4 minutes.

Balance, Gait, and Mobility (Including Locomotion)

Bed mobility was maximal assist of 1 with bed rails for side-to-side turning (Functional Status Score for the Intensive Care Unit [FSS-ICU] 2). She transferred from side-lying to dangling on the side of the bed with maximum assist of 1 (FSS-ICU 2). She maintained dangling with moderate assist of 1 (FSS-ICU 3) while being provided cues for breathing and relaxation techniques x 1 minute. OOB activities (eg, sit↔stand transfers, gait assessment) were not performed at this time (FSS-ICU 0). Her total FSS-ICU score was 7/35, Activity Measure for Post Acute Care (AM-PAC) 6 clicks basic mobility score was 7/24, and the ICU Mobility Scale (IMS) was 3. Mrs. Cantrell was able to use a visual analog scale to rate her pain as 6/10 at rest and 8/10 with activity.

Muscle Performance

MMT 1-2/5 throughout; ROM decreased bilateral shoulders, hips, knees, and ankles (especially dorsiflexion). Medical Research Council (MRC) strength sum score of 20/48 (see Chapter 4, Figure 4-3).

Evaluation

Mrs. Cantrell is an older, frail female currently hospitalized secondary to left SLT for COPD. She also presents with profound deconditioning and difficulty in weaning from mechanical ventilation. She demonstrated poor endurance as demonstrated by her vital sign and subjective responses to the examination in bed. She did have a slight drop in BP, which may reflect orthostasis. There were no complaints of lightheadedness but this could be masked by her c/o SOB. The decline in SpO_2 most likely reflects her limited pulmonary reserve, graft dysfunction, and severe deconditioning, but also an abnormal breathing pattern with anxiety and activity. The observed anemia may contribute to her SOB.

Diagnosis

The patient presents with severe activity limitations secondary to motor weakness and atrophy, limited pulmonary reserve, and challenged by profound SOB and anxiety related to prolonged bed rest and complications of multiple surgeries. The patient has intensive care unit–acquired weakness (ICU-AW), but deconditioning at baseline also probably contributes to her current presentation.

Prognosis

Slow, progressive daily therapy will optimize independence with functional activities during the weaning process. Prolonged physical therapy will be necessary to progress to ambulatory independence with appropriate cardiovascular and pulmonary responses. Outcomes are hopeful but guarded due to limited gas-exchanging capabilities of the transplanted lung, side effects of the pharmacological post-transplant regimen (eg, immunosuppressive medications), deconditioning with possible ICU-AW and limited pre-transplant aerobic capacity, as well as continued airway resistance of the native COPD lung and persistent pain from compression fractures. Her anxiety is being managed by medication prior to and following daily therapy and is a factor hindering her weaning from the ventilator.

Intervention

With transfer back to bed, Mrs. Cantrell required suctioning to clear the airway following transfer back to supine with splinted support for pain. Breathing exercises were instructed post-suctioning to allow her SOB, RR, and anxiety to decrease. Recommend coordinating therapy with pain medication delivery as well as daily therapy combined with progression of OOB tolerance. Therapy should focus on therapeutic exercises to improve motor strength, motor control, and ROM; mobility retraining to address impairments and activity limitations and enhance OOB abilities; pain management; and integumentary precautions. Breathing retraining and relaxation exercises will be key during progression of functional activities due to the patient's profound DOE and anxiety. Airway clearance is important to enhance ventilation and gas exchange and reduce the need for suctioning. Sitting edge of bed (EOB) and OOB should help with improving postural control, sitting balance, and cough effectiveness. Careful monitoring of laboratory data, vital signs, and subjective symptoms is important and may provide evidence of infection/rejection in the transplant patient.

Outcomes

Coordination of pain and anxiety medications was initiated after the initial examination. After 10 days, the reexamination status included moderate assistance of 1 with bed rail for bed mobility and transfer to EOB (FSS-ICU 3). She could sit at the EOB with supervision (FSS-ICU 5). Transferring to the bedside chair requires maximum assist of 1 by a stand-step-pivot transfer (FSS-ICU 2), supported standing with platform walker moderate assistance of 2 for 30 seconds x 3, and her OOB tolerance in supported chair 45 minutes twice per day with Hoyer lift back to bed. Mrs. Cantrell's VS responses were BP 152-164/80-92 mm Hg, RR 26-30 breaths/minute, HR 124-128 (sinus tachycardia), SpO_2 92% with standing and sitting (F_IO_2 0.4 [40%]) and pain 4-5/10 with activity. Her total FSS-ICU score was 15/35, the AM-PAC 6 clicks basic mobility score improved from 7 to 10/24 and her IMS was 5.

Mrs. Cantrell developed a compression fracture of L2 on day 26, resulting in low back pain limiting the weaning process and OOB mobility. Other complications included frequent pulmonary infections, renal insufficiency, HTN, and GI abnormalities (gastroparesis and malabsorption). Her physical therapy continued slowly, she was able to be weaned from the ventilator, her tracheostomy tube was removed prior to discharge to the inpatient rehabilitation unit 2.5 months after initiating physical therapy. The tracheostomy stoma did not close immediately following tube removal. This area was covered with gauze and she was progressing to self-occlude the stoma to help with cough effectiveness. Her breath sounds improved to distant right > left but clear to auscultation bilaterally. Her thoracic incision had healed with minimal keloid scarring and she was off contact isolation at the time of discharge to inpatient rehabilitation. She remained on pain medication due to persistent pain from compression fracture.

ICF Clinical Reasoning Tool Case Study Summary

Health Condition

HPI: Left SLT, cachexia, muscle weakness (possible ICU-AW), tracheostomy, acute lung allograft rejection, high-dose steroids, pseudomonas pneumonia, HTN, MRSA, candida in sputum, new onset atrial flutter and diabetes, compression fractures, *Clostridium difficile* with diarrhea, leukocytosis, hyponatremia, anemia, hypoxemia, anxiety
PMHx: End-stage COPD

Precautions/Contraindications

Pain, new onset atrial flutter and diabetes, contact precautions, ineffective cough, anxious, challenge to wean from MV, desaturates with activity, former smoker, dependent on oxygen prior to surgery, anxiety, infection risk due to immunosuppression

Body Structure and Function			*Activity/Task Limitations*			*Participation*		
Impairment/ Problem	*Tests and Measures*	*Intervention*	*Activity*	*Tests and Measures*	*Intervention*	*Participation*	*Tests and Measures*	*Intervention*
• Impaired airway clearance with ineffective cough • Impaired ROM and strength • Impaired gas exchange • Orthostatic hypotension • ↓ endurance • Weight below IBW • Pain • Abnormal lab values • Skin integrity • Impaired cognition • Challenging communication • Immunosuppression	• Chest assessment • VS including ROM/MMT • VS including SpO_2 and ECG • BMI • Pain/VAS • Lab values • BMI • Integumentary examination • CAM-ICU • Lab values	• Breathing exercises and education on coughing (splint incision, upright positioning) • Bedside ROM, progressive resistance interval training • Consult registered dietician and speech pathologist	• ADLs • Bed mobility • Transfers • Gait	• Functional task analysis • AM-PAC "6 Clicks" • FSS-ICU • IMS • RPE with activity • VAS with activity	• Progressive functional retraining following pulmonary rehab guidelines	• Unable to return home • Unable to help prepare for new grandchild	• MMSE • SF-36 • HADS • PHQ-9	• Continue physical therapy services • Consult social worker and occupational therapist

(continued)

ICF Clinical Reasoning Tool Case Study Summary (continued)

Personal Factors	*Other Considerations*	*Environmental Factors*
• Age: 55 y/o female • Awake and alert • Primary language: English • Married x 34 years, retired elementary teacher • 3 daughters • Husband truck driver on road for 6 days a week • I with ADLs prior to admission, increased time to complete tasks due to SOB • 60 pk/year smoker • Anxious and fearful of pain with movement, SOB		Home: • 2 stories, older brownstone • 5 steps to enter house; bedroom/bathroom 2nd floor, no handrail Hospital: • MV with tracheostomy, pneumatic compression stockings, arterial line, central venous line, resting BLE splints

HADS = Hospital Anxiety Depression Scale; HPI = history of present illness; I = independent; MMSE = Mini-Mental State Examination; MV = mechanical ventilator; NP = nasal prongs; pk/yrs = packs per years; PHQ-9 = Patient Health Questionnaire; PMHx = past medical history; RPE = rate of perceived exertion; SF = Short Form; VAS = visual analog scale.

Adapted from American Physical Therapy Association. *Guide to Physical Therapist Practice*. 3rd ed. http://www.apta.org/Guide/. Updated October 21, 2015. Accessed October 5, 2018 and *Towards a Common Language for Functioning, Disability and Health*. World Health Organization. www.who.int/classifications/icf/icfbeginnersguide.pdf. Published 2002. Accessed April 29, 2019.

Chapter Review Questions

1. Which of the following best represents the most common early complications of transplantation compared to complications after 1 year from time of transplant?
   a. Graft failure and infection
   b. Malignancy and lymphoma
   c. Bronchiolitis and CMV
   d. Acute rejection and non-lymphoma
2. Which of the following are the most appropriate rehabilitation goals in the initial stages of acute care following transplant?
   a. Initiate work retraining to lower anaerobic threshold and FSS-ICU score
   b. Improvement in Function in Sitting Test score and peak oxygen consumption
   c. Improve CAM-ICU score and Functional Independence Measure
   d. Improve airway clearance and functional mobility
3. Which of the following best represent the hemodynamic limitations to exercise in heart transplant recipients?
   a. Corticosteroids and development of diabetes
   b. Blunted heart rate response due to denervated heart
   c. Renal failure and hyperlipidemia
   d. Elevated oxygen consumption and exercise HR
4. Which of the following are some of the most common immunosuppression medication side effects following transplant?
   a. HTN, nephrotoxicity, risk for neoplasm, weight gain
   b. Fever, chills, nausea, anorexia, macular degeneration
   c. Hyperkalemia, weight loss, bone growth, gingival hypoplasia
   d. Depression, improved wound healing, myopathies, diabetes
5. Chronic rejection for heart and lung transplant present as which of the following?
   a. Glomerulopathy and bronchitis
   b. Vanishing bile duct syndrome and empyema
   c. Cardiac vasculopathy and BOS
   d. Ductopenic nephropathy and pulmonary edema

Answers: 1a, 2d, 3b, 4a, 5c

References

1. Cooper DKC. Christiaan Barnard and his contributions to heart transplantation. *J Heart Lung Transplant.* 2001;20(6):599-610.
2. Dalton ML. The first lung transplant. *Am J Surg.* 2004;70(4):364-365.
3. Miniati DN, Robbins RC. Heart transplantation: a thirty-year perspective. *Ann Rev Med.* 2002;53:189-205.
4. Harringer W, Haverich A. Heart and heart-lung transplantation: standards and improvements. *World J Surg.* 2002;26:218-225.
5. Shumway NE. Thoracic transplantation. *World J Surg.* 2000;24(7):811-814.
6. Radovancevic B, Frazier OH. Heart transplantation: approaching a new century. *Tex Heart Inst J.* 1999;26:60-70.
7. Versluis-Burlis T, Downs AM. Thoracic organ transplantation: heart, lung, and heart-lung. In: Hillegass EA, Sadowsky HS, eds. *Essentials of Cardiopulmonary Physical Therapy.* 2nd ed. Philadelphia, PA: WB Saunders; 2001.
8. O'Neill JO, Taylor DO, Starling RC. Immunosuppression for cardiac transplantation: the past, present and future. *Transplant Proc.* 2004;36(2 suppl):S309-S313.
9. Baran DA, Galin ID, Gass AL. Current practices: immunosuppression induction, maintenance, and rejection regimens in contemporary post-heart transplant patient treatment. *Curr Opin Cardiol.* 2002;17:165-170.
10. Banner NR, Yacoub MH. Cyclosporine in thoracic organ transplantation. *Transplant Proc.* 2004;36(2 suppl):S302-S308.
11. Braith RW, Edwards DG. Exercise following heart transplantation. *Sports Med.* 2000;30(3):171-192.
12. Scherer S. The transplant patient. In: Frownfelter D, Dean E, eds. *Principles and Practice of Cardiopulmonary Physical Therapy.* 3rd ed. Philadelphia, PA: Mosby- Year Book, Inc; 1996.
13. Smith JM, Weaver T, Skeans MA, et al. OPTN/SRTR 2017 Annual data report: intestine. *Am J Transplant.* 2019;19(suppl 2):284-322. doi: 10.1111/ajt.15277
14. Kreider M, Hadjiliadis D, Kotloff KM. Candidate selection, timing of listing, and choice of procedure for lung transplantation. *Clin Chest Med.* 32(2011)199-211.15.
15. Braun AT, Merlo CA. Cystic fibrosis lung transplantation. *Curr Opin Pulm Med.* 2011;17:467-472.
16. Lynch JP, Sayah DM, Belperio JA, Weigt SS. Lung transplantation for cystic fibrosis: results, indications, complications, and controversies. *Semin Respir Crit Care Med.* 2015;36:229-320.
17. Whitson BA, Hayes D. Indications and outcomes in adult lung transplantation. *J Thorac Dis.* 2014;6(8):1018-1023.
18. Ghant M, Jim B. Renal transplantation in advanced chronic kidney disease patients. *Med Clin N Am.* 2016;100(3):465-476.
19. Glicklich D, Vohra P. Cardiovascular risk assessment before and after kidney transplantation. *Card Rev.* 2014;22(4):153-162.
20. Krowka MJ, Wiesner RH, Heimbach JK. Pulmonary contraindications, indications and MELD exceptions for liver transplantation: a contemporary view and look forward. *J Hept.* 2013;59:367-374.
21. Maddur H, Bourdilon PD, Liangpunsakul S, et al. The role of cardiac catheterization and percutaneous coronary intervention in pre-operative assessment and management of patients prior to OLT. *Liver Transpl.* 2014;20(6):664-672.
22. Martinex-Palli G, Cardenas A. Preoperative cardiopulmonary assessment of the liver transplant candidate. *Ann Hepatol.* 2011;10(4):421-433.
23. Liver transplant. Mayo Clinic. http://www.mayoclinic.org/tests-procedures/liver-transplant/basics/how-you-prepare/prc-20014076. Updated March 19, 2019. Accessed March 19, 2019.
24. National Kidney Foundation. Evaluation for kidney transplant. www.kidney.org/atoz/content/kidney-transplant-evaluation. Accessed July 18, 2019.
25. Heart evaluation. Penn Medicine. www.pennmedicine.org/transplant/patient-care/transplant-programs/heart-transplant/transplant-process/evaluation.html. Accessed March 19, 2019.
26. Transplantation. National Kidney Foundation. https://www.kidney.org/atoz/content/pancreastx. Accessed March 19, 2019.
27. Levine SM. A survey of clinical practice of lung transplantation in North America. *Chest.* 2004;125(4):1224-1238.

28. Eberlein M, Garrity ER, Orens JB. Lung allocation in the United States. *Clin Chest Med.* 2011;32(2):213-222.
29. Pisani B, Mullen GM. Prevention of osteoporosis in cardiac transplant recipients. *Curr Opin Cardiol.* 2002;17:160-164.
30. Boehler A. Update on cystic fibrosis: selected aspects related to lung transplantation. *Swiss Med Wkly.* 2003;133:111-117.
31. Gilbert S, Dauber JH, Hattler BG, et al. Lung and heart-lung transplantation at the University of Pittsburgh: 1982-2002. In: Cecka PI, Teraski JM, eds. *Clinical Transplants* (pp 253-261). Los Angeles, CA: UCLA Immunogenetics Center; 2002.
32. McAnally KJ, Valentine VG, LaPlace SG, McFadden PM, Seoane L, Taylor DE. Effect of pre-transplantation prednisone on survival after lung transplantation. *J Heart Lung Transplant.* 2006;25:67-74.
33. UNOS. Transplant trends. https://unos.org/data/transplant-trends. Accessed July 1, 2019.
34. Changes to the lung allocation system. Organ Procurement and Transplantation Network. http://optn.transplant.hrsa.gov/news/changes-to-the-lung-allocation-system. Accessed March 19, 2019. Published February 17, 2015.
35. Lund LH, Edwards LB, Kucheryavaya AY, et al. The registry of the international society for heart and lung transplantation: thirty-first official adult heart transplant report-2014; focus theme retransplantation. *J Heart Lung Transplant.* 2014;33(10):996-1008.
36. Yusen RD, Edwards LB, Kucheryavaya AY, et al. The registry of the international society for heart and lung transplantation: thirty-first adult lung and heart-lung transplant report-2014; focus theme: retransplantation. *J Heart Lung Transplant.* 2014;33(10):1009-1023.
37. Goldfarb SB, Benden C, Edwards LB, et al. The registry of the international society for heart and lung transplantation; eighteenth official pediatric lung and heart-lung transplantation report-2015; focus theme: early graft failure. *J Heart Lung Transplant.* 2015;34:1255-1263.
38. Yusen RD, Edwards LB, Kucheryavaya AY, et al; International Society of Heart and Lung Transplantation. Registry of the International Society for Heart and Lung Transplantation: thirty-second adult lung and heart-lung transplant report-2015; focus theme: early graft failure. *J Heart Lung Transplant.* 2015;34:1264-1277.
39. Toyada Y, Toyada Y. Heart-lung transplantation: adult indications and outcomes. *J Thorac Dis.* 2014;6(8):1138-1142.
40. Kotloff KM, Thabut G. Lung transplantation. *Am J Respir Crit Care Med.* 2011;184:159-171.
41. Organ Procurement and Transplantation Network. Annual report. US Department of Health and Human Services. https://optn.transplant.hrsa.gov/data/view-data-reports/annual-report. Published 2017. Accessed July 18, 2019.
42. Mason DP, Thuita L, Nowicki ER, Murthy SC, Pettersson GB, Blackstone EH. Should lung transplantation be performed for patients on mechanical respiratory support? The US experience. *J Thorac Cardiovasc Surg.* 2010;139:765-73
43. Date H. Update on living-donor lobar lung transplantation. *Curr Opin Transplant.* 2016;16:453-457
44. Valapour M, Skeans MA, Smith JM, et al. OPTN/SRTR Annual Data Report 2014: Lung. *Am J Transplant.* 2016;16(suppl 2):141-168. doi:10.1111/ajt.1367145
45. Weill D, Benden C, Corris PA, et al. A consensus document for the selection of lung transplant candidates: 2014-an update from the pulmonary transplantation council of the International Society for Heart and Lung Transplantation. *J Heart Lung Transplant.* 2015;34:1-15.
46. Gottlieb J, Warnecke G, Hadem J, et al. Outcome of critically ill lung transplant candidates on invasive respiratory support. *Intensive Care Med.* 2012;38:968-975.
47. Hoopes CW, Kukreia J, Golden J, Davenport DL, Diaz-Guzman E, Zwischenberger JB. Extracorporeal membrane oxygenation as a bridge to pulmonary transplantation. *J Thorac Cardiovasc Surg.* 2013;145:862-868.
48. Chiumello D, Coppola S, Froio S, Colombo A, Del Sorbo L. Extracorporeal life support as bridge to lung transplantation: a systematic review. *Crit Care.* 2015;19:19. doi: 10.1186/s13054-014-0686-7
49. de Perrot M, Chaparro C, McRae K, et al. Twenty-year experience of lung transplantation at a single center: influence of recipient diagnosis on long-term survival. *J Thorac Cardiovasc Surg.* 2004;127(5):1493-1501.

50. Algar FJ, Alvarez A, Lama R, et al. Lung transplantation patients under mechanical ventilation. *Transplant Proc.* 2003;35(2):737-738.
51. Ferdinande P, Buryninckx F, Van Raemdonck D, Daenen W, Verleden G. Phrenic nerve dysfunction after heart-lung and lung transplantation. *J Heart Lung Transplant.* 2004;23(1):105-109.
52. Burns KE, Iacono AT. Incidence of clinically unsuspected pulmonary embolism in mechanically ventilated lung transplant recipients. *Transplantation.* 2003;76(6):964-968.
53. Lung transplant. National Heart, Lung, and Blood Institute. https://www.nhlbi.nih.gov/health/health-topics/topics/lungtxp/risks. Accessed March 19, 2019.
54. De Vlaminck I, Martin L, Kertesz M, et al. Noninvasive monitoring of infection and rejection after lung transplantation. *Proc Natl Acad Sci U S A.* 2015;112(43):13336-1341. doi: 10.1073/pnas.151749411255
55. Verleden GM, Vos R, Vanaudenaerde B, et al. Current views on chronic rejection after lung transplantation. *Transpl Int.* 2015;28(10):1131-1139.
56. Verleden GM, Raghu G, Meyer KC, Glanville AR, Corris P. A new classification system for chronic lung allograft dysfunction. *J Heart Lung Transplant.* 2014;33(2):127-133.
57. Vos R, Verleden SE, Verleden GM. Chronic lung allograft dysfunction: evolving practice. *Curr Opin Organ Transplant.* 2015,20:483-491.
58. Anile M, Diso D, Rendina EA, Venuta F. Airway anastomosis for lung transplantation. *J Thorac Dis.* 2016;8(suppl 2):S197-S203.
59. De Jonge N, Kirkels H, Lahpor JR, et al. Exercise performance in patients with end-stage heart failure after implantation of a left ventricular assist device and after heart transplantation. *J Am Coll Cardiol.* 2001;37:1794-1799.
60. Reinsma GD, ten Hacken NHT, Grevink RG, van der Bij W, Koeter GH, van Weert E. Limiting factors of exercise performance 1 year after lung transplantation. *J Heart Lung Transplant.* 2006;25:1310-1316.
61. Wickerson L, Mathur S, Brooks D. Exercise training after lung transplantation: a systematic review. *J Heart Lung Transplant.* 2010;29:497-503.
62. Nytroen K, Gullestad L. Exercise after heart transplantation: an overview. *World J Transplant.* 2013;3(4)78-90.
63. Squires R. Exercise therapy for cardiac transplant recipients. *Prog Cardiovascular Dis.* 2011;53:429-436.
64. Wilhem MJ. Long-term outcome following heart transplantation: current perspective. *J Thorac Dis.* 2015;7(3):549-551.
65. Chaudry H, Yip DS, Bush T, et al. Exercise performance increases coincident to body weight over the first two years following cardiac transplantation. *Clin Transplant.* 2011:25:685-688.
66. Langer D, Burtin C, Schepers L, et al. Exercise training after lung transplantation improves participation in daily activity: a randomized control trial. *Am J Transplant.* 2012;12:1584-1592.
67. Marconi C, Marzorati M. Exercise after heart transplantation. *Eur J Appl Physiol.* 2003;90:250-259.
68. Didsbury M, McGee RG, Tong A, et al. Exercise training in solid organ transplant recipients: a systematic review and meta-analysis. *Transplantation.* 2013;95:679-687.
69. Armstrong HF, Gonzalez-Costello J, Thirapatarapong W, Jorde UP, Bartels MN. Effect of lung transplantation on heart rate response to exercise. *Heart Lung.* 2015;44:246-250.
70. Fink G, Lebzelter J, Blau C, Klainman E, Aravot D, Kramer MR. The sky is the limit: exercise capacity 10 years post-heart-lung transplantation. *Transplant Proc.* 2000;32(4):733-734.
71. Toyoda Y, Guy TS, Kashem A. Present status and future prospectives of heart transplantation. *Circ J.* 2013;77:1097-1110.
72. Frazier OH, Myers TJ, Radovancevic B. The Heartmate left ventricular assist system. *Tex Heart Inst J.* 1998;25:265-271.
73. Mangini S, Alves BR, Silvestre OM, et al. Heart transplantation: review. *Einstein (Sao Paulo).* 2015;13(2):310-318.
74. Birati EY, Rame E. Post-heart transplant complications. *Crit Care Clin.* 2014;30:629-637.
75. Heart transplant. National Heart, Lung, and Blood Institute. https://www.nhlbi.nih.gov/health/health-topics/topics/ht/after. Accessed March 19, 2019.
76. Valantine H. Cardiac allograft vasculopathy after heart transplantation: risk factors and management. *J Heart Lung Transplant.* 2003;23(suppl 1):S187-S193.

77. Hayes D, Galantowicz M, Hoffman TM. Combined heart-lung transplantation: a perspective on the past and the future. *Pediatr Cardiol.* 2013;34:207-212.
78. Hart A, Smith JM, Skeans MA, et al. Kidney. Special Issue OPTN/SRTR Annual Data Report 2014. *Am J Transplant.* 2016;16(S2):11-45.
79. Chandran S, Vincenti F. Clinical aspects: focusing on key unique organ-specific issues of renal transplantation. *Cold Spring Harb Perspect Med.* 2014;4(2):a015644.
80. Ghanta M, Jim B. Renal transplantation in advanced chronic kidney disease patients. *Med Clin N Am.* 2016;100:465-476.
81. Mastas AJ, Smith JM, Skeans MA, et al. OPTN/SRTR 2012 Annual Data Report: kidney. *Am J Transplant.* 2014;14 (suppl 1):11-44.
82. Scheuber C. A review of organ transplantation: heart, lung, kidney, liver, and simultaneous liver-kidney. *Crit Care Nurse Q.* 2016;39(3):199-206. doi: 10.1097/CNQ.0000000000000115
83. Brenner BM, ed. *Brenner & Rector's: The Kidney.* 7th ed. Philadelphia, PA: WB Saunders; 2004.
84. Stuart FP, Abecassis, Dixon KB. *Organ Transplantation.* Georgetown, TX: Landes BioScience; 2000.
85. Lee J, Ordon M. Innovative applications of robotic surgery: renal allograft and autologous transplantation. *F1000Res.* 2016;5:ii. doi:10.12688/f1000research.7343.1
86. Vincenti F, Rostaing L, Grinyo J, et al. Belatacept and long-term outcomes in kidney transplantation. *New Enlg J Med.* 2016;374:333-343.
87. Rossi AP, Vella JP. Hypertension, living kidney donors, and transplantation: where are we today? *Adv Chronic Kidney Dis.* 2015;22(2):154-164.
88. Tholking G, Schuette-Nuetgen K, Kentrup D, Pawelski H, Reuter S. Imaging-based diagnosis of acute renal allograft rejection. *World J Transplant.* 2016;6(1):174-192.
89. Sagiv M, Rudoy J, Rotstein A, Fisher N, Ben-Ari J. Exercise tolerance of end-stage renal disease patients. *Nephron.* 1991;57(4):424-427.
90. Painter P, Messer-Rehak D, Hanson P, et al. Exercise capacity in hemodialysis, CAPD, and renal transplant patients. *Nephron.* 1986;42(1):47-51.
91. Painter PL, Hector L, Ray K, et al. A randomized trial of exercise training after renal transplantation. *Transplantation.* 2002;74(1):42-48.
92. Kim WR, Lake JR, Smith JM, et al. Liver. *Am J of Transpl.* 2016;16(suppl 2):69-98.
93. Farkas S, Hackl C, Schlitt HJ. Overview of the indications and contraindications for liver transplantation. *Cold Spring Harb Perspect Med.* 2014;4(5):ii. doi: 10.1101/cshperspect.a015602
94. Wan Song AT, Avelino-Silva VI, Arruda Pecora RA, et al. Liver transplantation: fifty years of experience. *World J Gastroenterol.* 2014;20(18):5363-5374.
95. Joshi D, Agarwal K. Role of liver transplantation in human immunodeficiency virus positive patients. *World J Gastroenterol.* 2015;21(43):12311-12321.
96. Townsend CM, ed. *Sabiston Textbook of Surgery.* 16th ed. Philadelphia, PA: WB Saunders; 2001.
97. Moon DB, Lee SG. Liver transplantation. *Gut Liver.* 2009;3(3):145-165.
98. Dansinger M. Life after your transplant: signs of rejection. WebMD. http://www.webmd.com/a-to-z-guides/life-after-transplant-signs-rejection. Published 2017. Accessed March 20, 2019.
99. Liver transplant: what to expect. Barnes Jewish Hospital. http://www.barnesjewish.org/Medical-Services/Transplant/Liver-Transplant/Liver-Transplant-Process/After-Liver-Transplant#Rejection. Accessed March 20, 2019.
100. Zieve D. Transplant rejection. *Medline Plus.* https://medlineplus.gov/ency/article/000815.htm. Published May 21, 2017. Accessed March 20, 2019.
101. Kaltsakas G, Antoniou E, Palamidas AF, et al. Dyspnea and respiratory muscle strength in end-stage liver disease. *World J Jepatol* 2013 February 27;5(2):56-63.
102. Feltracco P, Carollo C, Barbieri S, Pettenuzzo T, Ori T. Early respiratory complications after liver transplantation. *World J Gastroenterol.* 2013;19(48):9271-9281.
103. Vintro AQ, Krasnoff JB, Painter P. Roles of nutrition and physical activity in musculoskeletal complications before and after liver transplantation. *AACN Clin Iss.* 2002;13:333-347.
104. Kelly DA. Managing liver failure. *Postgrad Med J.* 2002;78:660-667.
105. Minemura M, Tajiri K, Shimizu Y. Systemic abnormalities in liver disease. *World J Gastroenterol.* 2009;15(24):2960-2974.

106. Kotarska K, Wunsch E, Jodko L, et al. Factors affecting exercise test performance in patients after liver transplantation. *Hepat Mon.* 2016;16(3):e34356.
107. van Ginneken BTJ, van den Berg-Emons RJG, Kazemier G, Metselaar HJ, Tilanus HW, Stam Hj. Physical fitness, fatigue, and quality of life after liver transplantation. *Eur J Appl Physiol.* 2007;100:345-353.
108. Bozbas SS, Eyuboglu F. Evaluation of liver transplant candidates: a pulmonary perspective. *Ann Thorac Med.* 2011;6(3):109-114.
109. Foroncewicz B, Mucha K, Szparaga B, et al. Rehabilitation and 6-Minute Walk Test after liver transplantation. *Transplant Proc.* 2011;43:3021-3024.
110. Galant LH, Ferrari R, Forgiarini LA, Monteiro MB, Marroni CA, Dias AS. Relationship between MELD severity score and distance walked and respiratory muscle strength in candidates for liver transplantation. *Transplant Proc.* 2010;42:1729-1730.
111. Painter P, Krasnoff J, Ascher N. Physical activity and quality of life in long-term liver transplant recipients. *Liver Transplant.* 2001;7:213-219.
112. Redfield RR, Rickels MR, Naji A, Odorico JS. Pancreas transplantation in the modern era. *Gastroenterol Clin North Am.* 2016;45(1):145-166.
113. Kandaswamy R, Skeans MA, Gustafson SK, et al. Pancreas. Special Issue: OPTN/SRTR Annual Data Report 2014. *Am J Transplant.* 2016;16(S2):47-68.
114. Mittal S, Johnson P, Friend P. Pancreas transplantation: solid organ and islet. *Cold Spring Harb Perspect Med.* 2014;4:a015610.
115. Shapiro AMJ. Islet transplantation in type 1 diabetes: ongoing challenges, refined procedures, and long-term outcome. *Rev Diabet Stud.* 2012;9(4):385-406.
116. Wrightson N, Blake A, English L. Care of the heart transplant patient. *Nurs Times.* 2002;98(28):34-37.
117. Kuntz K, Weinland SR, Butt Z. Psychosocial challenges in solid organ transplantation. *J Clin Psychol Med Setting.* 2015;22:122-135.
118. Rainer JP, Thompson CH, Lambros H. Psychotherapy theory, practice, training. *Psychotherapy (Chic).* 2010;47(3):403-412.
119. Coglianes EE, Samsi M, Liebo MJ, Heroux AL. The value of psychosocial factors in patient selection and outcomes after heart transplantation. *Curr Heart Fail Rep.* 2015;12:42-47.
120. Spaderna H, Smits JMA, Rahmel AO, Weidner G. Psychosocial and behavioural factors in heart transplant candidates-an overview. *Transpl Int.* 2007;20(11):909-920.
121. Maldonado JR, Sher Y, Lolak S, et al. The Stanford integrated psychosocial assessment for transplantation: a prospective study of medical and psychosocial outcomes. *Psychosom Med.* 2015;77(9):1018-1030.
122. Grover S, Sarkar S. Liver transplant-psychiatric and psychosocial aspects. *J Clin Exp Hepatol.* 2012;2(4):382-392.
123. Moreau A, Varey E, Anegon I, Cuturi M-C. Effector mechanisms of rejection. *Cold Spring Harb Perspect Med.* 2013;3:a015461.
124. Allison TL. Immunosuppressive therapy in transplantation. *Nurs Clin N Am.* 2016;51:107-120
125. Sykes M. Fundamentals of transplant immunology. In: Paul WE, ed. *Fundamental Immunology.* Philadelphia, PA: Lippincott Williams & Wilkins; 2003.
126. Yakupoglu U, Baranowska-Daca E, Rosen D, Barrios R, Suki WN, Truong LD. Post-transplant nephrotic syndrome: a comprehensive clinicopathologic study. *Kidney Int.* 2004;65(6):2360-70.
127. Solez K, Colvin RB, Racusen LC, et al. Banff '05 Meeting Report: differential diagnosis of chronic allograft injury and elimination of chronic allograft nephropathy ('CAN'). *Am J Transplant.* 2007;7(3):518-526.
128. Moini M, Schilsky ML, Tichy EM. Review of immunosuppression in liver transplantation. *World J Hepatol.* 2015;7(10):1355-1368.
129. Pellegrino B. Immunosuppression. *Medscape.* http://emedicine.medscape.com/article/432316-overview. Accessed March 20, 2019. Updated
130. Bamgbola O. Metabolic consequences of modern immunosuppressive agents in solid organ transplantation. *Ther Adv Endocrinol Metab.* 2016;7(3):110-127.
131. Munagala MR, Phancao A. Managing cardiovascular risk in the post solid organ transplant recipient. *Med Clin N Am.* 2016;100:519-533.

132. Early C, Stuckey L, Tischer S. Osteoporosis in the adult solid organ transplant population: underlying mechanisms and available treatment options. *Osteoporos Int.* 2016;27:1425-1440.
133. Yu TM, Lin CL, Chang SN, Sung FC, Huang ST, Kao CH. Osteoporosis and fractures after solid organ transplantation: a nationwide population-based cohort study. *Mayo Clin Proc.* 2014;89(7):888-895.
134. Zafar SY, Howell DN, Gockerman JP. Malignancy after solid organ transplantation: an overview. *Oncologist.* 2008;13:769-778.
135. Chapman JR, Webster AC, Wong G. Cancer in the transplant recipient. *Cold Spring Harb Perspect Med.* 2013;3:1015677.
136. Drugs.com. Accessed August 5, 2019.
137. Horber FF, Scheidegger JR, Grunig BE, Frey FJ. Evidence that prednisone-induced myopathy is reversed by physical training. *Clin Endocrinol Metab.* 1985;61(1):83-88.
138. Braith RW, Welsch MA, Mills RM Jr, et al. Resistance exercise prevent glucocorticoid-induced myopathy in heart transplant recipients. *Med Sci Sports Exerc.* 1998;30(4):483-489.
139. Scherer SA, Bookstien NA. Clinical perspective: framework and rationale for physical therapy management of lung transplant patients with osteoporosis. *Cardiopulmonary Phys Ther J.* 2001;12:75-82.
140. Colberg SL, Albright AL, Blissmer BJ, et al. Exercise and type 2 diabetes: American College of Sports Medicine and the American Diabetes Association: Joint Position Statement. *Med Sci Sports Exerc.* 2010;42(12):2282-2303.
141. Ligibel JA, Alfano CM, Courneya KS, et al. American Society of Clinical Oncology Position Statement on Obesity and Cancer. *J Clin Oncol.* 2014;32(31):3568-3574.
142. American Physical Therapy Association. *Guide to Physical Therapist Practice.* 3rd ed. http://www.apta.org/Guide/. Updated October 21, 2015. Accessed October 5, 2018.
143. Shen J, Townsend R, You X, et al. Pharmacokinetics, pharmacodynamics, and immunogenicity of belatacept in adult kidney transplant. *Clin Drug Investig.* 2014;34:117-126.
144. UNOS. Preparing your patients for changes to the lung allocation system. *Heart/Lung News.* https://unos.org/news/preparing-patients-changes-lung-allocation-system. Published January 19, 2014. Accessed July 18, 2019.
145. ISHLT Transplant Registry Quarterly Reports for Heart in North America. International Society for Heart and Lung Transplantation. https://ishltregistries.org/registries/quarterlyDataReportResults.asp?organ=HR&rptType=all&continent=4. Published January 5, 2018. Accessed July 18, 2019.

BIBLIOGRAPHY

Craig CR Stitzel RE. *Modern Pharmacology with Clinical Applications.* New York, NY: Little, Brown, and Co; 1997.

De Bonis M, Reynolds L, Barros J, Madden BP. Tacrolimus as a rescue immunosuppressant after heart transplantation. *Eur J Cardio-Thoracic Surg.* 2001;19(5):690-695.

Deglin, JH, Vallerand AH. *Davis's Drug Guide for Nurses.* 8th ed. Philadelphia, PA: FA Davis; 2003.

Harringer W, Haverich A. Heart and heart-lung transplantation: standards and improvements. *World J Surg.* 2002;26:218-225.

Janeway CA, Travers P, Walport M, Shlomchik M. *Immunobiology: The Immune System in Health & Disease.* 5th ed. New York, NY: Garland Publishing; 2001.

Karch AM. *Lippincott's Nursing Drug Guide.* Springhouse, PA: Lippincott Williams & Wilkins; 2004.

Mignat C. Clinically significant drug interactions with new immunosuppressive agents. *Drug Saf.* 1997;16(4):267-278.

Miniati DN, Robbins RC. Heart transplantation: a thirty-year perspective. *Ann Rev Med.* 2002;53:189-205.

Parekh K, Trulock E, Patterson GA. Use of cyclosporine in lung transplantation.*Transplant Proc.* 2004;36(2 suppl):S318-S322.

Parizel PM, Snoeck HW, van den Hauwe L, et al. Cerebral complications of murine monoclonal CD3 antibody (OKT3): CT and MR findings. *Am J Neuroradiol.* 1997;18(10):1935-1938.

Physicians' Desk Reference. 57th ed. Montvale, NJ: Thompson PDR; 2003.

Radovancevic B, Frazier OH. Heart transplantation: approaching a new century. *Tex Heart Inst J.* 1999;26:60-70.

Ritter JM, Lewis LD, Mant TG. *Textbook of Clinical Pharmacology*. London, United Kingdom: Edward Arnold Co; 1995.

Serkova N, Litt L, James TL, et al. Evaluation of individual and combined neurotoxicity of the immunosuppressants cyclosporine and sirolimus by in vitro multinuclear NMR spectroscopy. *J Pharmacol Exp Ther*. 1999;289(2):800-806.

Nursing 2011 Drug Handbook. 31st ed. Philadelphia, PA: Lippincott Williams & Wilkins; 2011.

Serkova N, Litt L, Leibfritz D, et al. The novel immunosuppressant SDZ-RAD protects rat brain slices from cyclosporine-induced reduction of high-energy phosphates. *Br J Pharmacol*. 2000;129(3):485-492.

Valantine H. Cardiac allograft vasculopathy after heart transplantation: risk factors and management. *J Heart Lung Trans*. 2004;23(suppl 1):S187-S193.

Appendix

Pharmacological Information: Transplantation Pharmacology

Corticosteroids

Action

Corticosteroids primarily inhibit inflammation in addition to suppressing immune responses by preventing production of vasoactive substances and cytokines. Corticosteroids inhibit accumulation of WBCs at inflammatory sites (eg, sites of rejection) by reducing the release of inflammatory mediators (eg, interleukins, tumor necrosis factor [TNF]) and inducing cell lysis. Additionally, corticosteroids limit phagocytosis and lysosomal enzyme release impairing leukocyte function. Corticosteroids suppress cell-mediated immune reactions and are the most widely used immunosuppressive agents. Corticosteroids are used for maintenance immunosuppression and induction, as well as for acute rejection.

Side Effects

CNS: Insomnia, nervousness, mood swings, hallucinations, depression

CV: Diaphoresis, rare tachycardia, hyperlipidemia

GI: Dyspepsia/heartburn, abdominal distention, increased appetite, diarrhea, constipation, peptic ulcers, gingival hyperplasia,

Miscellaneous: Nephrotoxicity, secondary renal vasoconstriction, osteopenia/osteoporosis, acne, facial flushing, delayed wound healing, infection risk, myopathy, muscle wasting, cataracts, amenorrhea, glucose intolerance, hyperkalemia, hypomagnesia, hyperuricemia, hypertrichosis, hirsutism, malignancy, hemolytic uremic syndrome.

Common Medications

Prednisone, methylprednisolone, prednisolone

Calcineurin Inhibitors

Action

Calcineurin inhibitors (eg, cyclosporine) reduce the activity of intracellular calcineurin phosphatase leading to a reduction in the production and release of several cytokines important for the proliferation, differentiation, and recruitment of lymphocytes (eg, interleukin 2, interleukin 3, interleukin 4, TNF). Cyclosporine is highly specific for inactivation of T lymphocytes.

Side Effects

CNS: Headache, dizziness, seizures, visual abnormalities, focal deficits, mild tremor, paresthesias

CV: HTN, dyspnea, hyperkalemia, hypercholesterolemia, thrombotic microangiopathy

GI: Nausea, vomiting, epigastric pain, diarrhea, anorexia

GU: Nephrotoxicity

Miscellaneous: Malignancy (eg, lymphoproliferative disease, skin neoplasms), myalgia/arthralgia, restless leg syndrome, post-transplant infection, hirsutism, gingival hyperplasia, thrombocytopenia, microangiopathic hemolytic anemia

Common Medications

Sandimmune (cyclosporine A); Neoral, Gengraf (cyclosporine-modified)

Tacrolimus

Action

A macrolide antibiotic that functions similarly to cyclosporine by binding intracellular proteins and inhibiting calcium dependent phosphatases. This limits T lymphocyte activation thereby suppressing immune mediated inflammatory responses.

Side Effects

CNS: Headache, dizziness, visual disturbances, decreased hearing, tinnitus, neurotoxicity, photophobia
CV: HTN, dyspnea, leg cramps, hyperglycemia, prolong QT/QTc, myocardial hypertrophy
GI: Nausea, vomiting, epigastric pain, perforation
GU: Nephrotoxicity
Miscellaneous: Hyperkalemia, infection risk, diabetes, increased serum creatinine and BUN, lymphoma

Common Medications

Prograf (tacrolimus); Envarsus XR, Astagraf XL, Hecoria (extended-release tacrolimus)

Purine Synthesis Inhibitors

Action

Purine synthesis inhibitors acts by blocking purine metabolism. The purines, adenine and guanine, are vital components for DNA synthesis. Purine synthesis inhibitors hinder DNA synthesis thereby limiting the proliferation of lymphocytes (eg, T and B cells).

Side Effects

CNS: Headache, insomnia (rare)
CV: HTN, anemia (less common with mycofenolate mofetil), peripheral edema
GI: Diarrhea, vomiting, dyspepsia, constipation, stomach area pain
Miscellaneous: Fever, leukopenia, neutropenia, infection risk, thrombocytopenia, bleeding

Common Medications

Imuran (azathioprine), Cellcept (mycofenolate mofetil), Myfortic (mycophenolate sodium)

Proliferation Signal Inhibitors (Mammalian Target of Rapamycin Inhibitors)

Action

Proliferation signal inhibitors suppress interleukin 2 (IL-2), a cytokine that promotes the proliferation, differentiation, and recruitment of T-lymphocytes, leading to immunosuppression.

Side Effects

CNS: None, unless combined with other medications
CV: HTN, thrombocytopenia, hyperlipidemia, anemia, angioedema, peripheral edema
GI: Diarrhea, GI distress, aphthous ulcers
Miscellaneous: Hepatic- and nephrotoxicity, acne, arthralgia, fever, weight gain, thrombocytopenia hypokalemia, impaired wound healing, graft thrombosis, pneumonitis, infection, worsening proteinuria with sirolimus.

Common Medications

Zortress (everolimus); Rapamycin, Rapamune (sirolimus)

Biologic Agents

Antilymphocyte Preparations

Action

Antilymphocyte preparations include immunoglobulins and antibodies developed from animals against human lymphocytes. The immunoglobulins or antibodies bind to circulating T lymphocytes leading to their inactivation or removal from the circulation, thus producing immunosuppression. Category includes polyclonal antibodies, murine monoclonal anti-CD 3 antibody, and humanized monoclonal anti-CD52 antibody.

Side Effects

CNS: Seizures, lethargy, decreased mental function, increased risk of CNS adverse effects with combination of indomethacin
CV: Occasionally dyspnea, apnea, chest pain, phlebitis, hypotension
GI: Occasionally nausea, vomiting, diarrhea
Miscellaneous: Increases incidence of rejection and viral infections (CMV), post-transplantation lymphoproliferative disorder, sensitization/serum sickness and "first-dose effect" (fevers, chills, mild hypotension, arthralgia, flu-like symptoms), anaphylaxis, thrombocytopenia, infection, pulmonary edema,anemia, idiosyncratic pancytopenia, autoimmune disorders, thrombocytopenia, thyroid disease

Common Medications

ATG, ATGAM (antithymocyte globulin); Orthoclone OKT3 (muromonab-CD3); Campath-1H (alemtuzumab)

Monoclonal Antibody Interleukin-2 Receptor Antagonists

Action

Monoclonal antibody IL-2 receptor antagonists prevent activation of the lymphocyte IL-2 receptor reducing proliferation, differentiation, and recruitment of this immune response cell type. Eliminates most B cells and is approved for some post-transplantation lymphoproliferative disease in organ transplant recipients.

Side Effects

CNS: Dizziness, tremor
CV: HTN, cough, dyspnea, hypotension, tachycardia
GI: Abdominal pain, diarrhea
Miscellaneous: Infection, edema, hypersensitivity reaction, bronchospasm, pulmonary edema

Common Medications

Daclizumab, Zenapax (dacliximab); Simulect (basiliximab)

Selective Co-Stimulation Blocker

Action

First in class selective co-stimulation blocker. Prevents T cell activation and proliferation and inhibits subsequent alloimmune responses post–organ transplantation.

Side Effects

CNS: Fever, headache, insomnia, anxiety, Guillain-Barré syndrome, dizziness
CV: Peripheral edema, HTN, hypotension
GI: Diarrhea, constipation, nausea, vomiting, abdominal pain
Miscellaneous: Serious infections, anemia, leukopenia, cough, upper respiratory infection, bronchitis, nasopharyngitis, dyspnea, arthralgia, back pain, diabetes, proteinuria, renal graft dysfunction, hematuria, increased serum creatinine, alopecia

Common Medications

LEA29Y, Nulojix (belatacept)

Chapter 15

Integumentary Disorders and Wound Management

Christine F. Ehlers, PT, CWS, CLWT

Wounds are defined as any injury to the integumentary system, one of the largest and most complex organs of the body. Wounds involve injury to the skin and damage to the underlying tissues. The integument not only withstands the abuses of the environment, but also is impacted directly and indirectly by other body systems and diseases. The purpose of this chapter is to develop wound care management skills by reviewing the anatomy of the integument, normal wound healing processes, methods of closure, risk factors and etiologies of specific integument abnormalities, and provide an overview of the interventions to achieve wound healing or closure. Wound management is complex and involves many professionals who provide different perspectives and skills to the patient care plan. Throughout the chapter, various professionals are mentioned but many more exist that play important roles such as the physician, surgeon, nurse, wound, ostomy, and continence nurse (WOCN), social services, occupational therapist, speech therapist, product vendors, and, most importantly, the patient and his or her support system. Physical therapists play a unique role with their knowledge of mobility and the impact of altering and changing functional movement and postures that may cause, as well as resolve, wounds. The physical therapist's knowledge of anatomy, wound healing, and modalities provide additional skills to offer to the patient and the wound care team to optimize wound management.

Anatomy of Skin and Surrounding Tissues

Multiple layers comprise the soft tissues of the skin and these layers vary in depth throughout the body. For example, the thigh includes a large muscle mass and the ability to support larger amounts of subcutaneous tissue compared to the heel where there is limited muscle and subcutaneous tissue. This variation is of great importance in pressure redistribution. The soft tissue layers do not stack in an even, linear fashion, but rather may be arranged irregularly. The skin is divided into 2 layers: the

Malone DJ, Bishop KL, eds. *Acute Care Physical Therapy: A Clinician's Guide, Second Edition* (pp 639-679).

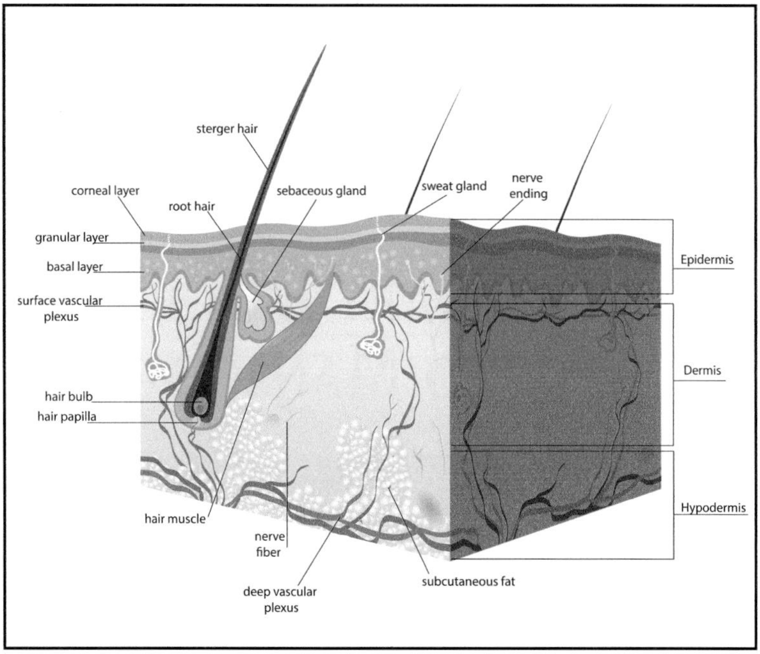

Figure 15-1. Structure of the skin showing the 2 layers: a superficial epidermis made of epithelial tissue, and a deeper dermis made of connective tissue. Beneath the skin is a layer of fatty tissue, the hypodermis. (Elen Bushe/Shutterstock.com)

epidermis and the dermis (Figure 15-1). The epidermis, the uppermost structure, is further divided into 5 separate layers:

1. Stratum corneum: Outermost layer
2. Stratum lucidum: Found in high-stress regions, such as palms of hands and soles of feet
3. Stratum granulosum
4. Stratum spinosum
5. Stratum germinativum or stratum basale: The reproductive layer that dips into the dermis covering hair follicles, sweat glands and sebaceous glands

The epidermis ranges from 4 to 6 mm in depth and can be as thick as 7 mm in regions of high stress, such as the soles of the feet and palms of the hands. The layers of the epidermis are graduated layers of cells that change shape from rounded in the basal layer to a flattened compacted upper layer. These skin layers serve to protect the underlying tissues keeping them hydrated, protected from microbes, keeping fluids and nutrients within the body, and responding to many external stimuli. The basement layer of the epidermis is the basal cell layer and is the site of regeneration of the epidermal layers (Figure 15-2). The basal layer dipping into the dermal layer determines if a wound is full- or partial-thickness. Partial-thickness indicates a portion of the dermis remains intact, including the basal layer, and allows for epidermal migration into the wound bed, which can accelerate wound healing significantly. Cell migration from basal layer to the stratum corneum, also termed the **horny layer**, is estimated to take from 28 to 32 days.

The dermal layer contains many active structures, including nerve endings, hair follicles, lymph vessels, capillaries, sweat glands, and sebaceous glands. These structures provide the active, protective, and sensory aspects to skin. The epidermis

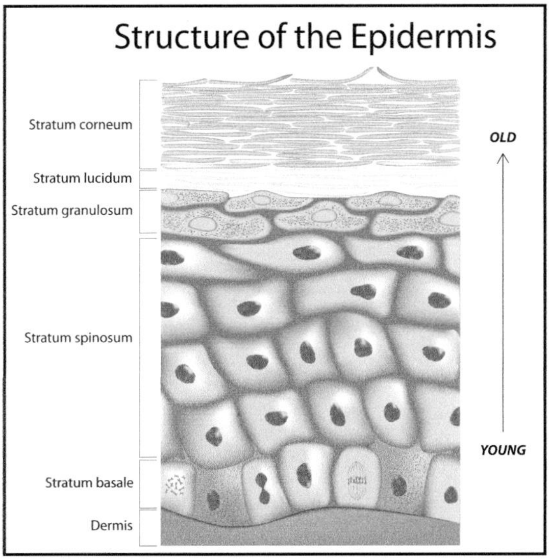

Figure 15-2. Epidermis of the skin. Note the change in shape from the deep basal layer to the superficial stratum corneum. (Alila Medical Media/Shutterstock.com)

and dermis are connected by rete pegs, a structural configuration that resembles a "tongue and groove" fit allowing for tight adherence of dermis to epidermis. This connection flattens with aging and increases the risk of skin tears, allowing separation of the dermal and epidermal layers.

There are additional layers found beneath the epidermis and dermis, which vary in thickness depending on the region of the body. The subcutaneous layer is the fatty layer that provides insulation, support, and cushioning to surrounding structures. Weight loss reduces this layer and can lead to increasing pressure and tissue breakdown in cachectic, malnourished, and mobility challenged individuals. Muscle can be found deep to the subcutaneous layer and generally has a good blood supply. The muscle layer and those layers more superficial can generally heal within 3 to 5 days under normal conditions. Tendons connecting muscle to bone need to remain hydrated to stay healthy and intact. Tendons are surrounded by a membrane, the peritenon, that helps maintain tendon moisture. Ligaments and tendons are highly fibrinous and generally white in color in the healthy state. The deepest structure tends to be bone, especially in the extremities. Bone is generally hard and white in color. Bone, tendon, and ligament generally heal within 6 to 8 weeks under normal conditions.

Wound Healing

Wound healing is a complex series of events involving many cell types and cellular responses to stabilize, debride, and heal the wound. Many products and modalities on the market address stimulation of particular cell types involved in the healing process. Understanding the wound healing process helps make effective clinical decisions in determining which products to prescribe to meet the wound care goals. Wound healing is categorized into 3 phases (Figure 15-3):

1. Inflammatory
2. Proliferative
3. Maturation/remodeling

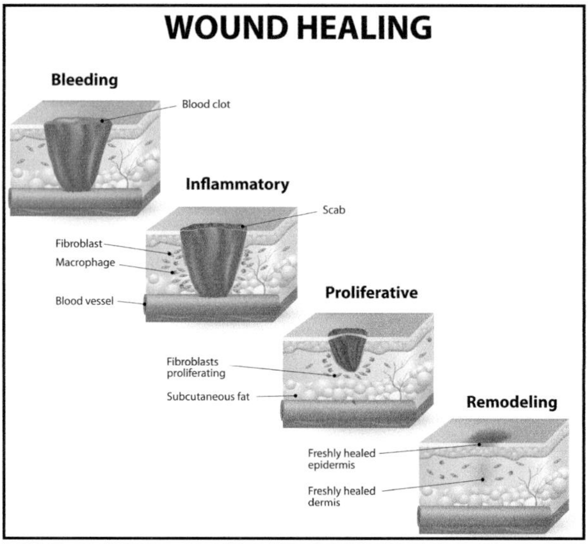

Figure 15-3. Stages of wound healing starting with hemostasis (blood clotting) and ending with remodeling. (Designua/Shutterstock.com)

The phases occur concurrently and the actual timeline each phase begins is debatable (Figure 15-4). For example, signs of all 3 phases have been identified in the first days after wounding and will be different for each individual.

The first response in normal healing to a wounded area is vasoconstriction to stabilize bleeding coupled with clot formation through platelet aggregation along the endothelium of the injured area (hemostasis). Once controlled, the phase of **inflammation** begins. Vasodilation occurs to allow an influx of neutrophils and monocytes. Neutrophils respond first to control local bacteria and aid debridement. Monocytes enter the wounded area and differentiate into macrophages. Macrophages clean up the wound site by phagocytosis and secrete growth factors and other chemotactic substances to communicate and attract other cells to initiate tissue repair. Clinical appearance of this phase will be edema (localized swelling), erythema (redness in and around the wound site), localized warmth of the tissues, and pain. The presence of necrotic tissue or debris signifies the wound is still in some phase of inflammation. Drainage in this phase is termed **exudate**. Exudate is the fluid that filters from the circulatory system into the wounded area. Exudate will have a milky appearance and have an increased viscosity.

The **proliferative phase** involves continued macrophage activity through the secretion of growth factors and chemotactic substances. Fibroblasts enter the wound site to deposit collagen and convert to myofibroblast. Myofibroblast possess contractile activity and serves to decrease the wound size. Endothelial cells form buds at the end of capillaries to create a vascular supply (angiogenesis) to the injured area. Clinical appearance of this phase includes granulation, reepithelialization, and wound contraction. Granulation tissue has a red cobblestone appearance on the wound surface and denotes the presence of capillary loops in the wound bed. Reepithelialization represents the migration of epidermal cells into the wound bed from the wound edges. The edges will change from cliff-like to beveled and resemble waves receding on the sand. Contraction is the visible presence of decreased wound size that can be measured. Drainage in this phase is termed **transudate**. Transudate is extravascular fluid with little protein and few cells. Transudate is clearer and less

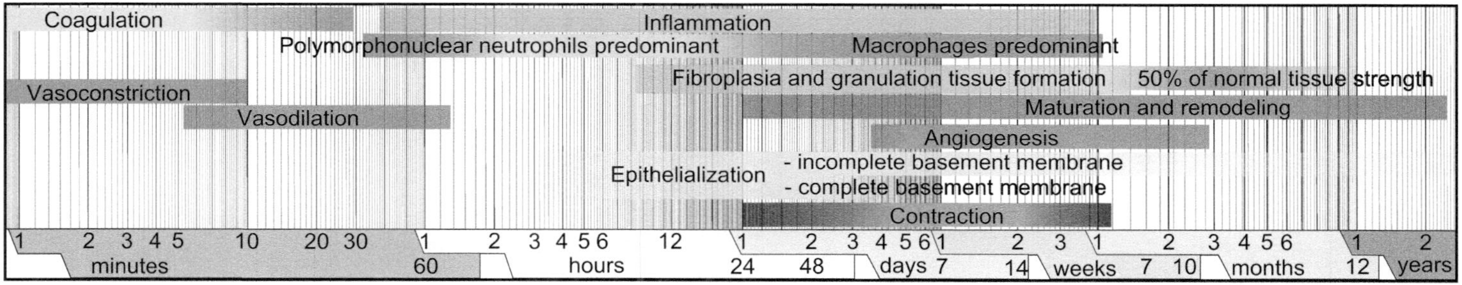

Figure 15-4. Approximate times of the different phases of wound healing. (Reprinted with permission from Häggström, Mikael. "Medical gallery of Mikael Häggström 2014." *WikiJournal of Medicine.* 1[2]. doi: 10.15347/wjm/2014.008. ISSN 20018762. Public Domain. Mikael Häggström, used with permission.)

viscous in composition. A balance between collagen deposition and breakdown is important during this phase to establish a strong, cosmetically appealing scar. Increased collagen production will form a hypertrophic, raised scar area called a **keloid scar**, and too little collagen production or too much collagen breakdown will create a weak scar that is easy to reinjure.

The **maturation/remodeling** phase is distinguished by the disappearance of a variety of cell types from the wound. Fibroblasts, which deposit collagen during the proliferative phase, exit and the collagen remodels from a disorganized mass to more ordered alignment with increased fibril diameter and compacted groupings. The visual appearance will be a shrinking and thinning of scar tissue while redness dissipates with the regression of the capillary beds. This phase can last as long as 2 years and is important to identify if applying scar treatment interventions.

It is important to be able to visually recognize the clinical signs of each phase in the wound bed. This recognition establishes and directs the wound care that is needed. Pressure redistribution, dressings, and modalities can be chosen to facilitate and advance the wound to the next phase of healing. Recognition of the phase of healing is also important to warn of wound regression. The therapist will need to identify the potential sources of the problem to halt wound breakdown.

Wounded tissue will never return to 100% tensile strength. It is estimated scar tissue can achieve only 75% of its former, uninjured strength. Wounded tissue will be more fragile and easily disrupted in the presence of pressure, shear, and friction. It is important during the patient examination to note any previously healed areas that may need extra care and protection. Injured areas will require protective equipment to diffuse pressure and prevent further injury.

Methods of Wound Closure

Open wounds can close in different methods and typically fall into 1 of 3 categories: primary, secondary, and delayed primary. **Primary closure** involves a linear lesion involving minimal to no tissue loss. It is easily approximated and closes easily. An example of primary wound closure is a postoperative incision. **Secondary closure** involves open areas with extensive tissue loss. Approximating wound edges is difficult to impossible. This type of wound will require intervention to form a granular bed, reepithelialization at the edges, and progressive contraction. **Delayed primary closure** involves a linear lesion that is left open to determine if abscesses or infections resolve and may be closed later or allowed to close on its own.

Wound closure occurs in the form of contraction and reepithelialization. It has been estimated that reepithelialization is limited up to 1 cm from the wound edge. This would then render wounds greater than 2 cm unable to close if only reepithelialization is available. Contraction plays a strong role in achieving and maintaining wound closure. Contraction in wounds gradually pulls the wound edges together to achieve closure. It is important to recognize where contraction is interrupted. Challenges to contraction may include direct pressure (eg, weightbearing on the wound), trauma (eg, heel wounds dragged over the sheets or bed, pushing the heel into a shoe), or indirect forces that manipulate the wound edges (eg, wound size in an edematous extremity will vary depending on the volume of the extremity). Wound contraction is challenging in wounds derived from pressure, especially in the feet, and wounds located around joints. Feet splay (ie, spread with pressure and weightbearing) naturally and this action will eliminate contraction and prolong, if not halt, wound closure. Another example is wounds in the calf area. These wounds tend to close faster when the patient is sitting and ambulating compared to prolonged supine positioning. Calf pressure is reduced in sitting and standing but increases in supine. The supine position leads to calf tissue spread and expansion and increased pressure disrupting wound contraction. Wounds around joints will need to be closely assessed and an appropriate compromise between function, range of motion (ROM), and wound closure will need to be determined.

Wound Examination

When working with a patient with a wound, a thorough examination needs to be completed. The physical therapist should include current and past medical history, laboratory testing, and radiology (as appropriate), social support, ROM, muscle strength, coordination, tone, balance, and sensation, as well as examining supine, seated, and standing mobility. Investigation of the home environment, communication, vision, hearing, durable medical equipment, and wound supplies should be included. Equipment evaluation, including seating (wheelchair and/or wheelchair cushion), orthotics (shoes, inserts, ankle-foot orthosis [AFO]), assistive devices (crutches, walker, cane), or prosthetic devices (above or below knee) can reveal contributing causative factors and specify needs for the wound healing plan of care and discharge planning. The individual should be observed in application and use of these devices. Additionally, bowel and bladder function in relation to wound location and cleanliness should be examined.

Observation of the wound should include the wound periphery and not just the wound itself. The wound periphery includes assessing for hair growth (present/absent), skin condition (moist, dry, scaly, maceration), callous (location and amount), scar tissue (present/absent, location), structural anomalies, particularly as it relates to wound location (scoliosis, Charcot foot), and bony prominences. Signs of other tissue damage or injury, such as bruising, abrasions, and scratches, should be noted. Look for specific signs to determine which phase of healing—inflammatory, proliferative or maturation—is most prominent. Use of complete and accurate wound documentation provides a clear picture of progress or regression. Table 15-1 provides more specifics on wound care terminology and examples of potential examination findings.

Documentation begins with the **physical location** of the wound. **Wound size** includes measuring the longest length and width as well as the direction and length of **undermining**, **tunneling**, or **sinus tracts**. **Types of tissues** in the wound (ie, viable, nonviable, eschar, slough, granulation, smooth) should be included. Different **classification systems** exist for different wound etiologies, including staging, color system, phase of healing, or depth using partial- or full-thickness. Staging is used for pressure wounds and will be discussed in the section on pressure. A simplistic method to document is to describe colors observed in and around the wound. Describe how much of each color in percentages is present within the wound. Color description can be used for the periphery describing how far from the wound edge is a specific color. Mention **notable structures** in and around the wound, including bone, ligament, tendons, joints, orifices, or hardware from previous surgeries and note how it will affect wound progression. Document any **unusual odors** detected as well as **drainage** type (exudate or transudate), color, and amount. In the presence of **edema**, girth measures of the involved and uninvolved areas should be performed. Extent of **induration** from wound edges tracks swelling in areas where girth measures are uninformative (trunk, hips, buttocks). Pulses should be examined, and pulse quality should be described (eg, weak/thready, strong) (see Table 1-10). Assessment of **pain** should also be included. Table 15-2 provides a list of examination items.

Wound examination should be performed at least weekly. These ongoing assessments can detail wound progression, stagnation, or decline. In the situation of wound stagnation or decline, the clinician must first determine if the patient and/or staff is adhering to the care plan. Second, check that all risk factors affecting healing are addressed and determine if risk factor modifications are successful or ineffective. Finally, assess specific wound treatments and determine if the plan of care

Table 15-1

WOUND EXAMINATION TERMINOLOGY

Location	*Term/Type*	*Definition/Tips*	*Graphic*	*Healing Phase*
Wound Drainage	Exudate	Can be amber, pink, green, but will have a milky base or purulence due to increased cellular waste; thicker in texture	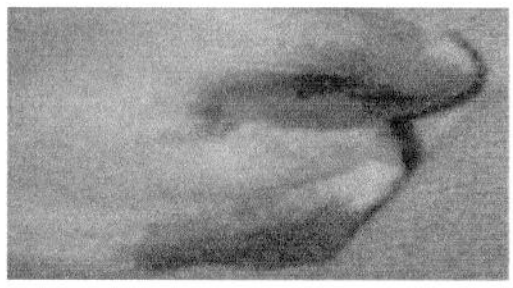	Inflammatory
	Transudate	Can be amber, pink, or yellow but will be clear; generally thinner		Proliferative
Tissues within the wound	Viable	Red or pink in color; can be smooth or uneven; tissue appears live	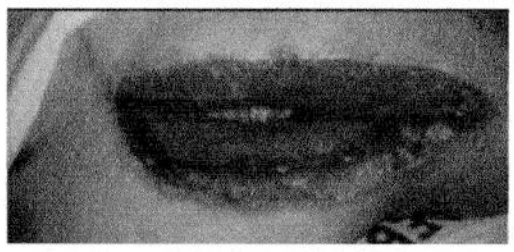	Inflammatory or proliferative
	Granulation	Red with a cobblestone texture; texture is presence of capillary loops	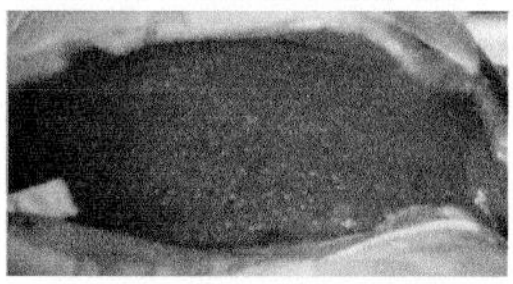	Proliferative
	Eschar	Dark, leathery or hard, dry tissue; minimally effected by moisture; a full-thickness wound; tissue is necrotic.	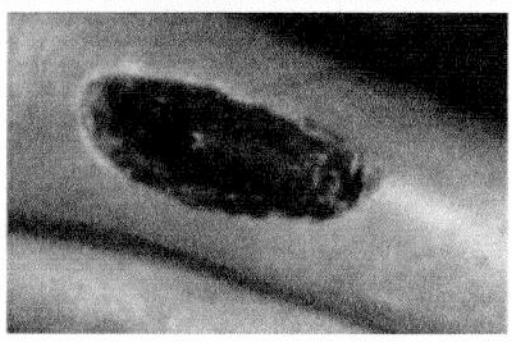	Inflammatory
	Slough	Moist necrotic tissue; can be soft or fibrinous; color can be yellow, gray, tan, or greenish	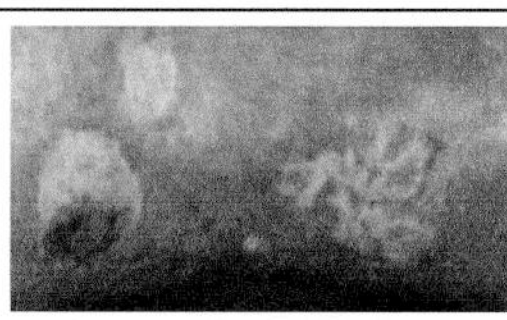	Inflammatory
	Dessication	Wound is dried out, crusty; will slow cell migration and function	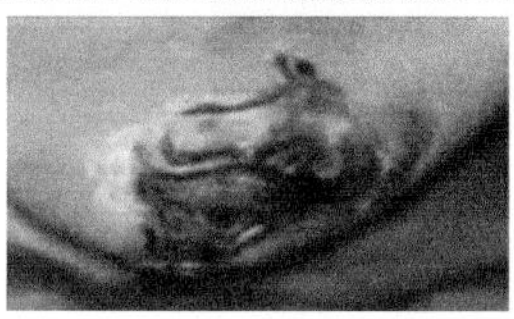	Inflammatory or proliferative

(continued)

Table 15-1 (continued)

WOUND EXAMINATION TERMINOLOGY

Location	*Term/Type*	*Definition/Tips*	*Graphic*	*Healing Phase*
Tissues within the wound	Hyper-granulation	Granulation tissue has developed to raise above the level of the epithelium; epithelial cells unable to migrate over and healing will be halted	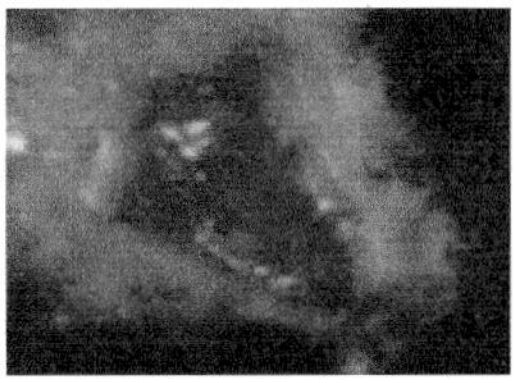	Proliferative
Wound edges	Denuded	Tissue breakdown due to skin exposure to toxic substances, often urine and feces; managed best by prompt cleaning and skin protection in incontinent episodes	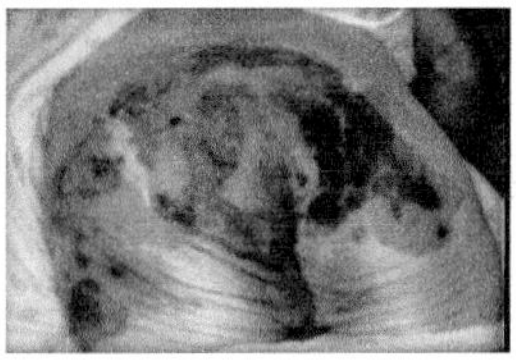	Inflammatory
	Demarcation	Clear definition between wound and periphery; positive sign body is able to isolate wound from viable tissue	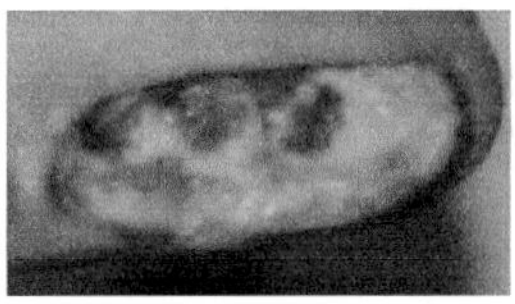	Proliferative and inflammatory
	Reepithelial-ization	Migration of epithelium into the wound bed; indicates a viable bed exists for epithelium to thrive	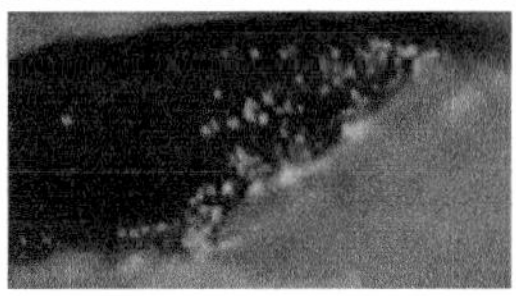	Proliferative *(continued)*

Table 15-1 (continued) WOUND EXAMINATION TERMINOLOGY				
Location	*Term/Type*	*Definition/Tips*	*Graphic*	*Healing Phase*
	Epiboly	Presents as a rounded or rolled edge in the wound; in migration, the epithelium was forced to double back on itself; wound healing will be halted if not corrected	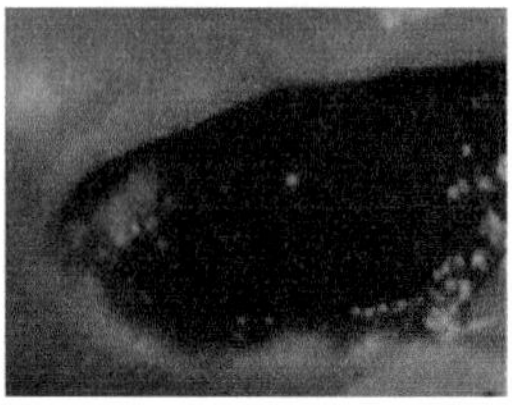	Proliferative
	Dehiscence	When the wound, particularly an incision, separates; unable to heal	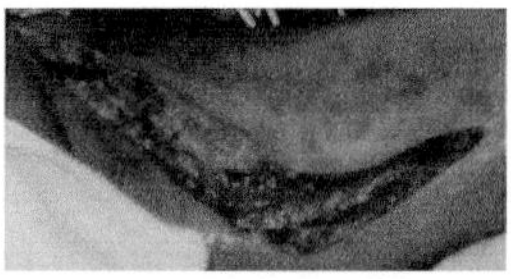	Inflammatory
Wound depths	Tunneling	Wound burrows into the tissues and connects with another wound; tract with 2 openings	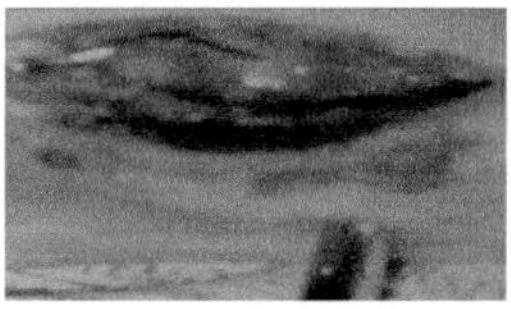	Inflammatory or proliferative
	Undermining	Wound extends beneath what is visible and spans either partially or all around wound edges; sign area experiences pressure and/or friction	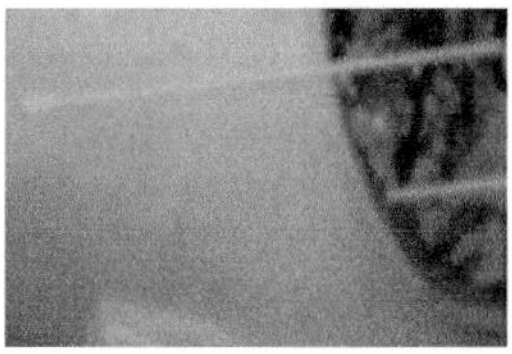	Inflammatory or proliferative
	Sinus tract	Wound burrows into tissues toward deeper structures; depths often cannot be visualized	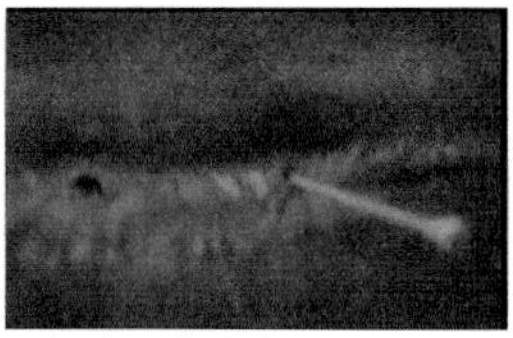	Inflammatory or proliferative

(continued)

Table 15-1 (continued)

WOUND EXAMINATION TERMINOLOGY

Location	*Term/Type*	*Definition/Tips*	*Graphic*	*Healing Phase*
Wound periphery	Induration	Determined by palpation, not visual appearance; hard feel in soft tissues; not bone or scar tissue; can be local edema or indicate an abscess in the tissues	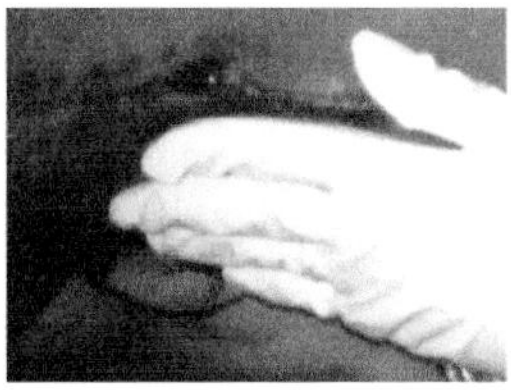	Inflammatory
	Erythema	Reddened discoloration at the wound edge; often tracked as a visual sign of resolving infection or pressure of the wound	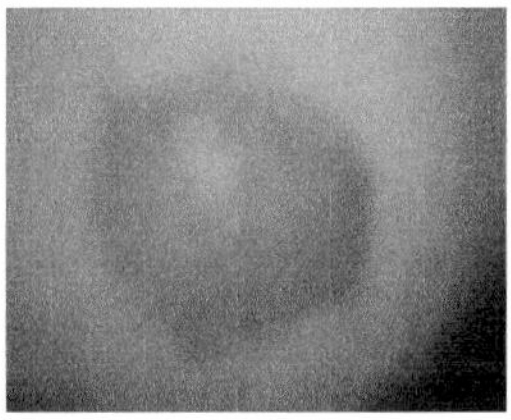	Inflammatory
	Maceration	Excess moisture at wound edges; overhydrates the epithelium causing these cells to easily rub off; halts closure or increases wound size if not managed; increased dressing absorption can help	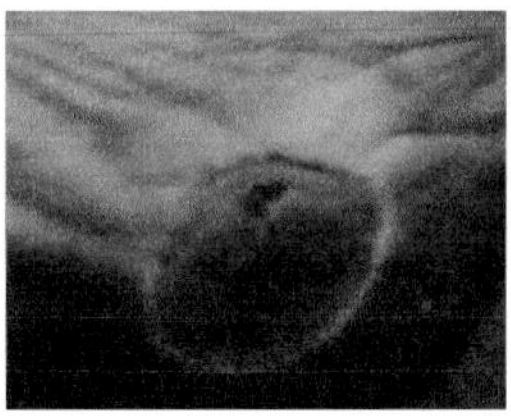	Inflammatory and proliferative
	Hemosiderin deposits	Dark staining located in the gaiter area of legs; sign of chronic venous insufficiency	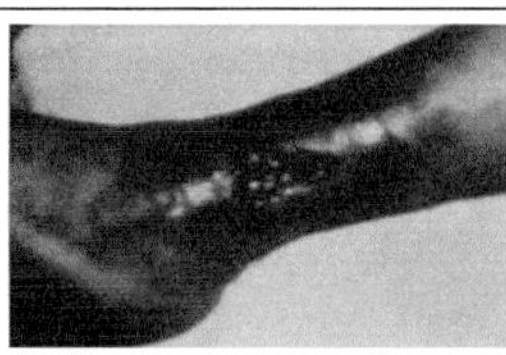	Present regardless of a wound

(continued)

Table 15-1 (continued) WOUND EXAMINATION TERMINOLOGY				
Location	*Term/Type*	*Definition/Tips*	*Graphic*	*Healing Phase*
	Excoriation	Linear lesions created by scratching; need to address source of irritation to control further wounds		Inflammatory

is addressing all aspect of the wound. If the wound does not progress in a 2-week period, a change is needed to facilitate wound healing.[1]

Wound Measurement

Comprehensive measures of the wound are important to appreciate progression or regression. Different methods exist ranging from volumetric measures to photographs. Metric measurements (centimeters and millimeters) give increased accuracy and increased ease in documentation. Photographs will need to have equal lighting, distance, and angle with each subsequent picture to accurately demonstrate wound progress. Other clinical measures are linear measures of length, width, and depth. Use of disposable rulers decreases cross-contamination. Take the longest measure in each direction. Wound tracing is another method, using a 2-ply clear plastic sheet and a permanent marker (Figure 15-5). Place the 2 stacked pieces of plastic over the wound and trace the entire wound and any notable tissues (granulation, eschar, slough), tissue formations (cluster of viable or nonviable tissue), or structures (bone, tendon, ligament). Plastic nearest the wound should be clipped away and discarded. The tracing can then be copied or measured and placed in the medical record.

Risk Factors

Wound healing involves a collaborative effort of internal and external factors to bring about closure. There are multiple known factors that impact wound healing. Some of these factors can be altered and controlled and others only noted or monitored. If all interventions are used correctly, healing progress should be seen in 2 to 4 weeks.[1] Lack of progression past this time frame may then classify the wound as chronic. Multiple factors contribute to the development of chronic wounds, such as age, mechanical stress, chemical stress, inadequate circulation, poor nutrition, ongoing infection, carcinoma, and diabetes. It is important to determine the presence of these risk factors as part of the wound assessment.

Age impacts multiple aspects of wound healing. Skin elasticity decreases with age, reducing the skin's ability to conform to stress. This is evident in wrinkling and sagging skin. Aging slows the turnover rate from the basal layer (stratum germinatum/basale) to the surface (stratum corneum) and with continual sloughing off at the surface layers, this creates a slower regeneration of the epidermal layer. Rete pegs, the tongue and groove connection of epidermis to dermis, flatten with aging. This

Table 15-2

PHYSICAL THERAPY EXAMINATION OF THE PATIENT WITH WOUNDS

Client history: Current and past medical history
Pertinent lab work: WBC, serum albumin, HbA1c
Social history: Any caregivers in house or available; are they able and willing to help?
Communication: Expressive and receptive
Home/living environment: Stairs, ability to mobilize using an assist device, clean, running water, and/or electricity
Hearing: If impaired, what other methods are needed to communicate?
Vision: If impaired, will this impact skin inspections or dressing changes?
Equipment: Assist devices they own or have available to them
Coordination: Does it impact wound acquisition or repair?
Range of motion: In general and around wound; how might it impact mobility or wound acquisition or healing?
Strength: In general; how does it impact wound acquisition or healing?
Balance: In general; does it impact wound acquisition or healing?
Sensation: Present or absent; results of monofilament testing; does it impact wound acquisition or healing (eg, lack of protective sensation will render client unable to detect if proper offloading is occurring)?
Tone: Does it impact wound healing or patient mobility?
Mobility: Assess all possible skills client has (eg, bed mobility, sitting, transfers, standing, gait); does it impact wound acquisition or healing?
Bowel/bladder function: Does it directly or indirectly effect the wound or patient safety?
Pain: In general and wound location; use a 0 to 10 pain scale
Wound location: Specific location on body; if in area of weightbearing, specify
Wound size: Length, width, and depth; if multiple wounds, use a body graph to shade the areas involved; note largest and smallest wound present
Undermining/tunneling/sinus tracts: Location and depth
Wound etiology: Pressure, arterial, venous, infection
Wound odor: Present or absent; does it impact social environment? (There are dressings available to address odor.)
Tissue types in wound: Necrotic, viable, eschar, slough, granulation tissue; tissue colors present may also be used
Wound drainage: Amount and type; does it impact wound healing (excess amounts cause peripheral maceration)?
Structures within wound: Presence of tendon, ligament, or bone; see or palpate should be noted
Periwound: Colors present, maceration, demarcation, tissue damage
Pulses and/or vascular tests: Present or absent and quality if present.

flattening reduces the adhesion of dermis to epidermis and increase the opportunity for skin injury, contusion, and tears.

Mechanical stress can involve direct, indirect, and repeated trauma. Direct pressure to the wound as in sitting, lying, or standing on a wound will prevent the edges from contracting or pulling together in the usual drawstring fashion. Indirect stress involves the skin and soft tissue around joints allowing motion. Movement around the joint will pull on wounds located near the involved joint. An example would be wounds over the patella or the elbow. Depending on location, this pulling can

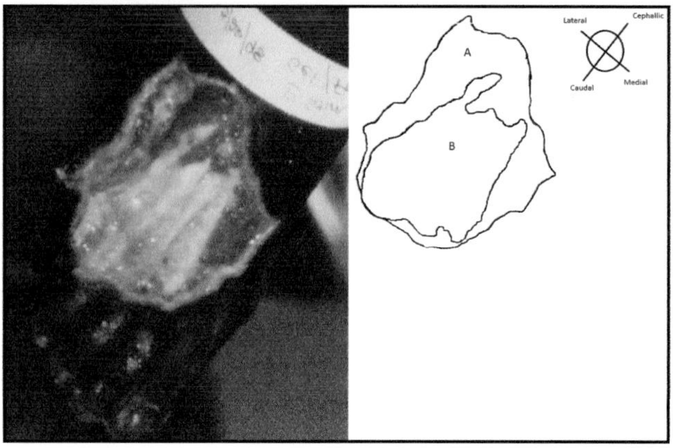

Figure 15-5. Example of wound tracing to measure the dimension of a wound as part of the wound examination.

impede or even halt wound closure. This indirect stress will need to be assessed and the physical therapist will need to determine if splinting or limiting motion will facilitate wound closure. If immobilization is needed, the joint should be placed in an optimal functional position (eg, ankle in neutral, wrist in slight extension). Individuals with limited mobility are at risk due to increased time on hardened surfaces creating excessive and repeated stress. Areas of particular concern include all bony prominences, such as the hips, sacrum, heels, back of skull, and ears (Figure 15-6). Shear and friction forces due to repeated dragging and rubbing on any area can cause wounds and negatively influence wound healing. It is important to inspect these areas regularly and alter these stresses to facilitate wound healing.

Chemical stress involves topical and enteral products that slow or stop wound healing. Drugs, such as steroids and immunosuppressive agents, are designed to decrease the inflammatory response, and a weakened inflammatory response will reduce chemotaxis and recruitment of cells that promote more advanced phases of healing. Chemotherapy is used to destroy cancerous cells but may not differentiate between cancerous and normal dividing cells. Topically, wounds can be treated with antibacterial creams and ointments (eg, Neosporin [neomycin/polymyxin B/bacitracin], bactroban, silvadene cream, bacitracin) to decrease surface bacteria delivered in a moisturizing agent. Antimicrobial and antiseptic creams and solutions (eg, silvadene cream, acetic acid, chlorpactin, Dakin's solution [sodium hypochlorite]) are applied to combat surface infections. Finally, anti-inflammatory creams and ointments (eg, triamcinolone acetonide, Temovate [clobetasol propionate], hydrocortisone) are used to reduce inflammatory reactions experienced in some dermatological conditions. In some cases, these additives are necessary and effective; however, they can also kill cells and slow or arrest wound healing. Prolonged administration overstresses the body as it needs to create more cells for wound healing. Another concern to prolonged exposure is bacteria can mutate leading to resistance. Before applying these products, determine what is happening in the wound. Does the wound need this extra assistance? Is there another method to achieve the same goal without random destruction? For example, wound cleansing can be accomplished with wound cleansers or normal saline instead of skin soaps or use dressings that promote autolysis instead of harsh chemical additives like Dakin's solution (a hypochlorite solution made from bleach) which promote destruction of necrotic tissue without harming viable cells. If a cytotoxic additive is needed, frequently assess the wound to determine if goals such as decreasing bacterial load or wound debridement are being achieved. Once goals are achieved, immediately discontinue use of the cytotoxic agent.

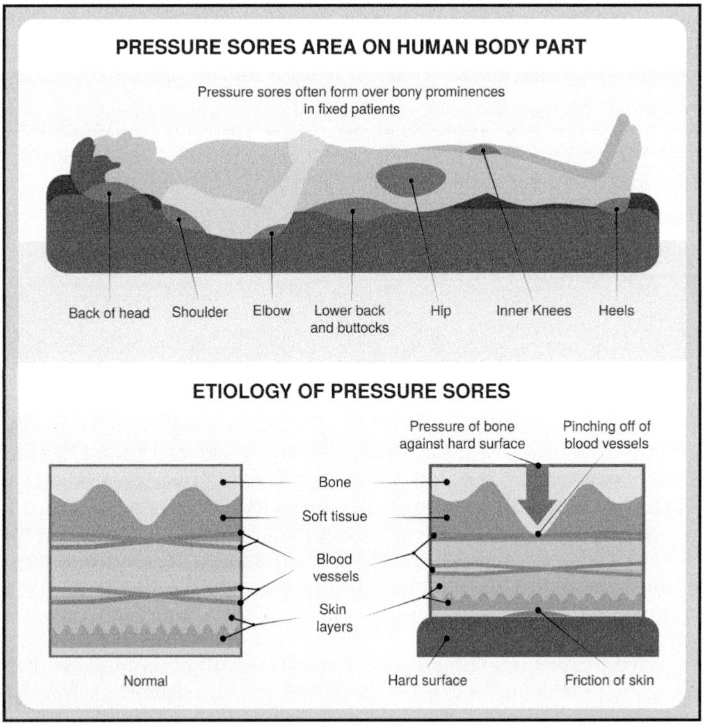

Figure 15-6. Areas of greatest pressure for the patient in bed. Note in the bottom panel how soft tissues are compressed between the hard surface of the bed and the patient's bony prominence. (Raccoonez/Shutterstock.com)

Adequate and consistent blood circulation is necessary to deliver cells and nutrients to the tissues. Arterial blood supply is discussed further in this chapter for more detail. **Oxygen** is a catalyst for many phases of wound healing. If blood oxygen levels are not adequate, healing will be delayed. An arterial blood gas (ABG; see Chapter 7) provides the most accurate measure, but is not feasible or indicated on a frequent basis. Pulse oximetry, using fingertip or earlobe probes, can evaluate peripheral oxygen saturation levels (normal $SpO_2 > 93\%$). Reduced oxygen saturation is seen predominantly in people with pulmonary diseases (eg, chronic obstructive pulmonary disease [COPD], pulmonary fibrosis) and heart failure. When monitoring oxygen saturation, pulse oximetry levels at rest and during activity should be assessed. Oxygen needs increase with activity and the individual may have adequate levels at rest but drop significantly when active. This drop on a repetitive basis can impair wound healing.

Nutrition status also impacts wound healing. Adequate calories, fluids, and supplements (eg, vitamins, minerals) are required for wound healing, and referral to a registered dietician may be essential. Nutritional decline could result from challenging food availability or food choices, decreased appetite, difficulty swallowing, and impaired digestion. If issues with chewing and swallowing are present, a speech therapist consult is beneficial. A dietician can assess nutrition related lab values, such as albumin, prealbumin, blood urea nitrogen, and other serum proteins. A dietician can also determine caloric needs, meal content, and supplements required to optimize healing. Frequent monitoring of oral intake and weight status is also informative. It should be remembered that overweight individuals can also be malnourished. Although losing weight is advantageous to the overall health of some patients, weight loss while trying to heal a wound may deplete necessary nutritional elements.

Systemic and **local infections** negatively impact wound healing. First, you must determine if the wound is clinically infected or colonized. Bacteria and microbes exist in all wounds and wounds are typically classified into 4 states:

1. Contamination
2. Colonization
3. Critical colonization
4. Infection

Contamination means bacteria are present, but are not proliferating, a phenomenon found in normal flora. **Colonization** is defined as bacteria that are present and proliferating, but not disrupting the host and surrounding tissues. **Critical colonization** describes the presence of proliferating bacteria that are disrupting only the local wound bed and arresting wound healing, but not considered clinically infected. The wound may appear healthy, but will not progress. **Infection** exists when the bacteria are proliferating and harming the host. Wound cultures will reveal over 100,000 (10^5) organisms per gram of tissue. Critically colonized and infected wounds may benefit from the use of systemic and/or topical medications. Caution needs to be exercised in type of medication and appropriate duration to be most effective. The gold standard for diagnosing wound infection is needle aspiration of the wound and biopsy of viable tissue near the wound bed. Collaborative consultation with the physician, physician's assistant, or nurse practitioner is necessary to obtain the needed tests and medication. Infection visually can be identified by inflammation. Infection differs from normal inflammation by a significant increase in white blood cells (WBCs) on serum lab values, feeling of general malaise, and possibly systemic elevation in temperature (fever).

Carcinoma can cause open wounds and a tissue biopsy is essential for accurate diagnosis. Treatment options will not follow common protocols as healing is altered. Wound healing can be negatively impacted because the body's resources necessary for wound healing may be depleted. In addition, many of the medical treatments for cancer (eg, chemotherapy, radiation therapy) negatively impact immune cell development and function and this will also negatively impact wound healing. Additional information is discussed in the section on dermatological diseases.

Diabetes does not cause wounds but increases the risks for acquiring a wound and impairs wound healing once a wound is present. Elevated blood glucose, over 110 mg/dL, increases the risk for atherosclerotic changes in the vasculature and decreases blood flow, especially to the distal lower extremities. A decrease of blood flow to bone (as seen in prolonged hyperglycemia) can soften bone causing Charcot foot deformities. Peripheral neuropathy leads to sensory and motor changes that increase the risk for repetitive trauma in the lower extremities. Repetitive trauma causes callous formation that easily split and crack, leading to small open wounds and opportunity for infection. Once tissue damage has occurred, impaired sensation prevents the individual from proper protection and offloading the wound, which obstructs wound contraction. Motor neuropathy results in claw and hammertoe deformities increasing ulceration with toes rubbing on the toe box of shoes. Blood glucose levels consistently above 200 mg/dL halt macrophage migration, suppressing normal wound healing. Nutritional status can be impaired by gastroparesis leading to abdominal discomfort, emesis, and reduction of oral intake. Retinopathy limits visual inspections of the feet and the capacity to change one's own wound dressings. Blood glucose control between 70 to 110 mg/dL is a primary goal for successful wound healing.

Etiologies, Diseases, or Conditions That Can Cause Wounds

In this section, each disorder is presented separately. It should be noted that many patients may have more than one disorder as part of their medical history. It is important that the gravity of each process is weighed on a case by case basis and a priority made to what needs to be handled first. In many cases, inadequate blood supply will need to be addressed first because an adequate blood supply is necessary for all phases of healing.

Arterial Insufficiency

Wounds occur due to a lack of adequate blood supply. Some common causes are atherosclerotic disease, arteriosclerosis obliterans, or, less frequently, trauma, entrapment syndromes, or acute embolic syndromes. Arterial wounds are commonly observed in the lower extremities (LEs) on or below the ankle and over bony prominences, particularly in areas of trauma, like the tips of toes and the malleoli. Lack of arterial circulation leads to deeper tissue damage. Clinically, arterial wounds appear "punched out" in appearance, pale in color, produce less drainage, and are painful, especially to touch. On interview, the patient may complain of pain that interferes with sleep. Elevation of the involved extremity will increase the pain and dangling the extremity off the bed provides relief. Ambulation can be limited because of claudication, a complaint of cramping, and pain after walking prolonged distances. Tissue ischemia results from inadequate blood flow to the exercising muscles causing the symptoms of claudication. Observation of the involved leg will reveal a limb pale in color and lacking hair growth, and the feet and toes may be cool to the touch. Palpation of the peroneal artery (located posterior to the lateral malleolus), posterior tibial artery (located posterior to the medial malleoli), and the dorsalis pedis artery (located on dorsum of the foot around base of first to third metatarsal) pulses can offer insight to actual blood flow of the extremity. Weak pulses or absence of pulses indicate potential peripheral arterial occlusive disease (PAOD). Additional testing can confirm the diagnosis of PAOD.

Noninvasive clinical tests can verify suspected peripheral arterial disease and determine if more invasive testing is needed. These following tests are used to assess the arterial supply to the limb. All that is needed is possibly a watch or stopwatch or extra physical assistance if the patient debility is severe.

Rubor of dependency can be assessed any time the foot is dangling below the level of the heart. This color change can be best observed on the bottoms of the feet. Darker skin colors may mask this alteration in color. The foot will appear red as if blushing. Physiologically, when the leg is dangling and blood is rushing to the toes, occlusion in the arteries interferes causing blood to shunt to the tissues instead of through the vessels. This sign is either present or absent.[2] **Venous filling time** assessment begins with the individual in supine. The patient's lower extremity should be held above the level of the heart. Assist the patient to a sitting position and begin the timer. Observe the dorsum of the foot while timing how long it takes for any vein to fill and distend above the surface. The first sign of distension ends the time. Physiologically, in supine the veins are not as engorged but in sitting the blood with gravity's assistance rushes to the feet engorging the veins. If occlusion is present in the arteries, the blood will be shunted and increase the time it takes for veins to fill with blood. Filling times greater than 20 seconds usually indicate severe occlusive disease.[1] **Capillary refill** is assessed in the toes. Press the great toe nail bed or tip of the toe until blanching (white discoloration) is observed. Release and assess in seconds how long it takes for usual color to return. Normal refill time is less than 3 seconds. Longer times may indicate arterial insufficiency. Capillary refill may not be a good indicator of proximal issues as it only alters surrounding tissues.[1] **Elevational pallor** is assessed with the patient in supine. The limb is elevated to 60 degrees above the heart and observed for color changes. Pale discoloration in lighter skin and gray hues in darker skin tones is significant. Normal circulation should reveal no color change. Change that occurs within 25 seconds indicates severe occlusive disease. Pallor within 25 to 40 seconds indicates moderate occlusive disease and pallor within 40 to 60 seconds indicates mild occlusive disease.[1] These tests give objective information to determine arterial insufficiencies based on peripheral changes. **Ankle Brachial Index** (ABI) will give numeric values to assess arterial blood flow and compare the LE pressure to upper extremity (UE) pressure, providing an indirect assessment of extremity perfusion. Equipment needed is a blood pressure cuff, a 5- to 7-MHz Doppler probe, and conductive gel. Apply the blood pressure cuff to the brachium, then, using palpation, locate the brachial artery. Apply gel and position Doppler probe at a 45-degree angle pointing in superior direction until the blood flow can be heard. Keep probe steady while inflating the cuff until the sound disappears. Deflate the cuff noting when the first sound returns. This is the brachial number. Apply the cuff to the midcalf and palpate the peroneal artery (posterior to lateral malleoli), posterior tibial artery (posterior to medial malleoli), or dorsalis pedis artery (dorsal aspect of mid foot). Apply gel and determine ankle number same as with brachial number. Divide ankle over brachial for the ABI.

- ABI 1.0 to 1.3: Normal range
- ABI 0.6 to 0.8: Borderline perfusion
- ABI $\leq$0.5: Severe ischemia; avoid compression; wound healing unlikely
- ABI $\leq$0.4: Critical limb ischemia
- ABI $\geq$1.3: Abnormally high range, typically because of calcification of the vessel wall in the patient with diabetes; toe cuff pressures more accurate

Restoration of blood flow is the first priority in arterial insufficiency, especially if severe enough to cause open wounds. This is typically accomplished through surgical interventions. It should be noted, not all occlusions can be revascularized and wound protection measures may need to be implemented. Nonsurgical treatments include appropriate dressings, offloading or pressure redistribution, electrical stimulation, wound protection, exercise training, and patient/family education. The severity of the disease will dictate the dressings needed. If circulation is poor (ABI $\leq$0.4) wound healing is impossible. Treatment options will be limited to protection and containment of bacteria. Wounds are left dry or covered with antimicrobial solutions to discourage bacterial growth. Amputation of digits or the limb may be necessary if limb salvage is not possible or the wound poses a threat to the peripheral tissue or overall patient health. Wounds present in areas with an ABI greater than 0.5 can be treated with dressings that provide moisture, as arterial wounds tend to be dry. These dressings will facilitate autolysis (self-debridement) of any necrotic tissue while supporting granulation, reepithelialization, and contraction. Exercise such as ankle pumps, lower extremity ROM, progressive resistive exercises, and walking or biking to the claudication threshold are beneficial activity choices. These activities may help increase the flow of lesser used collateral arteries over time. Proper skin cleansing with mild, nonirritating soaps or skin cleansers and the use of moisturizers can help prevent further ulceration due to cracking of dry skin. Assess if the wound contraction is eliminated due to pressure or pulling on the wound. Broken skin is much like broken bones. If pressure is placed on them continually, it cannot heal properly. Offloading or pressure redistribution of the wound area using proper fitting shoes may delay further wound damage and allow enhanced patient mobility by decreasing pressure and pain. Offloading devices, like the Multi Podus (AliMed) or custom-made splints, can help prevent and protect wounds, especially in the heels and toes. Assistive devices, including walkers and canes, combined with weightbearing restrictions may decrease or eliminate pressure on the foot or leg. Consider the patient's abilities, skills, comfort, safety, and possible limb salvage. A wheelchair might be needed if the patient is unable to safely mobilize. Wheelchairs offer more options in pressure relief and provide the patient greater independence and self-esteem than being bed bound.

Venous Insufficiency

Venous insufficiency is the ineffective return of blood to the heart, usually from the LEs. Visual inspection shows swelling of the legs with the possible presence of varicose veins and/or spider veins. Edema will increase when the legs are in a dependent position and decrease with elevation. A brown discoloration will appear over time, initially in patches progressing to circumferential coverage and located between the malleoli and lower to mid-calf, the gaiter area. This brown staining is termed **hemosiderin staining** and is caused by lysis of red blood cells in the tissues. Venous insufficiency wounds are typically below the knee and above or around the ankles, irregular in shape, and may produce excessive discharge. The discharge will decrease with better control of the edema through elevation and compression.

The underlying pathology for venous insufficiency is venous hypertension. Venous hypertension can be caused by obstruction, valve incompetence, and muscle pump failure or weakness. The common cause of venous obstruction is deep vein thrombosis (DVT). Other causes include pregnancy, obesity, congestive heart failure, ascites, tumors, or severe trauma to the leg. Obstruction blocks flow of the blood causing venous distention and leakage of deoxygenated blood into the interstitial tissues. Distention causes the vein leaflets to separate and not completely seal, permitting retrograde blood flow and venous pooling. Muscle pump failure is poorly understood, but may include inactivity, neuromuscular abnormalities, or musculoskeletal changes resulting from aging, arthritis, or a sedentary lifestyle. Though leakage is from the venous system, the reduction of interstitial fluid it the responsibility of the lymphatic system (see Lymphedema later in this section).

The optimal treatment option for venous insufficiency is 30 to 40 mm Hg of compression to control peripheral edema. Chronic edema leads to skin breakdown and in the presence of an existing wound, impairs wound healing. The pressure of the accumulated fluids flowing out to the wound plus the force of the excess fluid expanding the tissues keep the wound bed from closing or contracting. Successful treatment must first establish if the patient has adequate arterial circulation before compression is applied. An ABI greater than or equal to 0.8 is recommended. Compression applied to a limb with inadequate arterial flow can lead to limb ischemia and amputation. Compression at lower levels (20 mm Hg) has been used with ABI lower than 0.8 but must be closely monitored. Results are similar to higher compression but require a longer period of time. Second, patient compliance and ability to return for follow-up care must be known before embarking on compression.

Compression is offered in many forms. Three- and four-layer wrap systems are available to use with venous insufficiency in the presence of wounds, offering both compression and absorption of wound drainage.. These systems must be applied properly and are generally changed within 3 to 4 days after the first application, and weekly thereafter until wound closure is achieved. Wound dressings that provide absorption if used under compression will need to provide uniform depth to prevent pressure areas due to sporadic bulky spots. Venous insufficiency is a life-long problem for patients and requires ongoing treatment. Compression garments that can be washed and worn will be needed. Custom and off-the-shelf compression garments (eg, socks, stockings) are available and should be used anytime the patient's legs are in the dependent position. Ideally, these garments should be purchased 2 at a time, so a clean pair is available while the other is being cleaned. Garments should be purchased every 6 to 12 months based on manufacturer directions. Inelastic compression (eg, CircAid) has also proven helpful with a longer use life than elastic compression. Inelastic compression is a series of stiff straps and adjustable stiff sleeve that cover the edematous area and offer rigid support. Elastic and inelastic garments should be removed for bedtime, prolonged supine, and positions with legs elevated. Mechanical sequential compression pump systems are used at rest and will offer short-term compression, especially at the end of the day. These devices should be used in conjunction with compression garments that are worn during the day. Weight loss and LE elevation coupled with exercise will help decrease LE edema. Patients with ABI less than 0.8 should combine frequent elevation with exercise as the safest treatment option. ACE wraps (long stretch) bandages provide compression but over extended wear periods they will wrinkle and bunch causing pressure areas. ACE wraps require complete unwrapping and rewrapping, making them more useful for short durations (12 to 24 hours or less). Stockings are recommended because wrinkles and bunching are easier to identify and fix.

Lymphedema results from decreased return of the protein rich lymphatic fluid to the circulation, resulting from mechanical insufficiency or damage to the lymph system. All edema regardless of the etiology is due to failure of the lymph system. It is responsible for clearing all edema in the interstitial spaces, interstitial fluid does not reenter the vein at the peripheral level as previously thought. There are 4 stages in lymphedema: Stage 0—swelling not yet evident, Stage 1—edema is present, but resolves with elevation, Stage 2—elevation alone does not reduce tissue swelling and pitting is present, and Stage 3—dermal skin changes, elephantiasis including lobular folds. Lymphedema needs to be managed by therapists with knowledge in complete decongestive therapy (CDT). CDT typically involves 5 components: manual lymph drainage, compression (variable types based on stage of edema), exercise, skin care, and patient education to manage this life long disorder. Lack of proper management of the edema in the presence of a wound will render poor wound healing. Proper diagnosis and treatment of lymphedema is essential for positive outcomes.

Pressure

Pressure is defined as the amount of force applied perpendicular to a surface per unit area of application.[3] Pressure injuries are any lesion caused by unrelieved pressure resulting in damage of underlying tissue and are frequently observed in the mobility challenged. Wounds are found over bony prominences, as tissue compression is greatest in these areas (see Figure 15-6). Bony prominences normally include back of the skull, ears, shoulders, scapula, elbows, sacrum, ischial tuberosities, greater trochanters, knees, heels, metatarsal heads, and toes. In the presence of bony anomalies or deformities other area of pressure may exist. Pressure alone is not the only force involved in creating tissue injury. **Shear** stress results from the application of a force parallel to the surface of an object while the base of the object stays stationary (eg, buttocks positioned in a bed then the head of the bed is elevated causing a downward slide on fixed buttocks).[2] **Friction** is defined as action of one object rubbing against the other (eg, frequent motion of the heel sliding and dragging on the bed sheets with hip and knee flexion and extension).[2] Pressure injuries are characterized by undermining with damage nearest to bone. A cross section view of undermining would look like a vase with the wider portion in the structures below the epidermis and the narrow opening in the epidermis (Figure 15-7). As pressure alone is not the sole culprit in wounding, but also includes shear and friction, damage does not always occur at the site of bony prominences. The pressure injury staging system was developed to classify the degree of tissue damage observed (Table 15-3). Pressure injuries can be observed in a variety of patients from bed bound to ambulatory and these wounds need frequent monitoring and intervention to determine the source of the stressor and how to eliminate it.

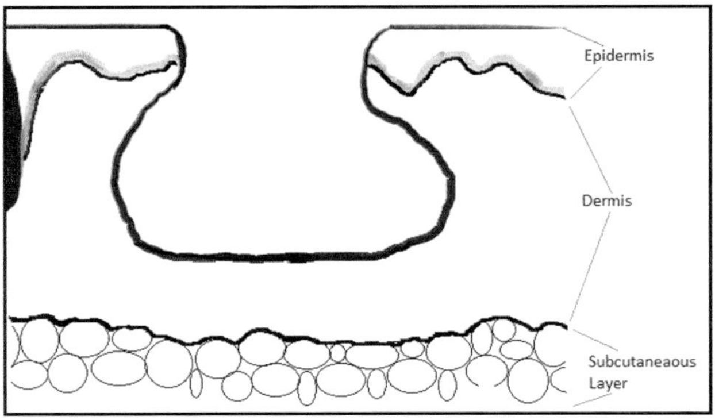

Figure 15-7. Cross-section of undermining.

The optimal treatment for pressure injuries is pressure redistribution, also called **offloading**. Pressure should be removed from the wound region with redistribution to the largest area possible. Two aspects of pressure redistribution will be reviewed: supine and sitting. Frequent position changes greatly decrease pressure. Supine patients should be turned every 2 hours with utilization of multiple positions. Options include supine, side-lying, prone (if tolerable), one-quarter side-lying, and one-quarter prone. If a wound is present, the patient should be positioned off the injury at all times. Assess the patient for any other problems that may prohibit certain positions and create a positioning program that includes all permissible options. Pillows and wedges can be used to maintain positions and to separate and cushion bony prominences, such as the knees. Specialized beds, mattresses, and overlays can be used. Many of these are pressure reducing or decreasing overall pressure, not relieving (complete reduction). One feature these devices offers is pressure distribution by conforming to all the body curves and surfaces as demonstrated in Figure 15-8. This equipment is not a replacement for good turning practices but can help prevent further ulceration. Special needs beds are also available. For example, bariatric beds are wider and sturdier in construction. Beds that convert to a sitting position promote upright positions in a mobility challenged patient. A patient's heels are more vulnerable and can breakdown even with good turning practices and pressure reducing devices. Heels are susceptible to breakdown because they carry large amounts of the LE weight on a small bony area and if neuropathy and/or arterial insufficiency are present, heel breakdown is highly probable. Pillows placed under the entire length of the calf leaving the heel suspended is an easy method of pressure redistribution. Heels are especially vulnerable in the client that has undergone recent LE orthopedic or vascular surgeries. It is important to educate these patients in heel floating, or complete suspension, using pillows to prevent ulceration. Splints can be made or purchased that will relieve all heel pressure by suspension. Some of these devices will also position the ankle in neutral to help prevent foot drop and plantar flexion contracture (eg, Multi Podus boot).

Sitting positions require additional considerations. Weight shifts in sitting should be performed every 15 minutes. Does the chair adequately fit the patient? Oversized chairs offer decreased UE and trunk support, causing significant lateral shifts and decreased leverage for weight shifts. Small chairs create additional pressure areas and can complicate transfers out of the chair. A chair/wheelchair with a firm seat and adequate seat cushion that provides good weight distribution without added pressures to bony prominences is ideal. Assess the patient's wound location and determine in what position the wound experiences the greatest pressure and avoid that position as much as possible. Sacral wounds are frequently mistaken for being acquired in sitting, and often the supine reclined position is the culprit. Assess the

Table 15-3

International NPUAP/EPUAP Pressure Ulcer Classification System

A pressure ulcer is localized injury to the skin and/or underlying tissue usually over a bony prominence, as a result of pressure, or pressure in combination with shear. A number of contributing or confounding factors are also associated with pressure ulcers; the significance of these factors is yet to be elucidated.

Category	*Description*
Stage I: Non-Blanchable Erythema 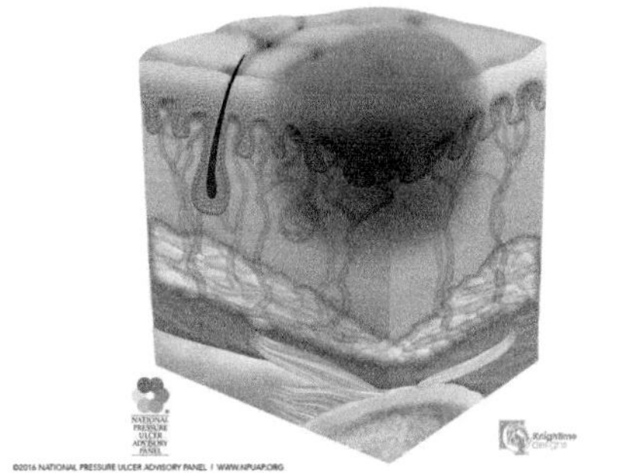	Intact skin with non-blanchable redness of a localized area, usually over a bony prominence. Darkly pigmented skin may not have visible blanching; its color may differ from the surrounding area. The area may be painful, firm, soft, warmer, or cooler as compared to adjacent tissue. Stage I may be difficult to detect in individuals with dark skin tones. May indicate at risk individuals (a heralding sign of risk).
Stage II: Partial-Thickness Skin Loss 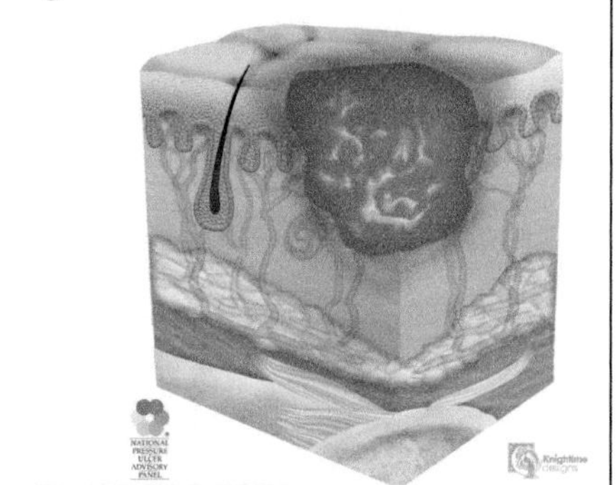	Partial-thickness loss of dermis presenting as a shallow, open ulcer with a red-pink wound bed without slough. May also present as an intact or open/ruptured serum filled blister. Presents as a shiny or dry shallow ulcer without slough or bruising.* This stage should not be used to describe skin tears, tape burns, perineal dermatitis, maceration, or excoriation. *Bruising indicates suspected deep tissue injury.
Stage III: Full-Thickness Skin Loss 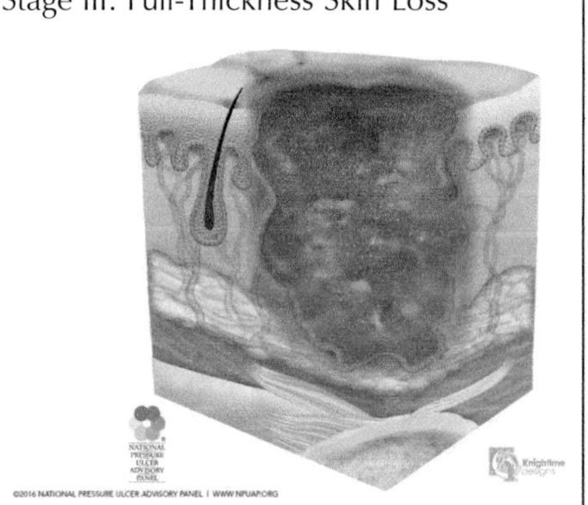	Full-thickness tissue loss. Subcutaneous fat may be visible but bone, tendon, or muscle are not exposed. Slough may be present but does not obscure the depth of tissue loss. May include undermining and tunneling. The depth of a Stage III pressure injuries varies by anatomical location. The bridge of the nose, ear, occiput, and malleolus do not have subcutaneous tissue and Stage III injuries can be shallow. In contrast, areas of significant adiposity can develop extremely deep Stage III pressure injuries. Bone/tendon is not visible or directly palpable. *(continued)*

Table 15-3 (continued)

INTERNATIONAL NPUAP/EPUAP PRESSURE ULCER CLASSIFICATION SYSTEM

Category	*Description*
Stage IV: Full-Thickness Tissue Loss 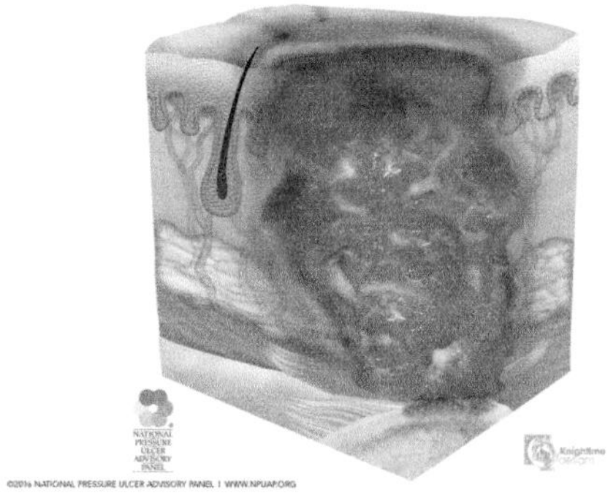	Full-thickness tissue loss with exposed bone, tendon, or muscle. Slough or eschar may be present on some parts of the wound bed. Often include undermining and tunneling. The depth of a Stage IV pressure ulcer varies by anatomical location. The bridge of the nose, ear, occiput, and malleolus do not have subcutaneous tissue and these ulcers can be shallow. Stage IV pressure injuries can extend into muscle and/or supporting structures (eg, fascia, tendon, joint capsule) making osteomyelitis possible. Exposed bone/tendon is visible or directly palpable.
Unstageable: Depth Unknown With Eschar 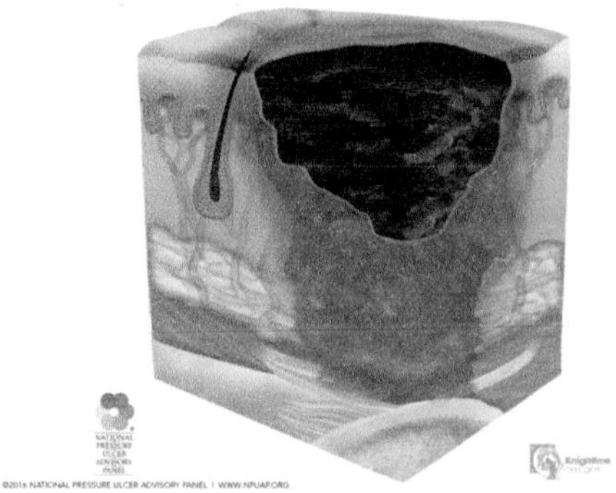	Full-thickness tissue loss in which the base of the ulcer is covered by slough (yellow, tan, gray, green, or brown) and/or eschar (tan, brown, or black) in the wound bed. Until enough slough and/or eschar is removed to expose the base of the wound, the true depth, and therefore Category/Stage, cannot be determined. Stable (dry, adherent, intact without erythema or fluctuance) eschar on the heels serves as the body's natural (biological) cover and should not be removed.
Suspected Deep Tissue Injury: Depth Unknown 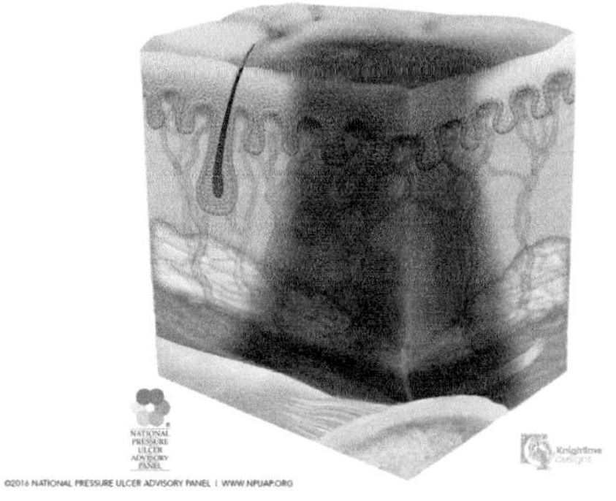	Purple or maroon localized area of discolored intact skin or blood-filled blister due to damage of underlying soft tissue from pressure and/or shear. The area may be preceded by tissue that is painful, firm, mushy, boggy, warmer, or cooler as compared to adjacent tissue. Deep tissue injury may be difficult to detect in individuals with dark skin tones. Evolution may include a thin blister over a dark wound bed. The wound may further evolve and become covered by thin eschar. Evolution may be rapid, exposing additional layers of tissue even with optimal treatment.

Figures reprinted with permission from National Pressure Ulcer Advisory Panel (NPUAP), European Pressure Ulcer Advisory Panel (EPUAP) and Pan Pacific Pressure Injury Alliance. *Prevention and Treatment of Pressure Ulcers: Quick Reference Guide.* Emily Haesler (Ed.). Cambridge Media: Perth, Australia; 2014.

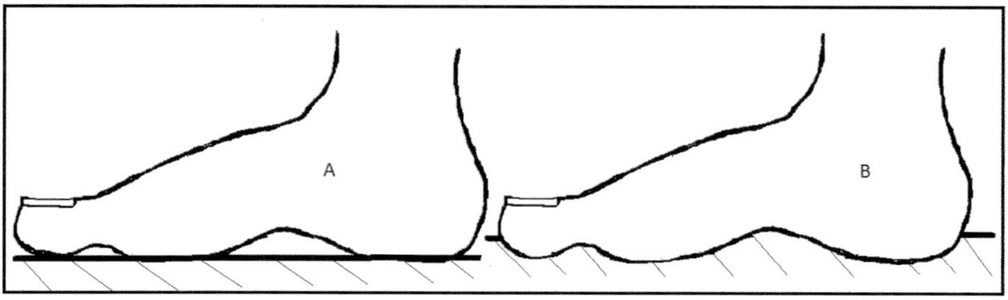

Figure 15-8. Example of pressure distribution. Note how the surface conforms to the entire foot in B providing optimal pressure distribution compared to A.

patient in sitting and determine if the wound is being compressed. If so, can alterations in the chair or chair cushion be made for proper fit, positioning, and pressure relief? If not, should the patient remain in bed until the ulcers heal? For patients who are wheelchair dependent, the physical therapist will need to assess the chair, cushion, and patient in the chair to determine if adjustments are needed to prevent repeated breakdown. Computerized pressure mapping systems are available to visually measure the effectiveness of the cushion and chair. This can be performed as a single assessment but is more informative to assess over the course of a day. Referral to a seating clinic is imperative for wheelchair dependent individuals. It will be a waste of resources to simply order them new equipment without a proper assessment. Over time bodies change in shape and pressure distribution; the chair must support these changes.

Additional tips to reduce pressure wounds include:

- Avoid dragging the patient for repositioning; lift the patient and/or use draw sheets.
- Good perineal hygiene; cleaning stool and urine from the skin as soon as possible; using appropriate cleansers to reduce rubbing on fragile skin; barrier ointments and creams to protect the skin can prevent breakdown and reduce pain.
- Strengthening and transfer training can help increase mobility and provides the patient the opportunity to independently manage his or her own turning, weight shifts, and toileting.
- Patient and family education will promote active participation in the patient's care for short- and long-term success.

Neuropathies

Neuropathic wounds are most common in patients with diabetes. Other causes of peripheral neuropathies include Hansen's disease, chronic alcoholism, latent syphilis, spinal cord injuries, and critical illness. This section will focus on diabetic neuropathies. The section on diabetes in Risk Factors describes many of the complications and challenges these patients face, including alterations in microvascular supply, sensory and motor neuropathy, Charcot deformities, and impaired immune function and wound healing (see Chapter 10). Peripheral neuropathies cause the patient to experience pain, and the absence of sensation in later stages may cause wounds to go undetected. Wounds are typically located around the nail beds, tips of toes, bony prominences, and plantar surfaces of the feet. Wounds may appear punched out, pale in color, and surrounded by callous due to repeated trauma.

Clinical assessments may include ABI, but results are limited because small vessel disease is not detected by ABI and inaccuracies are associated with atherosclerotic changes in the vessels. Toe cuff pressures may offer more useful information. Blood glucose and glycosylated hemoglobin monitoring are important laboratory value measures (see Chapters 2 and 10). Blood glucose control can be one of the most important factors for wound healing for the patient with diabetes. Sensation testing is imperative to identify the location and extent of the neuropathy. Monofilament testing will offer objective and specific assessment of peripheral sensation. The monofilament size used is 5.07 and this applies 10 g of pressure to the skin surface. A 5.07 monofilament assess protective sensation, the ability to detect contact with other objects. Testing is done only on intact skin, not the wound or over the callous, and multiple site testing is recommended as shown in Figure 15-9. The patient is asked to close his or eyes and the filament should contact the skin at a 90 degrees angle for approximately 1 second, buckle slightly on impact, then be quickly removed. The patient is asked to identify the location of the contact. Use an alternating rhythm and occasional fake contact to gain a genuine assessment. The inability to perceive the 10 g of force the monofilament applies is associated with clinically significant large-fiber neuropathy. Keep in mind this does not mean the patient feels nothing. Many times, patients can detect deep pressure, which fools the individual in to believing he or she has intact sensation. Vibration testing using a 128 Hz tuning fork should also be performed using the same locations as noted in Figure 15-9. Manual muscle testing of the LEs and reflex testing of the patellar and Achilles tendons assesses neuromuscular involvement.

Offloading or pressure redistribution of the immediate wound area is critical. Standing or weightbearing pressure redistribution devices range from splints, adapted postoperative shoes, cast boots, and custom fit shoes with custom fit inserts. These devices use material that reduce pressure at and around the wound site and conform to the curves and varying depths of the foot to distribute body weight over the largest possible area. The gold standard is total contact casting or total contact cast splints. This technique requires special clinician training. It offers optimal offloading of the wound area with contouring of the entire foot and leg and added stability at the ankle. Part of the superiority of casting over splinting involves the inability to remove the cast. Cast compliance can be 100%, but weekly assessment is necessary to ensure proper fit and wound management. Orthotists, pedorthists, and podiatrists can create custom shoes and inserts, but often prefer to wait for wound closure prior to provision of these custom devices. Custom shoes and inserts are permanent, long-term devices that require an exact fit and are difficult to alter if further wounds or amputations occur.

The physical therapist should also establish mobility needs and limit gait to basic needs (bed to chair, chair to bathroom, and use of wheelchair over gait) if wound healing is compromised. Walkers, crutches, and wheelchairs assist the patient in offloading the LE. The patient will need to be evaluated and trained in the proper use of the device on all terrain he or she will encounter. Proper footgear and assist devices may provide the optimal conditions to promote patient safety, stability, and wound closure. Many individuals with diabetes can develop nephropathy and kidney insufficiency leading to variable LE edema. Additionally, peripheral neuropathies can cause foot drop that can be controlled with the use of an AFO. Many AFOs are made of hard plastic and will not adjust to varying leg circumferences. Variable edema with lack of peripheral sensation can significantly increase the risk for pressure injury development with an AFO. Direct consultation with an orthotist clarifying these specific problems can yield a safe, custom-molded device. Patient and caregiver education in proper skin inspections is vital to prevent foot ulcers. Finally, callous must be kept trimmed and pliable to prevent further interference with wound contraction and further opportunities for infection. Wound dressings may need to provide moisture, unless an infection is present or if the wound is in the inflammatory phase of healing. If significant drainage is present, an absorptive dressing may be effective.

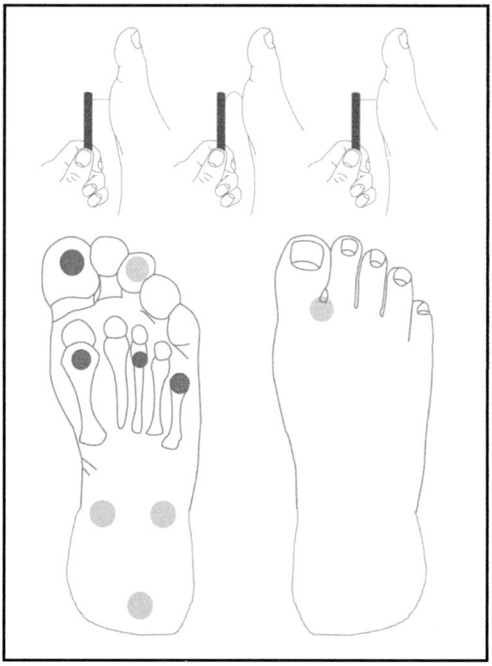

Figure 15-9. The 5.07 Semmes-Weinstein monofilament testing is performed on 10 sites (as shown) to evaluate all dermatomes of the foot. (Adapted with permission from Boulton AJ, Armstrong DG, Albert SF, et al. Comprehensive foot examination and risk assessment. *Diabetes Care.* 2008;31[8]:1679-1685.)

Dermatological Diseases

Dermatological lesions comprise many diseases that may include cancers, allergic reactions, immunological complications, insect bites, and factitious (self-inflicted) wounds. Clinically, these wounds are recognized because of a unique presentation and failure to respond to typical treatment options. These lesions are best diagnosed using skin and tissue biopsy and require management by specific medical professionals, such as a dermatologists, oncologists, or psychiatrist.

Treatment options of open wounds with dermatological issues may involve odor control, simple protection, or maintenance until the primary etiology can be controlled. An example is **pyoderma gangrenosum**, which is characterized by a blue-gray or battleship gray periwound, with lesions that are typically painful and begin after a local trauma, such as an ant bite, bee sting, or local abrasion. The wound quickly progresses to a larger, necrotic wound. Localized trauma to the area initiates the destructive process and may be exacerbated by repeated trauma. Typically, necrotic tissue will slow wound healing and should be removed. With pyoderma gangrenosum, debriding agents may worsen the wound. Anti-inflammatory and immunosuppressive agents are often prescribed. Moist wound healing principles can offer comfort and facilitate healing as the condition stabilizes. Other dermatologic lesions will have their own unique presentations and require specific interventions that may not follow conventional methods. It is important to understand the specific etiology and proper treatment to select the most efficacious intervention.

Burns

Burns are caused by 4 main sources: thermal, chemical, radiation, and electrical exposure. Burns are typically classified based on the depth of damage (Figure 15-10). Firs-degree burns are superficial and involve the epidermis only. Second

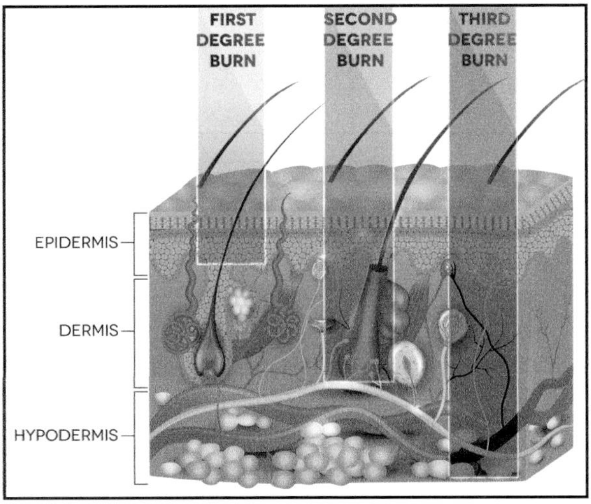

Figure 15-10. Simplified classification of skin burns. Note that second degree burns can be classified as superficial partial-thickness and full-thickness (see text for greater detail). (Tefi/Shutterstock.com)

degree burns are classified as superficial partial-thickness, involving the epidermis and upper layers of dermis and full-thickness, involving the epidermis and deeper regions of dermis. Third degree burns are full-thickness injuries involving the epidermis and complete destruction of the dermis. Finally, fourth degree burns are full-thickness damage extending to fascia, muscle, or bone.[1] Additional classification systems are used to estimate the size of the burn as a percentage of total body surface. One system is the rule of nines that divides the entire body into anatomic regions each representing 9% of the total body surface (Figure 15-11). This calculation works best with adults. Children under age 15 do not share the same proportions and the rule of nines is inaccurate. The Lund-Browder chart divides each body part into percentages and is suitable for children under 15, making it more accurate for variable ages. Partial- to full-thickness burns are measured with each system. These measures are initially used to assess fluid replenishment needs.

Initial treatment begins with medical stabilization and topical antimicrobials (eg, Silvadene cream) can be used to prevent additional infections. Once the patient is stable, other treatment options are begun, including skin grafting as needed. New advances continue to emerge in the areas of skin replacement (bioengineered skin), especially in burns involving extensive skin loss. Moist wound healing principles can facilitate wound healing and offer pain relief. Clinicians may continue to use antimicrobial creams until wound closure, even though these creams can slow wound healing. Newly healed burn wounds can easily dry and crack. Regular moisturizing with an appropriate cream or ointment is recommended. Lotions and some creams contain higher amounts of water and will not be effective. Higher solid contents in creams, butters, and ointments are needed. Hypertrophic scaring can be functionally limiting and cosmetically unappealing. Compression garments at 30 to 40 mm Hg are worn from the time of closure throughout the maturation phase of healing to shape and reduce hypertrophic scarring. Adhesive scar management sheets can provide local direct pressure to smaller or difficult areas (eg, cervical region). Compression must be continued over a 1- to 2-year period, the duration of the maturation phase, for maximal effectiveness. Soft tissue mobilization, ROM, strength, mobility, and gait training are important interventions. If immobilization of a joint is needed to facilitate wound healing, ensure the joint is in a functional position (eg, ankle dorsiflexion in neutral, wrist in slight extension). Working with the patient throughout the healing phases is imperative to maximize functional mobility.

Figure 15-11. Rule of 9s to estimate body surface area involved in burn injuries. (Blamb/Shutterstock.com)

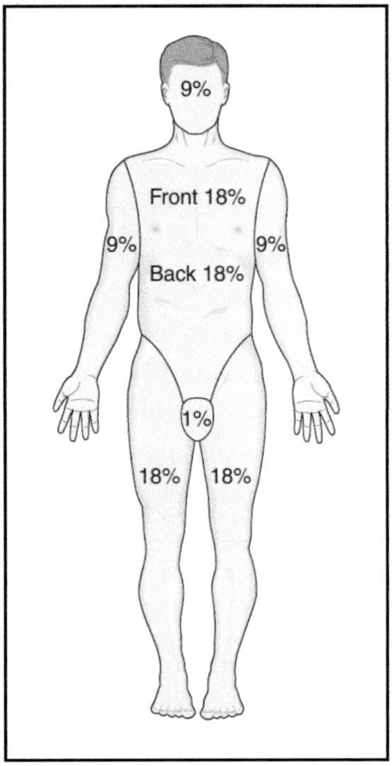

Surgical Incisions and Amputations

Surgical incisions were introduced in the section Method of Wound Closure, specifically primary wound closure. Most surgical incisions will close with minimal intervention. Stitches or staples are typically removed in 10 to 14 days, but, in some cases, surgeons may leave them in longer for patients with slower healing times, such as individuals with diabetes, the elderly, and those on prescribed corticosteroids. Skin glues and Steri-Strips (3M) are other alternatives to staples and sutures. New incisions should be kept clean and protected. The wound edges should remain approximated and an optimal moist environment provided. Wound contraction is impaired with excessive strain or pulling at or around the incision site and should be avoided. If bone, ligament, or tendons were incised, healing time duration is prolonged to 6 to 8 weeks. The physical therapists should discern which movements and activities of daily living (ADLs) may need to be altered or avoided to allow proper healing. One example is the sternotomy approach used in cardiac and thoracic surgeries. Patients who are overweight, have diagnosed diabetes, or have experienced prolonged mechanical ventilation, a perioperative infection, or increased weakness are at risk for sternotomy dehiscence. It may be prudent to limit UE weightbearing to afford proper bone healing in this population. Patients who require extensive UE function and weightbearing for mobility may have to find alternative or adaptive solutions.

Amputations involve the partial or complete loss of a limb or digit. The amputated region includes all involved damaged and nonviable tissue and may include adjoining viable tissue but should provide residual limb length to support a prosthesis if possible. Amputations of the leg include below knee amputation (BKA), where the foot and ankle are removed; above the knee amputation (AKA), where the foot, ankle, and knee joints are removed; and hip disarticulation, where the entire leg is removed up to the hip joint. Several approaches have been applied to the foot from individual digits, transmetatarsal amputation (TMA), the removal of the toes and a portion of the metatarsals, and ankle disarticulation, the removal of the foot at the tibial-calcaneus joint.

Common therapeutic interventions for the amputee include ROM to joints around the amputation site to ensure functional movement, strengthening exercises of the involved and uninvolved limb and UEs to prepare for altered mobility needs, and examination of balance in sitting and standing. Limb loss alters the center of gravity and may require extensive balance retraining in sitting and standing. Surgeons will have different protocols regarding prosthetic fitting, and the therapist must be familiar with each physician's preferences prior to initiating patient education and training. Prosthetic fitting usually includes waiting until the staples are removed, good wound tensile strength is established, and there is a stable limb circumference. ACE wraps initially after surgery help shape the residual limb but should be exchanged for stump shrinkers for ease of patient application and smooth fit. Stump shrinkers or ACE wraps conform to the residual limb and should be applied so greater pressure is provided distally to decrease edema and shape the residual limb in preparation for the prosthesis. Incorrect ACE wrapping techniques can damage the limb. ACE wraps will need to be changed up to 3 times per day to prevent wrinkling and avoid point specific pressure potentially causing tissue damage.

Extensive wounds, as seen in pressure and burn injuries, can be slow to heal or need assistance for closure. Skin and/or muscle grafting are available and performed by plastic surgeons. Full-thickness skin grafts are done for cosmetic purposes (eg, facial burns) and in areas of high stress (eg, feet, hands). Split-thickness skin grafts are used for larger coverage areas. Autologous skin grafts are harvested from the patient and common donor sites include the thigh and back. Muscle grafting procedures are used to fill deeper damaged areas. Grafting will require immobilization at the graft site to allow for graft, skin, and muscle adherence and viability. The physical therapist's role includes assisting in immobilization of surgical areas and placing any joints that will negatively impact the surgical site in neutral functional positions. The physical therapist should assess joints that are allowed to move for functional ROM and strength to prepare for current and future mobility needs (eg, transfers, gait, wheelchair mobility). While staples are present at the surgical site weightbearing on the site should be avoided. Once staples are removed and/or wound healing is deemed adequate, weightbearing and progressive ROM should be initiated. The surgical site should be continually assessed for integrity with progressively added stress (weightbearing and stretching). If the wound remains intact, continue to gradually progress, if regression or breakdown is detected, weightbearing and stretching need to be reassessed, and possibly stopped, until healing has progressed.

Debridement and Wound Healing

Necrotic tissue is dead matter within the wound bed (see Table 15-1). It provides a medium for bacteria to thrive and increases the risk for local and systemic infections. Additionally, necrotic tissue creates a physical barrier impeding wound closure. Necrotic tissue is not viable and appears yellow, gray, green, or black. Eschar is thick, tough, dead tissue that cannot be fully hydrated and indicates the wound is full-thickness in depth. Slough is dead tissue that remains moist or can be penetrated by moisture, if dried. Debridement of necrotic tissue enhances wound closure. Factors that need to be assessed to determine the safest, most effective debridement methods are:

- Is the patient prescribed anticoagulants?
- Is the blood supply adequate to support wound healing and management of an increased bacterial release?
- Do the institution policy and procedures and state practice acts support sharp debridement?
- Is further training needed before performing certain types of debridement?
- What is the difference between viable and nonviable tissue?
- What structures lie in and around the wound that need to be protected and avoided?
- Are the instruments sterile and suitable for the job?
- How can bleeding be stopped?

Mechanical debridement includes hydrotherapy and wound scrubbing using gauze-type dressings. This method is nonspecific and can damage viable tissues.

Autolytic debridement is the selective removal of necrotic tissue by the body's endogenous enzymes. It can be achieved by using moist wound dressings that support cell function. The process is slow and, in certain patient populations (eg, geriatric, malnourished, immunosuppressed), difficult to achieve because of reduced production of enzymatic cells. **Sharp** debridement uses sharp, sterile instruments (eg, scissors, scalpels, curettes) to remove necrotic tissue and reduce or shave callous. Sharp debridement is very specific and requires an appropriately trained health professional. Each profession is governed by its own state practice act and individuals need to determine their institution's policies and procedures prior to performance of sharp debridement. Sharp debridement can be contraindicated in patients on anticoagulation therapy as control of bleeding can be difficult. Should bleeding occur, the therapist should perform one of the following:

- Apply direct pressure and elevation up to 10 minutes
- Place silver nitrate sticks on the area of bleeding
- Apply an alginate or collagen dressing

Knowledge of the surrounding anatomy and recognizing the difference between viable and nonviable tissues are keys to performing efficacious debridement to avoid damaging other adjacent structures. Viable tissue bleeds, senses pain, and contracts (ie, moves when stimulated). Nonviable tissue is avascular, lacks sensation, and is noncontractile. Nonviable, necrotic soft tissue are the only types of tissue that can be removed by a physical therapist. **Enzymatic** or **chemical debridement** involves topical exogenous enzymes or chemical solutions to break down necrotic tissue. Products may be specific to the substrates they effect (eg, collagenase) or more broad and nonspecific (eg, Dakin's solution). The wound environment must also be considered. Collagenase works best in moist environments, so should not be covered by moist dressings that move the active ingredient away from the wound, and eschar will need to be incised or cross-hatched to the moist base to be most effective. Manufacturer's instructions provide guidance for the safest, approved methods for each product.

Dressings and Wound Healing

There are a large variety of wound dressings and this section will review general considerations and provide clinical tips to aid the decision-making process. Products are constantly evolving in content and efficacy. First, it is established that moist wound healing is the optimal environment.[1] The cells necessary for wound healing and soft tissues thrive in a moist environment. Moist wound healing uses dressings that support this environment and are widely researched and accepted practice.[4] Moisture and bacterial growth is a concern; however, studies support moist wound environments compared to conventional gauze dressings demonstrating reduced infection rates using moist wound healing.[5] Moisture balance is vital. Sloppy, wet wounds and crusty, dry wounds will slow wound healing. Too much moisture overhydrates the epidermal cells leading to peripheral maceration; too much moisture inhibits cell anchoring and stability, allowing cells to float away from the wound surface. Dry and crusty wound beds halt or slow cell mobility causing cells to seek moisture to survive and move. Wound characteristics (ie, amount of drainage, depth, location) and established goals should define wound needs and direct wound dressing choices. It is important to review the package insert of each product for specific use and application. Specialized dressings initially appear to cost more than traditional dressings; however, specialized dressings require less frequent dressing changes and the use of moisture will accelerate wound healing, decreasing the duration required for specialized dressing application. Other considerations when determining wound

Table 15-4

DRESSING GUIDE

Basic Dressing Categories	*Possible Properties*	*Forms*
Polyurethane films	Thin film, offers protection and holds other dressings in place	Sheets
Hydrocolloids	Mild absorption, strong adhesive and wound protection	Wafers, sheets
Hydrogels	Moisturizes	Sheets, gels
Foams	Absorbs	Sheets, ropes
Alginates	Absorbs	Sheets, ropes
Hydrofibers	Absorbs, can offer moisturize	Sheets, ropes
Cotton gauze	Dry and absorptive; provides a medium to offer moisture; can retract from tunnels or tracts; adheres/sticks to wound bed	Pads, rolls, rope
Collagen	Provides cells in wound bed matrix to anchor to, increase inflammation, thicken	Sheets, rope, loose granules, gels
Nonadherant sheets	Specialized plastic; does not stick, but allows drainage to pass through	Sheets

dressings are patient and caregiver preferences, ability to apply properly, and product availability. See Table 15-4 for basic dressing components and purposes.

MODALITIES AND WOUND HEALING

Modalities can impact wound healing either by assisting in debridement or providing stimulation of cells needed for wound healing. In this section, modalities will be listed and their impact on wounds discussed.

Ultrasound stimulates fibroblasts and macrophages, promotes angiogenesis, and reduces the inflammatory phase in wound healing. There are units created specific for wound applications (eg, the MIST [Celularity Functional Regeneration, LLC]).

Hydrotherapy aims to debride devitalized tissue, remove surface contaminants and promote circulation. It is contraindicated in dry gangrene wounds and in limbs with an ABIs less than 0.4. It is a nonselective form of mechanical debridement and works best in patients with extensive necrotic tissue. Whirlpool as an intervention is not recommended. Whirlpool predisposes the patient to risks of infection by cross-contamination and the variable water pressures and risk of thermal injury may damage viable and developing granulation tissue. Placing an extremity in a dependent position in warm water may worsen edema, especially in the patient with venous insufficiency. Other more selective forms of hydrotherapy should be utilized, such as directed wound irrigation or a pulsatile lavage. **Pulsatile lavage** is a fluid-based (usually normal saline) modality combined with suction applied directly to the wound bed to loosen necrotic tissue and aid in debridement. The unit delivers fluid at less than 15 psi of pressure. Higher pressures may drive bacteria into viable tissue. Many units supply cones or tubing delivery systems to cleanse various sized and shaped wounds. Specific infection control guidelines must be followed as well as manufacturer-prescribed equipment duration of use. To prevent bacterial proliferation while applying hydrotherapy, personal protective equipment must be used and may include waterproof gowns, shoe covers, gloves, eye protection, and face masks. Once the necrotic tissue is removed, hydrotherapy should be discontinued. It should be remembered that intact skin that is dry and cracking will worsen if moisturizers are not applied. Burn injuries, especially in the presence of large surface area wounds are prone to increased infection rates, so the water must remain mobile to reduce bacterial colonization.

Electrical stimulation has multiple effects on the wound. It augments circulation, wound contraction, and epidermal migration, reduces edema, and uses negative and positive polarities to attract cells to the wound. Electrical stimulation can be used in the presence of clean or necrotic tissue and research has demonstrated its efficacy.[1] High volt, pulsed current is used in wound healing with voltage in the 100 to 200 range. Polarity should vary throughout the treatment and protocols will vary from regular cycling (every 3 days) to change when observed progress slows. A wound healing naturally experiences polarity changes throughout the healing process. Electrical stimulation can be used throughout the healing process, not just as a "jumpstart" modality.

Hyperbaric oxygen increases tissue oxygen levels and enhances cellular activity. The patient must breathe 100% oxygen while being exposed to pressures greater than 1 atmosphere. This requires full body chambers, such as those used with divers for decompression sickness. Topical applications, such as single extremity units, do not offer the same benefits and are not considered in this category.

Negative-pressure wound therapy (NPWT), sometimes referred to as **vacuum-assisted closure** (VAC), uses negative pressure at the wound surface to pull excess fluids away from the wound, stimulates cellular activity, and supports wound contraction. NPWT has significantly changed and advanced wound care, reducing surgeries and accelerating wound healing rates for more extensively involved wounds. For optimal results, the wound should be 75% clear of necrotic tissue before use or actively being debrided with each dressing change.

Goal Setting in Wound Healing

A thorough understanding of the phases of wound healing and specifically understanding the clinical appearance of the wounds at each stage is imperative to be able to set tangible, accurate, and achievable wound goals. To set goals, determine the current stage of the wound and the presumed next phase with progressive healing. For example, recall that wounds in the inflammatory stage are erythematous, can contain necrotic tissue, and the edges may not be well defined or demarcated because of recent injury or infection. Granulation, reepithelialization, and contraction characterize the next phase of wound healing, the proliferative phase. Possible goals for the wound in the inflammatory phase might be clear definition or demarcation of wound edges, a reduction in necrotic tissue, a decrease in wound size, and/or the emergence of granulation tissue or peripheral reepithelialization, all signs of the proliferative phase. Use percentages or measurements to quantify wound progress. To determine a time frame, evaluate risk factors. If the individual has multiple risk factors and is noncompliant with risk factor modification or the care plan, progress will be delayed. Two weeks or more may be needed to accomplish small increments of change. If there are few risk factors and the patient adheres to the care plan, then significant progress can be made each week.

Case Study

Ms. Walker is a 68-year-old female who presented to her primary physician feeling generally fatigued and with a low-grade temperature of 99.6°F. Physician examination revealed right leg cellulitis and presence of a necrotic wound located over the plantar aspect of the right first metatarsal head. She has been admitted to the hospital with sepsis and right lower extremity (RLE) cellulitis with an open wound.

Patient/Client History

General Demographics, Social History, and Living Environment

Ms. Walker lives alone in a house with 3 steps and a rail to enter. Her daughter lives about 15 minutes away and checks in on her periodically. She is retired and widowed with no other children. She owns a cane and rolling walker that was her husband's. He passed away 5 years ago.

General Health Status, Social/Health Habits, and Family History

Ms. Walker was in her usual state of health and compliant with all oral medications.

Medical/Surgical History

Past medical history includes osteoarthritis, coronary artery disease (CAD) with coronary artery bypass grafting (CABG) of 2 vessels 2 years ago, gastroesophageal reflux disease (GERD), and diabetes type 2.

Current Condition

Ms. Walker had an aching pain in her foot and began to feel extremely fatigued. Her blood glucose remained elevated above 200 mg/dL for the past 2 days.

Activities and Participation

Ms. Walker has been independent will all mobility, ADLs, and instrumental activities of daily living (IADLs) and does not require use of an assistive device. She takes care of her home and shopping needs outside of the house. She is retired.

Other Clinical Tests

Highlights of her laboratory results include elevated WBC count at 14,000, decreased albumin of 2.8 mg/dL, and an elevated hemoglobin A1c of 8.1%.

Systems Review

Cardiovascular and Pulmonary

Resting supine in bed, her vital signs were heart rate (HR) 96 beats per minute (bpm)and regular, blood pressure (BP) 130/90 mm Hg, respiratory rate (RR) 15 breaths/minute, and SpO_2 97%.

Integumentary

The RLE has cellulitis extending over the foot to mid-calf and noticeable edema is present. There is a wound present on the plantar aspect of right first metatarsal head.

Musculoskeletal

ROM and strength appear to be normal.

Neuromuscular

Sitting and standing balance, both static and dynamic, were good.

Communication, Affect, Cognition, Language, and Learning Style

Ms. Walker speaks fluent English. She is fully alert and oriented to person, place, time, and situation. She demonstrates good eye contact and appropriate responses to all communication. She needs glasses to read and is a high school graduate. She can follow simple and complex commands.

Tests and Measures

Aerobic Capacity and Endurance

Vital signs (VS) demonstrated normal response to mobility assessment. After completion of physical examination and wound assessment HR 98 and regular, RR 16, SpO_2 99%, and BP 134/88. There was no shortness of breath (SOB) with activity. Mobility was limited due to the patient's inability to maintain non-weightbearing of right forefoot.

Assistive and Adaptive Devices

Ms. Walker had not previously used a standard or rolling walker, but might need one now to help offload the right forefoot. The rolling walker she owns will need to be assessed for proper fit and structural safety.

Balance, Gait, and Mobility (Including Locomotion)

Ms. Walker has demonstrated independence with bed mobility (Functional Independence Measure [FIM] 7) and requires minimal assistance with sit-to-stand transfers (FIM 4). She lacks proper sensation to offload the right forefoot; bears full weight with stand pivot transfer and ambulation up to 5 feet, with and without use of rolling walker. Gait was limited due to the patient's inability to actively keep weight off the forefoot. Stand pivot transfers to a chair or wheelchair may be necessary to keep right foot elevated. She may need to learn wheelchair mobility to mobilize to facilitate offloading and wound closure.

Ventilation and Respiration

SpO_2 was normal. Breath sounds are clear to auscultation throughout all fields.

Mental Function

Ms. Walker was alert, awake, and oriented x4. She followed commands easily but appeared fatigued. She has a Richmond Agitation Sedation Score (RASS) of 0.

Muscle Performance

Manual muscle testing was 5/5 except right ankle dorsiflexion, which was grossly 4/5. She was unable to maintain non-weightbearing of right foot or stand on right heel only.

Pain

She detects general pain in the foot, but nothing specific. She rates her pain as 3 out of 10 on the numeric pain scale. She notes no difference in pain with resting or standing position and this does not change with mobility.

Integumentary Integrity

Edema is present in the RLE with the ankle measuring 2.0 cm, forefoot 1.0 cm, and mid-calf 0.5 cm greater on the right compared to the left. Knee circumference is equal on both legs. Plantar aspect of right first metatarsal head has an open wound measuring 1.5 cm x 1.7 cm and 0.2 cm depth with bone palpable at the base. Eschar covers 50% of the wound, yellow slough covers 30%, and 20% is red viable tissue. Wound borders are 25% well-defined and 75% hazy edges. Moderate amount of yellow purulent drainage is identified in old dressings. Wound periphery reveals wound 100% surrounded by callous extending up to 1 cm from the edges. Note right first and second toes are edematous compared to toes 3 through 5. Hair growth is absent from mid-calf to toes of both legs.

Sensory Integrity

Reflex testing revealed equal response at Achilles tendons bilaterally. Monofilament testing, using 5.07 monofilament, revealed lack of protective sensation from mid-calf to toes of both feet.

Noninvasive Vascular Tests

Pulses are palpable at posterior tibialis and dorsalis pedis but are weak and limited by edema. Capillary refill using tip of right great toe revealed 5 seconds refill time. Venous filling time of RLE was 60 seconds. It was noticed in sitting that the plantar aspect of the right foot had a ruddy color. Considering this information, the physician ordered further vascular tests. An ABI of the RLE was 0.7 at the lateral ankle (posterior tibialis artery) and 0.5 along the dorsum of the foot (dorsalis pedis artery). Left lower extremity (LLE) was 1.0. Radiology testing indicated possible osteomyelitis of head of the first metatarsal.

Diagnosis

Ms. Walker has several risk factors that will impact wound healing, including diabetes, loss of protective sensation, decreased peripheral circulation, infection of wound and bone, increased age, and increased pressure and stress at the wound site. She has diabetes that has been poorly controlled, possibly due to infection or need to alter her medications. She needs glasses to read, but it is questionable how well she can visualize the wound. Location can be difficult to see especially if her flexibility is decreased and darker skin pigmentation can mask early signs of erythema. If she wears dark socks or stockings, she may not detect early signs of wound drainage in a dark garment. (Many individuals with peripheral neuropathy are advised to always wear light or white color socks as a method of early detection.) She developed a wound in a common location for increased stress with standing and ambulation. The first metatarsal head is usually a loadbearing joint. This wound likely began due to pressure, stress, and peripheral neuropathy. An object may have been in her shoe, or possibly she was wearing new shoes or the seam of her sock landed on a bony prominence and caused increased point pressure. Aging results in slower cell turnover and decreased fat pad depths in the feet increasing stress at bony prominences. An open wound began, and the wound then became infected. This was indicated by fatigue, fever, and uncontrolled elevated blood glucoses as well as the redness spreading up the RLE. In the hospital, she was administered IV antibiotics. It was also determined she has limited blood supply to the ankle and foot.

Prognosis

LE bypass graft surgery was performed and successfully provided adequate blood flow to the foot and ankle. Wound location provides many challenges in offloading and pressure redistribution. This wound location can also present challenges to secure dressings. Ms. Walker will need to follow up for ongoing wound care at a wound clinic if available. She may also need assistance from her daughter for help with dressing changes and ADLs.

Intervention

Offloading or pressure redistribution may be key for this wound to close. Hopping, even while using an assist device, may also cause similar pressure areas and wounds in the left foot. Many options exist to completely offload, such as a kneeler or knee sling attached to a walker or a knee scooter. If the patient has balance or space issues using the kneeler at home, postoperative shoes can be adapted to shift the weightbearing off the forefoot to the heel. A total contact cast boot or controlled ankle motion (CAM) boot are other options to secure and keep weight off the forefoot. Home environment, extremity strength, and ROM will need to be considered to choose the best option. Patients with similar wound locations are often issued wedge shoes that place the foot in dorsiflexion with weightbearing. It is important to determine if patients have adequate ROM to safely use these shoes. If ROM is inadequate, patients may fall with these shoes or shift the weight to be on the toes only.

Necrotic tissue present in the wound will hamper wound closure by supporting a bacterial load and the physical presence of the necrotic tissue will hinder cell migration. An adequate blood supply will need to be ensured before aggressive debridement can be safe and effective and discussion with the surgical team is indicated. Autolytic, mechanical, and sharp debridement are all options once the wound has an adequate blood supply. Peripheral callous will need to be pared until soft and supple to allow wound contraction. Hard callous will act like a picture frame, keeping the wound edges open.

Dressings will need to address not only absorption of excess moisture of the wound but will also have to stay secure in a high-stress area and offer a uniform depth to avoid uneven pressure distribution areas and to supplement offloading. The wound will need to be assessed at least weekly to determine effectiveness of wound healing and closure.

Modalities that may help are electrical stimulation and ultrasound to attract needed cells for debridement and closure. The NPWT devices tend to be more appropriate for deeper wound depths. If wound drainage cannot be controlled by conventional dressings and wound maceration is evident, then the NPWT may be a viable option, with caution to place the nipple attachment in an area of non-weightbearing; the NPWT needs to be assessed with offloading devices in place. If the osteomyelitis in the bone is not treatable by conservative management, the affected area of bone will need to be surgically removed. Offloading will be very important to ensure the wounds will close after surgery. Once wounds are closed, shoe inserts and adapted shoes may be needed, as well as an assist device for balance and safe mobility.

ICF Clinical Reasoning Tool Case Study Summary

Health Condition

HPI: Fevers with complaints of fatigue, RLE cellulitis, and right foot plantar wound (possible osteomyelitis); elevated WBC and HbA1C, decreased albumin; amputation of 1st metatarsal and toe
PMHx: Type 2 diabetes, osteoarthrtis, CABG x2, GERD

Precautions/Contraindications

Poorly controlled diabetes, active wound infection with edema and cardiovascular disease; NWB RLE

Body Structure and Function			Activity/Task Limitations			Participation		
Impairment/ Problem	*Tests and Measures*	*Intervention*	*Activity*	*Tests and Measures*	*Intervention*	*Participation*	*Tests and Measures*	*Intervention*
• Wound present with impaired wound healing • Poor diabetes control • Edema • Impaired sensation • Weak pulses • Muscle weakness • Poor nutrition status • Abnormal lab values	• VS including SpO_2 and ECG • Wound examination (including capillary refill, ABI) • ROM/MMT • Sensation testing using monofilament • Lab values • Pain/numeric scale	• Wound management • Order heel shoe • Education on fall risk, off-loading and NWB of RLE, signs and symptoms of infection • Frequent skin checks • Consult registered dietician	• ADLs • Bed mobility • Transfers • Gait	• Functional task analysis • FIM • TUG as appropriate • RPE	• Progressive functional training (emphasis on NWB & offloading of forefoot) • Determine walker type (standard, rolling) or wheelchair needed for discharge	• Unable to care for herself • Unable to be independent in her home	• DQoL	• Continue physical therapy services • Consult social worker • Family meeting to discuss discharge plans and need for future home physical therapy, equipment requirements, and wound treatment

(continued)

ICF Clinical Reasoning Tool Case Study Summary (continued)		
Personal Factors	*Other Considerations*	*Environmental Factors*
• Age: 68 y/o female • AAO x4; follows commands easily • Primary language: English • Widowed with 1 adult daughter; daughter visits weekly • Independent prior to admission		Home: • Lives alone; possible support from daughter • Ambulates independently Hospital: • Urinary catheter, IV, rolling walker

DQoL = Diabetes Quality of Life Measure; ECG = electrocardiogram; Hb = hemoglobin; HPI = history of present illness; IV = intravenous; MMT = Manual Muscle Test; PMHx = past medical history; RPE = rate of perceived exertion; TUG = Timed Up and Go; y/o = year old.

Adapted from American Physical Therapy Association. *Guide to Physical Therapist Practice*. 3rd ed. http://www.apta.org/Guide/. Updated October 21, 2015. Accessed October 5, 2018 and *Towards a Common Language for Functioning, Disability and Health*. World Health Organization. www.who.int/classifications/icf/icfbeginnersguide.pdf. Published 2002. Accessed April 29, 2019.

Outcomes

Following the surgery, Ms. Walker's blood glucose was better controlled using her oral medications. Her balance and mobility were optimized using the rolling kneeler and her local church built her a ramp to ease her entry and exit from her home. She also used a postoperative shoe with a 3- to 5-degree wedge to increase heel weightbearing with soft foam at the forefoot and thickened felt at mid- to hindfoot to increase contour conformity to increase weightbearing surfaces.

Ms. Walker was able to return home and is followed by home health services, including physical therapy, to assess proper offloading, wound care, and progress mobility and independence with ADLs. Her daughter checks by nightly to help with housekeeping, shopping, bathing, and meals.

Chapter Review Questions

1. What are the primary functions of the skin?
   a. Organ protection, sensory feedback, and production of Vitamin A
   b. Maintenance of fluid status, immune defense, and thermoregulation
   c. Vitamin D production, dissipation of heat, and immunoglobulin distribution
   d. Conservation of heat and cold, homeostasis of sodium, and barrier to microorganisms
2. What are the 3 phases of wound healing?
   a. Proliferation, infiltration, and granulation
   b. Reepithelialization, proliferation, and contraction
   c. Inflammation, maturation, and proliferation
   d. Contraction, granulation, and proliferation
3. A Stage III pressure injury is defined by:
   a. Non-blanchable redness of a localized area, usually over a bony prominence
   b. Involvement of the dermis only
   c. Full-thickness tissue loss without visible muscle, tendon, or bone
   d. Full-thickness tissue loss with visible muscle, tendon, or bone
4. Risk factors for poor wound healing are:
   a. Age, blood supply, diabetes, and mechanical stress
   b. Age, carbon monoxide, carcinomas, and dementia
   c. Age, kidney function, sensation, and colonization
   d. Age, capillary refill, chemotherapy, and presence of rubor on the plantar surface
5. Three noninvasive, clinical assessment tools of arterial blood flow are:
   a. Two-point discrimination, hair loss, pitting edema
   b. Vibratory test, line of demarcation, venous filling time
   c. Doppler ultrasound, Homan's sign, Well's criteria
   d. ABI, rubor of dependency, capillary refill

Answers: 1b, 2c, 3c, 4a, 5d

References

1. US Department of Health and Human Services. *Treatment of Pressure Ulcers, Clinical Practice Guideline, Number 15*. Rockdale, MD: AHCPR Pub; 1994.
2. Bryant RA, Nix DP. *Acute and Chronic Wounds: Current Management Concepts*. 3rd ed. St. Louis, MO: Elsevier; 2007.
3. International Review. Pressure ulcer prevention: shear, friction and microclimate in context. A consensus document. *Wound International*. https://www.woundsinternational.com/resources/details/international-review-pressure-ulcer-prevention-pressure-shear-friction-and-microclimate-context. Published September 2, 2010. Accessed March 21, 2019.
4. Baranoski S, Ayello EA. *Wound Care Essentials, Practice Principals*. 3rd ed. Philadelphia, PA: Lippincott, Williams & Wilkins; 2012.
5. Kerstein MD. Moist wound healing: the clinical perspective. *Ostomy Wound Manage*. 1995;41(7ASupp):37S-44S.

Bibliography

Baker LL, Chambers R, Demuth SK, Villar F. Effects of electrical stimulation on wound healing in patients with diabetic ulcers. *Diabetes Care*. 1997;20(3):405-412.

Bjork R, Hettrick H. Endothelial glycocalyx layer and interdependence of lynphatic and integumentary systems. *Wounds International*.https://www.woundsinternational.com/resources/details/endothelial-glycocalyx-layer-and-interdependence-of-lymphatic-and-integumentary-systems. Published May 2, 2018. Accessed August 19, 2019.

Burton CS. Venous ulcers. *Am J Surg*. 1994; 167(1A Suppl):37S-41S.

Clinician lists. http://www.choosingwisely.org/clinician-lists/#parent Society=American_Physical_Therapy_Association. Choosing Wisely. Accessed March 21, 2019.

Feeder JA, Kloth LC, Gentzkow G. Chronic dermal ulcer healing enhance with monophasic pulsed electrical stimulation. *Phys Ther*. 1991;71(9):639-649.

Field FK, Kerstein MD. Overview of wound healing in a moist environment. *Am J Surg*. 1994;167(1A):2S-6S.

Gates JL, Holloway GA. A comparison of wound environments. *Ostomy Wound Manage*. 1992;38(8):34-37.

Gentzkow GD. Electrical stimulation to heal dermal wounds. *J Dermatol Surg Oncol*. 1993:19:753-758.

Glover JL, Weingarten MS, Buchbinder DS. A 4-year outcome based retrospective study of wound healing and limb salvage in patients with chronic wounds. *Adv Wound Care*. 1997;10(1):33-38.

Gogia PP, Marquez RR, Minerbo GM. Effects of high voltage galvanic stimulation on wound healing. *Ostomy Wound Manage*. 1992;38(1):29-35.

Graff MK, Bryant J, Beinlich N. Preventing heel breakdown. *Orthop Nurs*. 2000;19(5):63-69.

Haisfield-Wolfe ME, Rund C. Malignant cutaneous wounds: a management protocol. *Ostomy Wound Manage*. 1997; 43(1):56-66.

Heyneman A, Vanderwee K, Grypdonck M, Defloor T. Effectiveness of two cushions in the prevention of heel pressure ulcers. *Worldviews Evid Based Nurs*. 2009;6(2):114-120. doi: 10.1111/j.1741-6787.2009.00153.x

Junkin J, Gray M. Are pressure redistribution surfaces or heel protection devices effective for preventing heel pressure ulcers? *J Wound Ostomy Continence Nurs*. 2009;36(6):602-608. doi: 10.1097/WON.0b013e3181be282f

Kloth LC, McColloch JM. *Wound Healing: Alternative in Management, Contemporary Perspectives in Rehabilitation*. 3rd ed. Philadelphia, PA: FA Davis; 2001.

Kraft JC, Treuting PM, Ho RJY. Indocyanine green nanoparticles undergo selective lymphatic uptake, distribution and retention and enable detailed mapping of lymph vessel nodes and abnormalities. *J Drug Target*. 2018;26(5-6):494-504.

Laing P. Diabetic foot ulcers. *Am J Surg*. 1994;167(1A suppl):31S-36S.

Lavery LA, Armstrong DG, Harkless LB. Classification of diabetic foot wounds. *Ostomy Wound Manage*. 1997;43(2): 44-53.

Leigh IH, Bennett G. Pressure ulcers: prevalence, etiology and treatment modalities: a review. *Am J Surg*. 1994;167(1A suppl):25S-30S.

McColloch J. Physical modalities in wound management: ultrasound, vasopneumatic devices and hydrotherapy. *Ostomy Wound Manage.* 1995;41(5): 30-32.

McColluch JM, Kloth LC, Feeder JA. *Wound Healing Alternative in Management.* 2nd ed. Philadelphia, PA: FA Davis; 1990.

Micholivitz SL, Wolf SL. *Therapeutic Ultrasound: Thermal Agents in Rehabilitation.* Philadelphia, PA: FA Davis; 1986.

Haesler, E, ed. *Prevention and Treatment of Pressure Ulcers: Quick Reference Guide.* Perth, Australia: Cambridge Media; 2014.

Nelson EA. Compression bandaging for venous leg ulcers. *Prof Nurse.* 1997;12(7 suppl):S7-S9.

Nelzen O, Bergqvist D, Lindhagen A. Long-term prognosis for patients with chronic leg ulcers: a prospective study. *Eur J Vasc Endovasc Surg.* 1997;13(5):500-508.

O'Meara S, Al-Kurdi D, Ologun Y, Ovington LG, Martyn-St James M, Richardson R. Antibiotics and antiseptics for venous leg ulcers. *Cochrane Database Syst Rev.* 2014;1:CD003557. doi: 10.1002/14651858.CD003557.pub5

O'Meara S, Cullum N, Nelson EA, Dumville JC. Compression for venous leg ulcers. *Cochrane Database Syst Rev.* 2012;11:CD000265. doi: 10.1002/14651858.CD000265.pub3

Ryan TJ. Wound dressing. *Dermatol Clin.* 1993;11(1):207-213.

Sheffet A, Cutryn AS, Louria DB. Applying electric and electromagnetic energy as adjuvant treatment for pressure ulcers: a critical review. *Ostomy Wound Manage.* 2000;46(2):29.

Staley M, Richard R. Management of the acute burn wound: an overview. *Adv Wound Care.* 1997;10(2):39-44.

Surman MW. An introduction to hyperbaric oxygen therapy for the ET nurse. *J Wound Ostomy Continence Nurs.* 1996;23(2):80-89.

Sussman C, Bates-Jensen B. *Wound Care: A Collaborative Practice Manual for Health Professionals.* 3rd ed. Philadelphia, PA: Lippincott, Williams & Wilkins; 2006.

Tompach PC, Lew D, Stoll JL. Cell response to hyperbaric oxygen treatment. *Int J Maxillofac Surg.* 1997;26(2):82-86.

Wiley TL. *A Dressing Application Guide for the Care of Wounds Using Moist Healing Principles.* London, United Kingdom: Smith & Nephew; 1989.

Willey T. Use a decision tree to choose wound dressing. *Am J Nurs.* 1992; 92(2):43-46.

Wong VK, Stotts NA. Physiology and prevention of heel ulcers: the state of science. *J Wound Ostomy Continence Nurs.* 2003;30(4):191-198.

Woo KY, Sibbald RG. The ABC's of skin care for wound care clinicians: dermatitis and eczema. *Adv Skin Wound Care.* 2009;22(5):230-236.

Appendix

Kathy Lee Bishop, PT, DPT, CCS and Daniel J. Malone, PT, PhD, CCS

Example of Acute Care/ICU Competency

Adapted from Advanced Acute Care Elective Doctor of Physical Therapy Program Department of Rehabilitation Medicine, Emory University School of Medicine.

	The following are categories from the written competency for the entry level evaluation and treatment in the intensive care unit (ICU)	Review of Written Material	Discussed and/or Asked Questions	Practiced Competency (practice test)	Pass/Date/ Initials of Tester (demonstrated ≥85% understanding)
I. Written Competency					
A.	*Examination*				
B.	*Sedation, Delirium, Medications*				
C.	*Line Identification*				
D.	*Electrocardiogram (ECG) Identification and Interpretation*				
E.	*Ventilation/Oxygenation*				
F.	*Intervention, Methods for Progression*				
G.	*Common Tests, Procedures, Surgeries*				

Malone DJ, Bishop KL, eds. *Acute Care Physical Therapy: A Clinician's Guide, Second Edition* (pp 681-712).

	The following are categories from the written competency for the entry level evaluation and treatment in the intensive care unit (ICU)	Review of Written Material	Discussed and/or Asked Questions	Practiced Competency (practice test)	Pass/Date/ Initials of Tester (demonstrated ≥85% understanding)
H.	*Rehabilitation Assessment Tools/Algorithms*				
I.	*Common Diseases/ Disorders*				
J.	*Universal Precautions and Infection Control*				
II. Practical					
A.	*Examination*				
1.	Establish therapist checklist: Entering and exiting patient room (organize session/safety); make a plan before entering the patient's room				
	i. Reviews medical record (eg, past medical history, history of present illness, hemodynamics, labs)				
	ii. Check orders/ clearance (eg, spine, weightbearing)				
	iii. Review any specific medical precautions for patient (parameters)				
	iv. Understand medications (eg, indications, potential side effects and impact on patient/physical therapy services)				
	v. Identify Richmond Agitation Sedation Scale (RASS) delirium scores				
	vi. Identify lines and tubes (eg, indications, precautions)				
	vii. Review patient information from last 24 hours (eg, hemodynamics, labs, diagnostic tests and procedures, delirium/sedation status, weaning from mechanical ventilation)				

	The following are categories from the written competency for the entry level evaluation and treatment in the intensive care unit (ICU)	Review of Written Material	Discussed and/or Asked Questions	Practiced Competency (practice test)	Pass/Date/ Initials of Tester (demonstrated ≥85% understanding)
	viii. Check with nurse and collaboratively determine patient appropriateness for physical therapy services				
	ix. Determine if patient has an artificial airway and requires mechanical ventilation? Determine mechanical ventilation settings and patient response (eg, assist control, pressure support, positive end expiratory pressure [PEEP], F_IO_2 [fraction of inspired oxygen], heart rate [HR], blood pressure [BP], respiratory rate [RR], oxygen saturation [SpO_2])				
	x. Describe at least 5 precautions before entering patient room				
	xi. What does the patient look like as you enter the room? What is your immediate observation/impression (eg, distressed, comfortable, position, in bed, equipment)?				
	xii. Identify and observe all monitors: Record baseline vital signs (VS) before you interact with patient; are any alarms sounding? Frequently recheck patient responses throughout session				
	xiii. Are family members or visitors present? Who should stay during session?				

	The following are categories from the written competency for the entry level evaluation and treatment in the intensive care unit (ICU)	Review of Written Material	Discussed and/or Asked Questions	Practiced Competency (practice test)	Pass/Date/ Initials of Tester (demonstrated ≥85% understanding)
	xiv. Set up ICU environment before moving patient (eg, is there sufficient length of tubing? can any lines/tubes be clamped before initiating session?)				
	xv. Describe exiting room process: Survey room; is patient safe? Are all monitors and alarms functioning? Are all lines/tubes properly functioning? Is the patient comfortable and appropriately draped? Do you need to debrief with medical team? Do you need to request updated orders or consults?				
2.	Describe universal precautions and infection control				
3.	Review medical record and documents per department policy				
4.	Assess and describe breathing pattern, RR, and cough				
5.	Assess pulses and determines HR and rhythm				
6.	Assess level of alertness, cognition, and ability to communicate				
7.	Assess skin color/ condition, temperature, nail beds/clubbing, vascular return/response				
8.	Assess BP				
9.	Assess orthopnea				
10.	Assess breathing pattern/shortness of breath (SOB)				

	The following are categories from the written competency for the entry level evaluation and treatment in the intensive care unit (ICU)	Review of Written Material	Discussed and/or Asked Questions	Practiced Competency (practice test)	Pass/Date/ Initials of Tester (demonstrated ≥85% understanding)
11.	Assess rate of perceived exertion (RPE)				
12.	Assess SpO_2				
13.	Auscultate for breath sounds, heart sounds, or interpret documented breath sounds or heart sounds				
14.	Assess tactile/vocal fremitus				
15.	Assess chest wall expansion				
16.	Assess endurance				
17.	Assess orthostatic signs				
18.	Complete gross range of motion (ROM), manual muscle testing (MMT), and balance, sensation screens				
19.	Implement appropriate outcome measures (eg, AM-PAC [Activity Measure for Post Acute Care], FIM [Functional Independence Measure], TUG [Timed Up and Go], 6MWT [6 Minute Walk Test])				
20.	Identify structural impairments, activity limitations, and participation restrictions				
21.	Identify primary diagnosis and medical/surgical comorbidities that may impact the plan of care				
B.	*Sedation/Delirium/Medications (Name at least 2 precautions for each)*				
1.	Describe the pros and cons of sedation				
2.	Perform Confusion Assessment Method for the Intensive Care Unit (CAM-ICU) and RASS as appropriate				

	The following are categories from the written competency for the entry level evaluation and treatment in the intensive care unit (ICU)	Review of Written Material	Discussed and/or Asked Questions	Practiced Competency (practice test)	Pass/Date/ Initials of Tester (demonstrated ≥85% understanding)
3.	Describe at least 2 ways to decrease delirium in the ICU				
4.	Name at least 2 medications for neuromuscular blockade				
5.	What does RASS stand for and how is this utilized in the ICU?				
6.	Describe impact of pain medications on delirium in the ICU				
7.	Describe the difference between pain management and sedation?				
C.	*Line/Tube Identification (Name indications and at least 2 precautions for each)*				
1.	Arterial line				
2.	Central venous line (ie, Swan-Ganz)				
3.	Peripheral intravenous (IV) line				
4.	Two types of dialysis ports (eg, hemodialysis, peritoneal)				
5.	Port-a-cath (Hickman)				
6.	Foley catheter				
7.	Peripherally inserted cardiac catheter (PICC)				
8.	Intracranial pressure device (eg, bolt, external ventriculostomy drain)				
9.	Nasogastric, gastronomy, jejunostomy tube				
10.	Rectal catheter/collection device				
11.	Hemovac (Jackson-Pratt)				
12.	Left (LVAS) or right (RVAS) ventricular assist system				
13.	Intra-aortic balloon pump (IABP)				

	The following are categories from the written competency for the entry level evaluation and treatment in the intensive care unit (ICU)	Review of Written Material	Discussed and/or Asked Questions	Practiced Competency (practice test)	Pass/Date/ Initials of Tester (demonstrated ≥85% understanding)
14.	Extracorporeal membrane oxygenation (ECMO)				
15.	Pacemakers (eg, transcutaneous, transvenous, external)				
16.	Permanent pacemaker and implantable cardioverter-defibrillator				
17.	External wearable cardiac defibrillator				
18.	ECG and electrodes				
19.	Epidural catheter				
20.	Patient-controlled analgesic pump and catheter				
21.	Lumbar drain				
22.	Chest tube (eg, mediastinal, pleural)				
23.	Waveform capnography				
24.	Noninvasive intermittent BP monitor				
D.	*ECG Identification and Interpretation (ie, impact on examination/interventions)*				
1.	Sinus rhythms				
	i. Normal sinus rhythm				
	ii. Sinus arrhythmia				
	iii. Sinus bradycardia				
	iv. Sinus tachycardia				
2.	Atrial rhythms				
	i. Premature atrial contraction				
	ii. Paroxysmal/atrial tachycardia				
	iii. Atrial flutter				
	iv. Atrial fibrillation				
3.	Heart blocks				
	i. First degree heart block				

	The following are categories from the written competency for the entry level evaluation and treatment in the intensive care unit (ICU)	Review of Written Material	Discussed and/or Asked Questions	Practiced Competency (practice test)	Pass/Date/ Initials of Tester (demonstrated ≥85% understanding)
	ii. Second degree heart block				
	a. Mobitz I (Wenckebach)				
	b. Mobitz II				
	iii. Third degree heart block				
4.	Junctional rhythms				
	i. Junctional escape rhythm				
	ii. Accelerated junctional rhythm				
	iii. Junctional tachycardia				
	iv. Premature junctional contraction				
5.	Ventricular rhythms				
	i. Idioventricular rhythm				
	ii. Ventricular tachycardia				
	iii. Ventricular fibrillation				
	iv. Premature ventricular contraction				
	v. Couplets, triplets, salvo				
	vi. Bigeminy, trigeminy, quadrigeminy				
	vii. Unifocal, multifocal				
6.	Asystole				
7.	Pacemakers (eg, atrial, ventricular, biventricular [cardiac resynchronization therapy])				
8.	Identify and describe possible impact of artifact on ECG analysis				
E.	*Ventilation/Oxygenation (ie, impact on examination/intervention)*				
1.	Validate SpO_2 measurement				
2.	Describe influences on SpO_2				
3.	Describe why supplemental oxygen is prescribed				

	The following are categories from the written competency for the entry level evaluation and treatment in the intensive care unit (ICU)	Review of Written Material	Discussed and/or Asked Questions	Practiced Competency (practice test)	Pass/Date/ Initials of Tester (demonstrated ≥85% understanding)
4.	Oxygen delivery devices (flow values–l/min and F_IO_2)				
	i. Nasal cannula				
	ii. High-flow nasal cannula				
	iii. Simple face or tracheostomy mask				
	iv. Venturi mask (face)				
	v. Face tent				
	vi. Non-rebreather mask				
	vii. Partial rebreather mask				
	viii. Manual ventilation bag				
	ix. Oxygen conservation devices (eg, Oxymizer system [Drive])				
	x. Endotracheal tube (ETT) or tracheostomy				
5.	Mechanical ventilation				
	i. Bilevel positive airway pressure (noninvasive positive pressure ventilation)				
	ii. Negative pressure devices (poncho/iron lung)				
	iii. Nasotracheal or oral ETT				
	iv. Identify rate, volume, pressure, PEEP, and F_IO_2				
	v. Identify cuff pressure via electronic medical record or flow sheet				
	vi. Identify "at lips or at teeth" markings on ETT				
	vii. Oral suction device (Yankauer)				
	viii. Sterile suction devices				

	The following are categories from the written competency for the entry level evaluation and treatment in the intensive care unit (ICU)	Review of Written Material	Discussed and/or Asked Questions	Practiced Competency (practice test)	Pass/Date/ Initials of Tester (demonstrated ≥85% understanding)
	ix. Oropharyngeal and nasopharyngeal airways				
	x. High-frequency oscillatory ventilation (HFOV)				
6.	Describe precautions for mobilizing patient with an artificial airway (eg, ETT, tracheostomy)				
7.	Identify location of mechanical ventilator alarms and describe reasons for high-/low-pressure and respiratory rate alarms				
8.	Describe and demonstrate assessment of patient tolerance to examination/ interventions for a patient who requires mechanical ventilation or supplemental oxygen				
9.	Describe purpose and precautions of manual ventilation				
10.	Describe benefits and precautions of portable ventilator use during mobilization				
11.	Demonstrate technique for turning on and shutting off oxygen cylinders (eg, e or h tank)				
12.	Describe purpose, precautions, and benefit of ECMO				
13.	Describe process for determining if patient should be transferred to portable mechanical ventilator				
14.	Describe process and reasoning for recommending oxygen titration during physical therapy interventions				

	The following are categories from the written competency for the entry level evaluation and treatment in the intensive care unit (ICU)	Review of Written Material	Discussed and/or Asked Questions	Practiced Competency (practice test)	Pass/Date/ Initials of Tester (demonstrated ≥85% understanding)
15.	Describe precautions for a patient who was recently extubated and/ or recently liberated from mechanical ventilation				
F.	*Physical Therapy Intervention/Methods for Progression*				
1.	Bed Exercise				
	i. Describe rationale for performing bed exercises and provide precautions as appropriate				
	ii. Demonstrate different types of exercises for position				
	iii. Describe and perform patient monitoring to determine the patient's response to the intervention				
2.	Semi-Fowler Position				
	i. Describe rationale for performing bed exercises and provide precautions as appropriate				
	ii. Demonstrate different types of exercises for position				
	iii. Describe and perform patient monitoring to determine the patient's response to the intervention				
3.	Dangling, Supported, Unsupported Edge of Bed				
	i. Describe rationale for performing bed exercises and provide precautions as appropriate				
	ii. Demonstrate different types of exercises for position				
	iii. Describe and perform patient monitoring to determine the patient's response to the intervention				

	The following are categories from the written competency for the entry level evaluation and treatment in the intensive care unit (ICU)	Review of Written Material	Discussed and/or Asked Questions	Practiced Competency (practice test)	Pass/Date/ Initials of Tester (demonstrated ≥85% understanding)
4.	Transfers, Standing, Out of Bed Activities				
	i. Describe rationale for performing bed exercises and provide precautions as appropriate				
	ii. Demonstrate different types of exercises for position				
	iii. Describe and perform patient monitoring to determine the patient's response to the intervention				
5.	Gait Training and Endurance Exercise				
	i. Describe rationale for performing bed exercises and provide precautions as appropriate				
	ii. Demonstrate different types of exercises for position				
	iii. Describe and perform patient monitoring to determine the patient's response to the intervention				
6.	Determining Patient Response and Progression				
	i. Describe and provide rationale based off patient's responses to the interventions for progression of the plan of care (eg, progressing from bed mobility and bed level exercises to dangling, edge of bed, transfers, gait and endurance training)				
	ii. Describe and provide rationale based off patient's responses for modifying the plan of care, including the prescribed frequency, intensity, and duration of therapy sessions				

	The following are categories from the written competency for the entry level evaluation and treatment in the intensive care unit (ICU)	Review of Written Material	Discussed and/or Asked Questions	Practiced Competency (practice test)	Pass/Date/ Initials of Tester (demonstrated ≥85% understanding)
	iii. Describe process for progressing supplemental oxygen delivery systems as functional level progresses				
	iv. Describe mobility protocols				
7.	Airway Clearance and Assistive Cough				
	i. Perform and describe benefit and rationale for pursed-lip breathing				
	ii. Perform and describe benefit and rationale for active cycle of breathing				
	iii. Perform and describe benefit and rationale of manual techniques, including chest percussion, vibration, and bronchial drainage				
	iv. Perform and describe types of assistive cough techniques, including the benefit and rationale for each				
	v. Describe protocol for suctioning via closed and open systems				
	vi. Describe precautions pre- and post-suctioning				
8.	Communication				
	i. Describe process with physician				
	ii. Describe process with patient's nurse and/or charge nurse				
	iii. Document examination/ intervention per hospital policy				
	iv. Describe role and responsibilities at team meetings				

	The following are categories from the written competency for the entry level evaluation and treatment in the intensive care unit (ICU)	Review of Written Material	Discussed and/or Asked Questions	Practiced Competency (practice test)	Pass/Date/ Initials of Tester (demonstrated ≥85% understanding)
	v. Describe process for family/significant other meetings				
	vi. Describe primary and alternative communication tools for patient				
G.	*Common Tests, Procedures, Surgeries (Describe procedure, indications, and precautions)*				
1.	Angioplasty (percutaneous transluminal coronary angioplasty [PTCA]/ percutaneous coronary intervention [PCI]) with or without stents (eg, bare metal stents, drug-eluting stents)				
2.	Ankle Brachial Index (ABI)				
3.	Arterial blood gases (ABG)				
4.	Blood transfusion				
5.	Bronchoscopy				
6.	Coronary artery bypass grafting (CABG)				
7.	Cardiac catheterization/ coronary angiography				
8.	Cardiac index				
9.	CardioMEMS HF System				
10.	Chest roentgenogram (x-ray)				
11.	Computed tomography (CT) scan				
12.	Dialysis: Hemodialysis, peritoneal, continuous renal replacement therapy (CRRT)				
13.	ECG (eg, transthoracic, transesophageal); stress or dobutamine				
14.	Electroencephalography (EEG)				

	The following are categories from the written competency for the entry level evaluation and treatment in the intensive care unit (ICU)	Review of Written Material	Discussed and/or Asked Questions	Practiced Competency (practice test)	Pass/Date/ Initials of Tester (demonstrated ≥85% understanding)
15.	Electromyography (EMG)				
16.	Electrophysiology studies				
17.	Exercise tolerance test				
18.	Exploratory laparotomy				
19.	Holter monitor				
20.	IABP				
21.	Implantable cardioverter-defibrillators (ICDs) and pacemakers				
22.	LVAS/RVAS				
23.	Lung volume reduction surgery				
24.	Magnetic resonance angiography (MRA), magnetic resonance imaging (MRI)				
25.	Mean arterial pressure (MAP)				
26.	Open reduction internal fixation (ORIF), external fixators, partial/total joint replacements				
27.	Orthotopic heart transplant				
28.	Pneumonectomy				
29.	Positron emission tomography (PET) scan				
30.	Pulmonary function testing (PFT)				
31.	SVO_2 (mixed venous oxygen saturation), SaO_2 (arterial oxygen saturation), SpO_2				
32.	Transcatheter aortic valve replacement (TAVR), transcatheter aortic valve implantation (TAVI)				
33.	Thallium scan (eg, pharmacologic/exercise)				
34.	Thoracentesis				
35.	Thoracotomy				

	The following are categories from the written competency for the entry level evaluation and treatment in the intensive care unit (ICU)	Review of Written Material	Discussed and/or Asked Questions	Practiced Competency (practice test)	Pass/Date/ Initials of Tester (demonstrated ≥85% understanding)
36.	Tracheostomy				
37.	Valve replacement/repair				
38.	Valvuloplasty				
39.	Ventilation perfusion scan				
40	Ventriculostomy				
41.	Wells Clinical Prediction Rule for deep vein thrombosis (DVT) and pulmonary embolism				
H.	*Rehabilitation Assessment Tools/Algorithms*				
1.	AM-PAC "6 Clicks," Acute Care Index of Function (ACIF), Barthel Index, FIM, Functional Status Score for the ICU (FSS-ICU)				
2.	Balance testing: Berg Balance Scale (BBS), Dynamic Gait Index (DGI), Functional Reach Test (FRT), Function in Sitting Test (FIST), TUG				
3.	CAM-ICU				
4.	Mini-Mental State Examination (MMSE), Montreal Cognitive Assessment (MoCA)				
5.	Medical Research Council (MRC) Scale for Testing Muscle Strength				
6.	Physical performance testing (5 Times Sit to Stand), Physical Function ICU Test-scored (PFIT-s), 2-/6MWT, TUG				
7.	RASS				
I.	*Common Disease/Disorders (Describe the following pathologies and impact on examination and intervention)*				
1.	Abdominal aortic aneurysm (AAA) or thoracic aortic aneurysm (TAA)				
2.	AIDS				

	The following are categories from the written competency for the entry level evaluation and treatment in the intensive care unit (ICU)	Review of Written Material	Discussed and/or Asked Questions	Practiced Competency (practice test)	Pass/Date/ Initials of Tester (demonstrated ≥85% understanding)
3.	Adult respiratory distress syndrome				
4.	Anemia				
5.	Asthma				
6.	Atelectasis				
7.	Basilar artery syndrome				
8.	Bronchiolitis obliterans				
9.	Bronchiolitis obliterans organizing pneumonia				
10.	CABG				
11.	Cardiac myxoma				
12.	Cardiac tamponade				
13.	Cardiomyopathy				
14.	Cerebrovascular accident (CVA)				
15.	Chronic bronchitis				
16.	Chronic obstructive pulmonary disease (COPD)				
17.	Compartment syndrome				
18.	Cor pulmonale				
19.	Coronary atherosclerosis (CAD)				
20.	Critical illness myopathy and polyneuropathy				
21.	Cystic fibrosis				
22.	DVT				
23.	Diabetes mellitus				
24.	Emphysema				
25.	Empyema				
26.	Esophageal varices				
27.	Flail chest				
28.	Flash pulmonary edema				
29.	Heart failure				
30.	Heterotrophic ossificans				
31.	HIV				

	The following are categories from the written competency for the entry level evaluation and treatment in the intensive care unit (ICU)	Review of Written Material	Discussed and/or Asked Questions	Practiced Competency (practice test)	Pass/Date/ Initials of Tester (demonstrated ≥85% understanding)
32.	Hypertension (HTN)				
33.	Hypertensive crisis				
34.	Leukemia				
35.	Locked-in syndrome				
36.	Lung cancer (small and non–small cell [SCLC/ NSCLC])				
37.	Lymphedema				
38.	Lymphoma				
39.	Malignant hypertension				
40.	Myocardial infarction				
41.	Myocardial ischemia (eg, angina, anginal equivalents)				
42.	Myositis ossificans				
43.	Necrotizing fasciitis				
44.	Obesity				
45.	Orthostatic hypotension				
46.	Osteopenia				
47.	Osteoporosis				
48.	Paget's disease				
49.	Pancreatitis				
50	Parkinson's disease				
51.	PCI/PTCA				
52.	Pericarditis				
53.	Peripheral vascular disease (PVD), peripheral arterial disease (PAD), peripheral venous disease, intermittent claudication				
54.	Pleural effusion				
55.	Pleuritis				
56.	Pneumocystis carinii pneumonia				
57.	Pneumocystis jirovecii pneumonia				

	The following are categories from the written competency for the entry level evaluation and treatment in the intensive care unit (ICU)	Review of Written Material	Discussed and/or Asked Questions	Practiced Competency (practice test)	Pass/Date/ Initials of Tester (demonstrated ≥85% understanding)
58.	Pneumonia (eg, aspiration, bacterial, viral), ventilator-associated pneumonia (VAP)				
59.	Pneumothorax (tension)				
60.	Pulmonary contusion				
61.	Pulmonary edema				
62.	Pulmonary emboli				
63.	Pulmonary fibrosis (interstitial)				
64.	Pulmonary hypertension				
65.	Renal failure (acute/ chronic)				
66.	Respiratory failure/distress (acute/chronic)				
67.	Rheumatic diseases				
68.	Systemic lupus erythematosus				
69.	Subcutaneous emphysema				
70.	TAVI/TAVR				
71.	Transient ischemic attack (TIA)				
72.	Transplants (eg, heart, lung, kidney, liver, pancreas)				
73.	Traumatic brain injury (TBI)				
74.	Tuberculosis				
75.	Watershed infarct				
76.	Pediatrics				
	i. Congenital heart defects (CHD)				
	ii. Diaphragmatic hernia				
	iii. Hyperbilirubenemia				
	iv. Meconium aspiration syndrome				

	The following are categories from the written competency for the entry level evaluation and treatment in the intensive care unit (ICU)	Review of Written Material	Discussed and/or Asked Questions	Practiced Competency (practice test)	Pass/Date/ Initials of Tester (demonstrated ≥85% understanding)
	v. Neonatal asphyxia				
	vi. Prematurity				
	vii. Spina bifida				
	viii. Transesophageal fistula				
J.	*Universal Precautions and Infection Control*				
1.	Describe your role in infection control				
2.	Describe at least 5 steps for infection control in the ICU				
3.	Define universal precautions				
4.	What is meant by droplet precautions?				
5.	What are airborne precautions?				
6.	What are contact precautions?				
7.	What is the benefit of a negative pressure room?				

Sample Acute Care/Intensive Care Unit Competency: Written Test

To pass the written competency section, the therapist must correctly answer over 85% of the questions. The questions are multiple choice. Circle the most appropriate answer. Note: The correct answer is indicated by an asterisk (*).

A. Examination

1. Which of the following is the best way to assess HR?
   a. Palpate radial pulse and external jugular vein
   b. Palpate pulse and read from ECG*
   c. Observe and read the rate off mechanical ventilator
   d. Observe arterial BP tracing on monitor
2. Which of the following is the best way to validate oxygen saturation?
   a. Palpate pulse and compare to pulse rate on pulse oximeter*
   b. Palpate pulse and assess respiratory rate on mechanical ventilation
   c. Observe ECG on monitor and compare with central venous pressure
   d. Observe ECG on monitor and assess the patient's perceived exertion on the modified Borg Scale
3. Which of the following is the best way to assess patient tolerance to evaluation or a treatment session?
   a. A change in mental status
   b. A change in lip color or nail polish color
   c. A change in baseline to activity/VS
   d. a, c*
4. A patient has developed the following changes during the examination: new onset S3, rales >1/3 up bilateral posterior lung regions, increased RR, positive accessory muscle use. Which of the following is most likely to be the diagnosis?
   a. Interstitial pulmonary fibrosis
   b. CHF*
   c. Cystic fibrosis
   d. Chronic bronchitis
5. Which of the following is the best possible diagnosis given these findings on assessment: patient status post (s/p) motor vehicle accident (MVA) with flail chest on the left confirmed by x-ray; tracheal deviation to the right, hyperresonant left chest to right with mediate percussion, distant breath sounds on auscultation left to right, decreased chest wall movement left to right, pale appearance, and rapid RR with accessory muscle use.
   a. Adult respiratory distress syndrome
   b. Pneumothorax*
   c. Pneumonia
   d. Pleural effusion

B. Sedation/Delirium/Medications

1. Mr. Jones has been in the ICU for 3 weeks. The electronic medical record flow sheet shows a poor sleep/wake cycle, he is requiring more sedation due to his fighting the ventilator (patient-ventilator dyssynchrony), and the nurses have noted full body shaking if he does not receive medications every 4 to 6 hours to calm him down. Which of the following would best describe what Mr. Jones may be experiencing?
   a. Withdrawal from opiates
   b. Severe pain
   c. Preexisting mental impairment
   d. Delirium*
2. What is meant by the ICU triad?
   a. Excessive over breathing on ventilator, severe tachycardia, generalized muscle weakness
   b. Intubation via an oral ETT, severe orthopnea, sleep deprivation
   c. Lack of homeostasis, inability to communicate, +score on Epworth Sleep Scale
   d. Delirium, agitation or unpleasant awareness, pain level*
3. Mr. Jones scored a +2 on the RASS. Which of the following best represents what this means for physical therapy examination and intervention?
   a. Patient combative; hold therapy today and discuss rationale with ICU team
   b. Patient lightly sedated; progress with therapy today
   c. Patient unarousable; hold therapy today and discuss rationale with ICU team
   d. Patient agitated; discuss with ICU team if therapy appropriate today and if patient requires additional sedation*
4. Mr. Jones scored a 0 on the RASS. Which of the following best represents what this means for physical therapy examination and intervention?
   a. Patient combative; hold therapy today and discuss rationale with ICU team
   b. Patient alert and calm; progress with therapy today*
   c. Patient unarousable; hold therapy today and discuss rationale with ICU team
   d. Patient agitated; discuss with ICU team if therapy appropriate today
5. Mr. Jones scored a +1 on the RASS. Which of the following best represents what this means for physical therapy examination and intervention?
   a. Patient combative; hold therapy today and discuss rationale with ICU team
   b. Patient alert and calm; progress with therapy today
   c. Patient unarousable; hold therapy today and discuss rationale with ICU team
   d. Patient restless but still appropriate for physical therapy services*

C. Line Identification

1. Which of the following is not a precaution when mobilizing a patient with a dorsalis pedis arterial line?
   a. Avoid weightbearing on the extremity with the arterial line
   b. Keep the transducer at heart level
   c. Avoid trunk flexion >90 degrees*
   d. Allow extra tubing to avoid dislodging arterial line when mobilizing
2. Which of the follow represents the only precaution/contraindication when mobilizing a patient with a PICC line?
   a. Avoid any type of ROM on the extremity 7 days after placement
   b. Allow the patient to have his or her BP measured in that extremity*
   c. Allow the patient to perform ADLs as tolerated
   d. Avoid out of bed (OOB) activities for 24 hours after placement
3. Which of the following is the best precaution for moving a patient OOB with a Foley catheter?
   a. Maintain the Foley catheter bag below the bladder*
   b. Drain the Foley catheter prior to transferring back to bed
   c. Allow extra tubing to be added to the catheter before transfers OOB
   d. All of the above
4. Which of the following best represents a precaution for mobilizing a patient with chest tubes?
   a. Check placement of tubes, security of tubes sutured to skin, move pleurovac out from under bed, do not open up foot rest on bottom of pleurovac, check for last dosage of pain medication
   b. Check placement of tubes, security of tubes sutured to skin, do not move pleurovac out from under bed, do not open up foot rest on bottom of pleurovac, check for last dosage of pain medication
   c. Check placement of tubes, security of tubes sutured to skin, move pleurovac out from under bed, open up foot rest on bottom of pleurovac, check for last dosage of pain medication*
   d. Check placement of tubes, loosen sutures on skin, move pleurovac out from under bed, open up foot rest on bottom of pleurovac, check for last dosage of pain medication
5. Which of the following is the most reasonable precaution during examination and intervention of a patient with a central venous catheter?
   a. Avoid excessive movement of the joint closest to the central line
   b. Avoid dislodging the central line by checking for tautness on line
   c. Avoid dislodging the central line by checking the level of the transducer
   d. a, b*

D. Electrocardiogram Identification

1. Which of the following is most likely the rhythm described: regular rate, unable to determine if P wave present, rate >150, QRS complex <.12 seconds?
   a. Supraventricular tachycardia*
   b. Ventricular tachycardia
   c. Idioventricular rhythm
   d. Sinus bradycardia
2. Which of the following best represents this rhythm: P wave in front of QRS complexes, PRI is normal, QRS complex is <0.12 seconds, rhythm is slightly irregular?
   a. Sinus rhythm with bundle branch block
   b. Sinus rhythm with bigeminy
   c. Sinus arrhythmia*
   d. Junctional escape rhythm
3. Which of the following best represents the rhythm that is likely to have an irregularly irregular pulse and negatively impact exercise tolerance?
   a. Atrial tachycardia
   b. Atrial fibrillation*
   c. Sinus arrhythmia
   d. Sinus bradycardia
4. Interpret the following electrocardiogram—determine the underlying rhythm.

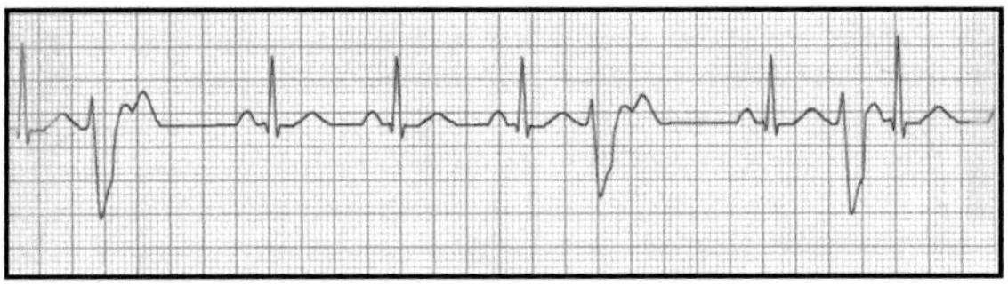

   a. Sinus rhythm*
   b. Sinus bradycardia
   c. Idioventricular rhythm
   d. Ventricular bigeminy
5. The abnormal depolarizations contained within the circle of the rhythm strip below indicates that:

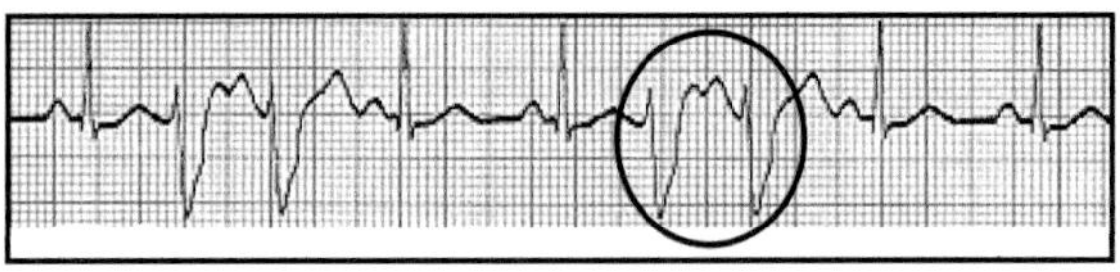

   a. There is an ectopic foci in the atria
   b. There is an ectopic foci in the atrioventricular node (ie, atrioventricular junction)
   c. There is an ectopic foci in the ventricles*
   d. You should not be concerned with this rhythm

E. Ventilation/Oxygenation

1. Which of the following is the most likely reason for the high-pressure alarm to go off on the mechanical ventilator?
   a. Disconnection
   b. An under-inflated balloon around the tracheostomy tube
   c. Coughing*
   d. Bronchodilation
2. Which of the following is most likely to be used as a supplemental oxygen delivery device when the patient with a tracheostomy is progressed for the first time off the mechanical ventilation for 1 hour?
   a. Nasal cannula
   b. Trach collar*
   c. Ambu bag (manual ventilator)
   d. Non-rebreather face mask
3. Which of the following best describes the reason to use 100% oxygen before, during, and following suctioning?
   a. To prevent pneumothorax
   b. To prevent dysrhythmias
   c. To prevent hypoxemia
   d. b, c*
4. Which of the following best represents how an assistive cough should be taught when the patient just had a right chest tube and a gastronomy tube placed yesterday?
   a. Cross one arm across anterior chest and one arm across abdomen with a blanket or pillow*
   b. Cross one arm across the anterior chest and one arm across abdomen without a blanket or pillow
   c. Perform abdominal thrusts with pain medication prior to treatment
   d. Request a nasopharyngeal airway be inserted followed by deep suctioning
5. Which of the following statements is the most true?
   a. A patient can set off a low-pressure alarm on a mechanical ventilator by coughing
   b. A patient can set off a high-pressure alarm on a mechanical ventilator by a disconnection
   c. A patient cannot breathe over and above an intermittent mandatory ventilation setting on a mechanical ventilator
   d. A patient can breathe over and above an intermittent mandatory ventilation setting on a mechanical ventilator*

F. Intervention/Methods for Progression

1. Mr. Jones is awake, alert, and has rested on the ventilator overnight. This is your first time in to examine Mr. Jones. The nurse tells you he has just been suctioned for a moderate amount of secretions and took a few minutes to stop coughing. Which of the following will be the most likely reason you choose to go ahead and evaluate his functional status today?
   a. His RR, breathing pattern, and HR have returned to his baseline prior to suctioning*
   b. His oxygen saturation is 89% compared to 100% during suctioning
   c. His BP is 20 mm Hg above his baseline from the nursing flow sheet and he has a headache
   d. His heart rhythm has changed to atrial fibrillation and he is complaining of lightheadedness
2. Mr. Jones is awake, alert, and has rested on the ventilator overnight. This is your third time treating Mr. Jones. The nurse tells you he has just been suctioned for a moderate amount of secretions and took a few minutes to stop coughing. Mr. Jones was reportedly agitated last night. Which of the following will be the most likely reason you choose not to progress his functional status today?
   a. He is having difficulty following 2-step directions during his ROM and bed mobility exercises (SpO_2 89% on 40% trach collar)
   b. He is not coughing during the ROM and bed mobility exercises (SpO_2 95% on 40% trach collar)
   c. He is having difficulty communicating and you notice accessory muscle use during his ROM and bed mobility exercises (SpO_2 84% on 40% trach collar)*
   d. He should not be seen at this time because of the agitation last night.
3. Mr. Jones is awake, alert, and has rested on the ventilator overnight. This is your third time treating Mr. Jones. The nurse tells you he has just been suctioned for a moderate amount of secretions and took a few minutes to stop coughing. Which of the following will be the most likely reason you choose to progress his functional status and activity level today?
   a. He is able to follow multi-step directions during his ROM warm-up exercises and his BP, SpO_2, RR, and breathing pattern have not varied from baseline*
   b. He reports feeling rested and his RR is 10 breaths/minute above resting, his systolic BP is 20 points above resting, and his HR is 20 beats above the resting value
   c. He is not able to follow more than 1-step commands, which is a change from his second treatment session, and his VS are deteriorating since he was suctioned
   d. His ECG shows new onset multifocal premature ventricular beats, and he is now complaining of sharp pain on inhalation

4. Of the following scenarios, which most likely represents how a therapist would determine positive progression in functional activity for Mr. Jones?
   a. VS response to activity, continued need for endotracheal suctioning, paradoxical breathing pattern during a 3-hour wean session, and lack of sleep
   b. VS response to activity, decreased need for endotracheal suctioning, no paradoxical breathing pattern during a 3-hour wean session, and adequate sleep*
   c. VS response to activity, continued need for endotracheal suctioning, paradoxical breathing pattern during any attempt to wean, and new crackles in right lower lung field
   d. VS response to activity, decreased need for endotracheal suctioning, no paradoxical breathing pattern during the first hour of the wean session, development of crackles in bilateral lower lung fields, and resting tachypnea

G. *Tests and Procedures*

1. Mr. Jones has been in the ICU for 3 weeks. Which of the following tests is helpful to determine the likelihood if the patient has a DVT?
   a. Wells Clinical Prediction Rule*
   b. Homan's sign
   c. Potassium concentration in blood serum
   d. Central venous pressure monitoring
2. Mr. Jones has thick green secretions, a persistent low grade temperature, coarse crackles over his right middle lobe (RML) and right lower lobe (RLL) region, limited chest wall expansion in the RML, RLL region, and + tactile fremitus along the right anterior middle and upper chest wall. Which of the following tests would be most likely to rule out pneumonia?
   a. Ventilation perfusion scan
   b. Cardiac catheterization
   c. ECG
   d. Chest x-ray*
3. The following lab work came back this morning on Mr. Jones to match his changing clinical signs: + creatine phosphokinase elevated, +troponins, +jugular venous distention, ST elevation in leads II, III, AVf. Which of the following medical tests (or procedures) would be most advantageous to identify the cause of the lab and clinical findings and intervene to prevent progression?
   a. Dobutamine stress ECG
   b. Thallium stress test
   c. Catheterization*
   d. EMG

4. Mr. Jones has been moved to a medical/surgical floor. He ambulated 25 feet with a rolling walker and minimal assistance of 1 this morning. You return to the room in the afternoon to progress his therapy and he complains of soreness in his right calf area. You note that his leg is swollen, red, and painful. Which of the following tests would be beneficial to perform before further therapy?
   a. ABI
   b. Cardiac index
   c. Ventilation perfusion scan
   d. LE ultrasound*
5. Mr. Jones has a PFT completed 1 week after being discharged from the ICU. While in the ICU, Mr. Jones required mechanical ventilation for 10 days. Which of the following measurements (compared to pre-hospitalization) would most likely be demonstrated by Mr. Jones on PFT?
   a. Decreased residual volume
   b. Increased NIF or MIP
   c. Decreased NIF or MIP*
   d. Increased inspiratory reserve volume

H. Rehabilitation Assessment Tools/Algorithms

1. Your patient is recovering from adult respiratory distress syndrome and you suspect that the patient may have ICU-acquired weakness (ICU-AW). The examination tool used to diagnose ICU-AW is:
   a. MRC examination*
   b. CAM-ICU
   c. RASS
   d. PFIT
2. Your patient is awake and alert with normal strength, but requires mechanical ventilation. An outcome measure to examine the patient's strength *and* mobility status that could be performed in the ICU would be:
   a. MRC examination
   b. CAM-ICU
   c. RASS
   d. PFIT-s*
3. On the MRC strength examination, Mr. Jones had 1/5 shoulder and hip strength, 2/5 elbow and knee strength, and 3/5 wrist and ankle strength. His sensation was intact, and he followed commands easily. What would he have scored on the MRC examination?
   a. 10
   b. 5
   c. 20
   d. 24*

4. A common examination tool to determine if delirium is present:
   a. Borg scale
   b. New York Heart Association classification
   c. MRC scale
   d. CAM-ICU*
5. Mr. Jones was reevaluated 12 days after initial ICU examination. At this time he could move his UEs against gravity, sit at the edge of the bed for 2 minutes supported, and required a Hoyer lift for daily transfers to the chair. What is the estimated level for him on the ICU Mobility Scale?
   a. Level I
   b. Level II
   c. Level III*
   d. Level IV

I. Common Diseases/Disorders

1. Mr. Jones presents with a barrel chest, diminished breath sounds throughout, minimal diaphragm excursion, hyper-resonant mediate percussion, dry, wheezy cough, hypertrophied accessory muscles, and an elevated resting RR and HR. Which of the following pathologies most likely represents these findings?
   a. Pneumonia
   b. Chronic bronchitis
   c. Pleural effusion
   d. COPD*
2. Mr. Jones presents with +accessory muscle use, +clubbing, cyanotic color in lips and nail beds, barrel chest, +thick purulent sputum, diffuse crackles, hyper-resonant mediate percussion, minimal diaphragmatic excursion, and +sweat test. Which of the following pathologies most likely represents these findings?
   a. Pulmonary edema
   b. Chronic bronchitis
   c. Cystic fibrosis*
   d. Asthma
3. Mr. Jones presents with +accessory muscle use, -clubbing, normal A-P diameter chest, frothy pink secretions, +orthopnea, +PND, +rales 2/3 B posterior lung fields, increased RR, and tachycardia. Which of the following pathologies most likely represents these findings?
   a. Pneumothorax
   b. Pulmonary edema*
   c. Pleural effusion
   d. Pneumonia

4. Mr. Jones is 6 hours postoperation for abdominal surgery for a benign tumor removal. He presents with –clubbing, normal lip and nail bed color, +crackles/rales B posterior bases, dry cough, and low grade temperature. Which of the following pathologies most likely represents these findings?
   a. Cystic fibrosis
   b. Bronchiectasis
   c. Atelectasis*
   d. Pulmonary fibrosis
5. Which of the following diagnoses is most likely to lead to a blunted HR response to an increase in activity?
   a. Adult respiratory distress syndrome
   b. Heart transplant*
   c. New onset diabetes
   d. Subcutaneous emphysema

J. Universal Precautions and Infection Control

1. Mr. Jones was admitted to a negative pressure room in the ICU. There is a closed room outside the patient's room. Which of the following best describes what this room is used for this patient?
   a. Donning gloves, gown, and appropriate face mask prior to entering room*
   b. Donning gloves and gown but the mask should be placed on the face after you enter the room
   c. Donning lab coat for identification of rehabilitation role in treatment of patient
   d. This room is used for private consultation with the family only.
2. Which of the following best represents when hand washing with soap and water should be used?
   a. After eating and shaking hands with the patient's family members but before you use the hand sanitizer
   b. After eating, going to the bathroom, or if any contact with bodily fluids*
   c. After eating but not after touching your hair or changing the patient's sheets.
   d. After eating, doffing gloves, and moving the patient's IV pole to the other side of the room
3. Which of the following best describes when gloves should be worn?
   a. When examining or performing an intervention in the ICU
   b. During suctioning and bronchial hygiene in the ICU
   c. During transfers onto the bed commode in the ICU
   d. All of the above*

4. Mr. Jones does not have any precautions posted outside his room. Which of the following is the best procedure you should follow when entering to examine, evaluate, and perform an intervention with Mr. Jones?
   a. Wash hands with soap and water and doff gloves
   b. Wash hands with soap and water and don a mask
   c. Use hand sanitizer in front of the patient and clean stethoscope before use.*
   d. Use hand sanitizer in front of the medical team and place clipboard on the patient's ventilator
5. As part of orientation and annual training, which of the following best represents steps as a health care professional to protect oneself and patients?
   a. Watch a video on universal precautions and pass a computerized competency test
   b. Participate in annual updates on infection control and universal precautions
   c. Take an annual health screening and keep all required vaccinations up to date
   d. All of the above*

Sample Answer Sheet: Acute Care/ Intensive Care Unit Written Competency

Staff Member Name: ____________________ *Score:* ____

A. Examination

1.	a. ___	b. ___	c. ___	d. ___
2.	a. ___	b. ___	c. ___	d. ___
3.	a. ___	b. ___	c. ___	d. ___
4.	a. ___	b. ___	c. ___	d. ___
5.	a. ___	b. ___	c. ___	d. ___

B. Sedation/Delirium/Medications

1.	a. ___	b. ___	c. ___	d. ___
2.	a. ___	b. ___	c. ___	d. ___
3.	a. ___	b. ___	c. ___	d. ___
4.	a. ___	b. ___	c. ___	d. ___
5.	a. ___	b. ___	c. ___	d. ___

C. Line Identification

1.	a. ___	b. ___	c. ___	d. ___
2.	a. ___	b. ___	c. ___	d. ___
3.	a. ___	b. ___	c. ___	d. ___
4.	a. ___	b. ___	c. ___	d. ___
5.	a. ___	b. ___	c. ___	d. ___

D. Electrocardiogram Identification

1.	a. ___	b. ___	c. ___	d. ___
2.	a. ___	b. ___	c. ___	d. ___
3.	a. ___	b. ___	c. ___	d. ___
4.	a. ___	b. ___	c. ___	d. ___
5.	a. ___	b. ___	c. ___	d. ___

E. Ventilation/Oxygenation

1.	a. ___	b. ___	c. ___	d. ___
2.	a. ___	b. ___	c. ___	d. ___
3.	a. ___	b. ___	c. ___	d. ___
4.	a. ___	b. ___	c. ___	d. ___
5.	a. ___	b. ___	c. ___	d. ___

F. Intervention/Methods for Progression

1.	a. ___	b. ___	c. ___	d. ___
2.	a. ___	b. ___	c. ___	d. ___
3.	a. ___	b. ___	c. ___	d. ___
4.	a. ___	b. ___	c. ___	d. ___

G. Tests and Procedures

1.	a. ___	b. ___	c. ___	d. ___
2.	a. ___	b. ___	c. ___	d. ___
3.	a. ___	b. ___	c. ___	d. ___
4.	a. ___	b. ___	c. ___	d. ___
5.	a. ___	b. ___	c. ___	d. ___

H. Rehabilitation Assessment Tools/Algorithms

1.	a. ___	b. ___	c. ___	d. ___
2.	a. ___	b. ___	c. ___	d. ___
3.	a. ___	b. ___	c. ___	d. ___
4.	a. ___	b. ___	c. ___	d. ___
5.	a. ___	b. ___	c. ___	d. ___

I. Common Diseases/Disorders

1.	a. ___	b. ___	c. ___	d. ___
2.	a. ___	b. ___	c. ___	d. ___
3.	a. ___	b. ___	c. ___	d. ___
4.	a. ___	b. ___	c. ___	d. ___
5.	a. ___	b. ___	c. ___	d. ___

J. Universal Precautions and Infection Control

1.	a. ___	b. ___	c. ___	d. ___
2.	a. ___	b. ___	c. ___	d. ___
3.	a. ___	b. ___	c. ___	d. ___
4.	a. ___	b. ___	c. ___	d. ___
5.	a. ___	b. ___	c. ___	d. ___

Abbreviations

Kathy Lee Bishop, PT, DPT, CCS

Δ	change
″	inches
(A-a) PO_2	alveolar to arterial oxygen gradient
+	plus
>	greater than
<	less than
μg/dL	micrograms per deciliter
6MWD	6 Minute Walk Distance
6MWT	6 Minute Walk Test
A & O	alert and oriented
A & P	auscultation and percussion
A & W	alive and well
A1AD	alpha-1 antitrypsin deficiency
A1C	glycosylated hemoglobin
AAA	abdominal aortic aneurysms
AACVPR	American Association of Cardiovascular and Pulmonary Rehabilitation
A-a gradient	alveolar to arterial oxygen gradient
AAO x 3	awake, alert, and oriented times 3 (person, place, time)
AAO x 4	awake, alert, and oriented times 4 (person, place, time, circumstance)
AAOS	American Academy of Orthopedic Surgeons
AAROM	active assistive range of motion
AAT	alpha-1 antitrypsin
ABC	airway, breathing, circulation
ABC	aspiration, biopsy, cytology
ABCD	Advanced Cardiac Life Support Survey: airway, breathing, circulation, differential diagnosis
ABCD	airway, breathing, circulation, disability

Malone DJ, Bishop KL, eds. *Acute Care Physical Therapy: A Clinician's Guide, Second Edition* (pp 713-738).

ABCD	asymmetry, borders, color, diameter
ABCDE bundle	awakening and breathing coordination, delirium monitoring and management, and early mobility bundle
ABE	acute bacterial endocarditis
ABG	arterial blood gas
ABI	acute brain injury
ABI	Ankle Brachial Index
ABO	blood type designation
ABPA	allergic bronchopulmonary aspergillosis
ABVD	doxorubicin, bleomycin, vinblastine, dacarbazine
ABX	antibiotics
A/C	assist control (ie, mode of mechanical ventilations)
ACA	anterior cerebral artery
ACB	active cycle of breathing
ACC	American College of Cardiology
ACDF	anterior cervical discectomy and fusion
ACE	angiotensin converting enzyme
ACEI	angiotensin converting enzyme inhibitor
Ach	acetylcholine
ACLS	advanced cardiac life support
ACOS	asthma–chronic obstructive pulmonary disease overlap syndrome
ACS	acute coronary syndrome
ACSM	American College of Sports Medicine
ACT	airway clearance technique
ACTH	adrenocorticotropin hormone
AD	autogenic drainage
ADDQoL	Audit of Diabetes-Dependent Quality of Life
ADH	antidiuretic hormone
ADL	activity of daily living
ADP	adenosine diphosphate
ADT	androgen deprivation therapy
AE	adverse events
AECOPD	acute exacerbation of chronic obstructive pulmonary disease
AED	automated external defibrillator
AF	atrial fibrillation
AFB	acid fast bacilli
AFL	atrial flutter
AFO	ankle foot orthosis
AFOP	acute fibrinoid-organizing pneumonia
AHF	acute heart failure
AHI	Apnea–Hypopnea Index
AHR	airway hyper-responsiveness
AI	aortic insufficiency
AI	aromatase inhibitors
AICA	anterior inferior cerebellar artery
AICD	automatic implanted cardioverter-defibrillator
AIDS	acquired immunodeficiency syndrome
AIP	acute interstitial pneumonia
AIS	Abbreviated Injury Scale
AIS	arterial ischemic stroke
AIVR	accelerated idioventricular rhythm
AJ	ankle jerk
AKA	above knee amputation
ALAD	acute lung allograft dysfunction
ALB	albumin

ALF	acute liver failure
ALF	assisted living facility
ALI	acute lung injury
ALIF	anterior lumbar interbody fusion
ALL	acute lymphoblastic leukemia
ALL	acute lymphocytic leukemia
ALL	allergy
ALL	anterior longitudinal ligament
ALND	axillary lymph node dissection
ALS	amyotrophic lateral sclerosis
ALT	alanine aminotransferase
AMA	against medical advice
AMI	acute myocardial infarction
AML	acute myeloid leukemia
AMP	adenosine monophosphate
AM-PAC	Activity Measure for Post Acute Care
AMS	acute myopathy syndrome
AMS	altered mental status
ANF	atrial natriuretic factor
ANP	atrial natriuretic peptide
ANS	autonomic nervous system
AoV	aortic valves
A-P	anterior-posterior
AP	action potential
APACHE II	Acute Physiology and Chronic Health Evaluation (ie, APACHE II score)
APLA	antiphospholipid antibodies
APTA	American Physical Therapy Association
APTT	activated partial thromboplastin time
AR	aortic regurgitation
ARAD	azithromycin-responsive allograft dysfunction
ARDS	adult respiratory distress syndrome
ARF	acute renal failure
AROM	active range of motion
ARVD	arrhythmogenic right ventricular dysplasia
AS	aortic stenosis
ASA	acetylsalicylic acid
ASD	atrial septal defect
ASHD	arteriosclerotic heart disease
ASIA	American Spinal Injury Association (ie, ASIA Impairment Scale)
ASPEN	American Society for Parenteral and Enteral Nutrition
AST	aspartate aminotransferase
AT	anterior tibial
AT	atrial tachycardia
ATN	acute tubular necrosis
ATP	adenosine triphosphate
ATPase	an enzyme that catalyzes the hydrolysis of ATP to ADP
ATPS	ambient temperature, pressure, saturated
A-V	arteriovenous
A-V fistula	arteriovenous fistula
AV	aortic valve
AV junction	atrioventricular junction
AV node	atrioventricular node
AV SEQ	atrioventricular sequential mode of pacemaker terminology
AVM	arteriovenous malformation

AVN	atrioventricular node
AVN	avascular necrosis
AVR	aortic valve replacement
AZT	azidothymidine
BAL	blood alcohol level
BAL	bronchoalveolar lavage
BBB	blood brain barrier
BBB	bundle branch block
BBS	bilateral breath sounds
BC	blood culture
BCA	bilateral carotid arteriogram
BCAA	branch chain amino acids
BCLS	basic cardiac life support
BCSVA	bilateral carotid subclavian vertebral arteriogram
BCx	blood culture
BD	bronchial drainage
BDI	Beck Depression Inventory
BE	barium enema
BE	base excess
BETS	blind endotracheal suctioning
BFA	bilateral femoral arteriography
BG	blood glucose
BGM	blood glucose monitor
BHR	bronchial hyperresponsiveness
BIBA	brought in by ambulance
BID	twice per day
Bio-LVR	biologic lung volume reduction
BiPAP	bilevel positive airway pressure
BiPAP	biphasic positive airway pressure
BKA	below knee amputation
BLE	bilateral lower extremity
BLS	basic life support
BLT	bilateral lung transplant
BM	bowel movement
BMD	bone mineral density
BMI	body mass index
BMP	basic metabolic panel
BMR	basal metabolic rate
BMS	bare metal stent
BMT	bone marrow transplantation
BNP	brain natriuretic peptide
BO	bronchiolitis obliterans
BOOP	bronchiolitis obliterans organizing pneumonia
BOS	bronchiolitis obliterans syndrome
BP	blood pressure
BPD	bronchopulmonary dysplasia
bpm	beats per minute
BPH	benign prostate hypertrophy
bpm	breaths per minute
BPPV	benign paroxysmal positional vertigo
BR	bed rest
BRAT	bananas, rice, applesauce, toast (refers to diet)
BRCA	breast cancer antigen
BRP	bathroom privileges

BS	breath sounds
BSA	body surface area
BSC	bedside commode
BSO	bilateral salpingo-oophorectomy
BTP	break through pain
BTVA	bronchoscopic thermal vapor ablation
BUE	bilateral upper extremity
BUN	blood urea nitrogen
BVM	bag valve mask
Bx	biopsy
C & S	culture and sensitivity
C	centigrade
Ca^{++}	calcium
CA	cancer
CABG	coronary artery bypass graft
CABS	coronary artery bypass surgery
CAD	coronary artery disease
CAM	complimentary alternative medicine
CAM-ICU	Confusion Assessment Method for the Intensive Care Unit
cAMP	cyclic adenosine monophosphate
CAO	conscious, alert, and oriented
CAP	community-acquired pneumonia
CAPD	continuous ambulatory peritoneal dialysis
CARES	Cardiac Arrest Registry to Enhance Survival
CAT	COPD Assessment Test
CAT	computed axial tomography (ie, CAT scan)
CAUTI	catheter-associated urinary tract infection
CAV	cardiac allograft vasculopathy
CAVH	continuous arteriovenous hemofiltration
CBC	complete blood count
CC	chief complaint
CCB	calcium channel blocker
CCE	clubbing, cyanosis, and edema
CCU	critical care unit
CD	cluster designation; cell surface proteins that characterize cell types (eg, CD4 T cells, CD8 T cells)
CDC	Centers for Disease Control and Prevention
C/D/I	clean, dry, and intact
CDT	catheter-directed thrombosis
CDT	complete decongestive therapy
CF	cystic fibrosis
CFTR	cystic fibrosis transmembrane conductance regulator
cGMP	cyclic guanosine monophosphate
CHADS2	congestive heart failure, hypertension, age >75 years, diabetes, prior stroke or transient ischemic attack
CHAL	central hyperalimentation
CHD	chronic heart disease
CHD	congenital heart disease
CHD	congestive heart disease
CHD	coronary heart disease
CHF	congestive heart failure
CHO	carbohydrates
CI	cardiac index
CI	cognitive impairment

CICU	coronary intensive care unit
CIDP	chronic idiopathic demyelinating polyradiculoneuropathy
CIDP	chronic inflammatory demyelinating polyneuropathy
CIM	critical illness myopathy
CIN	cervical intraepithelial neoplasia
CINMA	critical illness neuromuscular abnormalities
CIP	critical illness polyneuropathy
CIPN	chemotherapy induced peripheral neuropathy
CJD	Creutzfeldt-Jakob disease
CK	creatine kinase
CK-BB	creatine kinase bands specific to brain and neural tissue
CKD	chronic kidney disease
CK-MB	creatine kinase bands specific to heart muscle
CK-MM	creatine kinase bands primarily found in skeletal muscle
Cl^-	chloride
CL	cutaneous leishmaniasis
CLABSI	central line–associated blood stream infection
CLAD	chronic lung allograft dysfunction
CLIQ	Crohn's Life Impact Questionnaire
CLRD	chronic lower respiratory disease
cm	centimeters
cm H_2O	centimeters of water pressure
CM	cardiomyopathy
CMD	cardiac muscle dysfunction
CMV	controlled mechanical ventilation
CMV	cytomegalovirus
CNS	central nervous system
CO	carbon monoxide
CO	cardiac output
CO_2	carbon dioxide
COAD	chronic obstructive airway disease
COLD	chronic obstructive lung disease
COMT	catechol-o-methyl transferase (ie, COMT inhibitors)
COP	cryptogenic organizing pneumonia
COPD	chronic obstructive pulmonary disease
COTA	certified occupational therapy assistant
CP	chest pain
CPAP	continuous positive airway pressure
CPB	cardiopulmonary bypass
CPBP	cardiopulmonary bypass pump
CPET	cardiopulmonary exercise testing
CPK	creatine phosphokinase
CPM machine	continuous passive motion machine
CPN	central parenteral nutrition
CPR	cardiopulmonary resuscitation
CPRA	calculated panel reactive antibody
CPSS	Cincinnati Prehospital Stroke Scale
CPT	chest physical therapy
CPT	chest physiotherapy
CPX	cardiopulmonary exercise testing
CRC	colorectal cancer
CREST	calcinosis, Raynaud esophagus, sclerosis, telangiectasia
CRF	cancer-related fatigue
CRF	chronic renal failure
CRH	corticotropin-releasing hormone

CRI	chronic renal insufficiency
CRP	c-reactive protein
CRRT	continuous renal replacement therapy
CSA	cross-sectional area
CSF	cerebrospinal fluid
CSII	continuous subcutaneous insulin infusion
CSVT	cerebral sinovenous thrombosis
CT	chest tube
CT	computed tomography (ie, CT scan)
CTA	clear to auscultation
CTL	cytotoxic T lymphocyte (also called CD8 T Cells)
CTLO	cervical thoracic lumbar orthosis
CTO	cervical thoracic orthosis
CTPHE	chronic thromboembolic pulmonary hypertension
CTSIB	clinical test of sensory interaction on balance
CUS	compression ultrasound
CVA	cerebral vascular accident
CVAD	central venous access device
CVAHD	continuous arteriovenous hemodialysis
CVC	central venous catheters
CVD	cardiovascular disease
CVI	cerebrovascular insufficiency
CVP	central venous pressure
CVS	cardiovascular system
CVVHD	continuous venovenous hemodialysis
CWP	coal worker's pneumoconiosis
CWS	certified wound specialist
CX	circumflex artery
CXR	chest roentgenogram or x-ray

D-39	Diabetes-39 Questionnaire
DAD	diffuse alveolar damage
DAI	diffuse axonal injury
DALYs	disability-adjusted life years
DASH	dietary approaches to stop hypertension
DASH	Disabilities of the Arm, Shoulder, and Hand
DBP	diastolic blood pressure
DCD	donation after circulatory death
DCL	diffuse cutaneous leishmaniasis
DCM	dilated cardiomyopathy
DDD	dual chamber pacer
DES	diethylstilbestrol
DES	drug-eluting stent
DES	dry eye syndrome
DEXA	dual energy x-ray absorptiometry
DGF	delayed graft function
DHF	diastolic heart failure
DHF	dilated heart failure
DHP-1	Diabetes Health Profile
DHP-18	Diabetes Health Profile
DHS	dynamic hip screw
DHT	dihydrotestosterone
DHT	Dobhoff tube
D/I	dry, intact
DI	diabetes insipidus

DIC	disseminating intravascular coagulation
DIC	disseminating intravascular coagulopathy
DIEP	deep inferior epigastric perforator flap
DIMPS	dual isotope myocardial perfusion scans
DIP	desquamative interstitial pneumonia
DJD	degenerative joint disease
DKA	diabetic ketoacidosis
dl	deciliter
dL	deciliter
DLCO	diffusing capacity of carbon monoxide
DM	dermatomyositis
DM	diabetes mellitus
DMARD	disease modifying anti-rheumatic drugs
DMD	Duchenne muscular dystrophy
DME	durable medical equipment
DNA	deoxyribonucleic acid
DNAR	do not attempt resuscitation
DNI	do not intubate
DNR	do not resuscitate
DO2	delivery of oxygen
DOE	dyspnea on exertion
DPA	dorsalis pedis artery
DPG	diphosphoglycerate
DQoL	diabetes quality of life measure
DRS	dementia rating scale
DSA	digital subtraction angiography
DSA	donor specific antibodies
DSE	dobutamine stress echocardiogram
DT	delirium tremens
DTB	door to balloon
DTR	deep tendon reflex
DVT	deep vein thrombosis
D5W	5% dextrose in water
DW	dextrose in water
Dx	diagnosis
E coli	*Escherichia coli*
EBBS	equal bilateral breath sounds
EBL	estimated blood loss
EBM	evidence-based medicine
EBV	Epstein-Barr virus
EC	extracellular
$ECCO_2R$	extracorporeal carbon dioxide removal
ECF	extended care facility
ECF	extracellular fluid
ECG	electrocardiogram
ECLS	extracorporeal membrane oxygenation
ECMO	extracorporeal membranous oxygenation
ECOG	Eastern Cooperative Oncology Group Score
ECT	electroconvulsive therapy
ed	edition
ED	emergency department
EDD	esophageal detector device
EDH	epidural

EDH	extradural hematoma
EDP	end diastolic pressure
EDV	end diastolic volume
EEA	end-to-end anastomosis
EEC	endocervical curettage
EEG	electroencephalogram
EENT	ears, eyes, nose, throat
EF	ejection fraction
eg	for example
EGD	esophagogastroduodenoscopy
EKG	electrocardiogram
EMG	electromyography
EMS	emergency medical services
EMT	emergency medical technician
ENT	ears, nose, throat
EOB	edge of bed
EOM	extraocular movement
EP	electrophysiologist
EP	electrophysiology
EP	evoked potential
EPAP	expiratory positive airway pressure
EPO	erythropoietin
EPS	electrophysiology studies
ER	emergency room
ER	estrogen receptor
ERAS	enhanced recovery after surgery
ERCP	endoscopic retrograde cholangiopancreatography
ERV	expiratory reserve volume
ES	electrical stimulation
ESL	extracorporeal lithotripsy
ESLD	end-stage liver disease
ESLD	end-stage lung disease
ESR	erythrocyte sedimentation rate
ESRD	end-stage renal disease
ESS	Epworth Sleepiness Scale
ET	endotracheal
etc	et cetera
$ETCO_2$	end tidal carbon dioxide
ETOH	ethanol (ie, alcohol)
ETT	endotracheal tube
ETT	exercise tolerance test
EVD	external ventricular drain
Ex Fix	external fixation
Exam	examination
FACT-BMT	Functional Assessment of Cancer Therapy-Bone Marrow Transplant
FACT-E	Functional Assessment of Cancer Therapy-Esophagus
FAST	face, arm, speech, time to computed tomography scan
FB	foreign body
FBG	fasting blood glucose
FBS	fasting blood sugar
FDA	US Federal Drug Administration
$Fe3^{+}$	iron
FEF_{25-75}	mid expiratory flow rates

FET	forced expiratory technique
FEV_1	forced expiratory volume in one second
FFA	free fatty acid
FFP	fresh frozen plasma
FFR	fractional flow reserve
F_IO_2	fraction of inspired oxygen
FIM	Functional Independence Measure
FIST	Function in Sitting Test
FK506	tacrolimus
FOB	fiberoptic bronchoscopy
FOB	foot of bed
FOOSH	fall on outstretched hand
FOS	flight of stairs
FRC	functional residual capacity
FSH	follicle stimulating hormone
FSS-ICU	Functional Status Scale for the Intensive Care Unit
FTT	failure to thrive
FUO	fever of unknown origin
FVC	forced vital capacity
FWB	full weightbearing
Fx	fracture
FXN	function
g/dL	grams per deciliter
GABA	gamma-aminobutyric acid
GB	gallbladder
GBS	Guillain-Barré syndrome
GCA	giant cell arteritis
GCS	Glasgow Coma Scale
GCS	graduated compression stockings
GERD	gastroesophageal reflux disease
GFR	glomerular filtration rate
GGT	gamma glutamyl transferase
GH	growth hormone
GI	gastrointestinal
Glut4	glucose transporter protein 4
GnRH	gonadotropin releasing hormone
GN	glomerulonephritis
GOLD	Global Initiative for Obstructive Lung Disease
GSW	gunshot wound
GU	genitourinary
GVHD	graft-vs-host disease
GXT	graded exercise test
gyn	gynecological
H^+	hydrogen ion
H & H	hemoglobin and hematocrit
H & P	history and physical
H_2O	water
HA	headache
HAD	Hospital Anxiety and Depression (ie, HAD Scale)
HAI	hospital-acquired infection
HAL	hyperalimentation
HAP	hospital-acquired pneumonia

HAV	hepatitis A virus
Hb	hemoglobin
HbA1C	hemoglobin A1C (glycosylated)
HBO	hyperbaric oxygen
HBP	high blood pressure
HBV	hepatitis B virus
HCAP	health care–associated pneumonia
HCM	hypertrophic cardiomyopathy
HCO_3^-	bicarbonate
hct	hematocrit
HCT	hematocrit
HCTZ	hydrochlorothiazide
HCV	hepatitis C virus
HCVD	hypertensive cardiovascular disease
HD	hemodialysis
HD	Hodgkin disease (Hodgkin's lymphoma)
HDL	high density lipoprotein
HEENT	head, eyes, ears, nose, throat
HF	heart failure
HF-ACTION	Heart Failure-A Controlled Trial Investigating Outcomes of Exercise Training
HFCWC	high-frequency chest wall compression
HFCWO	high-frequency chest wall oscillation
HFJV	high-frequency jet ventilation
HFNC	high-flow nasal cannula
HFOV	high-flow oscillatory ventilation
HFpEF	heart failure with preserved ejection fraction
HFrEF	heart failure with reduced ejection fraction
HFS	hip fracture surgery
Hgb	hemoglobin
HH	hiatal hernia
HHNK	hyperosmolar hyperglycemic nonketotic
HIT	heparin-induced thrombocytopenia
HITT	heparin-induced thrombocytopenia complicated by thrombosis
HIV	human immunodeficiency virus
H-L Tx	heart lung transplant
HLA	human leukocyte antigen
HLT	heart lung transplant
HMG CoA	3-hydroxy-3 methyl glutaryl-coenzyme A
HMG CoA	hydroxy-methylglutaryl coenzyme A
HNCA	head and neck cancer
HNP	herniated nucleus pulposus
HO	heterotopic ossification
HOB	head of bed
HOH	hard of hearing
HPI	history of present illness
HPTX	hemopneumothorax
HPV	human papilloma virus
HR	heart rate
HRCT	high-resolution computerized tomography
HRQoL	health-related quality of life
HTN	hypertension
Hx	history
Hz	hertz

I & A	irrigating and aspirating
I & D	incision and drainage
IA	intra-arterial
IABP	intra-aortic balloon pump
IADL	instrumental activity of daily living
IBD	inflammatory bowel disease
IBDQ	Inflammatory Bowel Disease Questionnaire
IBM	inclusion body myositis
IBS	irritable bowel syndrome
IBW	ideal body weight
IC	inspiratory capacity
IC	intermittent claudication
IC	intracellular
ICA	internal carotid arteries
ICD	implantable cardioverter-defibrillator
ICDSC	Intensive Care Delirium Screening Checklist
ICH	intracerebral hemorrhage
ICH	intracranial hematoma
ICM	ischemic cardiomyopathy
ICP	intracranial pressure
ICS	intercostal space
ICU	intensive care unit
ICU-AW	intensive care unit–acquired weakness
IDDM	insulin dependent diabetes mellitus (type 1)
ie	that is
IE	infective endocarditis
IFN	interferons (ie, IFNα, IFNβ, IFNγ)
IgG, IgA, IgM, IgD, IgE	immunoglobulins (antibodies)
IHC	inhaled corticosteroid
IHD	ischemic heart disease
IHSS	idiopathic hypertrophic subaortic stenosis
IIP	idiopathic interstitial pneumonia
IJ	internal jugular
ILD	interstitial lung disease
IM	intramuscular
IMCU	intermediate care unit
IMN	intramedullary nail
IMR	intramedullary rod
IMT	inspiratory muscle training
IMT	intima-media thickness
IMV	intermittent mandatory ventilation
INH	isoniazid
INR	International Normalization Ratio
IO	intraosseous (ie, IO infusion)
IOLI	intraocular lens insertion
IP	interphalangeal
IP	intraperitoneal
IPAH	idiopathic pulmonary arterial hypertension
IPAP	inspiratory positive airway pressure
IPC	intermittent pneumatic compression
IPCD	intermittent pneumatic compression device
IPF	idiopathic pulmonary fibrosis
IPPB	intermittent positive pressure breathing

IPPV	intermittent positive pressure ventilation
IPS	Infection Probability Score
IR	ischemia-reperfusion
IRV	inspiratory reserve volume
IS	incentive spirometry
ISS	Injury Severity Score
IT	intrathecal
ITD	impedance threshold device
ITP	idiopathic thrombocytopenic purpura
IUD	intrauterine device
IV	intravenous
IVAC	infection-related ventilator-associated complication
IVC	inferior vena cava
IVCD	intraventricular conduction delay
IVP	intravenous pyelogram
IVUS	intravascular ultrasound
JP drain	Jackson-Pratt drain
JVD	jugular venous distention
JVP	jugular venous pressure
K^+	potassium
Kcal	kilocalorie
KCL	potassium chloride
KDPI	Kidney Donor Profile Index
kg/m^2	kilograms per meter squared
KPD	kidney paired donation
KS	Kaposi's sarcoma
KUB	kidney, ureter, and bladder (x-ray)
L/min	liters per minute
L4–L5	lumbar segments 4 through 5
LA	left atrium
LABA	long-acting beta 2 sympathomimetic agonists
LAD	left anterior descending
LAE	left atrial enlargement
LAHB	left anterior hemiblock
LAM	lymphangioleiomyomatosis
LAMA	long-acting muscarinic antagonists
LANA	Lymphology Association of North America
LAP	left atrial pressures
LAS	lung allocation score
LBBB	left bundle branch block
LBP	low back pain
LCA	left coronary artery
LCL	lateral collateral ligament
LCPD	Legg-Calve-Perthes disease
LCx	left circumflex artery
LD	lactate dehydrogenase
LDH	lactate dehydrogenase
LDL	low density lipoprotein
LDUH	low-dose unfractionated heparin
L/E	lower extremity
LE	lower extremity

LES	lower esophageal sphincter
LFA	left femoral arteriogram
LFT	liver function test
LGI	lower gastrointestinal
LH	luteinizing hormone
LIMA	left internal mammary artery
LIP	lymphoid interstitial pneumonia
LLE	left lower extremity
LLL	left lower lobe
LLQ	left lower quadrant
LLSB	lower left sternal border
LM	left main
LMA	laryngeal mask airway
LMP	last menstrual period
LMWH	low molecular weight heparin
LOC	loss of consciousness
LOCF	level of cognitive functioning
LOS	length of stay
LP	lumbar puncture
Lpa	lipoprotein (A) (Lpa1 = lipoprotein particle A1)
LPDA	left posterior descending artery
lpm	liters per minute
LPN	licensed practical nurse
LSO	lumbar sacral orthosis
LTAC	long-term acute care
LTCI	long-term cognitive impairment
LTx	liver transplant
LTx	lung transplant
LUE	left upper extremity
LUL	left upper lobe
LUQ	left upper quadrant
LV	left ventricle
LVAD	left ventricular assist devices
LVAS	left ventricular assist system
LVEDP	left ventricular end diastolic pressure
LVEF	left ventricular ejection fraction
LVESP	left ventricular end systolic pressure
LVH	left ventricular hypertrophy
LVR	lung volume reduction
LVRC	lung volume reduction coils
LVRS	lung volume reduction surgery
M & M	morbidity and mortality
mA	milliamperes
MA	medical assistant
MAAS	motor activity assessment scale
MABP	mean arterial blood pressure
MACE	major adverse cardiac event
MAE	moves all extremities
MAFO	molded ankle-foot orthosis
MALT	mucosal-associated lymphoid tissue
MAOI	monoamine oxidase inhibitor
MAP	mean arterial pressure
MARSA	methicillin- and aminoglycoside-resistant *Staphylococcus aureus*

MBSS	modified barium swallow study
MBTS	modified Blalock-Taussig shunt
MCA	middle cerebral artery
MCH	mean cell hemoglobin
MCH	mean corpuscular hemoglobin
MCHC	mean cellular hemoglobin content
MCHC	mean corpuscular hemoglobin concentration
MCL	medial collateral ligament
MCL	mucocutaneous leishmaniasis (also called espundia)
MCP	metacarpophalangeal
MCS	mechanical circulatory support
MCS	minimally conscious state
MCV	mean corpuscular volume
MD	medical doctor (ie, physician)
MD	muscular dystrophy
MDD	major depressive disorder
MDI	meter dose inhaler
MEF	maximal expiratory force
MELD	Model for End-Stage Liver Disease
MET	medical emergency team
MET	metastasis
MET	metabolic equivalent
mEq/L	milliequivalents per liter
Mg	magnesium
MG	myasthenia gravis
mg/dL	milligram per deciliter
MH	manual hyperinflation
MI	myocardial infarction
MICU	medical intensive care unit
min	minute
MIP	maximum inspiratory pressure (also called NIF)
misc	miscellaneous
mL	milliliters
mm	millimeter
MM	multiple myeloma
mmol/L	millimoles per liter
mMRC	modified Medical Research Council questionnaire
MMSE	Mini-Mental State Examination
MMT	Manual Muscle Test
MNG	multimodal goiter
mNIHSS	Modified National Institutes of Health Stroke Scale
MoCA	Montreal Cognitive Assessment
MOD	multiple organ dysfunction
MOF	multiple organ failure
Mono	monocyte
MOPP	mechlorethamine, vincristine, procarbazine, and prednisone
MPD	myeloproliferative disorder
MPS	myocardial perfusion scintigraphy
MPV	mean platelet volume
MR	mitral regurgitation
MRA	magnetic resonance angiography
MRC	Medical Research Council (sum scale)
MRCP	magnetic resonance imaging retrograde cholangiopancreatography
MRG	murmurs, rubs, and gallops

MRI	magnetic resonance imaging
MRM	modified radical mastectomy
MRND	modified radical neck dissection
MRSA	methicillin-resistant *Staphylococcus aureus*
MS	mental status
MS	mitral stenosis
MS	multiple sclerosis
MS04	morphine
MSCC	metastatic spinal cord compression
MSOF	multi-system organ failure
MTBI	mild traumatic brain injury
MTP	metacarpophalangeal
MTP	metatarsophalangeal
MUD	matched unrelated donor
MUGA	multigated acquisition (ie, MUGA imaging)
MUGA	multigated angiogram (ie, MUGA imaging)
MV	mechanical ventilation
MV	minute ventilation
MV	mitral valve
MVA	motor vehicle accident
MVC	maximal voluntary contraction
MVC	motor vehicle collision
MVC	motor vehicle crash
mVe	minute ventilation (RR x V_T)
MVO	mixed venous oxygenation %
MVR	mitral valve replacement
N/V	nausea/vomiting
Na^+	sodium
NaCl	sodium chloride
NAD	no apparent distress
NAS	no added salt
NASH	nonalcoholic steatohepatitis
NC	nasal cannula
NCCN	National Comprehensive Cancer Network
NCI	National Cancer Institute
NCV	nerve conduction studies
NG	nasogastric (ie, NG suction, NG tube)
NH3	ammonia
NHL	non-Hodgkin's lymphoma
NHP	Nottingham Health Profile
NICE-SUGAR	Normoglycemia in Intensive Care Evaluation and Survival Using Glucose Algorithm Regulation Trial
NIDDM	non–insulin dependent diabetes mellitus (type 2)
NIF	negative inspiratory force (also called MIP)
NIH	National Institutes of Health
NIHSS	National Institutes of Health Stroke Scale
NINDS	National Institute of Neurological Disorders and Stroke
NiPPV	noninvasive positive pressure ventilation
NIV	noninvasive ventilation
NK	natural killer (ie, NK cells)
NKDA	no known drug allergies
NLN	National Lymphedema Network
NM-ARF	acute neuromuscular respiratory failure

NMB	neuromuscular blockade
NMES	neuromuscular electrical stimulation
NMSC	nonmelanoma skin cancers
NO	nitric oxide
NODAT	new onset diabetes after transplantation
NOS	not otherwise specified
NOTA	National Organ Transplantation Act
NOTT	Nocturnal Oxygen Therapy Trial
NP	nurse practitioner
NPO	nil per os (nothing by mouth)
NPPV	noninvasive positive pressure ventilation
NRB	non-rebreather mask
NS	normal saline
NSAID	non-steroidal anti-inflammatory drug
NSCC	non–squamous cell carcinoma
NSCLCA	non–small cell lung cancer
NSIP	non-specific interstitial pneumonia
NSR	normal sinus rhythm
NSTEMI	non–ST segment elevation myocardial infarction
NSVT	non-sustained ventricular tachycardia
NT	nasotracheal
NTG	nitroglycerin
NTS	nasotracheal suctioning
NV	neurovascular
NWB	non-weightbearing
NYHA	New York Heart Association
O_2	oxygen
OA	osteoarthritis
OB	obliterative bronchiolitis
OGT	orogastric tube
OGTT	oral glucose tolerance test
OHT	orthotopic heart transplant
OLD	occupational lung disease
OM	otitis media
OM	obtuse marginal
OOB	out of bed
OPA	oropharyngeal airway
OPO	Organ Procurement Organization
OPTN	Organ Procurement and Transplantation Network
OR	operating room
ORIF	open reduction internal fixation
OSA	obstructive sleep apnea
OT	occupational therapy
OTC	over the counter
P	phosphate
P	phosphorus
PA	physician's assistant
PA	pulmonary artery
PAB	prealbumin
PAC	pulmonary artery catheter
PAC	premature atrial complex
PAC	premature atrial contraction

$PACO_2$	partial pressure of carbon dioxide in alveolar gas
$PaCO_2$	partial pressure of carbon dioxide in arterial blood
PAD	peripheral artery disease
PAD	premature atrial depolarization
PAF	platelet activating factor
PAF	paroxysmal atrial fibrillation
PAH	pulmonary arterial hypertension
PALS	pediatric advanced life support
PAO_2	partial pressure of oxygen in alveolar gas
PaO_2	partial pressure of oxygen in arterial blood
PAOD	peripheral arterial occlusive disease
PAP	pulmonary artery pressure
PAT	paroxysmal atrial tachycardia
PAOP	pulmonary artery occlusion pressure
PAWP	pulmonary artery wedge pressure
PBC	primary biliary cirrhosis
PBCT	peripheral blood cell transplantation
PBW	predicted body weight
PCA	patient-controlled analgesia
PCA	posterior communicating arteries
PCA	posterior cerebral artery
PCH	pulmonary capillary hemangiomatosis
PCI	percutaneous coronary intervention
PCO_2	partial pressure of carbon dioxide
PCN	penicillin
PCP	pneumocystis carinii pneumonia
PCP	primary care physician
PCR	polymerase chain reaction
PCWP	pulmonary capillary wedge pressure
PD	postural drainage
PD	Parkinson's disease
PD	peritoneal dialysis
PDA	patent ductus arteriosus
PDA	posterior descending artery
PDGF	platelet-derived growth factor
PDQ-39	Parkinson's Disease Quality of Life Questionnaire
PE	pulmonary emboli
PEA	pulseless electrical activity
PEEP	positive end expiratory pressure
PEFR	peak expiratory flow rate
PEG	percutaneous endoscopic gastrostomy (ie, PEG tube)
PEJ	percutaneous endoscopic jejunostomy (ie, PEJ tube)
PEP	positive expiratory pressure
PERL	pupils equal, round, reactive to light
PERRLA	pupils equal, round, reactive to light and accommodation
PET	positron emission tomography (ie, PET scan)
$PETCO_2$	partial pressure of end-tidal carbon dioxide
PFO	patent foramen ovale
PFT	pulmonary function test
PFIT	physical function intensive care unit test
PGD	primary graft dysfunction
pH	hydrogen ion concentration
PH	pulmonary hypertension
PHI	personal health information

PHI	protected health information
PHR	peak heart rate
PHQ-9	Patient Health Questionnaire-9
PICA	posterior inferior cerebellar artery
PICC	peripherally inserted central catheter
PID	pelvic inflammatory disease
PIJ	proximal interphalangeal joint
PJC	premature junctional complex
PJC	premature junctional complex
PL	pulmonary lymphangiectasia
PLB	pursed-lip breathing
PLF	posterolateral lumbar fusion
PLIF	posterior lumbar interbody fusion
PLL	posterior longitudinal ligament
PLT	platelets
PM	pacemaker
PM	polymyositis
PMBV	percutaneous mitral balloon valvotomy
PMD	primary medical doctor
PMH	past medical history
PMHx	past medical history
PMI	painless myocardial infarction
PMI	Pain Management Inventory
PMI	point of maximal impulse
PMV	Passy-Muir valve
PMV	prolonged mechanical ventilation
PNA	pneumonia
PND	paroxysmal nocturnal dyspnea
PNF	primary nonfunction
PNF	proprioceptive neuromuscular facilitation
PNS	parasympathetic nervous system
PO_2	partial pressure of oxygen
POBA	plain old balloon angioplasty
POC	point of care
POD	postoperative day
PONV	postoperative nausea and vomiting
POTS	postural orthostatic tachycardia syndrome
PPD	packs per day
PPD	purified protein derivative
PPE	personal protective equipment
PPH	primary pulmonary hypertension
PPI	proton pump inhibitors
PPM	permanent pacemaker
PPN	peripheral parenteral nutrition
PPV	pulse pressure variation
PR	progesterone receptor
pr	per rectum
PRA	panel reactive antibody
PRBC	packed red blood cells
PRE	progressive resistive exercise
PRI	PR interval of an electrocardiogram
PRIND	prolonged reversible ischemic neurologic deficit
PRN	as necessary
PROM	passive range of motion

PRV	post residual void
PS	pressure support (ie, mode of mechanical ventilation)
PS	Parkinsonism syndrome
PSA	prostate specific antigens
PSC	primary sclerosing cholangitis
PST	Persantine stress test
PSV	pressure support ventilation
PT	physical therapist
PT	posterior tibial
PT	prothrombin time
PTA	physical therapist assistant
PTCA	percutaneous transluminal coronary angioplasty
PTFE	polytetrafluoroethylene
PTH	parathyroid hormone
PTLD	post-transplant lymphoproliferative disorder
PTR	potential transplant recipient
PTS	post-thrombotic syndrome
PTSD	post-traumatic stress disorder
PTSS	post-traumatic stress syndrome
PTT	partial thromboplastin time
PTX	pneumothorax
PUD	peptic ulcer disease
PUO	pyrexia of unknown origin
PV	pulmonic valve
PVC	premature ventricular complex
PVC	premature ventricular complex
PVC	pulmonary vascular congestion
PVD	peripheral vascular disease
PVI	peripheral vascular insufficiency
PVR	pulmonary vascular resistance
PVT	percutaneous valve technologies
PVT	prosthetic valve thrombosis
PWB	partial weightbearing
PWP	pulmonary wedge pressure
Q	perfusion
QoL	quality of life
QRS	QRS interval of an electrocardiogram
QT	QT segment of an electrocardiogram
RA	rheumatoid arthritis
RA	right atrium
RA	room air
RAD	right axis deviation
RADS	dose of radiation
RAE	right atrial enlargement
RAGE	receptor for advanced glycation end products
RAKT	robotic-assisted laparoscopic kidney transplant
RAP	right atrial pressure
RAS	reticular activating system
RAS	restrictive allograft syndrome
RASS	Richmond Agitation Sedation Scale
RAV	repeated and verified
RBBB	right bundle branch block

RBC	red blood cell
RBILD	respiratory bronchiolitis interstitial lung disease
RCA	right coronary artery
RCT	randomized control trial
RDS	respiratory distress syndrome
REM	rapid eye movement
RF	renal failure
RF	respiratory failure
RF	rheumatic fever
RFA	right femoral arteriogram
RFA	right femoral artery
Rh	Rhesus blood factor
Rhabdo	rhabdomyolysis
RHD	rheumatic heart disease
RHR	resting heart rate
RICU	respiratory intensive care unit
RIFLE	risk, injury, failure, loss, end-stage kidney disease (criteria)
RIMA	right internal mammary artery
RIND	reversible ischemic neurologic deficit
RLE	right lower extremity
RLL	right lower lobe
RLQ	right lower quadrant
RML	right middle lobe
RN	registered nurse
RNA	ribonucleic acid
R/O	rule out
ROM	range of motion
ROS	review of systems
ROSC	return of spontaneous circulation
RPE	rate of perceived exertion
RPG	retrograde pyelogram
RPP	rate pressure product
RR	respiratory rate
RRE	round, regular, and equal
RRR	regular rate and rhythm
RRT	rapid response team
RRT	registered respiratory therapist
RS cell	Reed-Sternberg cell
RSV	respiratory syncytial virus
RT	respiratory therapist
r-tPA	recombinant tissue plasminogen activator
RUE	right upper extremity
RUL	right upper lobe
RUQ	right upper quadrant
RV	right ventricle
RV	residual volume
RVAD	right ventricular assist device
RVAS	right ventricular assist system
RVEDP	right ventricular end-diastolic pressure
RVF	right ventricular failure
RVH	right ventricular hypertrophy
RVP	right ventricular pressure
RVR	rapid ventricular response
RVT	renal vein thrombosis
Rx	treatment or prescription

S/P	status-post
s/p	status-post
S/S	signs and symptoms
SA node	sinoatrial node
SAH	subarachnoid hemorrhage
SAN	sinoatrial node
SAN	spinal accessory nerve
SaO_2	arterial oxygen saturation
SAPS	Simplified Acute Physiology Score
SAT	spontaneous awakening trial
SB	sinus bradycardia
SBAR	situation, background, assessment, recommendation
SBE	subacute bacterial endocarditis
SBMA	spinal bulbar muscular atrophy
SBO	small bowel obstruction
SBP	systolic blood pressure
SBS	short bowel syndrome
SBT	spontaneous breathing trial
SC	subcutaneous
SCA	spinocerebellar ataxia
SCA	sudden cardiac arrest
SCC	spinal cord compression
SCC	squamous cell carcinoma
SCD	sickle cell disease
SCI	spinal cord injury
SCID	severe combined immunodeficiency
SCIWORA	spinal cord injury without radiographic abnormality
SCLC	small cell lung cancer
SCM	sternocleidomastoid
SCUF	slow continuous ultrafiltration
$ScVO_2$	central venous oxygen saturation
SDH	subdural hematoma
SDH	subdural hemorrhage
SEM	systolic ejection murmur
SERMS	selective estrogen receptor modulators
SF-36	Short Form-36
SF-12	Short Form-12
SFA	superficial femoral artery
SG	Swan Ganz
SGA	small for gestational age
SGRQ	St. George's Respiratory Questionnaire
SGOT	serum glutamic-oxaloacetic transaminase
SH or SHx	social history
SHx	surgical history
SIADH	syndrome of inappropriate anti-diuretic hormone
SICU	surgical intensive care unit
SIDS	sudden infant death syndrome
SIMV	synchronized intermittent mandatory ventilation
SINS	Spinal Instability Neoplastic Score
SIP	sickness impact profile
SIRS	systemic inflammatory response syndrome
sit↔stand	transfer sitting to stand and return to sitting position
SK	streptokinase
SL	sublingual

SLC	single lumen catheter
SLE	systemic lupus erythematosus
SLEDD	slow/sustained low-efficiency daily dialysis
SLNB	sentinel lymph node biopsy
SLP	speech-language pathologist
SLR	straight leg raise
SLT	single lung transplant
SMA	spinal muscle atrophy
SMA	superior mesenteric artery
SMS	supramaximal stimulation
SND	selective neck dissection
SNF	skilled nursing facility
SNP	sodium nitroprusside
SNS	sympathetic nervous system
SOAP	subjective, objective, assessment, plan
SOB	shortness of breath
SOFA	sequential organ failure assessment
SOL	space occupying lesion
SOMI	sternal occipital mandibular immobilizer
SOT	solid organ transplant
SP	speech pathology
SPECT	single photon emission computed tomography
spiral CT	spiral computed tomography scan (corkscrew scan pattern)
SpO_2	oxygen saturation measured via pulse
SR	sinus rhythm
SRE	skeletal related events
SS-QOL	Stroke Specific Quality of Life Scale
SSE	soap suds enema
SSG	split skin graft
SSI	sliding scale insulin
SSLT	single sequential lung transplant
SSRI	selective serotonin reuptake inhibitor
SSS	sick sinus syndrome
ST	sinus tachycardia
staph	*Staphylococcus*
STD	sexually transmitted disease
STEMI	ST-segment elevation myocardial infarction
STMI	short-term memory impairment
strep	*Streptococcus*
STSG	split-thickness skin graft
supine↔sit	supine transfer to sitting
SV	saphenous vein
SV	stroke volume
SVC	superior vena cava
SVG	saphenous vein graft
SVO_2	mixed venous oxygen saturation
SVR	systemic vascular resistance
SVT	supraventricular tachycardia
SVV	stroke volume variation
Sz	seizure
T10–T12	thoracic segments 10 through 12
T_3	triiodothyronine
T_4	thyroxine

T & A	tonsillectomy with adenoidectomy
T & C	type and cross match
TAH	total abdominal hysterectomy
TAH	total artificial heart
TAVR	transcatheter aortic valve replacement
TB	mycobacterium tuberculosis
TBI	traumatic brain injury
TBW	total body water
TC	tracheostomy collar
TCA	transluminal coronary angioplasty
TCA	tricarboxylic acid cycle (Krebs cycle)
TCD	transcranial Doppler
TCDB	turn, cough, breath deep
TCN	tetracycline
TCP	transcutaneous pacing
TCT	thrombin clotting time
TD	tardive dyskinesia
TdP	Torsades de pointes
TEE	transesophageal echocardiography
TEN	total enteral nutrition
TENS	transcutaneous electric nerve stimulation
TEP	tracheosophageal puncture
TG	triglycerides
TGA	transposition of great arteries
TGF	tumor growth factor
TGV	transposition of great vessels
TH	thyroid hormone
THA	total hip arthroplasty
THINK	toxic situations and medications, hypoxemia, infection/sepsis, non-pharmacologic interventions, K^+ or other electrolyte interventions
THR	total hip replacement
TI	tricuspid insufficiency
TIA	transient ischemic attack
TID	3 times per day
TIMI	thrombolysis in myocardial infarction
TIPS	transjugular intrahepatic portosystemic shunt
TKA	total knee arthroplasty
TLC	therapeutic lifestyle changes
TLC	total lung capacity
TLC	triple lumen catheter
TLSO	thoracic lumbosacral orthosis
TM	tympanic membranes
TMA	transmetatarsal amputation
TMJ	temporal mandibular joint
TMR	transmyocardial revascularization
TNF	tumor necrosis factor
TNM	tumor/nodal/metastasis
TOF	Tetralogy of Fallot
TOF	train of four (impulse setting on stimulator to monitor neuromuscular blockade)
tPA	tissue plasminogen activator/alteplase recombinant
TPN	total parenteral nutrition
TPR	total peripheral resistance
TPR	temperature, pulse, and respiration

TR	tricuspid regurgitation
trach	tracheostomy
TRALI	transfusion-related acute lung injury
TRAM	transverse rectus abdominis myocutaneous flaps
TRH	thyroid releasing hormone
TRIT	triiodothyronine
trop	troponin
TS	type and screen
TSA	total shoulder arthroplasty
TSH	thyroid-stimulating hormone
TTE	transthoracic echocardiography
TTI	transthoracic impedance
TTP	thrombotic thrombocytopenic purpura
TUG	Timed Up and Go Test
TUIP	transurethral incision of the prostate
TUMT	transurethral microwave thermotherapy
TUNA	transurethral needle ablation
TUR	transurethral resection
TURP	transurethral resection of the prostate
TV	tidal volume
TV	tricuspid valve
TVH	total vaginal hysterectomy
TVP	transvenous pacing
TVR	tricuspid valve replacement
TWE	tap water enema
Tx	transplant
U/O	urine output
UA	urinalysis
UAC	umbilical arterial catheter
UBE	upper body ergometer
UBW	usual body weight
UC	ulcerative colitis
U/E	upper extremity
UE	upper extremity
UES	upper esophageal sphincter
UFH	unfractionated heparin
UGI	upper gastrointestinal
UI	urinary incontinence
UIP	usual interstitial pneumonitis
UNOS	United Network of Organ Sharing
UPDRS	Unified Parkinson's Disease Rating Scale
UQD	upper quarter dysfunction
URI	upper respiratory infection
URTI	upper respiratory tract infection
US	United States
US	ultrasound
USN	ultrasonic nebulizer
UTI	urinary tract infection
UUN	urinary urea nitrogen
UVC	umbilical venous catheter
V/Q	ventilation/perfusion
VA	visual acuity

VAC	ventilator-associated complication
VAD	ventricular assist device
VAE	ventilator-associated event
VA ECMO	venoarterial extra corporeal membrane oxygenation
VALI	ventilator-associated lung injury
VAP	ventilator-associated pneumonia
VAS	ventricular assist system
VAS	visual analog scale
VATS	video-assisted thoracoscopic surgery
VCA	vascularized composite allograft
(V_{df}/V_T)	physiologic dead space/tidal volume
VE	minute ventilation
VEGF	vascular endothelial growth factor
VF	ventricular fibrillation
VH	ventilator hyperinflation
VHD	valvular heart disease
VIDD	ventilator-induced diaphragmatic dysfunction
VILI	ventilator-induced lung injury
VKA	Vitamin K antagonist
VLDL	very low density lipoproteins
VO	verbal order
VO_2	oxygen consumption
VO_{2max}	maximal oxygen uptake
VOR	vestibulo-ocular reflex
VPAP	variable positive airway pressure
VRE	vancomycin-resistant enterococci
VRSA	vancomycin-resistant *Staphylococcus aureus*
VS	vital signs
VSD	ventricular septal defect
VSR	ventricular septal rupture
VT	ventricular tachycardia
V_T	tidal volume
VTE	venous thromboembolism
VTE	ventricular tachycardia event
VV ECMO	venovenous extra corporeal membrane oxygenation
W/U	work up
WBAT	weightbearing as tolerated
WBC	white blood cell
WCD	wearable cardioverter-defibrillator
WFL	within functional limits
WHO	World Health Organization
WN	well nourished
WNL	within normal limits
WOB	work of breathing
WPW syndrome	Wolff-Parkinson-White syndrome
XRT	radiation therapy
y/o	years old
yo	years old
Zn	zinc

Financial Disclosures

Dr. Joseph Adler has no financial or proprietary interest in the materials presented herein.

Dr. Heather Dillon Anderson has no financial or proprietary interest in the materials presented herein.

Dr. Esther H. Bae has no financial or proprietary interest in the materials presented herein.

Dr. Kathy Lee Bishop has no financial or proprietary interest in the materials presented herein.

Colleen Chancler has no financial or proprietary interest in the materials presented herein.

Christine F. Ehlers has no financial or proprietary interest in the materials presented herein.

David Fichandler has no financial or proprietary interest in the materials presented herein.

Dr. Zoher F. Kapasi has no financial or proprietary interest in the materials presented herein.

Dr. Daniel J. Malone has no financial or proprietary interest in the materials presented herein.

Dr. Lora Packel has no financial or proprietary interest in the materials presented herein.

Robin Stott-McNulty has not disclosed any relevant financial relationships.

Index

For Product Safety Concerns and Information please contact our EU representative GPSR@taylorandfrancis.com Taylor & Francis Verlag GmbH, Kaufingerstraße 24, 80331 München, Germany